AIDS AND
COMPLEMENTARY &
ALTERNATIVE
MEDICINE

Current Science and Practice

AIDS AND
COMPLEMENTARY &
ALTERNATIVE
MEDICINE

MEDICAL GUIDES TO
Complementary & Alternative Medicine

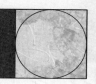

AIDS AND COMPLEMENTARY & ALTERNATIVE MEDICINE

Current Science and Practice

LEANNA J. STANDISH, ND, PhD, LAc
Director of Research, Bastyr University Research Institute
Bastyr University
Seattle, Washington

CARLO CALABRESE, ND, MPH
Research Professor
National College of Naturopathic Medicine
Portland, Oregon

MARY LOU GALANTINO, PT, MS, PhD
Professor of Physical Therapy, Richard Stockton College of New Jersey
Pomona, New Jersey
Clinical Specialist, University of Pennsylvania
Philadelphia, Pennsylvania

Series Editor **MARC S. MICOZZI**, MD, PhD
Executive Director, The College of Physicians of Philadelphia
Adjunct Professor of Medicine and Rehabilitation Medicine
University of Pennsylvania
Philadelphia, Pennsylvania

with 35 illustrations

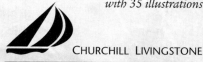

CHURCHILL LIVINGSTONE

A Harcourt Health Sciences Company
New York   Edinburgh   London   Philadelphia

CHURCHILL LIVINGSTONE
A Harcourt Health Sciences Company

The Curtis Center
Independence Square West
Philadelphia, Pennsylvania 19106-3399

NOTICE

Complementary and alternative medicine is an ever-changing field. Standard safety precautions must be followed, but as new research and clinical experience broaden our knowledge, changes in treatment and drug therapy may become necessary or appropriate. Readers are advised to check the most current product information provided by the manufacturer of each drug to be administered to verify the recommended dose, the method and duration of administration, and contraindications. It is the responsibility of the licensed prescriber, relying on experience and knowledge of the patient, to determine dosages and the best treatment for each individual patient. Neither the publisher nor the editors assume any liability for any injury and/or damage to persons or property arising from this publication.

Publishing Director: John A. Schrefer
Associate Editor: Kellie F. Conklin
Associate Developmental Editor: Jennifer L. Watrous
Project Manager: Karen Edwards
Design: Renée Duenow

AIDS AND COMPLEMENTARY & ALTERNATIVE MEDICINE:
CURRENT SCIENCE AND PRACTICE

ISBN 0-443-05831-8

Last digit is the print number: 9 8 7 6 5 4 3 2 1

Contributors

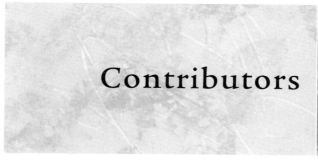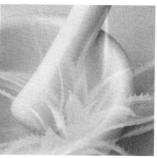

JOHN G. BABISH, PhD
Chairperson, BIONEXUS, Ltd
Ithaca, New York

ANNE E. BELCHER, PhD, RN, AOCN, FAAN
Professor and Director, Undergraduate Program
Department of Nursing
College of Health Professions
Thomas Jefferson University
Philadelphia, Pennsylvania

BARBARA BREWITT, PhD
Chief Scientific Officer, Biomed Comm, Inc
Visiting Staff Scientist, Department of Biological Structure
University of Washington
Seattle, Washington

CARLO CALABRESE, ND, MPH
Research Professor
National College of Naturopathic Medicine
President, Triangle Research Partners
Portland, Oregon

BRUNO CHIKLY, MD (France)
Laureat of the Medical Faculty of Paris
Associate Member of the American Academy
    of Osteopathy
Affiliated with the International Alliance of Healthcare
    Educators
Member of the International Society of Lymphology
Director of Lymph Drainage Therapy seminars
Scottsdale, Arizona

MISHA RUTH COHEN, OMD, LAc
Clinic Director, Chicken Soup Chinese Medicine
Research and Education Chair, Quan Yin Healing Arts
    Center
Faculty, Institute for Health and Aging
University of California, San Francisco
San Francisco, California

JAMES A. DUKE, PhD
Retired Economic Botanist
USDA
Senior Science Advisor
Nature's Herbs
Fulton, Maryland

SUNDAY T. EKE-OKORO, Dr Med Sc
Research Fellow
Physical Medicine and Rehabilitation
University of Medicine and Dentistry of New Jersey
Stratford, New Jersey

TIFFANY FIELD, PhD
Director, Touch Research Institutes
Pediatrics Department
University of Miami School of Medicine
Miami, Florida

MARY LOU GALANTINO, PT, MS, PhD
Professor of Physical Therapy
Richard Stockton College of New Jersey
Pomona, New Jersey
Clinical Specialist
University of Pennsylvania
Philadelphia, Pennsylvania

JON D. KAISER, MD
HIV Specialist, President, and Medical Director
Integrative Health Consulting, Inc
Faculty, Department of Medicine
University of California, San Francisco Medical School
Mill Valley, California

JEONGMIN LEE, PhD
Arizona Prevention Center
University of Arizona
Tucson, Arizona

RYAN HEATH LESS, MS (Oriental Medicine), LAc,
   DiplAc, DiplCH
Staff Acupuncturist, Healing Arts Department
Kripalu Center
Lenox, Massachusetts
Director, New England Acupuncture and Herb Clinic
Pittsfield, Massachusetts

XINFANG MA, MD, MPH
Laboratory Director
Illinois Department of Public Health
Springfield, Illinois

STEPHEN J. MERRILL, PhD
Professor of Mathematics
Department of Mathematics, Statistics, and Computer
   Science
Marquette University
Milwaukee, Wisconsin

ROBERT S. ROOT-BERNSTEIN, PhD
Professor of Physiology
Physiology Department
Michigan State University
East Lansing, Michigan

JOHN F. RUHLAND, ND
Naturopathic Medicine Faculty
Bastyr University
Seattle, Washington

ARTHUR D. SHATTUCK, LAc
NCCAOM
Physician of Oriental Medicine
Clinical Director
Wisconsin Institute of Chinese Herbology
Racine, Wisconsin

ELLEN SMIT, PhD, RD
Assistant Professor
Department of Social and Preventive Medicine
University at Buffalo, The State University of New York
School of Medicine and Biomedical Sciences
Buffalo, New York

LEANNA J. STANDISH, ND, PhD, LAc
Director of Research
Bastyr University Research Institute
Bastyr University
Seattle, Washington

ALICE M. TANG, PhD
Assistant Professor
Department of Family Medicine and Community Health
Tufts University School of Medicine
Boston, Massachusetts

JOHN E. UPLEDGER, DO, OMM, CST-D
President and Medical Director
The Upledger Institute, Inc.
Palm Beach Gardens, Florida

RONALD ROSS WATSON, PhD
Professor of Public Health, Family and Community
   Medicine, and Nutritional Sciences
Health Promotion Sciences
College of Public Health
University of Arizona
Tucson, Arizona

KOZO YOSHIKAWA, MD
Arizona Prevention Center
University of Arizona
Tucson, Arizona

This book is dedicated to AIDS doctors all over the world.

LJS

To AIDS-affected patients, whose daily spirit and ingenuity have provided uncountable scientific and moral lessons for us.

CC

This book is dedicated to my two children, Madison and Daniel, both of whom were conceived and born during the years of this book project.

MLG

Series
Introduction

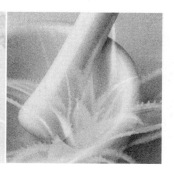

The aim of this Series is to provide clear and rational guides for health care professionals and students so they have current knowledge about:

- Therapeutic medical systems currently labeled as complementary medicine
- Complementary approaches to specific medical conditions
- Integration of complementary therapy into mainstream medical practice

Each text is written specifically with the needs and questions of a health care audience in mind. Where possible, basic applications in clinical practice are explored.

Complementary medicine is being rapidly integrated into mainstream health care largely in response to consumer demand but also in recognition of new scientific findings that are expanding our view of health and healing—pushing against the limits of the current biomedical paradigm.

Health care professionals need to know what their patients are doing and what they believe about complementary and alternative medicine. In addition, a basic working knowledge of complementary medical therapies is a rapidly growing requirement for primary care, some medical specialties, and the allied health professions. These approaches also expand our view of the art and science of medicine and make important contributions to the intellectual formation of students in health professions.

This Series provides a survey of the fundamentals and foundations of complementary medical systems currently available and practiced in North America and Europe. Each topic is presented in ways that are *understandable* and that provide an important *understanding* of the intellectual foundations of each system—with translation between the complementary and conventional medical systems whenever possible. These explanations draw appropriately on the social and scientific foundations of each system of care.

Rapidly growing contemporary research results are included whenever possible. In addition to providing evidence indicating when complementary medicines may be of therapeutic benefit, guidance is also provided about when complementary therapies should not be used.

This field of health is rapidly moving from being considered *alternative* (implying exclusive use of one medical system or another) to *complementary* (used as an adjunct to mainstream medical care) to *integrative medicine* (implying an active, conscious effort by mainstream medicine to incorporate alternatives on the basis of rational, clinical, and scientific information and judgment).

Likewise, health care professionals and students must move rapidly to learn the fundamentals of complementary medical systems to better serve their patients' needs, protect the public health, and expand their scientific horizons and understanding of health and healing.

MARC S. MICOZZI
Philadelphia, Pennsylvania
1997

Series Editor's Preface

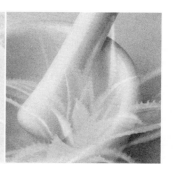

The book series, *Medical Guides to Complementary & Alternative Medicine*, is designed to provide the health professions with authoritative, credible information about therapeutic modalities and healing systems collectively known as *complementary and alternative medicine* (CAM). Existing titles in the series are organized by therapeutic system (e.g., Ayurveda, medical hypnosis, osteopathic medicine, chiropractic, acupuncture), following the organization of my basic text, *Fundamentals of Complementary and Alternative Medicine,* second edition, 2001, and by medical specialty practice (e.g., neurology, rehabilitation medicine). This title introduces a third category of text providing CAM approaches by medical condition. Together with the forthcoming title on alternatives in cancer, *AIDS and Complementary & Alternative Medicine* is the first to address the subject in this way. The editorial team consists of the leaders of the first NIH-funded grant to study the full scope of CAM approaches to AIDS, awarded to Bastyr University in Seattle, together with my colleague in the Department of Rehabilitation Medicine at the University of Pennsylvania. They provide the first systematic and credible review of this topic based on their experience with the NIH-sponsored epidemiological investigations, as well as their own clinical experiences.

People with AIDS represent a well-organized, vocal, and highly motivated group in the area of public health and public policy. Likewise, this volume provides a unique and useful resource as they continue to actively pursue therapeutic options and question medical scientific orthodoxy. One important question expresses doubt about the pathogenesis of AIDS. Although the "politically correct" decision was made by funding agencies several years ago to equate the clinical entity *AIDS* with the causative agent *HIV,* others, including a recent Nobel laureate, question the primary role of the virus. This volume addresses both those questions and concerns that highly toxic antiviral treatment for HIV infection may actually contribute to the pathogenesis of AIDS.

The global AIDS pandemic is testimony to the limits of the twentieth-century approach to control of infectious diseases. The nineteenth-century germ theory of disease led to great advancements in the treatment of bacterial infections with antibiotic "magic bullets." The eventual development of bacterial drug resistance turned magic bullets into "friendly fire." This problem of bacterial infections and the relative difficulty and expense of treating viral infections with drugs requires us to reexamine some of our century-old assumptions about the causes and control of infectious diseases.

A focus on host factors and selective stimulation and modulation of the immune system may represent useful new ideas that can help account for some of the clinical variability observed in infection, as well as compensating for the growing shortcomings of our long-term war against microbes. Many herbal remedies from Asian (e.g., Chinese medicine and Ayurveda) and Native American medical traditions have been observed to help modulate the immune system. Clearly, CAM has much to contribute to the support of AIDS patients, and people with AIDS have been quick to resort to these methods.

The health professions, as well as people with AIDS, have compelling reasons, rights, and needs to learn more about what CAM therapies have to offer in the treatment of AIDS—both to provide better and more affordable care to United States citizens and to expand our view of health and healing in American medicine. Because the rest of the world cannot afford conventional AIDS treatment, our renewed study of CAM may provide an opportunity to return a little of the wealth of medical knowledge we are obtaining from the health traditions of other cultures around the world.

MARC S. MICOZZI
Philadelphia, Pennsylvania
2001

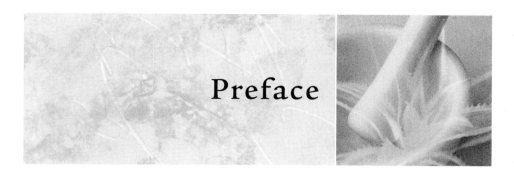

Preface

$\mathcal{I}$t's funny how things always seem to turn out for the best. In September 1998 this book was written and mailed to a publisher. The previous two years, 1996 to 1998, were a time when all of us involved in HIV research and clinical care were more and more certain that combination highly active antiretroviral therapy (HAART) was truly helping people with AIDS. Unforeseen developments resulted in our manuscript being assigned to new editors in 2000. They asked Dr. Calabrese, Dr. Galantino, and me if we were still interested in publishing this book. Somewhat reluctantly, we said yes. Our editors explained that we would need to update the book. After all, two critical years of AIDS science and medicine had elapsed. Updating the book was a daunting task, but we accepted, and the result is the appearance of this book 3 years after the original manuscript was written in 1998.

We are glad now that we were forced to look at the book and the field with fresh eyes. At the turn of the twenty-first century many wonderful and ominous things were happening in AIDS medicine and especially in combination HAART. We were asked to update our book at a time when it was obvious that conventional medicine, and the entire military industrial complex of which it is a part, had invented, developed, and tested the first truly important therapy for HIV infection and AIDS. This was a staggering achievement. Any doctor who has worked in the AIDS field has seen men and women dying of AIDS slowly get well enough to venture back into life from their homes, beds, and wheelchairs, return to graduate school or work, family, and a love life. Before the development of HAART, we had seen hundreds of people die despite our best efforts, but things in the West are different now. Some of our patients tell us confiden-

tially that they now have the damnable luxury of healthy persons: to suffer either ontological despair or the pain and beauty of a new love.

When we were finished with the first version of the book in 1998, it seemed that alternative medicine had failed in its mission to cure AIDS. We can remember feeling dispirited about the whole book project after the final draft was written and even worse when contemplating the revised update. After all, what was there to say at this point? That we were wrong about HIV not causing AIDS? That we were disappointed that we and the entire complementary and alternative medicine (CAM) community had produced such a disappointingly small, tattered array of controlled clinical studies? That we were disappointed in the paucity of research data despite approximately 70% of HIV-positive men and women across the United States using CAM to treat their HIV disease? How uninspiring to say in a book that none of the exciting, experimental CAM therapies that had so many supporters in urban politicized gay male culture have not panned out as dramatically useful therapies. Too many exciting CAM therapies, when examined closely, seemed to dissolve into nothing.

However, this was also a time when the side effects of HAART were discovered, and there was global consternation that over 97% of the world's HIV-infected persons had no access to HAART. Today's research and medical challenges of HIV/AIDS in the urban West are to develop HAART regimens that have fewer side effects and that better manage those side effects of HAART, which include diabetes, lipodystrophies, peripheral neuropathies, and hyperlipidemias.

Thankfully, our editors, Kellie Conklin and Jennifer Watrous, asked us to look at CAM in HIV/AIDS again and to do another complete search of the peer-reviewed biomedical literature. This rewriting process led us to a deeper understanding. We have a more mature perception of the role of CAM in the emerging integrative medicine movement that was in part inspired by the AIDS epidemic and the effective radical political organizing that occurred in minority communities across the United States.

Exciting basic science developments have been promoted by CAM AIDS research (for example, see Chapter 9). HIV/AIDS is an excellent research model for basic and clinical research, because it has reasonably correlated clinical and biological markers. Because of the unquestionable success of HAART, there is renewed justification for studying the anti-HIV effects of a combination of botanical and antiretroviral activity. Because of CAM research over the last decade, we now have preliminary evidence that certain nutritional, behavioral, botanical, and homeopathic approaches, as well as acupuncture, are effective in the treatment of several HIV-related conditions. We realized that the role has changed for alternative medicine, now more comfortably called *complementary medicine*. The role in HIV/AIDS is truly that of complementarity, and it is on this goal that CAM research should focus.

What do we know thus far? It is safe to suggest that we know the following from the past 15 years of CAM clinical research:

1. Suppression of HIV by a combination of antiretroviral drugs improves clinical and laboratory signs and symptoms of HIV infection and AIDS.
2. Those brave, although some thought foolish, CAM providers who advised their patients to delay use of AZT for as long as possible were correct. Many of those patients infected with HIV in the 1980s who eschewed AZT are alive today to benefit from the HAART regimens. Ironically, many of these regimens include the very AZT that was once so scorned.
3. There may be an important role for certain CAM therapies in managing some of the disease processes involved in HIV infection and in treating some of the adverse effects of HAART and prophylactic antibiotics.

We wish to thank the brilliant, committed men and women of the NIH, CDC, FDA, and the virological pharmaceutical companies for their staggering achievement in the development of HAART. We do not know what the total cost of this 10-year effort was between 1986 and 1996. We wonder what CAM researchers could claim as achievements today if similar resources and focus were put into CAM research in HIV/AIDS. We understand that the absence of financial incentives for natural products decreases entrepreneurial research, which is why the work of the NIH National Center of Alternative and Complementary Medicine (NCCAM) and its predecessor, the NIH Office of Alternative Medicine (OAM) is so important. The public needs to know about the safety and efficacy of CAM botanical, nutritional, and biological treatments. It will be up to the federal government to fund and direct this work at a national level.

We hope that this book will reinvigorate CAM research in HIV/AIDS. As we point out in this book, some promising avenues of basic and clinical research exist, but there still is much to do. Funding for research is now in place at the NIH. People with AIDS still need us. Let us proceed with vigor into the next decade of CAM research on HIV and AIDS.

LEANNA J. STANDISH
CARLO CALABRESE
MARY LOU GALANTINO

Acknowledgments

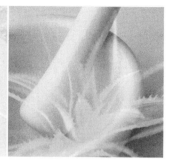

We warmly thank Heather Bradley for managing and coordinating this large and detailed project for 2 years. This book would never have happened without her competent and thorough dedication.

We also wish to thank the members of the scientific and technical staff of the Bastyr University AIDS Research Center. We are grateful to Cherie Reeves-Sperr, the Center's Project Manager, for 3 years of dedicated work that led to the most complete set of data regarding alternative medicine use among HIV-positive men and women in the United States. We also wish to thank Jose Berger, MF, Matt Brignall, ND, Jung Kim, and Langley Douglass for their expert literature and reference review work.

This project was made easier and more light-hearted by the constant support of Tove Hansen and Michele Bivins, our Administrative Assistants, and Maura Murphy, our Office Manager, who reminded us that we cold do this book and that it was worth doing.

We give grateful thanks to the brave men and women of the National Institutes of Health (NIH) Office of Alternative Medicine (OAM), who believed in the then-controversial concept that alternative medicine required investigation and supported Bastyr University's HIV/AIDS research with a grant: between 1994 and 1998. This study was supported by the NIH Office of Complementary and Alternative Medicine (OCAM), the National Institute of Allergy and Infectious Diseases (NIAID), and the NIH Office of Research on Women's Health (ORWH).

We especially want to acknowledge the hard-nosed dedication of the staff at the NIH OAM (now the National Center for Complementary and Alternative Medicine [NCCAM]). Our special thanks go to

Richard Nahin, PhD; Steven Groft, PhD; Wayne Jonas, MD; John Spencer, PhD; and Victoria Carper, MPA.

LJS

Deep thanks to Joe Pizzorno, ND, and the Board of Bastyr University, who provided the home where the groundwork was done; to my partners at the Bastyr University Research Institute, who were a fascinating and inspiring family; and to my co-editors, who made this book a wonderful experience. When you're headed in the right direction, all you need to do is keep going.

CC

"It is better to light one small candle than to curse the darkness"—Chinese Proverb

Many candles have been lighted throughout the HIV epidemic; many hopes and dreams for advances in various domains of integrative therapies. Those living with HIV disease ignited the way for my personal and professional exploration of complementary therapies, and I thank each person who presented their story and experience with me since the early 1980s. As this book evolved, I am grateful for the support of Marc Micozzi, MD, PhD, who envisioned this text in the series of complementary and alternative medicine books. I appreciate the dedication of my co-editors, Leanna Standish and Carlo Calabrese, for our discussions about the vision for this book and their continued commitment to research in complementary therapies. Technical support is the most crucial aspect in the logistics of such an endeavor, and I especially want to thank Heather Bradley, Carleen Finkle, Gwen Jones, and Amy Taylor—for without them, the organization and computer dynamics for the substrate of the book would not be forthcoming. Finally, I am grateful to my husband, David Pack, who knows my passion for this work and supports me unconditionally through it all.

MLG

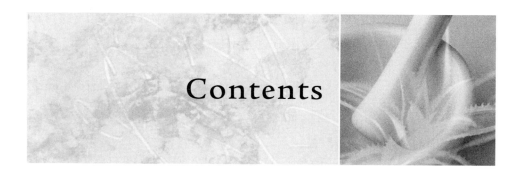

Contents

AIDS AND COMPLEMENTARY & ALTERNATIVE MEDICINE

Current Science and Practice

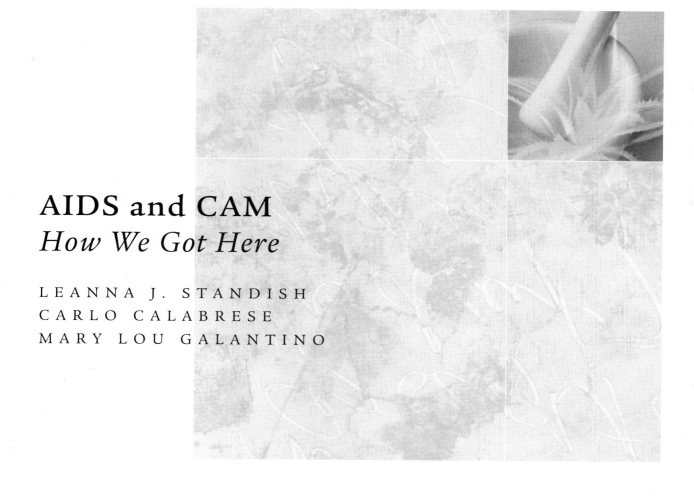

AIDS and CAM
How We Got Here

LEANNA J. STANDISH
CARLO CALABRESE
MARY LOU GALANTINO

The conventional and alternative medical communities responded to the AIDS epidemic in different ways. Conventional biomedical scientists and practitioners, as well as alternative medicine theorists and practitioners, sought and sometimes claimed medical solutions to human immunodeficiency virus (HIV) infection and acquired immunodeficiency syndrome (AIDS). The conventional biomedical community, including federal agencies, major universities, and the pharmaceutical industry, contributed enormous effort and money toward developing a synthetic drug or combination of drugs that would selectively destroy HIV in the infected host.

The alternative medicine community responded to AIDS differently. Some parts of the alternative medical community distrusted the pharmaceutical indus-

try, and some even questioned the theory that HIV causes AIDS. What was most significant for the development of the field of HIV/AIDS complementary and alternative medicine (CAM) was that practitioners were faced with HIV-positive and AIDS patients who were often desperately seeking help. Some patients came to CAM practitioners looking for miracle cures, while some sought help for HIV-related symptoms. Others sought alternative medicine to escape from the "HIV = AIDS = death" school of thought that seemed endemic in conventional medical settings in the early years of the epidemic. Some patients came to CAM practitioners looking for hope and camaraderie. As a result, many alternative practitioners felt called on to apply their modalities to HIV-infected patients. From the beginning of the American AIDS epidemic, more than a few alternative therapies claimed to "cure"

1

AIDS. Advocates from the HIV-infected community, health-care providers, and drug manufacturers claimed at times that certain botanicals, oxygenation therapies, Chinese herbal medicines, homeopathy, and bioelectromagnetic therapies could eradicate the virus, restore immune function, or both.

The CAM movement in the United States gained momentum over the last decade through its mobilization around the AIDS issue and in response to the needs of people living with HIV. Urban gay communities began organizing politically and socially around AIDS in the mid-1980s. Some CAM advocates and providers were part of both the interrelated American AIDS and gay sociopolitical movement in the major coastal cities of the United States. Strong advocates, often patients themselves, or politicized gay males spoke out in the AIDS or gay community media in favor of research in alternative medicine and in alternative therapies in particular.

Great achievements were made in the science of AIDS etiology and pathogenesis. A series of antiretroviral drugs were developed that lower viral counts to undetectable levels in peripheral blood samples using current technology of polymerase chain reaction (PCR) and branched-chain DNA amplification. Dramatic changes occurred in the health status of many HIV/AIDS patients starting in March 1996, when triple antiretroviral therapy (ART), including protease inhibitors (PIs), was made widely available to those HIV-infected patients who had a knowledgeable physician, medical insurance, or disposable income that could be spent on this therapy, which costs between $1000 to $2000 per month. At the June 1996 International AIDS Conference in Vancouver, British Columbia, international AIDS experts and members of the HIV-affected communities from all over the world admonished the medical community because combination ART although effective in suppressing HIV activity, was available only to 3% of patients worldwide who were infected with HIV. The remaining 97% of HIV-infected people live in countries where ART is typically inaccessible.

Combination ART was the first significant breakthrough in controlling the virus that presumably initiates the cascade of events that leads to deterioration of the immune system. Zidovudine (AZT) was the first antiretroviral drug approved by the Federal Drug Administration (FDA) in 1987 for the treatment of HIV. This was the beginning of the development of "highly active" ART (HAART). These useful antiviral (AV) drugs are not without their toxicities. AZT was the first nucleoside analog antiretroviral drug approved for use by the FDA. For many, AZT was without long-term clinical benefit. Some critics suggested that AZT made many HIV-positive patients worse and may even have hastened their demise. While this remains controversial, AZT is known to cause anemia, peripheral neuropathy (PN), and gastrointestinal (GI) complications in many patients.

It appears that the global HIV epidemic is accelerating. Disturbing epidemiological findings presented at the annual International AIDS Conferences suggest that the rate of HIV infection in Africa continues unabated. Currently, 90% of all HIV-infected people live in developing countries where combination ART is unavailable. It is estimated that between 30% to 40% of pregnant women in Harare, Zimbabwe, in subSaharan Africa are infected with HIV. It has been reported that 27% of Ugandan military personnel are infected with HIV. HIV infection rates increased in Russia by nearly 49-fold between 1991 and 1997.

The AIDS epidemic is not over and the need to evaluate alternative treatments for HIV/AIDS is undiminished. It is important to know if the claims that have been made for ozone, dinitrochlorobenzene (DNCB), Kemron, dehydroepiandrosterone DHEA, high-dose antioxidant vitamins, or electromagnetic (EM) therapies are valid. Despite the widespread use of CAM therapies by and for HIV/AIDS patients, very few of these therapies have been evaluated in randomized, controlled clinical trials (RCTs). Nevertheless, the number of alternative therapies used by HIV-positive Americans is astonishing.

Currently the most comprehensive description of alternative medicine use among HIV-positive Americans comes from the Bastyr University's Alternative Medicine Care Outcomes in AIDS (AMCOA) study. This nationwide observational study enrolled 1666 HIV-positive men and women between 1995 and 1997 who were self-identified users of alternative medicine for HIV/AIDS. Alternative medicine use was categorized into different types of providers, substances, and treatment activities garnered from the scientific literature, newsletters, clinicians, and buyers clubs. The cohort reported the use of a total of 1492 alternative treatments for HIV, many of which were administered or prescribed by 119 distinct CAM provider types.

Very few of these alternative therapies have been subjected to clinical evaluation. A systematic search of MEDLINE and AIDSLINE was performed by the

Bastyr University AIDS Research Center to locate RCTs published in peer-reviewed journals on CAM. Table I-1 presents a current summary of published RCTs for HIV/AIDS CAM therapies in use. Although 1492 alternative therapies are currently used by HIV-positive patients as of the year 2000, only 45 RCTs have been published, which evaluate only 24 of these therapies. The need for research is great indeed.

Over the last decade some of the philosophy and technology of alternative medicine has slowly been mainstreamed, and now many scientists, physicians, insurance companies, hospitals, and HMOs are

TABLE I-1

Randomized Clinical Trials (45) in HIV/AIDS Complementary and Alternative Medicine

This table represents all of the RCTs on CAM therapies for HIV published before 2001 in peer-reviewed journals, and although not journals published in the United States, they must have an English abstract. The table was compiled from MEDLINE and AIDSLINE searches, with the criteria for inclusion being that the studies be controlled and randomized. In some cases the studies were also placebo controlled.*

Treatment	Author	Number of subjects	Findings
Acemannan (Aloe)	Weerts (1990)	47 HIV+ patients	250 mg po qid for 24 weeks was not effective in reducing the hemotoxicity of AZT.
	Montaner (1996)	63 HIV+ males	400 mg po qid in patients taking AZT or ddI did not prevent CD4 decline or have significant effect on quantitative virology.
Acupuncture	Shlay (1998)	239 HIV+ subjects	14 weeks standardized acupuncture regimen was not effective in treating pain due to HIV-related PN.
Aerobic exercise	LaPerriere (1990)	50 asymptomatic gay males	5 weeks aerobic training, before notification of HIV-positive status, led to attenuation of detrimental immunological response associated with notification of HIV-positive status.
	Rigsby (1992)	37 HIV-1+ patients	12-week regimen, including aerobic and strength training, was associated with increased strength and cardiopulmonary function but not with changes in immune status.
	Stringer (1998)	34 HIV+ patients	6 weeks moderate or heavy training led to increased fitness and QOL measures but did not significantly affect immune function.
	Perna (1999)	28 HIV+ subjects	12 weeks laboratory-based aerobic exercise program led to an increase in CD4 cell counts as long as the individuals adhered to the exercise regimen.
Anaerobic exercise	Spence (1990)	24 HIV+ males with PCP	6 weeks resistance exercise training led to an increase in 13 of 15 anthropometric measures.

PCP, Pneumocystis carinii pneumonia; *ESR*, erythrocyte sedimentation rate; *CRP*, C-reactive protein; *IL-6*, interleukin-6; *PN*, peripheral neuropathy; *QOL*, quality of life; *SGA*, small for gestational age; *TMP-SMX*, trimethoprim-sulfamethoxazole.
*See Table I-1 references at the end of this chapter.

Continued

TABLE I-1

Randomized Clinical Trials (45) in HIV/AIDS Complementary and Alternative Medicine—cont'd

Treatment	Author	Number of subjects	Findings
Arginine/Omega 3 fatty acids	Pichard (1998)	64 HIV+ patients with CD4 >100/mm³	7.4 g arginine given with 1.7 g omega-3 fatty acid for 6 months did not lead to change in viral or immune measures. Both groups also received daily nutritional supplement.
Beta-carotene	Coodley (1996)	72 HIV+ patients	60 mg tid for 3 months did not lead to significant change in several measures of immune function. Both treatment and placebo groups received multivitamin supplement.
	Coodley (1993)	21 HIV+ patients	180 mg qd for 4 weeks led to significant increase in WBC count, % change in CD4, and % change in CD4:CD8 ratio. Absolute CD4 cell count elevated but not significantly.
Chinese herbs	Sankary (1989)	18 asymptomatic HIV+ males	50 mg Anginlyc tid had significant positive effect on CD4 cells and anti-p24 antibodies.
	Burack (1996)	30 HIV+, non-AIDS, CD4 of 200-499/mm³	28 tablets of a mixture containing 31 Chinese herbs showed insignificant improvement in QOL and decrease in symptoms.
	Weber (1999)	68 HIV+ adults	4 daily doses of a standardized preparation of 35 Chinese herbs did not improve QOL, clinical manifestations, plasma virus loads, or CD4 cell counts.
DHEA	Evans (1997)	16 HIV-1+	50 mg bid had no significant effect on ESR, CRP, or IL-6.
Ditiocarb sodium	Reisinger (1990)	60 HIV+ patients	24 weeks IV treatment significantly delayed disease progression. Benefits of oral treatment were not significant.
	Lang (1988)	83 HIV+ patients	16 weeks treatment significantly increased immune function and clinical status, while decreasing constitutional symptoms.
	HIV87 study group (1993)	1333 HIV+ patients	Risk of progression to AIDS was significantly higher in ditiocarb group than placebo group.
Folate/Vitamin B₁₂	Falguera (1995)	75 HIV+ patients with CD4<500/mm³ being treated with ART	15 mg qd folic acid, with monthly 1000 μg IM doses of B₁₂, did not reduce the risk of myelosuppression associated with AZT.
IMREG-1	Fiala (1991)	45 ARC patients	6 months treatment led to significantly reduced number of AIDS-defining events.

PCP, Pneumocystis carinii pneumonia; *ESR,* erythrocyte sedimentation rate; *CRP,* C-reactive protein; *IL-6,* interleukin-6; *PN,* peripheral neuropathy; *QOL,* quality of life; *SGA,* small for gestational age; *TMP-SMX,* trimethoprim-sulfamethoxazole.

TABLE I-1

Randomized Clinical Trials (45) in HIV/AIDS Complementary and Alternative Medicine—cont'd

Treatment	Author	Number of subjects	Findings
IMREG-1—cont'd	Gottlieb (1991)	143 ARC patients	Experimental group experienced fewer constitutional symptoms and slowed CD4 decline during 6 month trial.
L-carnitine	DeSimone (1994)	20 HIV+ patients	6 g/day for 4 months produced significant increases in CD4 counts and less substantial increases in CD8 counts.
Massage therapy	Birk (1996)	42 HIV+ patients	12 weeks massage therapy, with or without exercise training or stress management training, had no significant effect on immune function or QOL.
	Scafidi (1996)	28 neonates of HIV+ mothers	15 minutes massage therapy tid for 10 days was associated with increased weight gain and Brazelton performance scores.
Multivitamins	Fawzi (1998)	1075 HIV+ Tanzanian women 12-27 weeks gestation	Supplementation reduced risk of low birthweight, prematurity, SGA infants, and fetal death, as well as increasing counts of CD4, CD8, and CD3 cells.
	Fawzi (2000)	1083 HIV+ pregnant women	Vitamin A and multivitamin supplementation showed no effect on vertical transmission of HIV in utero or intrapartum and had no effect on birth weight of infants born HIV+.
N-Acetylcysteine	Akerlund (1997)	15 HIV+ patients with CD4<200/mm^3	800 mg qd did not significantly decrease risk of adverse reactions to pharmacological prophylaxis against PCP.
	Walmsley (1998)	238 HIV+ patients on TMP-SMX treatment	3 g/day did not show significant effect on TMP-SMX hypersensitivity.
	Breitkreutz (2000)	69 HIV+ patients, 40 with ART, 29 without ART	7 month double-blind placebo trial indicated that immunological function impairment may result from cysteine deficiency.
Ozone	Garber (1991)	14 HIV+ subjects with CD4 counts 200-400/mm^3	8 weeks ozone therapy did not significantly affect immune parameters or p24 antigen.
Peptide T	Simpson (1996)	81 HIV+ patients with DSP	12 weeks intranasal administration led to no change in symptoms of neuropathy or CD4 count.
	Heseltine (1998)	Trial size not indicated	6 mg/day did not product significant improvement in cognitive function.
Selenium/N-Acetylcysteine	Look (1998)	24 antiretroviral naïve HIV+ outpatients	600 mg tid of NAC given with 500 μg qd selenium, was associated with increase in CD4% but no change in glutathione levels or viral load.

Continued

TABLE I-1

Randomized Clinical Trials (45) in HIV/AIDS Complementary and Alternative Medicine—cont'd

Treatment	Author	Number of subjects	Findings
Stress management	Coates (1989)	64 HIV+ gay males	8 2-hr sessions and 1 all-day retreat led to significantly fewer sex partners in month of treatment but no change in lymphocyte numbers.
	Taylor (1995)	10 HIV+ asymptomatic males with CD4 <400/mm³	20 biweekly sessions led to improved mood, self-esteem, and T-cell counts through 1 month follow-up.
	Cruess (1999)	43 HIV+ males	10 weekly sessions of cognitive-behavioral stress management intervention can buffer against decrease in DHEAS.
	Antoni (2000)	73 HIV+ males	12 months of cognitive-behavioral stress management intervention produced significant increases in CD4 and CD8 cell counts, as well as improvement in self-reported anger, anxiety, and mood swings.
Support group	Goodkin (1998)	74 HIV+ and 45 HIV- gay males	10 weekly sessions were associated with significant increase in CD4 count, total T lymphocytes, cortisol levels, medication usage, and disease progression.
Thymopentin	Conant (1992)	91 asymptomatic HIV+ patients	50 mg SQ three times/week for 24 or 52 weeks led to insignificant reduction in disease progression.
Vitamin A	Kennedy (2000)	312 HIV+ pregnant females	5,000 IU/day with 30 mg beta-carotene and treatment of 200,000 IU at delivery did not produce significant decrease in HIV symptoms either prenatal or postnatal.
	Humphrey (1999)	40 HIV+ females of reproductive age	Single dose of 300,000 IU did not present significant clinical or immunological adverse effects.
	Semba (1998)	120 HIV+ IV drug users	Single dose of 200,000 IU had no effect on CD4 count or viral load at 2 and 4 weeks.
	Coutsoudis (1995)	118 children of HIV+ mothers in South Africa	Vitamin A (50,000-200,000 IU) given every 3 months reduced hospital admissions for diarrhea 77% and lowered overall morbidity in HIV+ infants.
Vitamin B₁₂	Navarette (1989)	49 subjects treated with AZT	1000 µg given weekly IM had no significant effect on MCV or Hb levels. Both groups received 50 mg folinic acid weekly IM.
Zinc	Ancarani (1993)	25 asymptomatic HIV+, CD4 <500/ml	200 mg zinc sulfate qd for 1 month significantly improved thymulin concentration, as well as CD4 and CD8 cells. Effects reversed within 2 months of treatment cessation.

PCP, Pneumocystis carinii pneumonia; ESR, erythrocyte sedimentation rate; CRP, C-reactive protein; IL-6, interleukin-6; PN, peripheral neuropathy; QOL, quality of life; SGA, small for gestational age; TMP-SMX, trimethoprim-sulfamethoxazole.

content with the inclusion of alternative medicine. Alternative medicine is now given the more benign and less controversial name of complementary and alternative medicine, and its acronym *CAM* is in common use. Alternative meant "instead of," or worse, "opposed to." Complementary means "to complete," implying at its best a cooperative co-management parallel to the biomedical mainstream, or at least a potential source of clinical ideas and theories. Some members of the CAM community suggest that while CAM never succeeded in curing anyone of AIDS, the nontoxic physiological, psychoemotional, and spiritual support provided by CAM therapists helps people live longer, perhaps long enough to benefit from recently developed HAART.

The AIDS epidemic had a significant effect on the history of science and medicine. The AIDS crisis generated, by the need for effective action, some of the clearest thinking among scientists and clinicians, and it forced the creation of new scientific vistas. Our understanding of the immune system was considerably advanced by insights provided from the study of AIDS patients and their cell systems. We now know much more about the immune system and the mechanisms that underlie both immune deficiencies and autoimmunity than we did fifteen years ago. We also know much more about nutrition, immunity, and psychoneuroimmunology (PNI), as well as the antibiotic treatment (and its limitations) of parasitic and bacterial infections.

The AIDS epidemic also changed the alternative medical community. Practitioners of Chinese and naturopathic medicine, as well as chiropractors, nutritionists, massage therapists, herbalists, homeopaths, and many others, responded to the needs of the HIV-positive community. For example, in the early days of the American AIDS epidemic, acupuncturists in San Francisco and New York were either called on or took it on themselves to help people with AIDS. There is now preliminary evidence that acupuncture may be an effective therapy for PN, a common manifestation of the disease (see Chapter 11).

In November 1997 the National Institutes of Health (NIH) published a Consensus Development Statement to provide health care providers, patients, and the general public with a responsible assessment of the use and effectiveness of acupuncture. Acupuncture is widely practiced in the United States as a therapeutic intervention. Whereas there are many studies of acupuncture's potential usefulness, many of these studies are of marginal design and provide equivocal results. The issue is complicated further by inherent difficulties in finding appropriate experiment controls, such as placebos or truly ineffective sham acupuncture treatment (see Chapter 1). Promising results emerged, for example, demonstrating the efficacy of acupuncture in nausea and vomiting that can occur in adults postoperatively and with chemotherapy. In conditions as diverse as addiction, stroke rehabilitation, headache, menstrual cramps, tennis elbow, fibromyalgia, myofascial pain, osteoarthritis, low back pain, carpal tunnel syndrome, and asthma, acupuncture is useful as an adjunct treatment in a comprehensive treatment program or even as an acceptable alternative. Further research is likely to expand evidence for the therapeutic potential of acupuncture.

CAM practitioners were asked by their patients to help handle some of the complex effects of the myriad of drugs they were prescribed, many of which have known toxicities. Many practitioners agree that combining CAM with good conventional medical care is the ideal. Evidence presented in Chapter 24 reflects this ideal.

The CAM community did not jump to any premature conclusions about the pathophysiology or effective treatment principles for HIV infection and AIDS. Future medical historians will write about the rapid scientific consensus that formed about the cause of "gay-related immune deficiency" (GRID) after Robert Gallo's announcement in 1984 of the discovery of HIV that preferentially affected T lymphocytes and caused AIDS. There is evidence that HIV is neither necessary nor sufficient in the etiology of AIDS, although most scientists agree that HIV is very closely associated with it.

Alternative theories of the origin and pathogenesis of AIDS helped shape many of the CAM therapies that are still used today. For example, the hypothesis that HIV infection occurs with other viruses, the so-called cofactor viruses, such as herpes simplex virus (HSV), hepatitis, human papillomavirus (HPV), and Epstein-Barr virus (EBV) (see Chapter 2), lead naturopathic physicians to emphasize early treatment to control or clear cofactor viruses.

Despite the current popularity of alternative medicine in industrialized nations, alternative medicine has not had an easy time. The entire field of CAM has many critics. The main and most valid criticism is that CAM treatments frequently lack supporting scientific evidence. However, a surprising amount of evidence exists for many of the commonly used HIV CAM therapies, such as antioxidants, multiple vitamins, acupuncture, massage, and others. The purpose of this book is to present some of that evidence.

In light of the successes of HAART, is there need for research, let alone a book, on alternative medicine in HIV/AIDS? Nevertheless, evidence shows that although combination ART is often effective in reducing viral replication, ART does not restore immune function. Many sessions of the International AIDS Conference held in Durban, South Africa, in June 2000 focused on immune restoration strategies, but only the bare beginnings of clinical approaches exist.

As we show in this book, a rational scientific basis exists for many of the complementary and alternative methods used to treat HIV/AIDS. For example, there is good evidence that vitamin and mineral therapies have positive effects on immune function and disease progression (see Chapters 4 and 5). Evidence also shows that several herbs have significant antiretroviral effects (see Chapter 6). One of the tasks of CAM is to develop a natural antiretroviral combination that interferes with HIV replication at multiple points in its life cycle. Preliminary evidence shows that homeopathically prepared substances have immunological and virological activity in vivo (see Chapter 9). Acupuncture techniques are shown to be clinically effective in several HIV-related complications (see Chapters 11 and 21).

In 1992 the NIH established the Office of Alternative Medicine (OAM) to study alternative medicine. The Congressional mandate for the OAM was to "screen and evaluate promising therapies from unconventional medical practices." The OAM established ten research centers in the United States to study alternative medicine in 1994 to 1997, including the Bastyr Center, through a 3-year cooperative agreement grant with the OAM and administered through the National Institute of Allergy and Infectious Disease Office of AIDS. Whereas scientific and political controversy surrounds the issue of alternative medicine and its application in HIV and AIDS, justification exists for federally funded research in this area. The justification for greater support for HIV/AIDS alternative medicine research falls within the following five areas:

1. The use of alternative medicine in the HIV-infected community is widespread, and yet the medical and scientific community knows little about either the safety or efficacy of most of these treatments. The media and the health products industry advertise sometimes intriguing or outrageous claims of efficacy for a variety of agents, modalities, and devices—claims that are largely unexamined.

2. Some of the more extreme therapies prescribed by CAM providers and self-prescribed by patients are potentially harmful. Moreover, little is known about the interaction of alternative medicines and conventional antiretroviral drugs and antibiotics. Studies recently found that *Hypericum perforatum,* an herb with purported AV effects popular in the HIV community, interacts with indinavir, one of the PIs, by more rapidly reducing the drug's concentration in the body, reducing its effectiveness (see references 152 and 153 in Chapter 20).

3. Currently there is no definitive treatment for the underlying immunological disorder that leads to clinical AIDS. Moreover, treatment for several of the AIDS-defining opportunistic infections (OIs) and neoplasms is as yet ineffective. Thus innovative strategies for the treatment of AIDS must be explored.

4. AIDS activist groups throughout the country continue to demand research in alternative approaches and alternative therapies.

5. Some evidence exists that a subset of alternative treatments may be effective and beneficial.

For these reasons the Bastyr University AIDS Research Center in Seattle opened in October 1994. Bastyr University specializes in clinical training in natural medicine. The Bastyr University AIDS Research Center screens and evaluates hundreds of CAM therapies, using an observational research design and studying a nationwide cohort of HIV-positive men and women who use CAM therapies.

Because there is no cure, justification exists for a continued effort by the CAM community to develop and test innovative therapies for HIV/AIDS. Some CAM practitioners have hypothesized that CAM has the potential to develop effective AV and immunoregulatory therapies that may have lower toxicity and more long-term benefits than currently available conventional therapies. Scientific progress requires diversity of thought. The alternative medicine community, including its most fringe aspects—perhaps because of its outliers—may hold new ideas about the genesis of both disease *and* health. Some of what we have learned has been applied to other serious health problems, particularly cancer.

Although antiretroviral pharmacological care of HIV-infected patients has advanced significantly in the last few years, these drugs are not without toxicities. Patients may only be able to tolerate them for a few years. Structured interruptions are being explored as a way to deal with the drug toxicities, but interruption is a compromise to viral suppression. Even without interruption, viral resistance can occur in patients despite continuous triple drug therapy.[1] For these reasons, failures in HAART are increasingly common.

Antiretroviral drugs are unavailable to 97% of the world's HIV-infected population due to their high cost. Utilization and development of traditional medicine may be the only health care AIDS patients receive in some parts of Africa and Asia. More research should be conducted to evaluate and develop less costly and less toxic AV and immune therapies. It is not impossible that findings from indigenous natural medicines may contribute to solving the AIDS problem even in the West.

There are effective tools of HIV disease management among alternative medical therapies. The AIDS problem is not over, and the work of the CAM scientific and medical community is not complete.

WHAT DOES CAM MEAN TO HIV/AIDS?

In this book, alternative medicine is defined as any treatment (substance or modality) used by or prescribed for HIV-positive patients that is not an FDA-approved pharmaceutical substance or device, or the use of FDA-approved substances or devices for indications and in doses not approved by the FDA for that agent or device. The NIH Office of Alternative Medicine offers a definition of CAM that revolves around professional use of a particular medical practice. A medical practice is considered highly CAM when it is not available in hospitals, not taught in medical schools, physicians are not typically trained in it, research funding is not available, the practice is not licensed in states, and insurance companies do not reimburse for it. Wayne Jonas, MD, the former Director of the NIH Office of Alternative Medicine, defines CAM as a "subset of medical and health practices that are not an integral part of conventional (Western) medicine."[2] Jonas also describes the spectrum of CAM by dividing CAM into three categories, depending on how integrated the practice is within conventional medicine. In Figure I-1, Jonas describes three areas of CAM as integrating areas, emerging areas, and frontier areas.

Recently published data show that an increasing number of Americans use some form of alternative medicine.[3,4] This rate is higher among the HIV/AIDS population. A number of studies suggest that over half of all HIV-positive gay or bisexual men are using alternative medical therapies; one of the most common is Chinese medicine.[5,6] Some estimates show that use of alternative medicine among HIV-positive adults is as high as 78%.[7] Despite their widespread use, most of these alternative therapies have not undergone adequate clinical evaluation.

Alternative therapy use in the HIV-infected community includes alternative health care providers, alternative substances, and alternative modalities. Licensed **alternative providers** include naturopathic physicians, chiropractors, acupuncturists, massage therapists, and hypnotherapists. Examples of commonly used **alternative substances** include *high dose vitamins, minerals, and antioxidants* administered both orally and intravenously (e.g., vitamin C, E, B$_{12}$, niacin, zinc, selenium, beta-carotene, *N*-Acetylcysteine); *botanical medicines* (e.g., SPV-30, aloe vera, *Carnivora, Glycyrrhiza glabra*, Hypericin, *Momordica charantia* or bitter melon, garlic, grapefruit seed extract, mistletoe); *biologicals* (DHEA, thymus gland fractions, PCM-4, peptide T, shark cartilage, transfer factor, antineoplastons); *pharmacologicals* (DNCB, hydrogen peroxide, naltrexone); and *homeopathics* (low dose interferon, 714X, nosodes, sarcodes and homeopathics listed in the *materia medica*). Commonly used **alternative modalities** include hyperthermia, therapeutic touch, remote healing, Chinese herbal medicine, EM microcurrent devices, acupuncture, and homeopathy. The list of alternative therapies used to treat HIV/AIDS grows monthly. To date, few have been subjected to evaluation for either safety or efficacy.

A second aspect of the meaning of CAM is worth mentioning. Several therapies are used within and by the conventional medical community, but by their intended use they are called alternative. For example, psychotherapy is claimed by 34.7% of the Bastyr University Alternative Medical Care Outcomes in AIDS (AMCOA) cohort (*n* = 1675) as a CAM therapy for HIV or AIDS. Conventional use of psychotherapy is widespread in North America and Europe. Its intended use in this context is to assist HIV-infected individuals in coping with the disease and making appropriate psychological adaptations to their condition. Another use of psychotherapy in the conventional medical setting is to treat anxiety and depression in HIV-positive

HOW INTEGRATED IS THE PRACTICE?

Frontier areas	Emerging areas	Integrating areas
• Frontier topics are those that challenge our conceptual and paradigmatic assumptions about the nature of biological or scientific reality. Examples include homeopathy, prayer, and healing practices such as therapeutic touch.	• Emerging CAM topics are those that involve common areas of interest for CAM and conventional medicine. Examples include acupuncture, herbalism (phytotherapy), and the use of high doses of combination nutritional supplements.	• Integrating topics are those often considered conventional but of interest to CAM practices. Examples include examining the mechanisms of action of popular dietary supplements, such as melatonin, DHEA, vitamins, minerals, antioxidants, and some behavioral medicine areas.

Figure I-1 The spectrum of CAM. (From Jonas W: *OAM: Investigating innovative approaches to health care, a report and plan for the Office of Alternative Medicine,* Bethesda, Md, 1998, National Institutes of Health.)

patients. The AMCOA study subjects also use psychotherapy as an intervention on the primary cause of the disease and to treat the immune deficit. The use of psychotherapy with the intention to "heal" HIV/AIDS would be considered an alternative medicine.

The addition of the word *complementary,* now in common parlance, implies that unconventional and conventional therapies and therapists can work best together. As alternative medicine becomes mainstream, the line between the two cultures is unclear. The use of multiple vitamins in therapeutic doses was once considered alternative but now is taken as common sense. Vitamin therapy is recommended by increasing numbers of conventionally trained physicians, as well as by alternative medicine practitioners. The increased use of multiple vitamin therapy was spurred on in part by the Barbara Abrams epidemiological study, showing how slowed progression to AIDS was associated with the use of daily multiple vitamins.[8]

What constitutes complementary and alternative medicine will be in constant flux, with new CAM therapies continuing to emerge and some CAM therapies being included in conventional care and reimbursed by third-party payers. Nevertheless, CAM by definition will continue to challenge the assumptions of the dominant medical culture, whatever those assumptions may be.

HOW THIS BOOK IS ORGANIZED

This book focuses on treatment. It also offers perspectives on etiology, pathogenesis, and on the methodological issues in evaluating whether CAM treatments work. The sections on treatments evaluate CAM approaches to treating the primary cause of HIV and central immune deficit, as well as treatments used to prevent and treat OIs and neoplasms. Contributing authors were sought whose clinical practice or scientific work encompassed clinical and laboratory outcomes that are important in understanding the experience of patients infected with HIV or those with AIDS, as well as the quantitative measures involved.

CAM treatments include numerous and sometimes overlapping categories. In 1992 the OAM categorized the field of CAM into seven areas that include (1) alternative systems of medical practice (e.g., traditional Chinese medicine, naturopathic medicine); (2) bioelectromagnetic applications; (3) diet, nutrition, lifestyle changes; (4) herbal medicine; (5) manual healing; (6) mind/body control; and (7) pharmacological and biological treatments. The integration of CAM and conventional medicine have been added as separate approaches to treatment. The chapters in this book represent some of the most current research in each of these seven areas of CAM in the treatment of HIV/AIDS.

HOW WE CHOSE THE TOPICS OF THIS BOOK

The Bastyr University AIDS Research Center identified 1492 CAM therapies used for HIV/AIDS. There is a discrepancy between available scientific evidence and the prevalence of use among people affected with AIDS. The task facing the scientific and medical CAM community is to distinguish useful CAM therapies from marketing "hype" and self-delusion on the part of both well-meaning clinicians and patients.

Early in its inception, the Bastyr AIDS Research Center[9] articulated the criteria by which HIV/AIDS alternative therapies were selected for evaluation, either by observational study or by clinical trial. Therapies were chosen that met one or more of the following criteria: (1) the particular CAM therapy was widely used; (2) patient or provider advocacy existed for the use of the therapy; (3) dramatic claims were made regarding the efficacy of the treatment; or (4) preliminary scientific evidence existed for the efficacy of the treatment. Sometimes attention is given to a CAM therapy that might be classified as an intellectual fad, or a "cure du jour." Examples were selected that have some scientific "staying power" or embody concepts persistent in CAM cultures.

The two alternative medical systems discussed in this book, naturopathic medicine and Chinese medicine, were chosen because both the American naturopathic and Chinese medical communities came forward at the beginning of the AIDS epidemic to offer help to people infected with HIV. These two medical systems generated the most comprehensive CAM treatment for HIV/AIDS. The chapters on the approach to treatment of HIV/AIDS by alternative medical systems demonstrate the complexity of therapeutic thinking. For example, only two treatment principles are applied in conventional FDA-approved HIV/AIDS treatments: (1) inactivate or destroy the virus, and (2) provide prophylaxis against OIs. Naturopathic medicine applies an array of principles to the treatment of HIV/AIDS (see Chapter 20). Chinese medicine diagnoses HIV-infected patients by an entirely different and more conceptually complex system than conventional biomedicine.

This book is not intended to offer comprehensive coverage of complementary and alternative medicine in HIV/AIDS. The intent is to provide some of the best examples of alternative perspectives and treatments for HIV/AIDS and to discuss some of the complex methodological issues pertinent to the scientific evaluation of CAM in AIDS or in any serious chronic disease. Not all evidence presented in this book for particular CAM approaches to HIV/AIDS is published in peer-reviewed scientific medical journals. The field of CAM in the treatment of HIV/AIDS research is in its infancy, and it is per-

haps premature to demand a surfeit of peer-reviewed papers from the CAM community. In the recent past, although ameliorated at present, a publication bias existed against CAM science, especially those approaches that do not conform to dominant biomedical theory about disease causation. Many CAM practitioners lack the research training necessary to execute well-designed research, let alone publish it or garner federal funding for it. Until recently there has been a dearth of funding for alternative medicine research. The availability of funding is growing but still lags behind the burgeoning interest in alternative medicine by both the public and the health care community.

CAVEATS

This book is not intended as a clinical cookbook nor as a patient self-care guide. It is an attempt to illustrate some CAM concepts as they relate to HIV/AIDS and to summarize the current state of science in the field. The central issue concerning CAM therapies used in HIV/AIDS is whether they are both safe and effective. It is often wrongly assumed that all natural substances and therefore most alternative therapies must be safe. Many CAM therapies derive from traditional medical systems that have been using particular herbs or medical procedures for centuries. Long-time traditional use can be taken as a suggestion of safety, but most therapies are not applied exactly as they have been traditionally applied. Other CAM therapies are more recently developed or invented, such as ozone, DNCB, and bioelectromagnetic therapies. Therefore we know less about short- or long-term consequences of their use. Ultimately, safety and efficacy should be established for each CAM therapy or combinations of CAM therapies in the same way that safety and efficacy are established for conventional pharmacologicals and procedures. Alternative medicine does not require an alternative science (see Chapter 1). With appropriate adaptations and modifications for the increased complexity of alternative medicine systems, such as combination therapy and acknowledgment of the significance of the placebo effect, the same standard scientific method should prevail. However, more sensitive measuring instruments may need to be developed, and methodologies may need to be refined. CAM takes it for granted that more may be going on in living systems than the currently-taught basic sciences might suggest.

THE CHANGING WORLD OF ALTERNATIVE MEDICINE

There will always be a medical frontier or "fringe" of medicine that is its leading growth edge. There will always be fringe practitioners, theorists, and experimentalists excluded from the dominant medical culture who are pioneers. Sociologists have long pointed out the value of fringe groups in any aspect of culture. As the current state of the science in HIV/AIDS alternative medicine is examined and reported, the field is changing. As parts of CAM are mainstreamed, new CAM therapies and practitioners arise to take over the pioneering fringe. This is as it should be.

References

1. Vella S et al: Recent advances in antiretroviral therapy of HIV infection, *J Biol Regul Homeost Agents* 11(1-2):60-63, 1997.
2. Jonas W: OAM: *Investigating innovative approaches to health care, a report and plan for the Office of Alternative Medicine,* Bethesda, Md, 1998, National Institutes of Health.
3. Eisenberg D, Kessler R, Foster C, et al: Unconventional medicine in the United States: Prevalence, costs, and patterns of use, *N Engl J Med* 328(4):248-252, 1993.
4. Eisenberg DM, Davis RB, Ettner SL, et al: Trends in alternative medicine use in the United States, 1990-1997: results of a follow-up national survey, *JAMA* 280(18):1569-1575, 1998.
5. Anderson WH et al: Patient use and assessment of conventional and alternative therapies for HIV infection and AIDS, *AIDS* 74:561-564, 1993.
6. O'Connor BB, Lazar JS, Anderson WH: Ethnographic study of HIV alternative therapies, Poster presentation, *Eighth Int Conf AIDS* 1992.
7. Mason F: *The complementary therapies project's HIV-treatment survey,* Toronto, Canada, 1995.
8. Abrams B, Duncan D, Hertz-Picciotto I: A prospective study of dietary intake and AIDS in HIV-seropositive homosexual men, *J Acquir Immune Defic Syndr Hum Retrovirol* 6(8):949-958, 1993.
9. Standish, LJ, Calabrese C, Reeves C, et al: A scientific plan for the evaluation of alternative medicine in HIV/AIDS, *Altern Ther Health Med* 3(2):58-67, 1997.

References for Table I-1

Multicenter, randomized, placebo-controlled study of ditiocarb (Imuthiol) in human immunodeficiency virus-infected asymptomatic and minimally symptomatic patients, The HIV87 Study Group, *AIDS Res Hum Retroviruses* 9(1):83-89,1993.

Akerlund B, Tynell E, Bratt G, et al: N-Acetylcysteine treatment and the risk of toxic reactions to trimethoprim-sulfamethoxazole in primary *Pneumocystis carinii* prophylaxis in HIV-infected patients, *J Infect* 35(2):143-147, 1997.

Ancarani F, Veccia S, Giacometti A, et al: Zinc therapy in HIV-infected subjects, *Int Conf AIDS* 9(1):493, 1993.

Antoni MH, Cruess DG, Cruess S, et al: Cognitive-behavioral stress management intervention effects on anxiety, 24-hr urinary norepinephrine output, and T-cytotoxic/suppressor cells over time among symptomatic HIV-infected gay men, *J Consult Clin Psychol* 68(1):31-45, 2000.

Birk TJ, MacArthur RD, McGrady A, et al: Lack of effect of 12 weeks of massage therapy on immune function and quality of life in HIV-infected persons, *Int Conf AIDS* 1996.

Breitkreutz R, Pittack N, Nebe CT, et al: Improvement of immune functions in HIV infection by sulfur supplementation: two randomized trials [see comments], *J Mol Med* 78(1):55-62, 2000.

Burack JH, Cohen MR, Hahn JA, et al: Pilot randomized controlled trial of Chinese herbal treatment for HIV-associated symptoms, *J Acquir Immune Defic Syndr Hum Retrovirol* 12(4):386-393, 1996.

Coates TJ, McKusick L, Kuno R, et al: Stress reduction training changed number of sexual partners but not immune function in men with HIV, *Am J Public Health* 79(7):885-887, 1989.

Conant MA, Calabrese LH, Thompson SE, et al: Maintenance of CD4[1] cells by thymopentin in asymptomatic HIV-infected subjects: results of a double-blind, placebo-controlled study, *AIDS* 6(11):1335-1339, 1992.

Coodley GO, Nelson HD, Loveless MO, et al: Beta-carotene in HIV infection, *J Acquir Immune Defic Syndr Hum Retrovirol* 6(3):272-276, 1993.

Coodley GO, Coodley MK, Lusk R, et al: Beta-carotene in HIV infection: an extended evaluation, *AIDS* 10(9):967-973, 1996.

Coutsoudis A, Bobat RA, Coovadia HM, et al: The effects of vitamin A supplementation on the morbidity of children born to HIV-infected women, *Am J Public Health* 85(8 Pt 1):1076-1081, 1995.

Cruess DG, Antoni MH, Kumar M, et al: Cognitive-behavioral stress management buffers decreases in dehydroepiandrosterone sulfate (DHEA-S) and increases in the cortisol/DHEA-S ratio and reduces mood disturbance and perceived stress among HIV-seropositive men, *Psychoneuroendocrinology* 4(5):537-549, 1999.

De Simone C, Famularo G, Tzantzoglou S, et al: Carnitine depletion in peripheral blood mononuclear cells from patients with AIDS: effect of oral L-carnitine, *AIDS* 8(5):655-660, 1994.

Evans TG, McArdle M: Effect of oral dehydroepiandrosterone (DHEA) administration on acute phase reactants in advanced HIV-1-infected patients, *Fourth Conference on Retroviruses and Opportunistic Infections* 144, 1997.

Falguera M, Perez-Mur J, Puig T, et al: Study of the role of vitamin B_{12} and folinic acid supplementation in preventing hematologic toxicity of zidovudine, *Eur J Haematol* 55(2):97-102, 1995.

Fawzi WW, Msamanga GI, Spiegelman D, et al: Randomised trial of effects of vitamin supplements on pregnancy outcomes and T cell counts in HIV-1-infected women in Tanzania, *Lancet* 51(9114):1477-1482, 1998.

Fawzi WW, Msamanga G, Hunter D, et al: Randomized trial of vitamin supplements in relation to vertical transmission of HIV-1 in Tanzania, *J Acquir Immune Defic Syndr* 23(3):246-254, 2000.

Fiala M, Cone LA, Sayre JW: Clinical benefits and recovery of delayed-type hypersensitivity in patients with AIDS-related complex treated with IMREG-1 or placebo, *Int J Immunopharmacol* 13(7):999-1004, 1991.

Garber GE, Cameron DW, Hawley-Foss N, et al: The use of ozone-treated blood in the therapy of HIV infection and immune disease: a pilot study of safety and efficacy, *AIDS* 5(8):981-984, 1991.

Goodkin K, Feaster DJ, Asthana D, et al: A bereavement support group intervention is longitudinally associated with salutary effects on the CD4 cell count and number of physician visits, *Clin Diagn Lab Immunol* 5(3):382-391, 1998.

Gottlieb MS, Zackin RA, Fiala M, et al: Response to treatment with the leukocyte-derived immunomodulator IMREG-1 in immunocompromised patients with AIDS-related complex. A multicenter, double-blind, placebo-controlled trial, *Ann Intern Med* 115(2):84-91, 1991.

Heseltine PN, Goodkin K, Atkinson JH, et al: Randomized double-blind placebo-controlled trial of peptide T for HIV-associated cognitive impairment, *Arch Neurol* 55(1):41-51, 1998.

Humphrey JH, Quinn T, Fine D, et al: Short-term effects of large-dose vitamin A supplementation on viral load and immune response in HIV-infected women, *J Acquir Immune Defic Syndr* 20(1):44-51, 1999.

Kennedy CM, Coutsoudis A, Kuhn L, et al: Randomized controlled trial assessing the effect of vitamin A supplementation on maternal morbidity during pregnancy and postpartum among HIV-infected women, *J Acquir Immune Defic Syndr* 24(1):37-44, 2000.

Lang JM, Touraine JL, Trepo C, et al: Randomised, double-blind, placebo-controlled trial of ditiocarb sodium (Imuthiol) in human immunodeficiency virus infection, *Lancet* 2(8613):702-706, 1988.

LaPerriere AR, Antoni MH, Schneiderman N, et al: Exercise intervention attenuates emotional distress and natural killer cell decrements following notification of positive serologic status for HIV-1, *Biofeedback Self-Regulation* 15(3):229-242, 1990.

Look MP, Rockstroh JK, Rao GS, et al: Sodium selenite and N-Acetylcysteine in antiretroviral-naive HIV-1-infected patients: a randomized, controlled pilot study, *Eur J Clin Invest* 28(5):389-397, 1998.

Montaner JS, Gill J, Singer J, et al: Double-blind placebo-controlled pilot trial of acemannan in advanced human immunodeficiency virus disease, *J Acquir Immune Defic Syndr Hum Retrovirol* 12(2):153-157, 1996.

Navarette MS, Gharakhanian S, Cardon B, et al: Vitamin B_{12} supplements in patients treated with zidovudine, *Int Conf AIDS* 5:338, 1989.

Perna FM, LaPerriere A, Klimas N, et al: Cardiopulmonary and CD4 cell changes in response to exercise training in early symptomatic HIV infection, *Med Sci Sports Exerc* 31(7):973-979, 1999.

Pichard C, Sudre P, Karsegard V, et al: A randomized double-blind controlled study of 6 months of oral nutritional supplementation with arginine and omega-3 fatty acids in HIV-infected patients, Swiss HIV Cohort Study, *AIDS* 12(1):53-63, 1998.

Reisinger EC, Kern P, Ernst M, et al: Inhibition of HIV progression by dithiocarb, German DTC Study Group, *Lancet* 335(8691):679-682, 1990.

Rigsby LW, Dishman RK, Jackson AW, et al: Effects of exercise training on men seropositive for the human immunodeficiency virus-1, *Med Sci Sports Exerc* 24(1):6-12, 1992.

Sankary T: Controlled clinical trial of anginlyc, Chinese herbal immune enhancer, in HIV seropositives, *Int Conf AIDS* 5:496, 1989.

Scafidi F, Field T: Massage therapy improves behavior in neonates born to HIV-positive mothers, *J Pediatr Psychol* 21(6):889-897, 1996.

Semba RD, Lyles CM, Margolick JB, et al: Vitamin A supplementation and human immunodeficiency virus load in injection drug users, *J Infect Dis* 177(3):611-616, 1998.

Shlay JC, Chaloner K, Max MB, et al: Acupuncture and amitriptyline for pain due to HIV-related peripheral neuropathy: a randomized controlled trial, Terry Beirn Community Programs for Clinical Research on AIDS [see comments], *JAMA* 280(18):1590-1595, 1998.

Simpson DM, Dorfman D, Olney RK, et al: Peptide T in the treatment of painful distal neuropathy associated with AIDS: results of a placebo-controlled trial, The Peptide T Neuropathy Study Group, *Neurology* 47(5):1254-1259, 1996.

Spence DW, Galantino ML, Mossberg KA, et al: Progressive resistance exercise: effect on muscle function and anthropometry of a select AIDS population, *Arch Phys Med Rehabil* 71(9):644-648, 1990.

Stringer WW, Berezovskaya M, O'Brien WA, et al: The effect of exercise training on aerobic fitness, immune indices, and quality of life in HIV-positive patients, *Med Sci Sports Exer* 30(1):11-16, 1998.

Taylor DN: Effects of a behavioral stress-management program on anxiety, mood, self-esteem, and T-cell count in HIV-positive men, *Psychol Rep* 76(2):451-457, 1995.

Walmsley SL, Khorasheh S, Singer J, et al: A randomized trial of *N*-Acetylcysteine for prevention of trimethoprim-sulfamethoxazole hypersensitivity reactions in *Pneumocystis carinii* pneumonia prophylaxis (CTN 057), Canadian HIV Trials Network 057 Study Group, *J Acquir Immune Defic Syndr Hum Retrovirol* 19(5):498-505, 1998.

Weber R, Christen L, Loy M, et al: Randomized, placebo-controlled trial of Chinese herb therapy for HIV-1-infected individuals, *J Acquir Immune Defic Syndr* 22(1):56-64, 1999.

Weerts D, De Wit S, Gerard M, et al: A phase II study of carrisyn (C) (Acemannan) alone and with AZT among symptomatic and asymptomatic HIV patients, *Int Conf AIDS* 6(3):203, 1990.

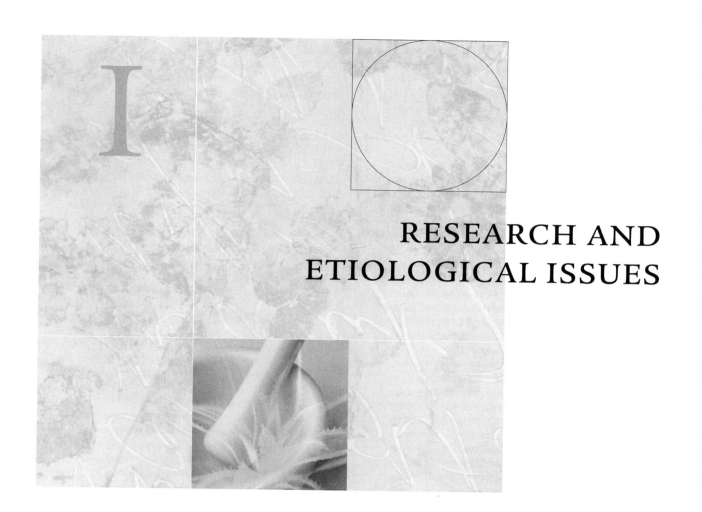

I

RESEARCH AND ETIOLOGICAL ISSUES

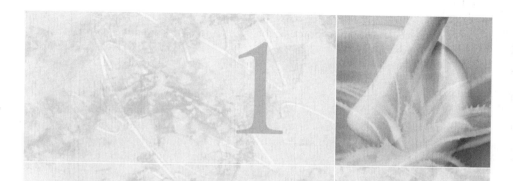

Research Issues in CAM and HIV/AIDS

CARLO CALABRESE

MARY LOU GALANTINO

Researchers have been increasingly interested in complementary and alternative medicine since the field was legitimized as an arena of investigation by the establishment in 1992 of the Office of Alternative Medicine (OAM) at the National Institutes of Health (NIH). Complementary and alternative medicine (CAM) use for all medical conditions is growing significantly in the United States and other countries. There is an increasing social impetus to determine the safety, effectiveness, and cost-effectiveness of CAM. A concomitant increase in public and private attention and funds is invested in research in this area. The first question the consumer asks is, "Does CAM work?" The medical professional asks, "Can CAM meet the standard of proof of modern research?" The following range of questions applies equally to all brands of medicine and contributes to evidence-based medical practice:

1. *Safety evidence*—Is the practice safe?
2. *Experimental evidence*—Is the practice efficacious when examined experimentally?
3. *Clinical practice evidence*—Is the practice effective when applied clinically?
4. *Comparative evidence*—Is it the best practice for the problem?
5. *Rational evidence*—Is the practice rational, progressive, and contributing to medical and scientific understanding?
6. *Demand evidence*—Do consumers and practitioners want the practice?
7. *Satisfaction evidence*—Is it meeting the expectations of patients and practitioners?

8. *Cost evidence*—Is the practice cost-effective?
9. *Meaning evidence*—Is the practice the right one for the individual?

The kinds of evidence listed should be part of a research agenda when possible, regardless of whether the clinical orientation is CAM or conventional.[1] The use of all these types is valuable not only to federal and state agencies that regulate practices and insurance companies that attempt to regulate health economics but also to caregivers and consumers using CAM. CAM adherents want more research done but meet obstacles early; CAM opponents feel that funding for research is unjustified and that the attention it brings merely gives consumers false hope. With the successes of protease inhibitors in the late 1990s, attention to CAM in the treatment of AIDS has relaxed somewhat, but the number of HIV-positive users did not significantly diminish and resurged with the emergence of the drawbacks of highly active antiretroviral therapy (HAART).

The difficulties of research in AIDS, whether in conventional or alternative medicine, are numerous. The putative causative agent—the human immunodeficiency virus (HIV)—is well protected and highly mutable. There are numerous contributory causes to the immunological pathogenesis. A number of blockable molecular targets have been identified in the virus, and some are being exploited pharmaceutically, but a cure is as yet out of reach. The search for a vaccine with an ability to effectively stimulate either an antibody or a cellular immunity against HIV has not yet been productive. The appropriate immunological targets for potentially supportive therapeutics have little consensus surrounding them. Stimulation of $CD4^+$ lymphocytes, for example, holds the potential danger of stimulating the production of the virus in infected cells, since the virus uses the replicative machinery of the cell itself. Some researchers hypothesize that the associated opportunistic infections (OIs) are precipitated by the senescence of the immune system, which is overstimulated from fighting the virus, and that further stimulation of the immune system would ultimately prove futile.[2]

The complications of the disease are numerous. Because separate drug regimens of varying effectiveness for each separate condition exist, distinguishing the effects of a single intervention is difficult. In addition, deleterious drug interactions are increasingly likely with additional treatments. Now that there are some effective therapeutics for HIV infection, the lo-

gistics and ethics of patient recruitment for clinical trials are compounded. Even when trials are conducted, the hard endpoints of viral load and $CD4^+$ lymphocyte levels are only substitute measures for the progress of the disease and the patient's quality of life (QOL). No studies have yet been done on the number of quality-adjusted life years saved by treatment of the putative causative infection by current antiretroviral therapy (ART) or for repair of the central immune deficit. Aside from these difficulties in AIDS research, greater problems exist in attempting to determine if CAM can play a role in ameliorating or even curing AIDS. Although the view exists that CAM research has no particular problems,[3] the research establishment is largely unable to affirm or deny the benefits of CAM in the treatment of AIDS.

Of the research domains—qualitative, laboratory, epidemiological, and clinical—of CAMs, we focus here on research on the evaluation of clinical outcomes. Clinical studies are the most problematic but also the most fruitful, definitive, and urgent. By necessity we must discuss the other research domains when their interrelationship with clinical studies is unavoidable.

THE PROMISE

The experienced CAM practitioner and other adherents answer the question "Does CAM work?" with an almost unequivocal "yes." Several studies have shown high rates of CAM use among HIV-positive persons. At Bastyr University a survey conducted of 120 self-described practitioners of alternative medicine revealed that these providers (MDs, NDs, DCs, acupuncturists, herbalists, and so forth) treat patients at all stages of HIV disease with a variety of CAM practices.[4] Over 90% of the surveyed providers of alternative therapies for HIV/AIDS claimed that their therapies were "somewhat" to "very effective" at all disease stages and on all disease measures, including symptom management (96%), maintaining QOL (98%), raising or maintaining $CD4^+$ lymphocyte levels (66%), slowing progression to AIDS (69%), and extending survival (73%). The providers in the survey were credentialed (80% held state licenses to practice), had substantial experience treating HIV disease (a mean of 6.5 years experience), and were generally willing and able to participate in studies that examined their claims. Some evidence shows that specific CAM treatments are effective in managing AIDS (see Chapter 20).

THE CHALLENGES

The Congressional mandate in the establishment of the OAM, now the National Center for CAM (NCCAM), was to screen and evaluate the most promising unconventional medical practices to develop reliable evidence as a guide to public policy. Given claims and preliminary evidence in the desperate situation of a worldwide pandemic, it is worthwhile to devote a small portion of societal resources to the fields of knowledge peripheral to orthodox approaches in response to the AIDS crisis. If this can be done, valuable treatments and approaches that would not otherwise be explored could be generalized to standard practice in AIDS medicine.

The Breadth of the Problem

To determine if CAM is effective, testworthy CAM practices must be standardized. Complementary and alternative medicines are immensely varied. There are perhaps 5000 plants in the world's herbal pharmacopeias, perhaps 2000 homeopathic remedies, hundreds of natural product medicinals, and at least hundreds of identifiable manipulative practices, dietary practices, psychospiritual approaches, and entire systems of medicine with their own nosologies and conceptions of etiology. In a thoroughgoing evaluation each of these would be parsed, and those relevant to AIDS would be tested. The breadth of content is not only theoretical. In our nationwide longitudinal observational study of 1689 HIV-positive people who were self-identified as using alternative medicine for HIV/AIDS, we categorized possible alternative treatments into different types of providers, substances, and treatment activities garnered from scientific literature, newsletters, clinicians, and buyers clubs.[5] We felt that we were being comprehensive in listing 21 alternative provider types, 86 substances, and 46 treatment activities and were amazed to see our participants add an additional 98 provider types, 1124 substances, and 236 treatment activities to the list. Thus between October 1995 and December 1997, the cohort reported the use of a total of 1492 alternative treatments provided by 119 different provider types for HIV disease. In addition to this imaginative and gritty response, alternative approaches to the AIDS epidemic are being developed simultaneously under urgent circumstances in intellectually and economically divergent cultures throughout the world. This book barely scratches the surface in providing an overview of the field's possibilities.

The Lack of Preliminary Bibliographical Data

A bibliographical search of the accumulated scientific literature is usually the beginning of the pursuit of potentially worthwhile treatments. Unfortunately, the literature on CAM is sparse. Literature on AIDS treatments is especially poor since AIDS is a new disease without the centuries of empirical experience of traditional healers frequently found in CAM treatments. The paucity of CAM literature is due partly to past publication bias against alternative medicine. Peer-review boards are composed of conventionally trained scientists who reject submissions that present a contradiction to the orthodox scientific knowledge base. Orthodoxies as systems are necessarily well organized to resist evidence of theoretically aberrant experiences. Although this prejudice may be overcome by several lines of evidence cogently presented to editors, such a scientific campaign is unlikely for most CAMs that do not have the cadres of scientists needed to design and perform the many experiments that are necessary to overcome divergent orthodox scientific opinion. Simultaneously, there is little resistance to the publication of poorly designed studies refuting claims of the effectiveness of alternative treatment. Recently, a first-rank medical journal, as evidence against CAM effectiveness, published a study designed by a fourth-grade student and a well-known opponent of alternative medicine. They performed an experiment refuting a tenet not even held by the alternative treatment therapy that was purported to be studied.[6] The scientific media has been much more receptive to discussion and evidence in CAM in the last few years, but the accumulation of studies is still small. The more germane problem regarding the lack of CAM data at this point is the lack of CAM research capacity.

The Lack of Research Infrastructure

Investigation in CAM practice has suffered from a relative lack of trained scientists and a lack of funding arising from corporate pharmaceutical research. Modern pharmaceutical research depends on patentability for profitability, and CAMs typically fail the legal tests for patentability. Thus molecular pharmaceutical medicines have the proper economic incentives for development by profit-driven industries while taking advantage of federal- and foundation-funded investigator-driven basic science. Although drug manufacturers are tempted by the economic carrot, they are also driven by regulatory necessity. CAM research incentives are missing at both ends of the process.

Basic research infrastructure for CAM is also missing in the nonprofit development arena because in recent history, applications for funding for research studies, research training, and research facilities for alternative medicine were likely to be rejected by scientific review boards of foundations and the Public Health Service (PHS). Review boards are composed of scientists who are dedicated to an orthodox body of knowledge. Clearly the theory and practice from which CAMs spring are not orthodox by definition. Despite an activist climate in favor of CAM treatments in AIDS research and high CAM use among AIDS patients, the NIH budget had no significant funding of the study of alternative medicine for AIDS until the establishment of Bastyr University's AIDS Research Center in 1994. Federal research dollars devoted to AIDS make it the number-one disease in funding per-disease-caused death at about 12% of the 1997 NIH budget. The 3% of OAM's 1997 budget of $12 million devoted to CAM in the treatment of AIDS was thus 0.0003% of the NIH AIDS budget in the best annual funding scenario in modern history. In Great Britain the situation is somewhat better, but alternative medicine research recently received only 0.08% of National Health Service (NHS) research spending.[7]

Finally, the impetus to do research is not universal among alternative advocates. Some CAM practitioners, although true believers in alternative medicine, feel that they have nothing to prove. Others, who are more inclined to the real-time study of their own therapies, may choose case histories and observational studies as ethically preferable to more convincing methods that are seen as objectifying and manipulating patients. The scientific and ethical interface is a subtle one in modern medical research and has taken decades, even centuries, to develop its safeguards. Its mores are learned through institutional enculturation and experience in applying ethical principles to particular scientific problems. Ethical boards for research have only recently become common in CAM institutions.

Ethics

The Nuremberg trials of 1946 defined the ultimate responsibility of the physician to engage only a well-informed, consenting patient in experimental procedures (Nuremberg Code of 1947). Similar ethical standards were promulgated worldwide with the Declaration of Helsinki in 1964. The Belmont Report (1975), on which US human research policy rests, emphasized the difference between therapeutic research and research unrelated to improving the patient's state of health (the principle of beneficence) and respecting the autonomy of the subject. These principles are no less applicable to research with human subjects for CAM as for conventional medicine. Yet ethical regulation of research arose from social values, including the clinical values of medical practice. The CAM professions are developing an ethical research structure, including institutional misconduct policies and ethical review boards, consistent with both their own professional context and current ethical controls for medical research that permits research consistent with CAM practice.[8]

Ethical control depends partly on preliminary safety information. What constitutes evidence of acceptable risk may be at issue between the two cultures, with animal testing and Phase I trials typically required by conventional authorities versus the evidence of common use usually presented by CAM practitioners. A design standard that calls for the need to withhold a known effective treatment may also make some CAM investigations impossible when seen from the point of view of conventional medical institutions. Some investigators suggest developing alternative trial designs to resolve current conflicts between the ethics and science even of conventional drug trials.[9]

However, the autonomy of patients who reject or fail conventional interventions also needs to be respected. Such patients may provide a volunteer pool for the investigation of CAMs. When the patients are children or other dependent individuals, their lack of autonomy compounds the ethical issue in clinical study, since others may need to make the crucial decisions for them. Yet in the case of pediatrics, pressure is growing to test treatments in children if the treatments are to be used in children.[10] The principle of beneficence in this instance precludes research that does not bear the possibility of therapeutic advantage for the subject. The problem of pediatric trials is common to both CAM and conventional medicine but may prove more difficult to solve with CAM.

Methodological Difficulties in CAM

Clinical research methodology has some difficulties with several characteristics of CAMs. Study designs can often accommodate these difficulties, but they must be well understood before research credible to all stakeholders will have been done.

Variability of CAM Interventions

Besides the contextual problems of the paucity of literature, funding, competent investigators, and other structural impediments in the field, inherent methodological difficulties exist in alternative medicine research. One is the variability of specific CAM interventions. Since replicability is a hallmark of the scientific method, specifically what is tested—whether a substance, a treatment procedure, or a system of practice—needs to be defined, described, and stabilized so that it can be delivered reliably from patient to patient and study to study so that one can make a generalization about the results. Funders of research intend to shape social policy by the results of their support, and they need some assurance of replicability. But in the history of research in alternative medicine, the definition of a practice has typically been ad hoc per study and has varied with the perspectives and affiliations of authors, making metanalyses futile.[11] The standards of complementary medicine tend to be organic and in flux, which is to be expected of a nascent science and industry. From the manufacturing practices for botanical preparations to educational standards for acupuncturists, the definitions and qualities of most CAMs have not achieved anything approaching consensus.

Botanical medicine, as an example, represents a relatively simple problem of nonstandardization among alternative medicines. With herbs it is quite possible to perform a single-agent controlled trial in a specific disease, but numerous choices need to be made regarding the intervention. Problems in studies begin with the verification of plant species used, conditions under which the plant is grown and harvested, and the storage and stability of active compounds. There are choices of whether to use the whole plant, particular parts, various crude extracts, or a specific chemical constituent that may be concentrated in various ways and to varying degrees of purity. Crude fresh extracts, to which many clinical herbalists are partial, are susceptible to deterioration. In the most sophisticated systems of botanical medicine preparation, a product

is standardized for a number of ingredients—for some guaranteeing a minimum concentration and for others a maximum concentration. This is true of the *Ginkgo biloba* extract, for example, which has been the most studied.[*]

Standardizing constituents may present complications. For instance, active ingredients in plants are often classes of molecules, like polysaccharides, saponins, or terpenes, which are difficult to distinguish in biological activity. Different compounds in a single species may have similar or possibly complementary effects, such as the polysaccharides and isobutylamides in *Echinacea* spp. During in vitro assays that guide fractionation of the crude extract toward a single active molecule, it is not uncommon for activity to increase but then diminish as an identified molecular species reaches greater purity, as was the case with the terpenes of *Andrographis paniculata,*[†] which have an influence in cell signaling. When such problems are addressed, these levels of standardization test the industrialization of botanical medicine rather than its roots and do not answer the questions of whether the more commonly used crude extracts or powdered herbs produce the hoped-for clinical benefits.

The problems in botanical research are compounded in other fields of CAM research. Nutrition, for example, can be divided into dietary practices and nutritional supplements. Studies in dietary interventions are demanding. The gold standard for dietary intervention is a residential facility to maintain adherence to the therapeutic regimen, which is an expensive solution, and recruits may be difficult to find. Other populations with controllable diets include the armed forces, prisons, retirement homes, and schools, but ethical review would need to be vigorous. Often in dietary studies a long observation time is needed because diets are often intended as preventives or restoratives, for which clinical outcomes would take a length of time to observe. Finding an appropriate comparison control may also be difficult. Nutritional supplements may be simple (e.g., individual nutrients such as vitamins, minerals, or other single-molecule agents) or complex interventions. Individual nutrients are well known and have been evaluated in general human health for many years. When they are efficacious, they are likely to work in a carefully selected clinical population with idiosyncratic genetically or

---

*Egb761, Schwabe GmbH.
†AndroVir, Paracelsian, Inc.

environmentally determined needs. Therefore clinical study typically calls for either extensive diagnostic studies or very large numbers of subjects (as relatively few will show clinical response). Complex nutritional supplements are special foods like probiotics (live, purportedly health-enhancing bacteria) or algae. Studies in these types of interventions have complications similar to botanical medicine studies.

Nonmaterial Interventions: Procedural, Verbal, and Behavioral Medicine

Both botanical medicine and nutrition are material interventions that, although there are difficulties involved, frequently have well-accepted research models. An adaptation of pharmaceutical clinical research methods may be made with some compromises. Nonmaterial interventions, such as manipulation, exercise, acupuncture and other forms of point work, or psychospiritual treatment, are more problematic. Some simple improvements in clinical research methods have gradually been accepted by both critics and adherents of various CAMs. A blind experiment can be maintained if the therapist and the assessor of health status and outcome see the subject independently. To increase the certainty that a treatment is given every chance to be effective, a rater whose expertise is similar to that of the therapist determines whether the treatment has been correctly applied. For example, two osteopathic doctors trained in the same approach to CranioSacral Therapy see the subject in succession. One treats the subject and the other determines if the subject has improved according to the tenets of the practice before the subject goes on to biopsychosocial medical evaluation. Controls may be difficult to select if a blind experiment is the goal. But progress has been made, even in acupuncture,[12] which has been notoriously difficult to blind. Placebo controls may be difficult to choose, such as with bed rest or eating more vegetables. Randomization to a waiting list or standard care is available, although the level of placebo effect will differ if the two interventions are grossly different or are delivered in different contexts. The increasingly popular electromagnetic (EM) treatments should be easy to test against a placebo as their immediate effects are not apparent to the subject, and the magnetic field can simply be turned off or the magnets removed and replaced by a look-alike. A subject determined to find out what treatment he or she is using, however, can figure it out under most circumstances, if he or she has time and opportunity.

CAM use of psychotherapies may be said to be those that are "off label" for psychotherapy, that is, intended to have effects on physical rather than on mental illnesses. It may be easier to perform tests of hypotheses related to such uses of psychotherapy, since measures of physical disease may be more reliable than psychological outcome measures. The preceding considerations on the variability of the intervention apply.

It is difficult to control the application of a particular psychological intervention because its application is hard to separate from the effect of the therapist. The specificity of practitioner-patient interaction is also troublesome if the experimenter, rather than the therapist, determines the result of the particular psychotherapy; this may result from the extended exposure and greater rapport that is established between therapist and patient. With few exceptions, little has been done on health outcomes consequent to psychological interventions in AIDS (see Chapter 18).

If psychotherapy is expanded to include spiritual interventions (such as personal prayer, meditation, or religious practice or belief), an arena often of significant interest to CAM holistic practitioners and adherents, the research record on interventions is practically nil. The use of spiritual experience is likely to be idiosyncratic or culture specific. Definitions of spirituality in medical literature refer to hope and meaning, a personal relationship with God,[13] serenity,[14] connectedness—all perhaps related to the patient's state of consciousness. A number of thinkers bemoan the lack of definition in this area.[15] Although efforts to present cogent, broadly acceptable definitions are made,[16,17] they have not been widely successful. Only in the fourth edition of the *Diagnostic and Statistical Manual-IV (DSM-IV)* (1995) was the possibility of a religious or spiritual problem even recognized.[18] In medical literature, most references to spirituality come from the nursing field. Relatively little interest has been displayed in the effect of different spiritual interventions on health. Although some traditional medicine practitioners seek to promote spirituality among AIDS patients[19] and some relate the hardiness of people with AIDS to their spirituality,[20] almost none seriously consider the possibility of a spiritual intervention,[21] and no recent studies have considered the effect of spiritual intervention on health outcome in AIDS. Usually, spirituality in AIDS is seen as a coping mechanism.[22]

Another aspect of the spiritually therapeutic refers not to the influence of a patient's internal states on health outcomes but to the intentional therapeutic action, not mediated by language or any well-known material force, of one individual on another. This is sometimes called *psychic* healing or simply *healing*. Prayer for a patient by others may also be included here.[23] Variations may include Therapeutic Touch (TT), laying on of hands, Reiki, Johrei,[24] psychic surgery, mental healing, and other types of paranormal healing. If the intent is to determine if these techniques have an effect on disease, there exist no more particular difficulties to researching studies other than are already addressed here. Design differences may be called for if the therapists were special versus ordinary people or if the healing energy is directed or willed versus invoked (as from God or spirits).

Homeopathy bridges material and nonmaterial interventions. Several treatment approaches exist in homeopathy: constitutional prescribing, acute treatment, proprietary combinations, nosodes, Bach Flower Remedies, Schussler Cell Salts, and so forth. In classical constitutional homeopathic theory, treatment outcome is exquisitely sensitive to the precise remedy chosen for an individual, and prescription errors may be frequent. An extensive case history must be taken and a remedy found before prescription. Then the prescriber proceeds from the clinical outcomes to determine if the correct remedy was chosen. Thus only expert prescribers should be research clinicians, and the likelihood of frequent prescription errors must be considered in design.

Combination Treatment

As complex as these problems are, they pale in the face of the tendency among experienced herbalists, for example, of all cultures to use botanical medicines in combinations individualized for a particular case. This almost universal practice of combination treatments complicates, by order of difficulty, the research problems of standardization, clinical indications, therapeutic targets, and potential toxicities. Individualization and combination are ubiquitous among alternative medicine practices. In a condition with the broad impact and variable expression of AIDS, they are almost inevitable. The tendency toward eclectic combination culminates in therapies such as magnetically enhanced homeopathic remedies (MEHR), in which the interaction of therapeutic cultures (with intriguing preliminary evidence in HIV disease in its favor) results in homeopathically potentized herbal preparations that are injected into the patient at spe-

cific points through a magnetic field. Combination treatment may be critical to the success of those regimens that use them. Single natural agents may have a true effect small enough that a very large patient sample size would be required to detect a difference. Several agents acting together, however, especially if by different mechanisms, may have a cumulative or synergetic effect of a size that may be more readily detectable in clinical trials. Combination treatment may also give the CAM practitioner additional latitude in choosing the correct remedy for a patient's condition, thereby increasing the success rate of treatment. The possibility of adverse events (AEs), however, may rise with combinations.

Individualization

The specificity of the constitutional homeopathic remedy introduces the idea of individualization of treatment regimes. Individualization means that remedies are not prescribed solely on the basis of a single disease category but on other characteristics of the patient. Such characteristics may be transient or constitutional, or they may be chosen as representative of the entire constellation of the patient's health problems and health strengths. The lack of fit between a person's health syndrome and a conventional disease model—expressed perhaps in the inability or reluctance of a conventional practitioner to diagnose a particular health problem—may be the very reason a patient turns to CAM. If a medical system does not recognize an entity, it is unlikely to have an effective therapy for it. The complaint will be managed as something else, resulting in ineffective treatment while exposing the patient to the side effects of the applied treatment. Conversely, a medical system that provides an adequate explanatory model for a patient's experience of his or her symptoms, their origin, and their aggravators and ameliorators has a better chance of having effective treatment or condition management. Thus individualization of treatment is a strength of CAM rather than merely a research problem. If the need for individualization where it is called for in the CAM therapeutic system is neglected in research design, the design will fail to apply the CAM as practiced and will fail to evaluate its potential benefit. A hallmark of medical science is replicability of results obtained with the same intervention. It may be that conventional scientists are reluctant to engage in methods that evaluate an individualized treatment because using such methods implies a rejection of the fundamental doctrine of replicability. In reality, however, no two cases are alike, and the effort to treat patients and their health as if they were engineering materials is a bare approximation of reality—a convenience for practitioners and their body of knowledge.

Medical Systems

The most extreme examples of combination treatment, and concomitantly the most difficult research problems, arise when entire medical systems are to be evaluated. Oriental medicine is an interlocking set of systems with a long history and a well-developed and highly specific body of theory. Some difficulties in acupuncture research have been mentioned. But acupuncture is not practiced alone; rather it is a physical therapy of Chinese medicine. The entire practice includes herbs (commonly in combination), foods, and other physical treatments. Chinese medicine has ramified throughout Asia, Europe, and North America with different styles developing such as traditional Chinese medicine (TCM), Five Element, Japanese acupuncture, and Kanpo. In any of these, the nosology (the array of described pathology) does not coincide with Western pathology. A Western audience, especially a scientific one, is rarely impressed by a superior treatment to correct "Stomach/Spleen disharmony" especially if intermediate markers may be tongue and pulse diagnosis. Proper treatment needs to be individualized and based on the Oriental diagnosis instead of on the diagnosis of AIDS. It is possible to approximately translate syndromes of one system into those of another, but it must be understood that this will decrease the likelihood of applying the correct treatment from one system (Oriental) when its diagnosis is compromised by guidance from principles of a second system (Western). Translation may take place by assigning a Western disease to several Oriental syndromes and then choosing the appropriate treatment for the patient's particular expression of the Western disease. Treatment algorithms that indicate specific Oriental treatments for the Oriental diagnoses that overlap Western diseases may be developed by expert Oriental practitioners who have cross-training in Western medicine. Similarly addressed would be Ayurveda, Unani, the whole practices of shamans and curanderas,[25] and other animistic and vitalistic traditions. Naturopathy, osteopathy, and chiropractic, although removed somewhat in practice from their historical origins, also need to be treated as whole systems.

Thus treatments from systems of medicine are combined and individualized based on the rules of the alternative practice being studied rather than on an allopathic approach to conventional Western disease entities. An allopathic approach implies directly contravening or suppressing a disordered physiological parameter or infectious agent. It is an approach that provides impressive results, at least in the short run, partly because substitute measures for human health improvement are derived from the reductionistic components within its theoretical underpinnings. Alternative practitioners frequently refer to a rationale of balancing, modulation, supporting, and detoxification. Quantifiable measures for these possibly metaphorical goals have not been developed. Despite the lapse of good measures for such outcomes, distorting a practice to fit current research or disease models and measures models may miss possible benefits of CAMs. CAMs that are not evaluated by their own principles cannot be confidently discarded as useless.

Holism

Holism in health research refers to all parameters of human health: physical, psychological, spiritual, social, and environmental. In a research model, holism may be applied to the intervention, as well as to the outcomes. An intervention intended to respond only to a disease entity is not a holistic response nor is it holistic to measure only disease-specific outcomes. While a truly holistic model must contain the reductionistic components to examine the relationship between parts and wholes, questions emerging from a holistic paradigm would be difficult to investigate in vitro. CAM adherents often claim that particular CAMs affect broad parameters of human function such as energy level, immune function, healing capacity, and sense of well-being. They are theorized to have less symptom-specific amelioration but more general health benefits. These kinds of outcomes are difficult to measure yet will have great impact on human suffering, as well as important economic effects in the use of health care and lost productivity.

Since holism implies a reference to the whole of life, studies that intend to measure such values may require extended trials (and substantial expense). When a health care practice is intended to affect the whole being and guide a person toward optimal health, a failure to measure whole health outcomes is a failure to fully evaluate the CAM under investigation. Some critics say that a holistic paradigm cannot be researched at all because research is necessarily reductionistic.[26] To investigate holistic practice, many compromises in the reductionistic gold standard need to be made. If there is to be a reasonable approach to the investigation of holistic medicine, at least one side of the intervention-outcome variables of scientific experimentation needs to be holistically conceived. Fortunately, the development of broad holistic health-outcome measures has advanced since the 1970s. Multifactorial holistic interventions, however, have been rarely investigated, and related proposals have suffered from even greater discrimination by research establishments than have simple materially based CAMs.

Intention

A confounder in a clinical trial is an apparent therapeutic effect that is attributable to a factor associated with the treatment rather than to the test treatment itself. Confounding is a risk inherent to all research. It is why randomization, blinding, and objective measures are valuable in distinguishing therapeutic differences among medications. The most honest scientists may have conscious or unconcious behaviors that modify study results. However, an important confounder that is integral to some CAMs is intentionality. The scientific literature may refer to this as mental or psychic healing and does not always attribute it to ordinary practitioners. Little is written on the capacity of intention to influence physical outcomes; in fact, critics implicitly reject the idea based on Cartesian mind-body duality. Nevertheless, a number of studies indicate its existence.[27,28] Studies of the effect of prayer are also relevant here[23] and raise the possibility that specific kinds of intentionality may make a difference. Studies that blind the practitioner and patient decrease or eliminate the possibility that intentionality will contribute to a positive outcome. Yet CAM theories explicitly accommodate bonding and expectation as contributors to outcome.[29] Intentionality, if it is effective at improving health outcomes, is a difficulty only for research. In clinical practice, therapist intention, if actually efficacious at improving health outcomes, is a wholly nontoxic intervention exercised by all healers—it is in fact the sine qua non of healers.

It is well accepted that orthodox medical care is practiced in a medical culture where practitioners and patients have certain roles and expectations that rein-force expected outcomes. Qualitative ethnographical research is needed to understand the consequences of diverse explanatory models and meanings of health and illness for patient-provider communication, adherence with professional recommendations, and satisfaction with care.[10] Some studies indicate that good physician-patient communication results in better medical outcomes.[30] Various alternative medicine systems have a culture with similarly reinforcing behaviors and beliefs for expected outcomes. Those who refuse to be randomized may likely have a therapeutic orientation that works synergistically with the physical effects of a preferred medicine. The tests of real interest to policymakers are not simply those that determine whether a CAM practice works for anyone to whom it is applied, but those that determine whether it works (and is cost-effective) among those who choose it. A study design that could determine the value of the availability of alternative care in those who choose it rather than when it is assigned is to randomize to either randomization to alternative versus conventional care or to a choice of alternative or conventional care. Such a four-group trial would compare the effects of the different treatments among those who chose them versus those who were assigned to them.

SOME RESPONSES TO THE PROBLEMS

Current circumstances present a wide field of choices to study in CAM medicine, few of which have much preliminary or distinguishing data. When this is combined with the paucity of research resources, picking the right questions—significant, answerable, and feasible to investigate—is a high art. A few principles suggested here may increase the quantity of significant research in CAMs.

Define the Interventions

First, definition and description are needed to identify and render various therapies replicably deliverable. Descriptive and qualitative research, although perhaps not as satisfying or as politically popular as outcomes testing, is necessary for serious investigation of individual treatments, systems, and approaches. Ongoing definition informs the conventional research establishment (e.g., NIH, PHS, medical academics, and the pharmaceutical and health insurance industries) so that the integration of CAMs with the dominant medical research and practice paradigm is facilitated. It allows CAM practitioners to focus on interventions that are replicable and transferable. These are the only interventions that are likely to be adopted in the increasingly industrialized—and now incorporated—health system.

Screen the Possibilities to Select the Best Candidates

Asking the right question is always the most difficult problem in research. This is especially true for CAM, since its research questions need to be refined. All of the problems of doing research in conventional biomedicine apply, without the guidelines that biomedical theory has built over the last two centuries. Although some CAM interventions are obvious choices for testing in other medical conditions, fewer such indicators exist in AIDS partly because it is a new disease without a long history of traditional treatment.

In general, clinical screens must be used to generate worthwhile hypotheses for further testing. Clinical outcomes are more relevant at this point than clinical mechanisms for three reasons: (1) we do not know the clinical mechanisms for most CAMs, (2) we may not have the tools to measure the mechanisms unique to alternative medicines, and (3) the interaction questions are often too complex to parse.

Once a commitment to clinical methods is made, a balance of tools should be favored that has a broad perspective (e.g., qualitative research, observational studies, small comparison trials) rather than just a focus on a few narrow, randomized trials. When with a new field, it is useful to begin with a wide-angle detection system that changes facultatively to a high-precision instrument to test specific examples as supportive evidence emerges. High assurance at first pass is not needed; rather, a ranked order of likely positive effects for the greatest health benefit provides the best guidance.

Use All of the Methods of Science

One of the most important research methods to pursue is the single-agent randomized, controlled trial (RCT). Single-agent RCTs provide empirical scientific evidence. Controlled clinical trials are the only legal basis for the Federal Drug Administration (FDA) to conclude that a new drug has shown "substantial evidence of effectiveness." Many RCT studies can be done now and have sufficient preliminary data to justify controlled trials, such as many of the interventions cited in this volume. Many questions can and should be addressed by RCTs. RCTs have the highest internal validity of any clinical research method. Studies that use randomization to eliminate selection bias and blinding to reduce nonspecific effects provide strong evidence, if results are significantly positive, that a well-defined medication is better than a placebo or an active control in the carefully selected population.

Although the RCT is the gold standard of medical research, by now it is well accepted that RCTs cannot answer all questions.[31] In the evaluation of alternative medicine the RCT can be entered too early, before the intervention is standardized and the right population is identified for sampling. RCTs are also expensive, such as the $4.5 million the NIH awarded in 1997 for a trial of St. John's wort (Hypericum perforatum) for depression ($n = 300$). Such expenditures cannot be made for many CAM interventions. Since funding in CAM research is limited, the value of small trials, open trials, case series, and case studies should be recognized. A controlled trial generally requires four times the number of subjects as an open trial to detect the same therapeutic difference in an outcome measure. Although the validity of the answer is less certain, several open trials can be conducted for the same expense and difficulty of one randomized trial. Because preliminary information is needed to select the best possibilities for more stringent trials, such design compromises are reasonable in early studies.

Many research designs are not frequently used but provide good information in early stages of investigational programs. Single-patient studies have reached a high level of sophistication and minimize risk to subjects.[32-34] Observational studies can track the outcomes of a number of therapies simultaneously,[5] and time-series studies have been developed for office practice and applied to CAM treatments.[35] When the medicine and mechanisms are not well-defined, a best-case series method, such as the one adopted by the National Cancer Institute (NCI) for novel therapies, will be useful. The investigation of remarkable cases, such as reports of retroconversion to seronegativity, may provide excellent leads for follow-up.[36] Case controls on hardy patients may indicate beneficial health characteristics and behaviors.[20] Open trials are valuable in AIDS research, which has hard objective endpoints such as viral load, $CD4^+$ lymphocyte levels, the expression of uncommon infections, and survival. The methodology of the RCT is undergoing rapid evolution to accommodate patient preferences, which is an important issue in CAM research.[37,38] For treatments that call for adaptation of medications, such as homeopathy, response-adaptive design theory may contribute.[39] Contrary to what many alternative practitioners believe, good research designs are available even for nonmaterial interventions.[3] Of course, funding review committees need to be as open to the possibilities of alternative trial designs as CAM researchers.

The many clinical cases under everyday CAM treatment are not evaluated in a consistent way. The high use of CAM for the treatment of AIDS is a great opportunity for community-based observational studies that scan users for associated benefits.[5] These indicators can then be tested further in clinical trials. Such studies are also valuable for scanning for possible harm, thus providing a great deal of information about a wide research field before turning to controlled (and expensive) randomized trials. Although the debate in conventional medicine argues over whether to allow or encourage patient access to CAM, ethics are local and should address the context in which they are applied.[40] Thus ethical issues are reduced in complexity. Similarly, regulatory issues in observational screening studies are also much reduced.

The World Health Organization (WHO) (1948) defined *health* as a "state of complete physical, mental, and social well-being and not merely the absence of disease or infirmity, maximizing patients' mental, physical, and social functioning."[41] The two most frequently operationalized parts of this definition of whole health are (1) a sense of well-being and (2) functionality. The emphasis on performance distinguishes functional status from other aspects of health-related QOL. A number of validated instruments for assessing sense of well-being now exist, such as the Quality of Well-Being Scale (QWB), the Symptom Distress Scale, and the Present State Examination. Instruments assessing functionality include the Karnofsky Performance Scale, the Sickness Impact Profile (SIP), the Instrumental ADL (IADL), Neurobehavioral Function: An ADL Rating Scale, the Katz Index of Activities of Daily Living, and the Functional Independence Measure (FIM). More sophisticated instruments attempt to address both the functioning and well-being dimensions of health simultaneously, most notably the several manifestations of the Medical Outcomes Survey—Short Form (MOS—SF 30, 36, 38, and 56), the Dartmouth COOP Functional Health Assessment Charts, Health Status Measures for Adults, and the QOL Instrument. Spiritual outcomes, or the individual's sense of fitness in the universe and his or her personal interface with the grand mysteries of being, are less studied than other spiritual clinical correlates. A review of the literature on spirituality demonstrates the use of only one scale used to measure Spiritual Well-Being (SWB). Ellison and Paloutzian (1982) designed the SWB scale, which consists of 20 items designed to measure religious well-being (RWB) and existential well-being (EWB).

More physical measures require further research as well. For example, instrumentation needs further development to measure whole-body responses to subtle influences, such as changes in low energy emissions from the body in response to Qigong.[42] Although the concentration here is on clinical work, all domains of medical research—basic science, clinical and epidemiological studies, and appropriate animal studies—have their respective strengths and should be pursued.

Test by Methods That Do Not Distort CAM Practice

Most health research is oriented to products, patents, and profits. The FDA system of drug regulation was developed to both restrain and encourage the pharmaceutical industry in its current economic environment. It works quite well for molecular medical approaches with novel molecules but not for many CAMs because of the issues previously cited. Pharmaceutical firms now fund 2.5 times as much clinical research as the NIH, and both sources of research funds are devoted essentially to products or devices. Researchers have relatively little interest in CAM procedures or combination treatments, and virtually no research exists in CAM systems such as Ayurveda and naturopathy. The current environment does not encourage medical advances that are not economically protected. After doing the necessary descriptive research on CAMs, research methods should be chosen that least interfere with the CAM practices to be studied instead of distorting CAM practices to fit models of research intended for patentable drugs. The medicine needs to be delivered in context, and broad measures of health and well-being are required to evaluate its outcomes. For some studies in individualized medicines, treatment could be determined by algorithm, but for others, using expert CAM practitioners for the more complex multimodality treatments may be a necessity. The practitioner could be considered as the intervention for a trial of a medical system. A Delphi panel of CAM practitioners could select a common treatment for a selected population sample. All of the methodologies that are appropriate to the evaluation of CAM practices have not yet been developed. Innovative designs, which CAM practitioners assert do not distort practice, will be needed instead of conventional designs, which produce high-validity answers to the wrong questions.

Reduce the Obstacles to More CAM Research

CAM clinician-scientists who have the incentive and ability to perform research studies are rare at present. The pool of researchers educated in both CAM and research methods needs to be increased, and CAM practitioners should be targeted for research traineeships. To develop CAM research infrastructure, the funding share for CAM needs to be increased, something which is occurring in the United States as the NIH National Center for CAM garners increased attention from Congress. The development of research capacity funded at CAM academic institutions is especially valuable because future research in these institutions will stay focused on CAMs rather than be diverted to more lucrative conventional drugs.

Regulation is somewhat of a deterrent to small trials. The FDA requires an investigational new drug (IND) application if a disease endpoint is being studied and toxicity data even in cases with a long history of human use. An intermediate standard for proceeding with a trial in a historical remedy for which no drug indication or regulatory protection is being sought should be explicitly implemented by the FDA.

The biases that continue to pervade the current research establishment[43] need to be further ameliorated. A temporary affirmative action program may be needed to appoint practitioners and researchers who are deeply familiar with CAMs to funding and publication review panels. Every research study, especially a clinical one, is a network of compromises. The compromises relevant to the issues raised in this chapter may seem arbitrary to those who are unfamiliar with CAM. Those compromises needed to protect the integrity of the medicine being tested should be defended, as well as those made to meet other needs in a particular study. To choose where to invest research dollars, consider the traditional CAM literature, academic centers, and experienced practitioners, as well as the much more common in vitro screens of traditional (not conventional) medicines.

Persistence Is Required

Finally, patience is in order. This is not easy to hear during the AIDS crisis. The CAM field is broader than the current field of conventional medicine and simultaneously holds multiple worldviews. Important questions will not be answered overnight. To realistically appraise the possibilities of CAM, social, scientific, and intellectual changes need to be made to the structure of research activities. A CAM research system created and disappearing overnight in response to politics, marketing, or clinical fads would be particularly destructive. There is good reason to continuously dedicate a portion of the social allocation of scientific resources to exploring alternative medicine. CAM may prove to be a valuable partner with conventional allopathic, reductionistic, and molecular approaches to health care. The fundamental intentions of allopathic medicine will be enhanced by alternative perspectives in the human response to health threats.

References

1. Spencer JW: Essential issues in complementary/alternative medicine. In Spencer JW, Jacobs JJ, editors: *Complementary/alternative medicine: an evidence-based approach,* St Louis, 1999, Mosby.
2. Pommier JP, Gauthier L, Livartowski J, et al: Immunosenescence in HIV pathogenesis, *Virology* 231(1): 148-154, 1997.
3. Vickers A: Methodological issues in complementary and alternative medicine research: a personal reflection on 10 years of debate in the United Kingdom, *J Altern Complement Med* 2(4):515-524, 1996.

4. Calabrese C, Wenner C: Treatment of HIV-positive patients with complementary and alternative medicine: a survey of practitioners, *J Altern Complement Med* 4(3):281-287, 1998.

5. Standish LJ, Calabrese C, Reeves C, et al: A scientific plan for the evaluation of alternative medicine in the treatment of HIV/AIDS, *Altern Ther Health Med* 3(2):58-67, 1997.

6. Rosa L, Rosa E, Sarner L, et al: A close look at therapeutic touch, *JAMA* 279:1005-1010, 1998.

7. Ernst E: Regulating complementary medicine: only 0.08% of funding for research in NHS goes to complementary medicine, *BMJ* 313(7061):882, 1996 (letter).

8. Gatterman MI: A patient-centered paradigm: a model for chiropractic education and research, *J Altern Complement Med* 1(4):371-386, 1995.

9. Parsons CD, Grubb IR: Tensions between the science and ethics of HIV clinical drug trials: social constructions of the trial, *Int Conf AIDS* 11(1):238 (abstract no. Tu.B.523), 1996.

10. Kemper KJ, Cassileth B, Ferris T: Holistic pediatrics: a research agenda, *Pediatrics* 103:902-909, 1999.

11. Anonymous: Defining and describing complementary and alternative medicine, Panel on definition and description, CAM Research Methodology Conference, April 1995, *Altern Ther Health Med* (2):49-57, 1997.

12. Zaslawski C, Rogers C, Garvey M, et al: Strategies to maintain the credibility of sham acupuncture used as a control treatment in clinical trials, *J Altern Complement Med* 3(3):257-266, 1997.

13. Swanson CS: A spirit-focused conceptual model of nursing for the advanced practice nurse, *Issues Compr Pediatr Nurs* 18(4):267-275, 1995.

14. Roberts KT, Whall A: Serenity as a goal for nursing practice, *Image J Nurs Sch* 28(4):359-364, 1996.

15. Goddard NC: "Spirituality as integrative energy": a philosophical analysis as requisite precursor to holistic nursing practice, *J Adv Nurs* 22(4):808-815, 1995.

16. Dyson J, Cobb M, Forman D: The meaning of spirituality: a literature review, *J Adv Nurs* 26 (6):1183-1188, 1997.

17. Pehler SR: Children's spiritual response: validation of the nursing diagnosis spiritual distress, *Nurs Diagn* 8(2):55-66, 1997.

18. Turner RP, Lukoff D, Barnhouse RT, et al: Religious or spiritual problem: a culturally sensitive diagnostic category in the *DSM-IV*, *J Nerv Ment Dis* 183(7):435-444, 1995.

19. Peri TA: Promoting spirituality in persons with acquired immunodeficiency syndrome: a nursing intervention, *Holist Nurs Pract* 10(1):68-76, 1995.

20. Carson VB: Prayer, meditation, exercise, and special diets: behaviors of the hardy person with HIV/AIDS, *J Assoc Nurses AIDS Care*, 4(3):18-28, 1993.

21. Hodges RD, Scofield AM: Is spiritual healing a valid and effective therapy? *J R Soc Med* 88(4):203-207, 1995.

22. Guillory JA, Sowell R, Moneyham L, et al: An exploration of the meaning and use of spirituality among women with HIV/AIDS, *Altern Ther Health Med* 3(5):55-60, 1997.

23. Targ E: Evaluating distant healing: a research review, *Altern Ther Health Med* 3(6):74-78, 1997.

24. Bihari B: Johrei in the treatment of HIV/AIDS, *Int Conf AIDS* 10(2):65 (abstract no. 537B), 1994.

25. Krippner S: A cross-cultural comparison of four healing models, *Altern Ther Health Med* 1(1):21-29, 1995.

26. Elbaz G: Holism: the other voice of AIDS activism, *Int Conf AIDS* 10(1):396 (abstract no. PD0193), 1994.

27. Benor DJ: *Healing research: holistic energy medicine and spirituality,* Munich, 1993, Helix Verlag GmbH.

28. Schlitz M, Braud W: Distant intentionality and healing: assessing the evidence, *Altern Ther Health Med* 3(6):62-73, 1997.

29. Wirth DP: The significance of belief and expectancy within the spiritual healing encounter, *Soc Sci Med* 41(2):249-260, 1995.

30. Stewart MA: Effective physician-patient communication and health outcomes: a review, *CMAJ* 152(9):1423-1433, 1995.

31. Rabeneck L, Viscoli CM, Horwitz RI: Problems in the conduct and analysis of randomized clinical trials: are we getting the right answers to the wrong questions? *Arch Intern Med* 152(3):507-512, 1992.

32. Kiene H, von Schon-Angerer T: Single-case causality assessment as a basis for clinical judgment, *Altern Ther Health Med* 4(1):41-47, 1998.

33. Barlow DH, Blanchard EB, Hayes SC, et al: Single-case designs and clinical biofeedback experimentation, *Biofeedback Self Regul* 2(3):221-239, 1977.

34. Guyatt GH, Keller JL, Jaeschke R, et al: The *n*-of-1 randomized controlled trial: clinical usefulness, our three-year experience, *Ann Intern Med* 112(4):293-299, 1990.

35. Keating JC Jr, Giljum K, Menke JM, et al: Toward an experimental chiropractic: time-series designs, *J Manipulative Physiol Ther* 8(4):229-238, 1985.

36. Weibo L, Ruixing W, Chongfen G, et al: A report on 8 seronegative converted HIV/AIDS patients with traditional Chinese medicine, *Chin Med J* 108(8):634-637, 1995.

37. Feine JS, Awad MA, Lund JP: The impact of patient preference on the design and interpretation of clinical trials, *Community Dent Oral Epidemiol* 26(1):70-74, 1998.

38. Rucker G: A two-stage trial design for testing treatment, self-selection and treatment preference effects, *Stat Med* 8(4):477-485, 1989.

39. Rosenberger WF, Lachin JM: The use of response-adaptive designs in clinical trials, *Control Clin Trials* 14(6):471-484, 1993.

40. Christakis NA: Ethics are local: engaging cross-cultural variation in the ethics for clinical research, *Soc Sci Med* 35(9):1079-1091, 1992.

41. World Health Organization, Regional Office for the Western Pacific: *Research guidelines for evaluating the safety and efficacy of herbal medicines,* Bangkok, 1993, WHO.

42. Godik EE, Gulyaev YV: Functional imaging of the human body: dynamic mapping of physical EM fields signals a breakthrough in medical diagnostics, *IEEE Eng Med Biol Mag Dec* 21-29, 1991.

43. Resch KI, Ernst E, Garrow J: A randomized controlled study of reviewer bias against an unconventional therapy, *J R Soc Med* 93:164-167, 2000.

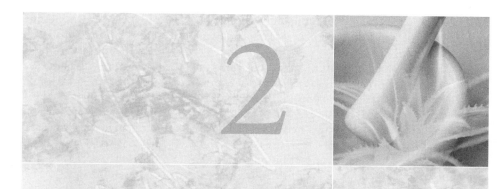

Etiology and Pathogenesis of AIDS

ROBERT S. ROOT-BERNSTEIN
STEPHEN J. MERRILL

INTRODUCTION

Science progresses through the constant interplay between theory and experience, which may occur in several ways. One employs a recursive process, in which a researcher creates a theory to explain a set of observations; makes predictions and tests them through further observation; modifies the theory in light of any new data; and makes new predictions. Two problems with this method are (1) that progress is incremental and (2) fundamental assumptions are infrequently challenged by observation. Data that support a theory are always easier to find than data that challenge it. Consequently, flaws in recursively tested theories often go unrecognized for extended periods of time. One alternative is to use a dialectical method in which a

thesis is contradicted by an antithesis with the goal of creating a new, more powerful synthesis. Unfortunately, dialectical methods are more likely to result in polarization of the issues, which leads to controversy that cannot be resolved, rather than a synthetic leap forward. A second, more workable alternative generates a wide range of tentative, competing explanations at the outset of research. Each explanation makes widely different predictions, which are used to create tests that can differentiate between their explanatory powers. The advantage of this method is that the researcher can quickly narrow down the types of theories most likely to suffice for any particular problem and simultaneously be assured that crucial assumptions underlying the different theories are tested against one another. The disadvantage is that the researcher must keep an open mind and take care not to become attached to a particular explanation in advance of relevant data.

All three methods are used to address acquired immune deficiency syndrome (AIDS). Mainstream researchers, comprised mainly of virologists, defined the standard approach to AIDS early in the epidemic when they focused on finding a new virus. Their underlying assumption was that a new disease required a new disease agent. The discovery of human immunodeficiency virus (HIV) in 1983 confirmed their expectations and set the course of AIDS research firmly on the track of the one disease agent/one disease/one treatment dogma that served Western medicine for nearly a century. Advances in AIDS research stemmed largely from the incremental, recursive development of the HIV theory, which states that HIV is both necessary and sufficient to account for the degeneration of the immune system as AIDS progresses. The HIV theory is the only theory to garner significant funding so far.

From the outset, some researchers were not convinced that HIV had the characteristics necessary to cause AIDS. These researchers range from Papadopulos-Eleopulos and her colleagues, who claim that HIV is an artifact of virological isolation methods that do not satisfy any of the criteria necessary for the identification of a new virus, to Nobel Prize winner Kary Mullis, who believes that HIV exists but has nothing to do with AIDS.[1] The most notable contrarian is Peter Duesberg. Duesberg, a virologist, believes that the existence of HIV has been demonstrated formally but doubts its pathogenicity. He adopts a dialectical approach to the HIV hypothesis, claiming that HIV is a "pussycat" that cannot cause disease. Many of Duesberg's early criticisms were cogent and gained widespread attention, spurring some important tests of the HIV theory. His failure to pose an alternative explanation for AIDS, however, presented a stumbling block to further progress. His theory that drug use, including antiretroviral drugs such as AZT, causes AIDS has neither gained acceptance nor generated any corroborative research results to date.[2]

A third group of investigators employing the multiple hypotheses approach to AIDS has also existed from the outset of the epidemic. They were led by Joseph Sonnabend, who noted even before HIV was isolated that the discovery of any new disease agent would have to be placed in the context of multiple immunosuppressive agents encountered by all individuals who contracted HIV and developed AIDS. Sonnabend pointed out the politically unacceptable observation that gay men and intravenous (IV) drug abusers who contracted HIV were also characterized by multiple, concurrent infections from sexually transmitted diseases (STDs); chronic infections from viruses known to be immunosuppressive, such as herpesviruses, cytomegalovirus (CMV), and hepatitis viruses; very high rates of antisemen antibodies that cross-reacted with and killed T cells; and the use of drugs, such as heroin, morphine, cocaine, and nitrite inhalants that have immunomodulatory effects. Consequently, Sonnabend argued that HIV might play any of several roles in AIDS: (1) it might be necessary and sufficient to cause AIDS; (2) it might be necessary but not sufficient; or (3) it might be an opportunistic infection (OI) taking advantage of an already compromised immune system.[3-5] We follow Sonnabend's lead by adopting the multiple hypotheses method.[6-8]

Consequently, we focus on the predictions that allow one theory to be distinguished from another and the phenomena that one would expect to observe, depending on which theory is correct. We also summarize the data that have been accumulated by an ever-growing number of investigators suggesting that there is more to AIDS than HIV.

ALTERNATIVE THEORIES

Standard textbook accounts of AIDS pathogenesis describe a process in which HIV infects CD4$^+$ T lymphocytes (hereafter referred to as T cells), macrophages, and dendritic cells, creating a persistent, low-level infection that slowly wears down the immune system over time. The exact mechanisms of cellular death are still the subject of intense investigation that includes possibilities such as HIV-triggered apoptosis (programmed cell death), direct cellular killing, and indirect cellular killing due to observed increases in cytokines, tumor necrosis factor (TNF), and related molecules.[9,10] Some investigators note that HIV proteins have significant homologies to human proteins, including class II major histocompatibility complex (MHC II) proteins and that most people with AIDS develop autoantibodies against T-cell determinants. These observations led to the hypothesis that HIV may trigger an autoimmune process in which B cells produce antibodies against HIV that cross-react with and kill T cells.[11-15] Other investigators note that HIV proteins have significant homologies with various nerve toxins, suggesting that the dementias associated with HIV infection may result from the buildup of toxic protein fragments from HIV.[16]

The key implications of the theory that HIV is both necessary and sufficient to cause AIDS (hereafter, the HIV-only theory) are as follows: (1) we are all at equal risk of HIV infection and AIDS, (2) everyone exposed to an equal dose of HIV should have an equal chance of chronic infection, (3) everyone infected with HIV should (within probabalistic variability) progress to AIDS at the same rate as everyone else, and (4) the only way to stop the progress of AIDS is to stop HIV.[9,10]

The second theory we consider is the cofactor theory, which has two major versions. The first version of cofactor theory retains the basic premises of the HIV-only theory and adds the prediction that the rate of AIDS development after HIV infection is determined by the presence or absence of specific cofactors. HIV infection requires that a potential T-cell host be in an activated or stimulated state,[17] and HIV replication requires that the infected T cell be stimulated.[18,19] Although HIV-only theories suggest that HIV creates its own stimulated lymphocytes, many investigators believe that the necessary activation can be achieved by other factors. These cofactors may be other viral, bacterial, or parasitic infections, as well as exposure to allogeneic antigens such as those found in blood and semen.[4,6,7] Broadening the definition of cofactors to include any factors or conditions that can change the natural history of HIV infection expands the cofactor list to include immunosuppressive drugs, malnutrition, or anything else that has a profound effect on immune function.[6,7] Thus this type of cofactor theory suggests that individuals with different post-HIV-infection risks have different natural histories of infection and as a result progress to AIDS at different rates. Conversely, the treatment of cofactor infections and conditions has a pronounced effect on development of AIDS. We call this the cofactor-promoted HIV theory.

A second version of cofactor theory argues that HIV is necessary but not sufficient to cause AIDS. Those who favor this approach to understanding AIDS argue that in the absence of cofactor exposures, HIV is neither able to infect people nor able to replicate within individuals once infection has occurred. This cofactor theory also posits that the cofactors play an essential role in establishing the immune status

and susceptibility to HIV before exposure. Thus healthy individuals are unlikely to become infected with HIV, and HIV-infected individuals who can eliminate existing cofactor risks and avoid future ones may be able to drive their HIV infection into latency. In contrast to the cofactor-promoted HIV theory, the risk of infection is determined by cofactor exposure. Both theories postulate that the rate of progress to AIDS after HIV infection is determined by cofactor presence, but since cofactors are *necessary* and not just modulatory, elimination of cofactors should be as effective at stopping AIDS as is treatment of HIV.[4,6,7] We call this the cofactors-required HIV theory.

A final theory should also be considered both to cover all the possibilities and to establish the null hypothesis. We must consider the possibility that HIV is neither necessary nor sufficient to cause AIDS. In this case two different explanations of AIDS are possible. First, HIV may be one of many immunosuppressive agents present in people who develop AIDS, having no greater or lesser bearing on pathogenesis than any of the others. Second, HIV is simply another OI typical of significant immune dysfunction but is actually secondary to the causes of AIDS. The implications are that AIDS is either the result of a single causative agent that has not yet been discovered or a multifactorial disease caused by an accumulation of immunological insults over time. In the second case it should be possible to demonstrate that people at risk for AIDS develop severe immune suppression either before exposure to HIV or in its complete absence. A significant number of people who have developed AIDS without being infected by HIV should exist, and the nature of the immunosuppressive risks encountered by these individuals should provide strong clues to the true causes of AIDS.[1,2] Thus treatment of HIV would be of secondary importance in preventing AIDS. We call this the non-HIV theory.

One caveat is in order when considering cofactor and non-HIV theories. A significant difference exists between the symbiotic interactions of disease agents, synergistic interactions, and progressive accumulation theories. In a symbiotic interaction, both agents are necessary for functionality. For example, Shope discovered in 1931 that swine flu in pigs is caused by a combination of a virus and a bacterium, neither of which is pathogenic in pigs by itself.[20] This case is quite different from that observed in the synergism between alcohol and barbiturates. Alcohol and barbiturates are each capable of causing death in large quantities but can cause death when taken together in relatively small amounts. Their effects are *more than additive*. Synergism in turn must be contrasted with progressive accumulation of exposures to immunosuppressive agents, in which the effects would be purely additive. According to a cumulative exposures or an antigenic overload theory of AIDS, immune destruction is the simple result of immunological depletion.[4,5,21-24] Thus we must consider the possibility that the dose of HIV and the dose of any putative cofactors are critical factors in determining the outcome of infection. Large doses of HIV may not require cofactors, but cofactors may greatly potentiate HIV activity or even cause infection with otherwise noninfective doses of HIV (an effect compatible with either a cumulative exposures theory or a synergistic theory). On the other hand, HIV may require cofactors (a symbiotic theory) along the lines of Shope's swine flu model in pigs. Synergistic theories also do not eliminate the logical possibility that a sufficient dose of cofactors might be capable of inducing acquired immunosuppression, just as alcohol or barbiturates are, in large enough doses, each capable of inducing death. The point is that not all alternative theories of AIDS are mutually exclusive, and therefore no single set of data will suffice to differentiate one theory from another.

CRITICAL STUDIES DIFFERENTIATING THE THEORIES

The critical information required to differentiate one theory from another can be summarized into the following categories: (1) tests of the null hypothesis (i.e., what evidence exists for AIDS without HIV?); (2) data concerning average rates of progression of different risk groups from HIV infection to AIDS; (3) clinical and epidemiological studies of the influence of specific cofactors on the progression of HIV infection; (4) laboratory studies of the influence of cofactors on HIV activity in vitro; (5) data concerning risk of HIV infection that depends on the nature of the exposure or health status at time of exposure to HIV; and (6) studies of the effect of treatment of cofactor risks on progression to AIDS.

First, we must test the null hypothesis by determining whether HIV is necessary to cause AIDS. The standard approach to this question is to point to large-scale clinical studies of people in high-risk groups for AIDS, such as gay men and hemophiliacs, that compare the incidence of AIDS in the presence and absence of HIV. All such studies unanimously conclude that HIV is necessary to cause AIDS because people without HIV infections have never developed severe immunosuppression or AIDS in any of these studies.[9,10,25] The only reason that the issue can reasonably be raised at present is that a very small number (much less than 1% of AIDS cases even by Duesberg's[2] most optimistic count) of idiopathic cases resembling AIDS in individuals with no evidence of HIV infection continuously turn up. Most of these cases are subsumed under the rubric of idiopathic CD4$^+$ T-cell lymphopenia (ICL), in which helper T-cell counts drop below 300 and OIs, Kaposi's sarcoma (KS), or central nervous system (CNS) lymphoma ensues.[26,27]

Unfortunately, the meaning of these cases is open to several interpretations. One is that as yet unidentified causes of immune suppression much rarer than HIV exist. According to this interpretation, HIV is the cause of AIDS, and exceptional cases have exceptional causes. Studies of hospitalized patients, blood donors, and HIV-negative people in West Africa all suggest that ICL is indeed an exceptional syndrome.[28-30] ICL has, however, been found to occur at significantly higher rates among sexual partners of HIV-infected individuals and others at risk for AIDS than among the general population.[31] These results suggest two additional interpretations. One is that these idiopathic cases disprove the HIV theory.

Duesberg and his colleagues[1,2] interpret all cases of ICL to support the thesis that HIV does not cause AIDS. The HIV theory, however, cannot be disproved by the simple observation of exceptions. Idiopathic versions exist for virtually every disease. Acquired immunosuppression may have several causes, HIV being only one of the most common. Evidence that some forms of acquired immunosuppression occur in the absence of HIV does not invalidate the HIV-only theory any more than the evidence that pneumonia can be caused by *Pneumocystis carinii* disproves the theory that pneumonia can also be caused by *Mycoplasma pneumoniae*. An additional step is necessary: to demonstrate that AIDS is caused by some agent or agents that are present not only in people infected with HIV but also in those with idiopathic immunosuppression. This second step has not been carried out successfully at present.

The fact that lymphopenia occurs much more frequently among those at risk for AIDS than among the general population suggests yet a third possibility, which is that HIV is the primary cause of AIDS but that cofactors associated with immunosuppression in AIDS may, in rare circumstances, synergize to create an AIDS-like symptom in the absence of HIV. In this case significant immunosuppression should be evident in some individuals exposed to putative AIDS cofactors in the absence of HIV infection. This is in fact the case for many people at risk for HIV, although the resulting immunosuppression is rarely sufficiently severe to result in OIs.[6,7] These cofactors may increase susceptibility to HIV and, under unusual circumstances, progress to AIDS independent of HIV. However, we will proceed on the basis that HIV is necessary to cause AIDS because all existing data are currently consistent with that proposition. We will concentrate instead on the question of whether HIV is sufficient.

Data concerning the rate of progression to AIDS after HIV infection can help to differentiate the HIV-only theory from cofactor theories. Different risk groups have widely different exposure rates to infectious and STDs, antibiotic use, immunomodulatory drugs, malnutrition, allogeneic stimuli such as semen or blood products, and preexisting medical impairments.[6,7] If cofactors affect progression from HIV infection to AIDS, then these different exposures should translate into observable rate differences. However, if HIV is both necessary and sufficient to account for AIDS, then no risk-group difference should be apparent. Weiss[9] has in fact claimed that people in all risk groups do progress to AIDS at the same rate (an average of 10 years from HIV infection to AIDS). The one exception that Weiss admits is young hemophiliacs, who survive somewhat longer (and whom he conjectures may start with higher numbers of T cells than older individuals have). Weiss concludes that cofactors play an insignificant role in AIDS pathogenesis. Root-Bernstein,[32] however, performed a more extensive study of available data and found, contrary to Weiss, that significant differences exist between rates of progression in risk groups. The rate of progression among young hemophiliacs is even slower than Weiss reported, averaging more than 20 years. Transfusion patients, whose date of infection is known, progress significantly faster than gay men or older hemophiliacs (averaging about 6 years from HIV infection to AIDS). People who contract HIV during a transplant operation and are subsequently immunosuppressed for thera-

peutic reasons develop AIDS on average within 2½ years,[33] and infants infected with HIV either serorevert or develop AIDS on average within 6 months. (Figure 2-1)[32] Additional studies confirm that rates of progression to AIDS differ by risk group.[34-38] Notably, elderly individuals (over the age of 60) have an increased rate of progression to AIDS compared with other population groups.[39] Thus little doubt exists that cofactors play some role in AIDS pathogenesis.

Clinical and epidemiological studies of AIDS progression give a more precise picture of AIDS pathogenesis that also suggests pivotal roles for cofactors. Once again, if HIV were responsible for all aspects of immune pathology in AIDS, then the presence or absence of other immunomodulatory diseases or agents would be expected to be irrelevant to AIDS progression, but this is not the case. Immune stimulation providing a broad source of activated macrophages and T cells is now generally considered to be a dominant feature of AIDS pathogenesis.[35,40-42] In addition, T-cell activation is shown to be a more important indicator of shorter survival than is HIV plasma burden or virus chemokine receptor usage (viral tropism).[43] A wide range of infectious agents are also known to infect T cells and macrophages, causing immunosuppression independent of HIV. These include CMV, hepatitis viruses (HBV and HCV), human T-lymphotropic viruses (HTLVs) types I and II, human herpesvirus (HSV, HHV-2, or HHV-6), and mycoplasmas. All of these infectious agents are highly associated with and actively produced and excreted by people infected with HIV. There is no reason to think that their immunosuppressive activity is eliminated simply because HIV is present, and there is every reason to believe that activation of these agents results in increased immunosuppression. The agents identified as cofactors of HIV infection, either through stimulation or suppression, are presented in Table 2-1.

Evidence showing increased rates of progression from HIV infection to AIDS associated with particular cofactors is widespread. CMV clearly speeds the rate at which HIV progresses to AIDS,[44,45] activates HIV-1 expression in coinfected chimpanzees,[46] and encodes a chemokine receptor used by HIV as a cofactor for lymphocyte entry. Other herpesviruses encode similar receptors.[47] Other infections commonly associated with AIDS that also increase disease progression include HHV-6,[48,49] HTLV-II,[50,51] hepatitis viruses,[52,53] tuberculosis,[54,41] febrile episodes of herpes zoster (HZ),[55] and malaria.[56]

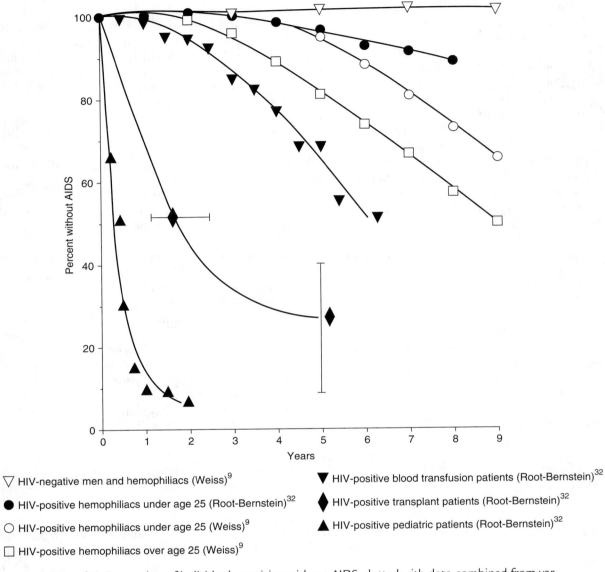

▽ HIV-negative men and hemophiliacs (Weiss)[9]

● HIV-positive hemophiliacs under age 25 (Root-Bernstein)[32]

○ HIV-positive hemophiliacs under age 25 (Weiss)[9]

□ HIV-positive hemophiliacs over age 25 (Weiss)[9]

▼ HIV-positive blood transfusion patients (Root-Bernstein)[32]

◆ HIV-positive transplant patients (Root-Bernstein)[32]

▲ HIV-positive pediatric patients (Root-Bernstein)[32]

Figure 2-1 Proportion of individuals surviving without AIDS plotted with data combined from various European and North American studies. (See Root-Bernstein[32] for details of all studies.) Note that no study of HIV-positive transplant patients larger than 25 patients was performed so that statistical variation in reported AIDS-free survival times varies much more widely than in studies of other risk groups. To indicate variation, bars were added to the transplant patient points to indicate the range of reported data, and the points themselves were drawn from a large study of 22 patients by Lang et al, 1991. Note the tailing off of AIDS risk with increasing length of AIDS-free time in infants and transplant patients.

TABLE 2-1

Identified and Potential HIV Cofactors

Agent	In vivo evidence	In vitro evidence	Agent	In vivo evidence	In vitro evidence
Viruses			*Vaccines*		
Adenoviruses		x	Influenza	x	
Influenza	x		Pneumococcal	x	
Cytomegalovirus	x	x	Tetanus toxoid	x	
Epstein-Barr		x			
Hepatitis C	x		*Drugs*		
Herpes simplex-1	x		Opiates	x	x
Herpes simplex-2	x	x	Cocaine	x	x
Herpes simplex-6	x	x	Inhalant nitrites	x	
Human foamy virus		x			
HTLV-1		x	*Immunological Alloantigens*		
Varicella-zoster	x		Blood transfusions	x	
			Clotting factors	x	
Bacteria			Semen	x	x
Gardnerella vaginalis		x			
M. avium complex	x		*Malnutrition*	x	
M. tuberculosis	x				
Mycoplasmas	x				
T. pallidum (Syphilis)	x	x			
Mastitis	x				
Protozoa					
P. carinii	x				
Giardia lamblia (Giardiasis)	x				
P. falciparum (Malaria)	x	x			

Adapted from Root-Bernstein, 1992, Wahl, Orenstein, 1997; Cytomegalovirus from Kovacs et al, 1999, Perez et al, 1998; Herpes simplex-2 from Perez et al, 1998; Herpes simplex-6 from Emery et al, 1999; Human foamy virus from Marino et al, 1995; Varicella-zoster from Alliegro et al, 1996; *G. vaginalis* from Hashemi et al, 1999; Mycoplasmas from Al-Hathi et al, 1999, Grau et al, 1998, Perez et al, 1998; *T. pallidum* (in vivo) from Otten et al, 1994, Kourmans et al, 2000; *T. pallidum* (in vitro) from Theus et al, 1998; Mastitis from Semba et al, 1999; *P. falciparum* (in vitro) from Hoffman et al, 1999; *P. falciparum* (in vitro) from Xiao et al, 1998; Opiates and Cocaine from Gorenbladh, Gunue, 1989, Weber, 1990; Alloantigens from Root-Bernstein, 1993, Root-Bernstein, DeWitt, 1995; Malnutrition from Chlebowski et al, 1995, Coursoudis et al, 1995.

Some infections alter the probability of primary HIV infection. The most clear-cut examples are STDs that result in open sores, thereby promoting HIV entry to the blood and immune systems and simultaneously producing immune system activation.[57] People actively excreting Epstein-Barr virus (EBV) in urine or saliva are more likely to seroconvert than those with latent infections or who have never been infected.[58-60] EBV also allows HIV to infect B cells, a process that further destroys immune function.[61-63] Both chlamydia infections[64] and helminths[65] also increase the probability of acquiring HIV.

A significant number of studies have failed to find any cofactor effect of some of these agents. All of the negative studies suffer, however, from having examined antibody prevalence rather than active infection. Since nearly every person at risk for AIDS has been exposed to CMV, EBV, and herpesviruses[7] and probably carries them latently, antibody prevalence is intrinsically unable to statistically distinguish between those at risk for AIDS and those with AIDS, or between those progressing quickly with AIDS and those progressing slowly. We do not therefore consider antibody prevalence studies to be useful in this context. To determine whether an infectious agent is promoting HIV activity requires measurement of that agent's production or excretion. Most studies of the effect of active infection with a cofactor on the rate of progression to AIDS show significant effects. In addition, if the cumulative effect of many agents involved in active infection is most significant in altering the progression rate, demonstrating that any one agent significantly causes this effect may be difficult.

Laboratory studies also implicate an important role for cofactors in AIDS pathogenesis. As noted, HIV requires activated T cells to infect and replicate, and elaborate schemes were devised by some AIDS researchers to explain how HIV could act as a self-stimulating infection, but laboratory evidence shows that HIV rapidly becomes latent or disappears altogether when T cells from a healthy individual are exposed to it. Laboratory models of HIV infection employ either specially susceptible leukemia cells or cells stimulated with viruses, mitogenic agents, or various drugs.[18,66,67] Not only can we assume that similar requirements are present in living human beings, but evidence exists that many people exposed to HIV do in fact eliminate their infection without producing antibodies.[68-70]

Laboratory studies show that the same agents that increase the rate of progression to AIDS also have a significant effect on HIV infectivity, replication, and pathogenicity in vitro. Both influenza[31] and tetanus toxoid[71] inoculations markedly increase HIV replication and serum levels of HIV in infected individuals, and tetanus toxoid has the same effect in vitro.[71] These results clearly show that when T cells are activated, HIV replication and infectivity increase. Thus any agent that stimulates T-cell activity can be expected to stimulate HIV activity as well, a critical observation that must be considered in the development of any new AIDS therapy. In addition to T-cell stimulation being directly responsible for the modulation of HIV replication, the infective ability of that virus is partially controlled by chemokine receptors. These receptors are cofactors for HIV infection of a susceptible cell and are modulated by the stimulatory agents identified earlier. The role of these receptors in the process of HIV infection is reviewed in Fauci[25] and Cohen et al.[72]

One final type of immunological factor—autoimmune processes—must also be considered, since it can both stimulate T cells and cause immune suppression by means of direct cell killing. People with AIDS have been known to develop a large number of different autoimmune diseases and at rates that are often hundreds of times higher than that of the general population. These diseases range from arthritis and demyelinating processes to autoimmune liver and kidney disease, as well as Sjögren's syndrome.[6,73] Perhaps most confounding is the observation that most people with AIDS develop autoantibodies directed against their own T cells and that in most cases these autoantibodies are cross-reactive with autologous antigens such as semen.[74] Most hemophiliacs who develop AIDS also develop very high levels of anti-B-cell autoantibodies. Thus it is not incorrect to characterize a significant portion of AIDS pathology as resulting from an autoimmune process against the immune system itself. What role this autoimmune process plays in providing an appropriate niche for HIV within the immune network has yet to be determined. It is not known what triggers these autoimmune phenomena. Some investigators believe that HIV is at fault, since HIV has proteins that mimic MHC-II proteins.[11-16] Other researchers have evidence that the autoimmunity may result from repeated exposure to alloantigens, such as sperm, semen, leukocytes, or blood.[74-80] Others suggest that autoimmunity results when the immune system is overwhelmed by specific combinations of agents.[6,7,74]

Three experiments are particularly notable. The first was performed by Kion and Hoffmann,[81] who showed that mice who develop a spontaneous lupus-like disease also develop an antibody repertoire typical of HIV-positivity—without ever having been exposed to HIV. Stott[82] reported similar findings in HIV-negative macaques. More recently, Ter-Grigorov et al[83] created a new model of AIDS in mice by inoculating them with large doses of paternal lymphocytes. The mice develop dramatic depletions of CD4+ cells, progressive impairment of immune responses, and Kaposi's-like sarcomas or terminal B-cell lymphomas—in the absence of any known retroviral exposure. The researchers have not ruled out the possibility that an endogenous retrovirus is activated by their experimental procedure; however, since the disease is transmissible by serum from one animal to another. Much of what we have taken to be evidence of immune impairment caused by progressive HIV infection may in fact be the result of non-HIV processes. HIV may be taking advantage of these other processes, thus acting as a synergistic or opportunistic rather than a strictly pathogenic agent.

In addition to clinical and laboratory evidence that cofactors play a significant role in AIDS pathogenesis, studies of who is at risk for infection also suggest a role. This model may explain a number of exceptional observations concerning HIV transmissibility. For example, it is well established that significant differences in susceptibility to HIV exist. Patients exposed to HIV via a blood transfusion seroconvert more than 60% of the time,[84] whereas persons exposed to HIV via a single dose of contaminated factor concentrate seroconvert about 5% of the time.[85] Health care professionals exposed percutaneously to HIV seroconvert only 0.3% of the time.[86] Although part of the difference in transmission may be due to HIV dose, another major difference between people in high-risk groups and the typical health care professional is that rates of putative cofactors for HIV are hundreds to thousands of times higher among the at-risk groups.[7]

Interactions between HIV and cofactors have an important implication. Because HIV requires activated lymphocytes to infect and replicate and because many of the cofactor infections just described also use lymphocytes to infect and replicate, AIDS progression should be manifested not only by increased HIV viremia but also by increased cofactor viremia. In essence, a vicious cycle should be initiated in which each virus primes further activity of the other. This is in fact the case. EBV and CMV viremia are both accurate markers for disease progression.[87-93] Measures of autoimmune processes such as circulating immune complexes and lymphocytotoxic antibodies have also been found to accurately predict AIDS progression.[5,68,94-99] Notably, both viral infections and autoimmune processes result in release of interferons (IFs), interleukins (ILs), TNF, and other chemokines often mistakenly attributed solely to HIV activity.[5,7,25,100] Thus any attempt to argue that HIV is the sole, necessary cause of AIDS must measure not only HIV but control for other immunologically active agents and processes. Only rarely are such controls run by those studying the role of HIV in AIDS, and thus any conclusions drawn by such uncontrolled studies must be suspect in light of the data just summarized.

One final type of evidence also argues against an HIV-only theory of AIDS pathogenesis. The treatment or elimination of putative cofactors for HIV often slows progression to AIDS significantly. Many studies suggest that elimination of ongoing risk factors that continuously reexpose individuals to HIV and its putative cofactors can slow progression to AIDS or result in rare seroreversions (i.e., loss of HIV-positivity). Thus people who stop using addictive drugs,[101,102] people who stop engaging in high-risk sexual behaviors,[103-105] and hemophiliacs who are switched from impure factor concentrates to those with a high-purity factor,[106-108] all experience significant improvements in clinical measures of disease progression. Nutritional changes to correct metabolic dysfunctions have also been found to improve survival and increase longevity of people infected with HIV.[109,110] Most importantly, many studies find that treatment of cofactor infections delays AIDS onset and progression. These include prophylaxis against mycobacteria,[111] treatment of CMV,[112-114] treatment of malaria,[115] and the recently discovered anti-EBV and anti-hepatitis benefits of so-called antiretroviral drugs.[116-119]

The only possible conclusion that can be drawn from these laboratory and clinical studies is that AIDS pathogenesis involves more than just HIV. Therefore theories of AIDS and treatments for AIDS must both take into account factors other than HIV if they are to be accurate and effective.

MATHEMATICAL AND STATISTICAL MODELS OF AIDS

Mathematical and statistical models of AIDS can be used in addition to experimental and clinical studies to investigate and compare theories of AIDS pathogenesis. Such models are generally of two basic types: (1) models of the epidemiological behavior of the epidemic, and (2) models of the effect of HIV and cofactors on the immune system. We consider both types.

Quantitative descriptions of the AIDS epidemic beyond descriptive analysis of the data (e.g., graphs, histograms, and computations of averages) necessarily involve the use of mathematical and statistical models. These models are actually an assortment of assumptions and simplifications that reflect the collective understanding and disposition of the investigators concerning the natural history of the disease and how it is spread. Different researchers propose different models by necessity, as each individual brings to the problem his or her unique educational experience and worldview—a mathematician sees the problems as primarily mathematical and a virologist views the same problems as an exercise of virological methods.

Difficulties with models of the AIDS epidemic come from the nature of the available data. First, there is never enough data, failing in either quality, quantity, or both. Gaps in the data record make necessary additional assumptions concerning what the data would look like if it *had* been collected. This process is equivalent to creating a line drawing from a "dot-to-dot" children's picture. If sufficient data (dots) and how these data relate to one another (the dot order) is available, then each person draws essentially the same conclusions (the line drawing). If, however, the data are too sparse or relationships between the data sets are not known, assumptions must add additional dots to the picture and specify the relationship between the new and original dots. Each different collection of new dots and numbering (assumptions) gives rise to different line drawings—all of which are consistent with the original dots. In other words, different assumptions can result in different quantitative predictions based on the same data.

An illuminating discussion of such differences can be seen in early computations of the mean time to AIDS (i.e., the mean of the latency or incubation time distribution). Assuming that the time to AIDS followed a commonly used distribution in reliability and survival analysis—a simplified Weibull distribution—a mean latency of 4 to 5 years was computed by examining parameter values of the distribution that gave the best fit to available data. This mean latency was widely believed to be a useful estimate. It was later shown that if a more general form of the Weibull distribution was assumed, such as a distribution that contained more parameters than the simplified one, the values of the parameters leading to the best fit to the *same* data set corresponded to a mean latency time of *200 years*.[120] The two distributions fit that data equally well. The differences in these estimates for the mean latency indicate the difficulties in using models to fill in the gaps when the data are too sparse and the care needed in using and interpreting those estimates.

Second, data are always uncertain. For instance, a long and highly variable time exists between HIV infection and discovery of an immune response to this exposure detected through an AIDS test. A highly variable period of time (the incubation time) from initial HIV infection to the clinical diagnosis of AIDS also exists. The resulting uncertainty in quantities like the "number of infected individuals" have made many models, which may have been based on adequate assumptions, unable to successfully forecast the future size of the epidemic. Kault[121] states:

Mathematical models of the AIDS epidemic have not been able to give accurate predictions about the size of the epidemic because it is not possible to obtain sufficiently accurate measurements of the factors that enable HIV transmission.

Using the previous analogy, this problem corresponds to uncertainties in the position and number of the original dots. This observation dictates that not all questions can be resolved by modeling methods. The effect of such uncertainties in AIDS epidemiological data is fully discussed in DeGruttola and Lagakos.[120]

Given a set of assumptions (i.e., a model) and appropriate data, estimates and predictions in the form of graphs and tables result. A seemingly contradictory observation is that if a set of assumptions gives rise to incorrect predictions (and the data uncertainty is small) at least one assumption was incorrect or the simplification was unjustified. If a forecast or prediction is confirmed (additional data dots did not invalidate the line drawing), the only conclusion is that the assumptions and simplifications are consistent with the data—but the validity of the assumptions is not directly tested. The preceding discussion shows that science progresses when a model fails (i.e., something thought to be true is not), while success of a model only demonstrates consistency of the ideas with the current data. The power of a mathematical or statistical model is that the logical consequences of a set of assumptions are revealed. If these consequences are not confirmed by data and observations, then the assumptions must not have been correct.

Thus models can be used as an important tool in the scientific process. Theories (i.e., models) are proposed and tested, resulting in new and improved theories. Unfortunately, models that fail are rarely published, so inconsistencies in assumptions and current belief (i.e., the dogma) are not always recognized.

Mathematical and statistical models of the AIDS epidemic have been used to forecast the extent of disease spread, probe the understanding of the nature of transmission of HIV through the various transmission modes, identify significant subgroups and describe the transmission within and between these subgroups, and estimate quantities such as the incubation time in different infected groups. Several collections, reviews, and monographs of this work are available.[122-130] These efforts indicate the wide range of epidemiological modeling of AIDS and technical difficulties in this type of research.

Discoveries made on the basis of epidemiological models often show that a simpler model cannot fit the known data but adding one suspected feature to the model can. Typical examples include the discoveries that a high-risk core group is needed to fit early epidemic data,[131] high risk of HIV transmission is concentrated in a relatively brief period of primary infection,[131] antiviral (AV) therapy can increase the number of AIDS cases,[132] infectivity changes with time,[133] and careful descriptions of partner formation are necessary to make accurate predictions for sexual transmission of HIV.[134]

Several studies exist in which the model used in the epidemiological study shed additional light on immune pathogenesis. Weyer and Eggers[135] observed that within each risk group the growth of the epidemic was initially exponential with approximately the same rate (but each was shifted in time to different starting points). They noted that the spread within any group must be independent of the nature of sexual activity or drug use—those factors determining the time at which the epidemic enters the group but not the rate of spread within the group. Through a mathematical model, they demonstrated that if an infectious cofactor was present, this same pattern results. Without the assumption of an infectious cofactor, different rates of spread in the groups are predicted. HIV has stayed largely within specific high-risk groups defined at the beginning of the epidemic (e.g., gay men; IV drug abusers; people exposed to blood and blood products; and populations in which malnutrition, STDs, and parasites are endemic), demonstrating that differential rates of HIV spread are the rule rather than the exception. Thus theory and epidemiology agree that cofactors appear to play a critical role in the transmission of AIDS.

The relationship between tuberculosis (TB) and HIV is a recent concern for health professionals, especially since HIV infection increases the number of identified cases of TB.[136] Active TB infection also increases the rate of HIV disease progression.[54] A proposed mechanism for the increased rate of immune deterioration was proposed by Placido et al,[137] who showed that viable *Mycoplasma tuberculosis* increases rates of apoptosis of alveolar macrophages in AIDS patients. Apoptosis does not increase with HIV alone. The microenvironment in the lungs of TB patients may also be rich in cytokines, which stimulate HIV replication.[138]

Hepatitis B is implicated as a cofactor in two ways. First, Twu et al[53] make a case for an increased number of HIV seroconversions in active HBV-infected individuals, after controlling for sexual behavior and changes in disease over time. This suggests that either an existing active HBV is a cofactor that helps to establish HIV infection after exposure or that HBV is a surrogate for other factors that perform that function. A second form of interaction is seen in an increased disease severity in children infected with both HIV and hepatitis.[52] Similar results have been recognized with coinfection with HTLV-II.[50]

Striking evidence for the role of cofactors in disease progression comes from two fronts. First, Alliegro et al[55] report that incidents of fever associated with HZ infection are associated with an acceleration of the progression to AIDS, suggesting that the increased stimulation of T cells associated with acute herpes episodes can increase viral replication in an existing HIV infection. Second, physicians treating malaria have noticed an increased progression of HIV in infected patients.[56] The relationship between malaria and HIV promises to be similar to that of TB and HIV.[139]

Mathematical models of HIV infection are used to investigate the interaction of HIV with the immune system, the effect on the disease process of the development of diversity in the HIV genome, the effect of drug treatments, and the role of stimulatory cofactors. These studies tend to be more theoretical in nature than the epidemiological modeling, since that work is motivated by collected data. Equivalently detailed data concerning HIV infection within individuals are not generally available.

A difficulty with using mathematical models as tools to study disease mechanisms is that to obtain results from a model, a larger number of assumptions and simplifications must be advanced. Many of these assumptions and simplifications are technical (and usually ad hoc), such as "the blood is a well-mixed medium," whereas others deal specifically with aspects of the theories being tested. Since the output of a model depends on the collection of all assumptions and simplifications made, including the technical ones, a direct and unambiguous comparison of theoretical alternatives is not possible. This difficulty is not unfamiliar to medical researchers, since in vivo experiments involving animal models must deal with the applicability to humans.

They must answer the question, "Does the result depend on the species chosen?"

In a sense, though, the models have been successful in their failures. Data that appear after the model has been published sometimes point out that the collection of assumptions on which the model is based was incorrect. For instance, all of the early models of the interaction of HIV with the immune system (about 20 of them) used standard assumptions about disease progression taken from other theories of epidemics and immunology and predicted that kinetics for CD4 T-cell counts would either drop quickly to zero (usually within a year or two) or reach an equilibrium (chronic and permanent) state with no progression after that point. All have since been shown to be incorrect after recognition of the near-linear decline in CD4 counts over most of the period of HIV infection.[140,141] The failure of such a large variety of these early models suggests that some process unlike those employed when modeling other diseases is needed to successfully describe AIDS. In other words, something other than the HIV-only theory is needed.

A second example of the failure of a model is the idea of a diversity threshold,[142] which tried to describe the role of the high mutation rate of HIV. Under this theory, the immune response can control an HIV infection until the diversity threshold in the number of HIV quasi-species present is reached, at which time there are too many antigens for the immune response to deal with and the system begins to collapse. Although consistent with the understanding (the dots) at the time it was written, the theory was recognized as false with the recognition of the extraordinary scale of the diversity and the stable viral loads through most of the disease period.[143]

The most direct demonstration that the HIV-only theory may not be tenable is found in Anderson, Ascher, and Sheppard.[144] They demonstrate that even with the most generous of assumptions, the tap and drain view of HIV progression cannot be possible. The tap and drain model,[10,145,146] the current dogma, proposes that direct (cytopathic) killing of CD4+ T cells by HIV, which is slightly faster than normal homeostatic mechanisms can replace, is primarily responsible for the progression of HIV infection. The argument made by Anderson, Ascher, and Sheppard is that replacement is several magnitudes larger than any possible killing rate by HIV—and that for most of the HIV infection period, the virus cannot be shown to be cytopathic in vivo. Mechanisms and factors other than

HIV alone must be involved in the process. The authors mention several feasible hypotheses that are consistent with current data. Grossman et al[42,147] view the goal of the immune response to HIV as primarily one of trying to come to terms with a chronic or parasitic infection. The deterioration or anergy (i.e., unresponsiveness) of the system arises from an "overadaptation of lymphocytes and accessory cells to the infectious agent(s)." Merrill and Radke[148] show that the linear decline in T cells and the distribution of the slopes of these declines are consistent with a slow decline of immune effectiveness as immune activation grows. Ascher and Sheppard[149,150] propose that T-cell signals generated by the interaction of HIV with CD4 lead to excess immune activation, which results in a negative selection for CD4+ T cells. All three models contain a central role for pathology generated by an excess activation of T cells.

One way that activation enters this system is through cofactors, as previously discussed. The results of these epidemiological models make reasonable the hypothesis that cofactors are essential for the natural disease course seen in HIV infection. That is, without externally supplied activation, the disease process cannot proceed. Root-Bernstein and Merrill[8] used a mathematical model to study the effects of cofactors in an HIV infection. The results surprisingly suggest that if cofactors are absent, no infection by HIV is possible if the dose of virus is small (e.g., a needle stick). Moreover, susceptibility to HIV increases with increasing cofactor load,. Thus this model helps to explain the previous observation that people in different risk groups for HIV infection seroconvert at different rates following a single HIV exposure. If cofactors are necessary to the transmission of HIV, then those at highest risk of infection from a single exposure will be persons already immunologically compromised by a large number of immunological insults, whereas healthy individuals with low numbers of activated T cells and an insignificant antigen load should have a low susceptibility to HIV.

Another striking implication of the cofactor-necessary model is that the nature of the AIDS epidemic becomes not a function of HIV prevalence, but rather a complex function of the interaction of HIV with cofactors. Thus HIV may have existed at very low levels in human populations for hundreds or thousands of years before its recognition because the conditions for its widespread transmission did not exist. It is critical to realize that the HIV epidemic followed closely behind epidemics of other sexually transmitted diseases and hepatitis viruses, as well as the innovation of disposable needles and syringes, vast increases in blood transfusions, and the use of blood-derived products. In a symbiotic or synergistic model, the effects of increasing these other factors would create a multiplicative effect on the incidence of HIV transmission, since people who acquired HIV would almost invariably also have the coinfections necessary to facilitate HIV transmission to others.[32] Conversely, medical and public health interventions that lower the cofactor incidence in a community will also have a multiplicative effect on lowering the incidence of HIV. Thus the efficacy of safer-sex measures and clean needle exchange programs may be due only partly to direct prevention of HIV exposure and, more importantly, to the concomitant intervention in the transmission of cofactors necessary for HIV transmission. If this is true, then we should observe that the AIDS epidemic disappears in populations that lower their cofactor risks. Conversely, HIV will remain endemic among high-risk groups characterized by high levels of cofactor exposures.

IMPLICATIONS FOR RESEARCH, PREVENTION, AND TREATMENT

Of the AIDS theories outlined in the first section of this chapter, two seem to be untenable. It is not likely that AIDS occurs in the absence of HIV. (This statement does not eliminate the possibility of acquiring significant immunosuppression in the absence of HIV but suggests that such immunosuppression can be properly classified as something other than AIDS.) Conversely, no compelling evidence exists that HIV alone can produce AIDS. No individual who has developed AIDS has been shown to be free of putative cofactors, whereas the vast majority have been shown definitively to be exposed to putative cofactors. We are therefore left with some type of cofactor theory as the most likely explanation for AIDS. The problem is which type: (1) cofactor-modulated HIV or (2) cofactors-necessary HIV? Are we talking about a symbiotic interaction, synergistic interaction, or a progressive accumulation (antigenic overload) theory? Finally, what is the role of autoimmune processes in these theories? Are such processes an almost ubiquitous side effect of AIDS or one of its causes? At this time it is not possible to give a definitive answer to these questions, in large part because the exclusive focus of the medical community on HIV has resulted in a general failure to see the many other processes that are part of AIDS pathogenesis.

Ignorance is not necessarily bad as long as it is recognized and carefully circumscribed.[151] In this instance, unanswered questions should become the springboards for future research. Laboratory and clinical investigators alike need to bear in mind the kinds of studies and data that will clarify outstanding questions. For example, very few studies exist correlating progression to AIDS with antigenic load as measured either by parameters of viral or bacterial antigens in blood or excretions, or by looking at general immune parameters. Despite data suggesting that CMV and EBV antigenemia are excellent markers for disease progression, no one has yet determined whether such viral antigen expression directly correlates with p24 HIV antigenemia or other HIV-derived correlates of AIDS development. Thus we have no idea whether HIV antigenemia precedes and stimulates the expression of other infectious agents or vice versa, or whether the two occur in tandem.

A related issue concerns the systemic effects of antiretroviral therapies. All current research assumes that the sole effect of such therapies is to lower HIV expression. Recently various nucleoside analogs designed to inhibit HIV replication have been found to inhibit the replication of cofactor viruses. Many nucleoside agents, including ddA, didanosine (ddI), and lamivudine (3TC), a common ingredient in antiretroviral cocktails, are extremely effective against hepatitis viruses and EBV.[116-119] Conversely, ganciclovir and foscarnet, which were designed as anti-herpesvirus agents and used to treat CMV and genital herpes, significantly lower HIV antigen levels in treated patients.[114] Because many antiretrovirals are effective leukocyte inhibitors, all T-cell, macrophage, and dendritic cell infections might respond to such agents. If this is true (and it could easily be tested in the laboratory by looking at the effect of drugs on mixed infections in vitro), then it might make sense to change the selection criteria for novel AIDS therapies from those that are highly specific for HIV or particular cofactor viruses to those that are broadly effective against any immune system infection, including HIV.

To accurately test any drug before it is used by human beings, however, it is necessary to establish viable animal models. Although AIDS models involving viruses analogous to HIV exist (e.g., simian immunodeficiency virus, feline immunodeficiency virus, murine immunodeficiency virus), significant differences also exist between human AIDS and these animal versions. Cofactor theories, whether they are synergistic, symbiotic, or progressive accumulation, suggest quite different and as yet untested animal models. No one has tested the effects of coinfecting chimpanzees and macaques, for example, with combinations of HIV, CMV, HTLV, and HHV-6, for example. No one has attempted to recreate in an animal exactly what happens to a human being who undergoes surgery, is exposed to multiple blood transfusions containing viruses such as CMV, EBV, and HCV, undergoes hours of anesthesia, and is given morphine, steroids, and other drugs postoperatively, in addition to encountering HIV. The effect of multiply exposing an animal anally to HIV contained in semen while the animal is simultaneously affected by antibiotics, nitrite inhalants, and various STDs (as occurred frequently in gay bath houses before the safe sex era) has never been reproduced. No one knows what effect chronic drug addiction, malnutrition, and multiple STDs has on the susceptibility of animals to HIV. Nor are these ludicrous experiments. It is worth considering that healthy rats, rabbits, and dogs are totally resistant to *Candida albicans* and *P. carinii* infections but become completely susceptible when immunosuppressed with steroids and other immunosuppressive agents.[152-154] In addition, a new animal model for EBV infection has recently been discovered in rhesus monkeys, which may provide a means to investigate the interactions between EBV and HIV.[155]

Clearly some interventions can ethically be attempted on people at risk for AIDS even if such animal models are not developed. These include lifestyle interventions that lower the risk of contracting any putative cofactor and lessen the probability of infection following exposure to HIV and its development into AIDS. Therapies directed at cofactor infections or the elimination of ongoing immunomodulation factors, such as drug use and malnutrition, can also be implemented. Therapies that reduce cofactor risks without activating the immune system may be particularly useful. These may range from exercise, meditation, and counseling to drugs that mediate cytokine functions.

Finally, since autoimmune diseases are virtually ubiquitous in AIDS patients, and since no effective treatments for any human autoimmune diseases exist, there is a possibility that even if clinicians learn how to control HIV and prevent retrovirally produced immune dysfunction, most (if not all) people with AIDS will continue to die of untreatable autoimmune complications unrelated to immunosuppression. If autoimmunity is a major cause of immune dysfunction as well, then treatments designed to stop HIV may have little or no effect on long-term immunosuppression either. It is therefore crucial that the role of autoimmune processes in AIDS pathogenesis be clarified and a major effort made to determine the causes and treatments of the entire range of such processes. Such an effort would not only benefit hundreds of thousands of people with AIDS but millions of other people suffering from autoimmune diseases as well.

It is worth remembering that AIDS itself is no more unique than any other disease. Whatever we know about disease in general must be applied to understanding and treating AIDS and, conversely, anything new we learn about AIDS and its effective treatment must be applied as broadly as possible to the understanding of other diseases. Thus understanding AIDS will have far greater consequences than controlling AIDS; it may influence the paradigm by which we understand disease.

References

1. Duesberg PF, editor: *AIDS: virus- or drug-induced?* Boston, 1996, Kluwer Academic Publishers.
2. Duesberg PF: *Inventing the AIDS virus,* Washington, DC, 1996, Regnery Press.
3. Sonnabend JA, Saadoun S: The acquired immunodeficiency syndrome: a discussion of etiologic hypotheses, *AIDS Res* 1:107-120, 1984.
4. Sonnabend JA, Witkin SS, Portillo DT: A multifactorial model for the development of AIDS in homosexual men, *Ann N Y Acad Sci* 437:177-182, 1984.
5. Sonnabend JA: AIDS: An explanation for its occurrence in homosexual men. In Ma P, Armstrong D, editors: *AIDS and opportunistic infections of homosexual men,* Stoneham, Mass, 1989, Butterworth.
6. Root-Bernstein RS: Do we know the cause(s) of AIDS? *Perspect Biol Med* 33:480-500, 1990.
7. Root-Bernstein RS: *Rethinking AIDS: the tragic cost of premature consensus,* New York, 1993, Free Press.
8. Root-Bernstein RS, Merrill SJ: The necessity of cofactors in the pathogenesis of AIDS: a mathematical model, *J Theor Biol* 187:135-146, 1997.
9. Weiss RA: How does HIV cause AIDS? *Science* 260:1273-1279, 1993.
10. Ho D: Viral counts count in HIV infection, *Science* 272:1123-1125, 1996.

11. Andrieu JM, Even P, Venet A: AIDS and related syndromes as a viral-induced autoimmune disease of the immune system: an anti-MHC II disorder, Therapeutic implications, *AIDS Res* 2:163, 1986.

12. Golding H, Robey FA, Gates FT III, et al: Identification of homologous regions in human immunodeficiency virus I gp41 and human MHC class II beta 1 domain, I. Monoclonal antibodies against the gp41-derived peptide and patients' sera react with native HLA class II antigens, suggesting a role for autoimmunity in the pathogenesis of acquired immune deficiency syndrome, *J Exp Med* 167:914-923, 1988.

13. Ziegler JL, Stites DP: Hypothesis: AIDS is an autoimmune disease directed at the immune system and triggered by a lymphotropic retrovirus, *Clin Immunol Immunopathol* 41:305-313, 1986.

14. Dalgliesh AG, Wilson S, Gompels M, et al: T-cell receptor variable gene products and early HIV-1 infection, *Lancet* 339(8797):824-828, 1992.

15. Susal C, Kropelin M, Daniel V, et al: Molecular mimicry between HIV-1 and antigen receptor molecules: a clue to the pathogenesis of AIDS, *Vox Sang* 65:10-17, 1993.

16. Bjork RL Jr: HIV-1: seven facets of functional molecular mimicry, *Immunol Lett* 28:91-96 (with discussion 97-99), 1991.

17. Zack JA, Arrigo SJ, Weitsman SR, et al: HIV-I entry into quiescent primary lymphocytes: molecular analysis reveals a labile latent viral structure, *Cell* 1:213-222, 1990.

18. Zagury D, Benard J, Leonard R, et al: Long term cultures of HTLV-III infected cells: a model of cytopathology of T-cell depletion in AIDS, *Science* 231:850-853, 1986.

19. Zack JA, Cann AJ, Lugo JP, et al: AIDS virus production from infected peripheral blood T cells following HTLV-I-induced mitogenic stimulation, *Science* 240:1026-1029, 1988.

20. Shope E: Swine influenza, I-III, *J Exp Med* 54:349-385, 1931.

21. Muller H, Takeshita M: Immunohistochemical characterization of HIV- and non-HIV-associated lymph node tuberculosis, *Verh Dtsch Ges Pathol* 75:166-170, 1991.

22. Sjamsoedin-Visser L J, Heijnen C J, Zegers B J, et al: Defective T suppressor–inducer cell function in human immune deficiency virus-seropositive hemophilia patients, *Blood* 72:1474-1477, 1988.

23. Michilany J, Mattos AL, Michilany NS, et al: Acquired immune deficiency syndrome (AIDS) in Brazil: necropsy findings, *Ann Pathol* 7:15-24, 1987.

24. Hood AF, Farmer ER, Weiss RA: Clinical conferences at the Johns Hopkins hospital: Kaposi's sarcoma, *Johns Hopkins Medical J* 151:222-230, 1982.

25. Fauci AS: Host factors and the pathogenesis of HIV-induced disease, *Nature* 384:529-534, 1996.

26. Santamauro JT, White DA: Respiratory infections in HIV-negative immunocompromised patients, *Curr Opin Pulm Med* 2:253-258, 1996.

27. Heredia A, Hewlett IK, Soriano V, et al: Idiopathic CD4[+] T lymphocytopenia: a review and current perspective, *Transfus Med Rev* 8:223-231, 1994.

28. Djomand G, Diaby L, N'Gbichi JM, et al: Idiopathic CD4[+] T-lymphocyte depletion in a west African population, *AIDS* 8:843-847, 1994.

29. Castelino DJ, McNair P, Kay TW: Lymphocytopenia in a hospital population—what does it signify? *Aust N Z J Med* 27:170-174, 1997.

30. Busch MP, Valinsky JE, Paglieroni T, et al: Screening of blood donors for idiopathic CD4[+] T lymphocytopenia, *Transfusion* 34:192-197, 1994

31. O'Brien TR, Diamondstone L, Fried MW, et al: Idiopathic CD4[+] T lymphocytopenia in HIV-seronegative men with hemophilia and sex partners of HIV-seropositive men, Multicenter Hemophilia Cohort Study, *Am J Hematol* 49:201-206, 1995.

32. Root-Bernstein RS: Five myths about AIDS that have misdirected research and treatment, *Genetica* 95:111-132, 1995.

33. Lang PP, Niaudet P, Groupe Cooperatif de Transplantation de l'Ile de France: Update and outcome of renal transplant patients with human immunodeficiency virus, *Transplant Proc* 23:1352-1353, 1991.

34. Eskild A, Magnus P, Brekke T, et al: The impact of exposure group on the progression rate to acquired immunodeficiency syndrome: a comparison between intravenous drug users, homosexual men, and heterosexually infected subjects, *Scand J Infect Dis* 29:103-109, 1997.

35. Bentwich Z, Kalinkovich A, Weisman Z: Immune activation is the dominant factor in the pathogenesis of African AIDS, *Immunol Today* 16:187-191, 1995.

36. Eskild A, Magnus P, Sohlberg C, et al: A comparison of the progression rate to acquired immunodeficiency syndrome between intravenous drug users and homosexual men, *Scand J Soc Med* 22:309-314, 1994a.

37. Eskild A, Magnus P, Sohlberg C, et al: Slow progression to AIDS in intravenous drug users infected with HIV in Norway, *J Epidemiol Community Health* 48:383-387, 1994b.

38. Wolfs TF, Wolf F, Breederveld C, et al: Low AIDS attack rate among Dutch haemophiliacs compared to homosexual men: a correlate of HIV antigenaemia frequencies, *Vox Sang* 57:127-132, 1989.

39. Medley GF, Anderson RM, Cox DR, et al: Incubation period of AIDS in patients infected via blood transfusion, *Nature* 328:719-720, 1987.

40. Wahl SM, Orenstein JM: Immune stimulation and HIV-1 viral replication, *J Leukoc Biol* 62:67-71, 1997.

41. Goletti D, Weissman D, Jackson RW, et al: Effect of *Mycobacterium tuberculosis* on HIV replication: role of immune activation, *J Immunol* 157:1271-1278, 1996.

42. Grossman Z, Bentwich Z, Herberman RB: From HIV infection to AIDS: are the manifestations of effective immune resistance misinterpreted? *Clin Immunol Immunopathol* 69:1-13, 1993.

43. Giorgi JV, Hultin LE, McKeating JA, et al: Shorter survival in advanced human immunodeficiency virus type 1 infection is more closely associated with T-lymphocyte activation than with plasma virus burden or virus chemokine coreceptor usage, *J Infect Dis* 179:859-870, 1999.

44. Sabin C, Phillips A, Elford J, et al: The progression of HIV disease in a haemophilic cohort followed for twelve years, *Br J Haematol* 83:330-333, 1993.

45. Sabin C, Phillips AN, Lee CA, et al: The effect of CMV infection on progression of human immunodeficiency virus disease in a cohort of haemophiliac men followed up to 13 years from seroconversion, *Epidemiol Infect* 114:361-372, 1995.

46. Castro BA, Homsy J, Lennette E, et al: HIV-1 expression in chimpanzees can be activated by CD8$^+$ cell depletion or by CMV infection, *Clin Immunol Immunopathol* 65:227-233, 1992.

47. Pleskoff O, Treboute C, Brelot A, et al: Identification of a chemokine receptor encoded by human cytomegalovirus as a cofactor for HIV-1 entry, *Science* 276:1874-1878, 1997.

48. Knox KK, Carrigan DR: Active HHV-6 infection in the lymph nodes of HIV-infected patients: in vitro evidence that HHV-6 can break HIV latency, *J Acquir Immune Defic Syndr Hum Retrovirol* 11:370-378, 1996.

49. Blazquez MV, Madueno JZ, Jurado R, et al: Human herpesvirus-6 and the course of human immunodeficiency virus infection, *J Acquir Immune Defic Syndr Hum Retrovirol* 9:389-394, 1995.

50. Eskild A, Samdal HH, Heger B: Coinfection with HIV-1/HTLV-II and the risk of progression to AIDS and death, The Oslo HIV Cohort Study Group, *APMIS* 104:666-672, 1996.

51. Visconti A, Visconti L, Bellocco R, et al: HTLV-II/HIV-1 coinfection and risk for progression to AIDS among intravenous drug users, *J Acquir Immune Defic Syndr Hum Retrovirol* 6:1228-1237, 1993.

52. Antipa C, Ruta S, Cernescu C, et al: Immunological disorders of increasing severity in children with AIDS associated with hepatitis B and C infections, *Rom J Virol* 46:3-8, 1995.

53. Twu SJ, Detels R, Nelson K, et al: Relationship of hepatitis B virus infection to human immunodeficiency virus type 1 infection, *J Infect Dis* 167:299-304, 1993.

54. Whalen C, Horsburg CR, Hom D, et al: Accelerated course of human immunodeficiency virus infection after tuberculosis, *Am J Respir Crit Care Med* 151:129-135, 1995.

55. Alliegro MB, Dorrucci M, Pezzotti P, et al: Herpes zoster and progression to AIDS in a cohort of individuals who seroconverted to human immunodeficiency virus, Italian HIV Seroconversion Study, *Clin Infect Dis* 23:990-995, 1996.

56. Bagla P: Malaria fighters gather at site of early victory (news), *Science* 227:1437-1438, 1997.

57. Padian NS, Shiboski SC, Glass SO, et al: Heterosexual transmission of human immunodeficiency virus (HIV) in northern California: results from a ten-year study, *Am J Epidemiol* 146:350-357, 1997.

58. Diaz-Mitoma F, Ruiz A, Flowerdew G, et al: High levels of Epstein-Barr virus in the oropharynx: a predictor of disease progression in human immunodeficiency virus infection, *J Med Virol* 31:69-75, 1990.

59. Ferbas J, Rayman MA, Kingsley LA, et al: Frequent oropharyngeal shedding of Epstein-Barr virus in homosexual men during early HIV infection, *AIDS* 6:1273-1278, 1992.

60. Lucht E, Biberfeld P, Linde A: Epstein-Barr virus (EBV) DNA in saliva and EBV serology of HIV-1-infected persons with and without hairy leukoplakia, *J Infect* 31:89-194, 1995.

61. Zhang RD, Guan M, Park Y, et al: Synergy between human immunodeficiency virus type 1 and Epstein-Barr virus in T-lymphoblastoid cell lines, *AIDS Res Hum Retroviruses* 13:161-171, 1997.

62. Poulin L, Paquette N, Moir S, et al: Productive infection of normal CD40-activated human B lymphocytes by HIV-1, *AIDS* 8:1539-1544, 1994.

63. Scala G, Quinto I, Ruocco MR, et al: Epstein-Barr virus nuclear antigen 2 transactivates the long terminal repeat of human immunodeficiency virus type 1, *J Virol* 67:2853-2861, 1993.

64. Schattner A, Hanuka N, Sarove B, et al: *Chlamydia trachomatis* and HIV infection, *Immunol Lett* 49:27-30, 1994.

65. Bentwich Z, Weisman Z, Moroz C, et al: Immune dysregulation in Ethiopian immigrants in Israel: relevance to helminth infections? *Clin Exp Immunol* 103:239-243, 1996.

66. Lemaitre M, Guetard D, Henin Y, et al: Protective activity of tetracycline 3 analogs against the cytopathic effect of the human immunodeficiency virus in CEM cells, *Res Virol* 141:5-10, 1990.

67. Sarngadharan MG, Markham PD: The role of human T-lymphotropic retroviruses in leukemia and AIDS. In Wormser, GP, editor: *AIDS—acquired immune deficiency syndrome—and other manifestations of HIV infection*, Park Ridge, N.J., 1987, Noyes Publications.

68. Clerici M, Giori JV, Chou CC, et al: Cell-mediated immune response to human immunodeficiency virus (HIV) type in seronegative homosexual men with recent sexual exposure to HIV-1, *J Infect Dis* 165:1012-1019, 1992.

69. Urnovitz HB, Clerici M, Shearer GM, et al: HIV-1 antibody serum negativity with urine positivity, *Lancet* 342:1458-1459, 1993.

70. Clerici M, Shearer GM: The T_H1-T_H2 hypothesis of HIV infection: new insights, *Immunol Today* 15:575-581, 1994.

71. Stanley SK, Ostrowski MA, Justement JS, et al: Effect of immunization with a common recall antigen on viral expression in patients infected with human immunodeficiency virus type 1, *N Engl J Med* 334:1222-1230, 1996.

72. Cohen OJ, Kinter A, Fauci AS: Host factors in the pathogenesis of HIV disease, *Immunol Rev* 159:31-48, 1997.

73. Morrow WJ, Isenberg DA, Sobol RE, et al: AIDS virus infection and autoimmunity: a perspective of the clinical, immunological, and molecular origins of the autoallergic pathologies associated with HIV disease, *Clin Immunol Immunopathol* 58:163-180, 1991.

74. Root-Bernstein RS, DeWitt SH: Semen alloantigens and lymphocytotoxic antibodies in AIDS and ICL, *Genetica* 95:133-156, 1995.

75. Hoff C, Peterson RDA: Does exposure to HLA alloantigens trigger immunoregulatory mechanisms operative in both pregnancy and AIDS? *Life Sci* 45:iii-ix, 1989.

76. Hoff C, James WC, Hester RB, et al: Signs of cellular immunosuppression correlate with HLA-DR phenotypes in healthy HIV-negative homosexuals: preliminary findings, *Hum Biol* 63:129-135, 1991.

77. Naz RK, Ellauri M, Phillips TM, et al: Antisperm antibodies in human immunodeficiency virus infection: effects on fertilization and embryonic development, *Biol Reprod* 42:859-868, 1990.

78. Mathur S, Goust J-M, Williamson HO, et al: Cross-reactivity of sperm and T-lymphocyte antigens, *Am J Reprod Immunol* 1:113-118, 1981.

79. Mavligit GM, Talpaz M, Hsia FT: Chronic immune stimulation by sperm alloantigens: support for the hypothesis that spermatozoa induce immune dysregulation in homosexual males, *JAMA* 251:237-241, 1984.

80. Witkin SS, Sonnabend JA: Immune responses to spermatozoa in homosexual men, *Fertil Steril* 39:337-342, 1983.

81. Kion TA, Hoffmann GW: Anti-HIV and anti-MHC antibodies in alloimmune and autoimmune mice, *Science* 253:1138-1140, 1991.

82. Stott EJ: Anticell antibody in macaques, *Nature* 353:393, 1991.

83. Ter-Grigorov VS, Krifuks O, Liubashevsky E, et al: A new transmissible AIDS-like disease in mice induced by alloimmune stimuli, *Nat Med* 3:37-41, 1997.

84. Ward JW, Bush TJ, Perkins HA, et al: The natural history of transfusion-associated infection with human immunodeficiency virus, *N Engl J Med* 321:947-968, 1989.

85. Ludlum CA, Tucker J, Steel CM, et al: Human T-cell lymphotropic virus infection type III (HTLV-III) infection in seronegative hemophiliacs after transfusions with factor VIII, *Lancet* ii:233-236, 1985.

86. Henderson DK, Fahey BJ, Willy M, et al: Risk for occupational transmission of human immunodeficiency virus type 1 (HIV-1) associated with clinical exposures, *Ann Intern Med* 113:740-746, 1990.

87. Biggar R J, Anderson HK, Ebbesen P, et al: Seminal fluid excretion of cytomegalovirus related to immunosuppression in homosexual men, *Br Med J* 286:2010-2012, 1983.

88. Drew WL, Mills J, Levye J, et al: Cytomegalovirus infection and abnormal T-lymphocyte subset ratios in homosexual men, *Ann Intern Med* 103:61-63, 1985.

89. Fiala M, Cone LA, Chang C-M, et al: Cytomegalovirus viremia increases with progressive immune deficiency in patients infected with HTLV-III, *AIDS Res* 2:175-181, 1986.

90. Rinaldo CR Jr, Kingsley LA, Ho, M, et al: Enhanced shedding of cytomegalovirus in semen of human immunodeficiency virus-seropositive homosexual men, *J Clin Microbiol* 30:1148-1155, 1992.

91. Rahman MA, Kingsley LA, Berinig MK, et al: Reactivation of Epstein-Barr virus during early infection with human immunodeficiency virus, *J Clin Microbiol* 29:1215-1220, 1989.

92. Munoz A, Carey V, Saah AJ, et al: Predictors of decline in CD4 lymphocytes in a cohort of homosexual men infected with human immunodeficiency virus, *J Acquir Immune Defic Syndr Hum Retrovirol* 1:396, 1988.

93. Sumaya CV, Boswell RN, Ench Y, et al: Enhanced serological and virological findings of Epstein-Barr virus in patients with AIDS and AIDS-related complex, *J Infect Dis* 154:864, 1985.

94. Zarling JM, Ledbetter JA, Sias J, et al: HIV-infected humans but not chimpanzees have circulating cytotoxic T lymphocytes that lyse uninfected CD4+ cells, *J Immunol* 144:2992-2998, 1990.

95. Daniel VR, Weimer R, Schimpf K, et al: Autoantibodies against CD4+ and CD8+ T lymphocytes in HIV-infected hemophilia patients, *Vox Sang* 57:1172-1176, 1989.

96. Ozturk GE, Kohler PF, Horsburgh CR, et al: The significance of antilymphocyte antibodies inpatients with acquired immune deficiency syndrome (AIDS) and their sexual partners, *J Clin Immunol* 7:130-133, 1987.

97. Stricker RB, McHugh TM, Moody MJ, et al: An AIDS-related cytotoxic autoantibody reacts with a specific antigen on stimulated CD4+ cells, *Nature* 327:710-713, 1987a.

98. Stricker RB, McHugh TM, Marx PA, et al: Prevalence of an AIDS-related autoantibody against CD4+ T cells in humans and monkeys, *Blood* 70:127A, 1987b.

99. McDougal JS, Hubbard M, Nicholson JKA, et al: Immune complexes in the acquired immunodeficiency syndrome (AIDS): relationship to disease manifestation, risk group, and immunologic defect, *J Clin Immunol* 5:130, 1985.

100. Fauci AS: Multifactorial nature of human immunodeficiency virus disease: implications for therapy, *Science* 262:1011-1018, 1993.

101. Groenbladh L, Gunne L: Methadone-assisted rehabilitation of Swedish heroin addicts, *Drug Alcohol Depend* 24:31-37, 1989.

102. Weber R, Ledergerber W, Opravil M, et al: Progression of HIV infection in misusers of injected drugs who stop injecting or follow a programme of maintenance treatment with methadone, *Br Med J* 301:1361-1365, 1990.

103. Fribourg-Blanc A: Deux observations d'annulation spontanee d'une seropositive HIV, *Med Mal Infect* 4:216-218, 1988.

104. Burger H, Weiser B, Robinson WS, et al: Transient antibody to lymphadenopathy-associated virus/human T-lymphotropic virus type III and T-lymphocyte abnormalities in the wife of a man who developed the acquired immunodeficiency syndrome, *Ann Intern Med* 103:545-547, 1985.

105. Farzedegan H, Polis MA, Wolinsky SM, et al: Loss of human immunodeficiency virus type 1 (HIV-1) antibodies with evidence of viral infection in asymptomatic homosexual men, *Ann Med* 108:785-790, 1988.

106. Hilgartner MW, Buckley JD, Operskalski EA, et al: Purity of factor VIII concentrates and serial CD4 counts, *Lancet* 341:1373-1374, 1993.

107. Mannucci PM, Gringeria A, De Biasi R, et al: Immune status of asymptomatic HIV-infected haemophiliacs: randomized, prospective, two-year comparison of treatment with high-purity or an intermediate-purity factor VIII (FVIII), *Thromb Haemost* 67:310-313, 1992.

108. Gomperts ED, De Biasi R, De Vreker R: The impact of clotting factor concentrates on the immune system in individuals with hemophilia, *Transfus Med Rev* 6:44-54, 1992.

109. Chlebowski RT, Grosvenor M, Lillington L, et al: Dietary intake and counseling, weight maintenance, and the course of HIV infection, *J Am Diet Assoc* 95:428-432, 1995.

110. Coutsoudis A, Bobat RA, Coovadia HM, et al: The effects of vitamin A supplementation on the morbidity of children born to HIV-infected women, *Am J Public Health* 85:1076-1081, 1995.

111. Kallenius G, Hoffner SE, Svenson SB: Does vaccination with bacille Calmette-Guerin protect against AIDS? *Rev Infect Dis* 11:349-351, 1989.

112. Jacobson MA: Current management of cytomegalovirus disease in patients with AIDS, *AIDS Res Hum Retroviruses* 10:917-923, 1994.

113. Markham A Faulds D: Ganciclovir: an update of its therapeutic use in cytomegalovirus infection, *Drugs* 48:455-484, 1994.

114. Balfour HH Jr, Fletcher CV, Erice A, et al: Effect of foscarnet on quantities of cytomegalovirus and human immunodeficiency virus in blood of persons with AIDS, *Antimicrob Agents Chemother* 40:2721-2726, 1996.

115. Kalyesubula I, Musoke-Mudido P, Marum L, et al: Effects of malaria infection in human immunodeficiency virus type 1-infected Ugandan children, *Pediatr Infect Dis* 16:876-881, 1997.

116. Balzarini J, Kruining J, Wedgewood O, et al: Conversion of 2',3'-dideoxyadenosine (ddA) and 2',3'-dideoxyadenosine (d4A) to their corresponding aryloxyphosphoramidate derivatives markedly potentiates their activity against human immunodeficiency virus and hepatitis B virus, *FEBS Lett* 410:324-328, 1997.

117. Rahn JJ, Kieller DM, Tyrrell DL, et al: Modulation of the metabolism of beta-L-(-)-2', 3'-dideoxy-3'-thiacytidine by thymidine, fludarabine, and nitrobenzylthioinosine, *Antimicrob Agents Chemother* 41:918-923, 1997.

118. Colledge D, Locarnini S, Shaw T: Synergistic inhibition of hepadnaviral replication by lamivudine in combination with penciclovir in vitro, *Hepatology* 26:216-225, 1997.

119. Mar EC, Chu CK, Lin JC: Some nucleoside analogs with antihuman immunodeficiency virus activity inhibit replication of Epstein-Barr virus, *Antiviral Res* 28:1-11, 1995.

120. DeGruttola V, Lagakos S: Epidemic models, empirical studies, and uncertainty. In Castillo-Chavez C, editor: *Mathematical and statistical approaches to AIDS epidemiology,* New York, 1989, Springer-Verlag.

121. Kault DA: Modeling AIDS reduction strategies, *Int J Epidemiol* 24:188-197, 1995.

122. Anderson RM: The role of mathematical models in the study of HIV transmission and the epidemiology of AIDS, *J Acquir Immune Defic Syndr Hum Retrolvirol* 1:241-256, 1988.

123. Anderson RM: Mathematical and statistical studies of the epidemiology of HIV, *AIDS* 3:333-346, 1989.

124. Jager JC, Ruitenberg EJ, editors: *Statistical analysis and mathematical modeling of AIDS,* Oxford, UK, 1988, Oxford University Press.

125. Castillo-Chavez C, editor: *Mathematical and statistical approaches to AIDS epidemiology,* New York, 1989, Springer-Verlag.

126. Hethcote HW, Van Ark JW: *Modeling HIV transmission and AIDS in the United States,* New York, 1992, Springer-Verlag.

127. Jewell NP, Dietz K, Farewell VT: *AIDS epidemiology: methodological issues,* Boston, 1992, Birkhäuser-Boston.
128. Nicolosi A, editor: *HIV epidemiology: models and methods,* New York, 1993, Raven Press.
129. Kaplan EH, Brandeau ML, editors: *Modeling the AIDS epidemic: planning, policy, and prediction,* New York, 1994, Raven Press.
130. Brookmeyer R, Gail MH: *AIDS epidemiology: a quantitative approach,* Oxford, UK, 1994, Oxford University Press.
131. Bailey NTJ: The use of operational modeling of HIV/AIDS in a systems approach to public health, *Math Biosci* 107:413-430, 1991.
132. Hethcote HW: Modeling AIDS prevention programs in a population of homosexual men. In Kaplan EH, Brandeau ML, editors: *Modeling the AIDS epidemic: planning, policy, and prediction,* New York, 1994, Raven Press.
133. Shiboski S: Statistical interpretation of data from partner studies of heterosexual HIV transmission. In Kaplan EH, Brandeau ML, editors: *Modeling the AIDS epidemic: planning, policy, and prediction,* New York, 1994, Raven Press.
134. Stigum H, Magnus P, Bakketeig LS: Effect of changing partnership formation rates on the spread of sexually transmitted diseases and human immunodeficiency virus, *Am J Epidemiol* 145:644-652, 1997.
135. Weyer J, Eggers HJ: On the structure of the epidemic spread of AIDS: the influence of an infectious coagent, *Zentralbl Bakteriol* 273:52-67, 1990.
136. West RW, Thompson JR: Modeling the impact of HIV on the spread of tuberculosis in the United States, *Math Biosci* 143:35-60, 1997.
137. Placido R, Mancino G, Amendola A, et al: Apoptosis of human monocytes/macrophages in *Mycobacterium tuberculosis* infection, *J Pathol* 181:31-38, 1997.
138. Garrait V, Cadranel J, Esvant H, et al: Tuberculosis generates a microenvironment enhancing productive infection of local lymphocytes by HIV, *J Immunol* 159:2824-2830, 1997.
139. Xiao L, Qwen SM, Rudolph DL, et al: *Plasmodium falciparum* antigen-induced human immunodeficiency virus type 1 replication is mediated through induction of human necrosis factor-α, *J Infect Dis* 177:437-445, 1998.
140. Phillips AN, Elford J, Sabin C, et al: Pattern of CD4+ T-cell loss in HIV infection, *J Acquir Immune Defic Syndr Hum Retrovirol* 5:950-951, 1992.
141. Sheppard HW, Lang W, Ascher MS, et al: The characterization of nonprogressors: long-term HIV-1 infection with stable CD4+ T-cell levels, *AIDS* 7:1159-1166, 1993b.
142. Nowak MA, Anderson RM, McLean AR, et al: Antigenic diversity thresholds and the development of AIDS, *Science* 254:963-969, 1991.
143. Sheppard HW, Ascher MS, Krowka JF: Viral burden and HIV disease, *Nature* 364:291, 1993a.
144. Anderson RW, Ascher MS, Sheppard HW: Direct HIV cytopathicity cannot account for the CD4 decline in AIDS in the presence of homeostasis, *J Acquir Immune Defic Syndr Hum Retrovirol* 17:245-252, 1998.
145. Stein DS, Drusano GL: Modeling of the change in CD4 lymphocyte counts in patients before and after administration of the human immunodeficiency virus protease inhibitor indinavir, *Antimicrob Agents Chem* 41:449-453, 1997.
146. Amadori A, Zamaechi R, Bianchi L: CD4:CD8 ratio and HIV infection: "the tap and drain," *Immunol Today* 1996:414-417, 1996.
147. Grossman Z, Herberman RB: T-cell homeostasis in HIV infection is neither failing nor blind: modified cell counts reflect an adaptive response of the host, *Nature Med* 3:486-490, 1997.
148. Merrill SJ, Radke RR: A stochastic model of the generation of diversity in HIV infection, *J Immunol Meth* (in press).
149. Ascher MS, Sheppard HW: AIDS as immune system activation II: the panergic imnesia hypothesis, *J Acquir Immune Defic Syndr Hum Retrovirol* 3:177-191, 1990.
150. Sheppard HW, Ascher MS: The relationship between AIDS and immunologic tolerance, *J Acquir Immune Defic Syndr Hum Retrovirol* 5:143-147, 1992.
151. Witte MH, Kerwin A, Witte CL, et al: A curriculum on medical ignorance, *Med Educ* 23:24-29, 1989.
152. Akker S, Van Den G, Goedbloed E: Pneumonia caused by *Pneumocystis carinii* in a dog, *Trop Geogr Med* 12:54-58, 1960.
153. Burke RA, Good RA: *Pneumocystis carinii* infection, *Medicine* 52:23-51, 1973.
154. Sheldon WH: Experimental pulmonary *Pneumocystis carinii* infection in rabbits, *J Exp Med* 110:147-159, 1959.
155. Moghaddam A, Rosenzweig M, Lee-Parritz D, et al: An animal model for acute and persistent Epstein-Barr virus infection, *Science* 276:2030-2033, 1997.

Suggested Readings

Al-Harthi L, Roebuck KA, Olinger GG, et al: Bacterial vaginosis-associated microflora isolated from the female genital tract activates HIV-1 expression, *J Acquir Immune Defic Syndr* 21:194-202, 1999.
Emery VC, Atkins MC, Bowen EF, et al: Interactions between beta-herpesviruses and human immunodeficiency virus in vivo: evidence for increased human immunodeficiency viral load in the presence of human herpesvirus-6, *J Med Virol* 57:278-282, 1999.
Grau O, Tuppin P, Slizewicz G, et al: A longitudinal study of seroreactivity against *Mycoplasma penetrans* in HIV-infected homosexual men: association with disease progression, *AIDS Res Hum Retroviruses* 14:661-667, 1998.

Hashemi FB, Ghassemi M, Roebuck KA, et al: Activation of human immunodeficiency virus type 1 expression by *Gardnerella vaginalis, J Infect Dis* 179:924-930, 1999.

Hoffman IF, Jere CS, Taylor TE, et al: The effect of *Plasmodium falciparum* malaria on HIV-1 RNA blood plasma concentration, *AIDS* 13:487-494, 1999.

Kovacs A, Schluchter M, Easley K, et al: Cytomegalovirus infection and HIV-1 disease progression in infants born to HIV-1-infected women, Pediatric Pulmonary and Cardiovascular Complications of Vertically Transmitted HIV Infection Study Group, *N Engl J Med* 341:77-84, 1999.

Marino S, Kretschmer C, Brandner S, et al: Activation of HIV transcription by human foamy virus in transgenic mice, *Lab Invest* 73:103-110, 1995.

Otten MW Jr, Zaidi AA, Peterman TA, et al: High rate of HIV seroconversion among patients attending urban sexually transmitted disease clinics, *AIDS* 8:549-553, 1994.

Perez G, Skurnick JH, Denny TN, et al: Herpes simplex type II and *Mycoplasma genitalium* as risk factors for heterosexual HIV transmission: report from the heterosexual HIV transmission study, *Int J Infect Dis* 3:5-11, 1998.

Root-Bernstein RS: HIV and immunosuppressive cofactors in AIDS, *J Immunol Immunopharmacol* 12:256-262, 1992.

Semba RD, Kumwenda N, Hoover DR, et al: Human immunodeficiency virus load in breast milk, mastitis, and mother-to-child transmission of human immunodeficiency virus type 1, *J Infect Dis* 180:93-98, 1999.

Theus SA, Harrich DA, Gaynor R, et al: *Treponema pallidum,* lipoproteins, and synthetic lipoprotein analogues induce human immunodeficiency virus type 1 gene expression in monocytes via NF-kappaB activation, *J Infect Dis* 177:941-950, 1998.

Ward JW, Bush TJ, Perkins HA, et al: The natural history of transfusion-associated infection with human immunodeficiency virus, *N Engl J Med* 321:947-968, 1989.

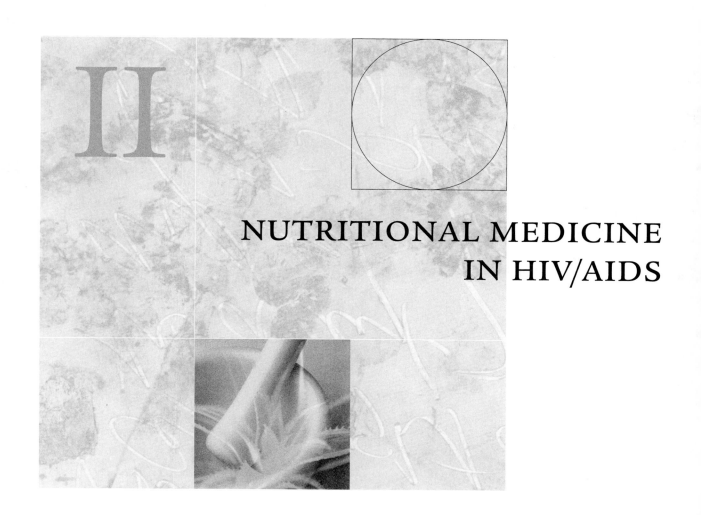

NUTRITIONAL MEDICINE IN HIV/AIDS

Introduction to Nutritional Approaches to HIV/AIDS

LEANNA J. STANDISH

utrition is the most extensively researched of all the diverse areas of complementary and alternative medicine (CAM) in the treatment of HIV/AIDS. This extensive research uses not only in vitro methods but also observational and clinical studies in HIV-infected humans. Numerous papers have been published studying the in vitro immunological and virological effects of single nutrients. Most of the human studies focus on measuring serum and cellular levels of nutrients, such as minerals, vitamins, and antioxidants, thought to be pertinent to HIV disease progress. Many studies suggest that the levels of important nutrients are lower in people infected with HIV and that these levels correlate with disease progression.[1-3]

Results from several epidemiological studies suggest that deficiencies of certain nutrients, such as vitamin A, may be associated with a poor immune status and that higher intakes of micronutrients at baseline were associated with higher $CD4^+$ T-cell counts. Longitudinal observational studies of HIV-positive cohorts suggest that slowed disease progression is associated with an increased intake level of certain nutrients. Tang et al[4] conducted an epidemiological study of 281 HIV-positive men, which provided evidence that certain dose ranges of dietary micronutrient intake of vitamins B_1, B_2, B_6, C, and niacin were associated with slowed disease progression, whereas high doses of zinc and vitamin A were associated with faster progression to AIDS. In another epidemiological study, Abrams prospectively examined the link between baseline dietary intake and development of AIDS in 296 HIV-positive men over a 6-year period. Higher intake of micronutrients at baseline was associated with higher CD4[+] T-cell levels. In the same study, daily multivitamin use was associated with a reduced risk of AIDS and a reduced baseline risk of low CD4[+] T-cell counts.[5] In 1996 Tang et al reported that intake of beta-carotene at 2 times the required daily amount was associated with increased survival in HIV-positive persons.[6] The HIV Epidemiology Research Study (HERS) reported on correlates of nutritional status in a cohort of 626 women (426 HIV-positive, 199 HIV-negative). Among HIV-positive patients, higher levels of ferritin and lower levels of B_{12}, zinc (Zn), and selenium (Se) were associated with lower CD4[+] T-cell levels.[7] Vitamin A deficiency was associated with lower CD4[+] T-cell levels among both HIV-positive and HIV-negative intravenous drugs users ($n = 179$). Among HIV-positive subjects, vitamin A deficiency was associated with increased mortality.[8] Serum vitamin A appears to be related to vertical transmission rates of HIV infection in African women. Semba et al (1994) studied 300 HIV-positive mothers in Africa and found that the rate of transmission was much greater in women who had low vitamin A levels; rates ranged from 32% in the women with the lowest vitamin A levels to 7% in women with the highest levels.[9]

Although the in vitro and epidemiological literature point to correlations between specific nutritional deficiencies, immunological status, progression, and transmission rates, it is uncertain if supplementation makes a positive difference. The current literature suggests that nutritional deficiencies are associated with decreased immune indices and higher risk for disease progression. The literature does not specify if additional supplementation above RDA levels increases immune indices or slows progression. A review of the literature elucidating how deficiencies of micronutrients, such as vitamin A, beta-carotene, Se, vitamin E, Zn, B vitamins, and magnesium (Mg), relate to clinical and laboratory measures of HIV disease illustrates the need for nutritional supplementation in HIV disease.[10-12]

Since evidence of nutritional deficiencies in HIV-infected individuals exists, many clinicians and consumers in the HIV-infected community have concluded that oral administration of mega-doses of vitamins, minerals, and antioxidants, such as N-Acetylcysteine (NAC), will slow progression of the disease. Surprisingly few human nutritional supplementation trials have been published. Controlled supplementation studies are needed to address whether oral supplementation of nutrients that are low in HIV-infected people or vitamins whose intake appears to be associated with slower disease progression in epidemiological studies significantly alters immunological status and viral load. Vitamin C, for example, is the most common alternative medicine reported by the Bastyr University AIDS Research Center's cohort of 1666 HIV-positive men and women. Yet vitamin C has not been evaluated in even a single clinical trial. Despite the fact that vitamin C is often taken in high doses by HIV-positive individuals, no controlled human studies have yet been done. Some in vitro research suggests that ascorbate can suppress HIV replication in both chronically and acutely infected T-cells.[13]

With the exception of the effects of vitamin A supplementation on HIV vertical transmission rates in pregnant women in Africa, the results of the few controlled clinical trials of single nutrients given in high oral doses to HIV-positive human subjects living in the United States have been disappointing. However, ample evidence from observational studies shows that even in US HIV-positive populations, vitamin and mineral supplementation is associated with decreased morbidity and mortality, although the relationships between some micronutrients and disease progression are complexly nonlinear.

The next two chapters focus on the topic of nutritional approaches to HIV/AIDS, both written by key researchers in the field. Chapter 4 reviews nutritional deficiencies in AIDS patients and provides a science-based rationale for adjunctive nutritional therapy during all stages of HIV infection. Chapter 5 reviews the literature on antioxidant deficiencies in HIV-positive individuals and discusses the current literature on the effects of high-dose antioxidant supplementation on immune indices and disease progression.

References

1. Patrick L: Nutrients and HIV: part one—beta-carotene and selenium, *Altern Med Rev* 4(6):403-413, 1999.
2. Patrick L: Nutrients and HIV: part two—vitamins A and E, zinc, B vitamins, and magnesium, *Altern Med Rev* 5(1):39-51, 2000.
3. Patrick L: Nutrients and HIV: part three—N-Acetylcysteine, alpha-lipoic acid, L-glutamine, and L-carnitine, *Altern Med Rev* 5(4):290-305, 2000.

4. Tang A, Graham NMH, et al: Dietary micronutrient intake and risk of progression to AIDS in HIV-1 infected homosexual men, *Am J Epidemiol* 138(11):937, 1993.

5. Abrams B, Duncan D, Hertz-Picciotto, I: A prospective study of dietary intake and AIDS in HIV-seropositive homosexual men, *J Acquir Immune Defic Syndr Hum Retrovirol* 6(8):949-958, 1993.

6. Tang AM, Graham NM, Saah AJ: Effects of micronutrient intake on survival in human immunodeficiency virus type 1 infection, *Am J Epidemiol* 143(12):1244-1256, 1996 (abstract We.B.182).

7. Smith, Graham, Flynn, et al: *XI Int Conf AIDS* Jul 1996 (abstract We.B.182).

8. Semba RD, Graham NMH, Caiaffa WT, et al: Increased mortality associated with vitamin A deficiency during human immunodeficiency virus type 1 infection, *Arch Intern Med* 153:2149-2154, 1993.

9. Semba RD, Miotti PG, Chiphangwi JD, et al: Maternal vitamin A deficiency and mother-to-child transmission of HIV-1, *Lancet* 343:1593-1597, 1994.

10. Patrick L: Nutrients and HIV: part one—beta-carotene and selenium, *Altern Med Rev* 4(6):403-413, 1999.

11. Patrick L: Nutrients and HIV: part two—vitamins A and E, zinc, B vitamins, and magnesium, *Altern Med Rev* 5(1):39-51, 2000.

12. Patrick L: Nutrients and HIV: part three—N-Acetylcysteine, alpha-lipoic acid, L-glutamine, and L-carnitine, *Altern Med Rev* 5(1):290-305, 2000.

13. Harakeh S, Jariwalla RJ, Pauling L: Suppression of human immunodeficiency virus replication by ascorbate in chronically and acutely infected cells, *Proc Natl Acad Sci U S A* 87:7245-7249, 1990.

Nutritional Deficiencies in AIDS Patients

A Treatment Opportunity

JEONGMIN LEE

KOZO YOSHIKAWA

RONALD ROSS WATSON

ABSTRACT

Immune dysfunction resulting from infection with the human immunodeficiency virus (HIV) is a major health threat to populations in North America and throughout the world. Since HIV-infected persons in industrialized nations can survive a previously life-threatening infection through the use of effective medical therapies, malnutrition and wasting are becoming central issues in the health care plans of long-term survivors. Nutrition is a fundamental intervention in both the early and the ongoing treatment of HIV disease. Nutrition therapy, in coordination with other medical interventions, can extend and improve the quality and quantity of life in individuals infected with HIV and those living with acquired immune deficiency syndrome (AIDS).

Medical nutrition therapy involves an assessment of nutritional status and treatment. Research on the relationship between nutrition and HIV infection is essential for understanding the mechanisms of wasting and for determining the effectiveness of medical nutrition therapy. This chapter uses currently published research papers to review the mechanisms and consequences of malnutrition in HIV/AIDS patients.

INTRODUCTION

An individual's nutritional status influences morbidity and mortality (M&M) in many diseases, regardless of the disease process. Nutrition should be central in the treatment of HIV infection because of the chronic nature of HIV and the numerous related opportunistic infections (OIs) that affect the digestive tract. Because undernutrition adversely affects immune defenses in people who do not have HIV, nutritional deficiencies in HIV-infected people accelerate the development of severe immunodeficiency. Although it has been poorly studied, nutritional supplementation may therefore overcome nutritional deficiency and immunosuppression in AIDS. Recently vitamin E deficiency was identified in HIV-infected people.[1] Another study showed that vitamin E replacement slowed the development of immune deficiency.[2,3] An associated editorial concluded that more research is needed on the benefits of vitamin supplementation to slow the loss of immune defenses and promote well-being in HIV-infected persons and that supplementation should start now while research is underway.[4] Therefore we reviewed vitamin and mineral deficiencies in AIDS patients and concluded that they are prevalent and should be treated, since they accentuate immune damage.

A macronutrient deficiency such as wasting, a common occurrence in HIV disease, is a protein-calorie malnutrition and is caused by inadequate calorie and protein intake, absorption, or use. The resulting loss of weight and muscle mass is directly associated with a deterioration in health and increased mortality. The loss of lean body mass (LBM) is associated with a greater incidence of OIs, further deterioration in immune function, and poorer nutritional status.[5] Because malnutrition has a direct impact on immune function, maintaining the nutritional status of the HIV-infected patient is a central concern.

MACRONUTRIENT DEFICIENCY AND PROGRESSION TO AIDS

Energy Expenditure

Resting energy expenditure (REE) correlated positively with the presence of HIV infection. REE was 10% higher in stable HIV-positive subjects and AIDS patients than in healthy controls.[6,7] Grunfeld found that REE was higher in HIV-positive patients, AIDS-related complex (ARC) patients, and AIDS patients who did not have concomitant OIs than it was in healthy controls, as long as the patient's oral intake was sufficient to maintain body weight (BW).[8] This finding contrasts

with AIDS patients who had concomitant infections, which resulted in increased REE, decreased oral intake, and weight loss. There was no compensatory decrease in REE, as might be expected with decreased oral intake. Failure to regulate REE as an adaptation to anorexia or malabsorption is often stated as the major cause of weight loss in individuals with AIDS. However, total energy expenditure (TEE) in HIV-infected patients was not significantly different from that in healthy controls but was decreased slightly in weight-stable AIDS patients.[6] With a spectrum of REE for hospitalized ARC and AIDS patients without malabsorption or uncontrolled infection,[9] 6% were hypometabolic, 26% were normal-metabolic, and 68% were hypermetabolic. Hypermetabolism is characteristic of cachexia (i.e., muscle wasting, inefficient use of energy, and loss of LBM), as seen in cancer and other chronic disease states, whereas hypometabolism is an appropriate compensatory response to starvation and protein-energy malnutrition.

It is unclear if weight loss correlates with the metabolic rate, since some studies show a decrease in energy expenditure during periods of weight loss.[8,10] Although REE increased in HIV-positive and AIDS patients, changes in weight correlated not with REE but with caloric intake.[8] The most common physiological causes of hypermetabolism, such as pregnancy, adolescence, and exercise, do not usually lead to wasting, perhaps because of higher caloric intake and metabolic adaptation.[11] The etiology of possible hypermetabolism remains unclear, since increased hormones or tumor necrosis factor (TNF) were not found in patients with high REE.[12,13] Whether or not chronic hypermetabolism occurs, frequent fevers associated with secondary infections in HIV-infected patients may result in short-term increased REE.[5] Malignancy may also raise REE.[14] It is, however, unclear if hypermetabolism is sufficient to cause wasting in the absence of other processes, although hypermetabolism may occur in some HIV-infected patients.[11]

Body Weight and Composition

Body wasting, particularly loss of body cell mass (BCM), is an increasingly prevalent AIDS-defining condition and is an independent risk factor for death in HIV-infected patients. Although they had the same BW as the controls, HIV-positive male patients had less BCM, greater potassium depletion, less intracellular water, more extracellular water, decreased serum proteins (e.g., albumin, retinol-binding protein [RBP]), and decreased total iron binding capacity (TIBC). This depletion occurred to a greater extent in the patients with diarrhea. Compared with normal values, body fat was also depleted but was similar to that of a control group of healthy homosexual males. Loss of body fat was found even in the earlier stages of HIV infection and was more severe than loss of BCM. Female patients had a larger decrease in body fat than male patients, whereas males showed a greater relative depletion of BCM than body fat. In more stable ambulatory patients with AIDS, however, weight loss was not associated with reductions in LBM, body fat, or total water, and the explanation for weight loss was unclear.[15]

In a follow-up retrospective study of wasted AIDS patients during the 100 days before death, BCM (decreased 50%) was reduced out of proportion to weight loss (decreased 33%).[16] In patients who died within 100 days of a body composition measurement, those with the lower BCM died sooner. Specifically, a loss of 37% of BW was associated with death. This study revealed that the progression of wasting was independent of body fat changes but was associated with loss of BCM. Thus a patient could have a normal BW yet a low BCM and still be at risk for death due to malnutrition.

Pathophysiology of Malnutrition in HIV Disease

A number of possible etiologies of weight loss in HIV infection exist. HIV wasting syndrome also may be multifactorial in etiology.[17] Multiple etiologies may be present in a single patient. The most likely etiologies can be divided into the broad categories of (1) decreased food intake, (2) malabsorption, (3) alterations in metabolism, (4) cytokine effects, (5) endocrine dysfunction, (6) steroids and growth hormones, (7) primary muscle disease, and (8) alcohol abuse.

Decreased Food Intake

Decreased food intake may result from anorexia or nausea secondary to medications, systemic illness (mediated by cytokines), neurological disease, or oral or esophageal pathology (e.g., dry mouth, odynophagia, ulcers, or malignancy).[18] Taste and smell loss due to medications, oral pathology such as candidiasis, and peripheral or central nervous system (CNS) disease are well documented in HIV-infected patients. These chemosensory abnormalities can impair food intake and contribute to wasting. Additionally, fatigue, dementia, and peripheral myoneuropathies influence a patient's ability to obtain food. Monetary considerations also play a role. Dependence on other people to prepare or purchase food may also limit a debilitated patient's intake.

Malabsorption

Oral, esophageal, stomach, pancreatic, biliary, hepatic, and small and large intestine pathology can influence the absorption of nutrients. Malabsorption, chronic diarrhea, or both may be secondary to infections, malnutrition, medications, enzyme deficiencies, malignancies, and HIV enteropathy.[19] Diarrhea is found in over 50% of AIDS patients with pathogens, including *Cytomegalovirus,* herpes simplex virus, adenovirus, *Salmonella, Shigella, Campylobacter, Clostridium difficile, Mycobacterium avium-intracellulare, Giardia, Entamoeba, Cryptosporidium, Microsporidium,* and *Isospora.*[19] Gastrointestinal dysfunction, especially malabsorption, is prevalent in advanced HIV infection, with or without identifiable pathogens. Villous abnormalities are frequent in these HIV-infected individuals, and small intestinal dysfunction has been demonstrated by abnormal D-xylose absorption tests, Schilling tests, C-14 glycocholate absorption, and the presence of steatorrhea.[13,20] Small intestinal pathology or pancreatic insufficiency may lead to fat malabsorption, weight loss, and depletion of fat-soluble vitamins in HIV-infected persons. Fat malabsorption occurred in 48% of a range of HIV-infected patients using a C-14 triolein breath test.[21]

Although severe malabsorption is limited to patients who have advanced HIV disease with CD4+ T-cell counts <100 and usually <50 cells/ml, overt malabsorption has not been described in early HIV infection. However, studies indicate that subclinical malabsorption may play a role in early HIV disease without evidence of diarrhea. The D-xylose test was abnormal in 25% of patients with early HIV disease,[22] and the lactulose mannitol permeability test was abnormal in 16%.[23] In addition, the hypometabolic status and reduced glucose cycling in clinically stable AIDS patients could be explained by subclinical malabsorption.[15,24] Hypochlorhydria has been found in 74% of AIDS patients[25] and is a permissive factor for enteric infections and bacterial overgrowth of the small intestine.[26] Furthermore, hypochlorhydria decreased the absorption of certain micronutrients such as folate and iron.[27] Lactase or other disaccharidase deficiency has also been reported in AIDS patients.

Altered Metabolism

Evidence exists for both hypermetabolism and hypometabolism in HIV-infected patients. The cachexia associated with cancer or concomitant inflammation has been related to the production of TNF.[28] Therefore the cachexia that occurs in HIV-positive persons also may be related to excess TNF production. This hypothesis has not yet been proven. Another study showed enhanced TNF production from peripheral blood mononuclear cells (PBMCs) of healthy subjects who had been starved for 6 days.[29] The intricate relationship between cytokine production, metabolic disturbances, viral burden, and weight loss in HIV-infected individuals is not completely understood. Increased futile cycling of substrates, energy use, and heat production exist without a net gain in product (such as fat oxidation and synthesis, triglyceride hydrolysis, and reesterification). In murine AIDS lipid levels in tissues and oxidation increase significantly.[30] Cytokine production also has metabolic consequences. For example, TNF enhances hepatic lipogenesis and very low density lipoprotein (VLDL) release, inhibits adipocyte lipoprotein lipase, and enhances adipocyte lipolysis. The result is that fatty acids (FAs) mobilize peripherally to the liver to be made into VLDLs and circulate but are not stored or used for energy. Other cytokines (e.g., IL-1β, IL-6, IFN-α, and IFN-γ) may synergize with TNF to enhance this cycle, as well as glucose futile cycles and proteolysis. This results in cachexia. Synergistic interactions are especially important during secondary OIs in HIV-positive persons.

Studies regarding basal blood levels of TNF, IL-1β, and IFN-α in HIV-positive patients are conflicting.[31] Wasting has not been directly proportional to circulating blood levels of triglycerides, free FAs, TNF, or IL-1β.[32] However, levels of IFN-α correlate positively with serum triglycerides.[33] TNF and IL-1 are produced by PBMC and monocyte cell lines infected in vitro with HIV-1 or PBMC isolated from HIV-positive patients.[34] Some researchers speculate that increased TNF production is related to the stage of disease; PBMC from patients with ARC or AIDS produce more TNF than those from patients with an asymptomatic infection.[35]

Cytokines

Elevated levels of certain cytokines, particularly TNF, may be responsible for the wasting and weight loss seen in AIDS patients.[36,37] However, several studies report elevations of TNF, particularly in symptomatic patients, while others do not.[38,39] In murine AIDS there is a significant increase in circulating TNF and T_H2 cell cytokines such as IL-6 but no change in muscle mass.[40] In a group of 33 HIV-positive outpatients, elevated TNF levels did not correlate with weight loss or increased metabolic rate.[41] Serum assays of TNF often are not sensitive or accurate enough to detect elevations, particularly since TNF is secreted in a pulsatile fashion.[38,39]

Either TNF or other cytokines could cause weight loss or HIV wasting syndrome by a number of mechanisms. TNF, and possibly IL-1, may induce anorexia. Alternatively, TNF may affect lipid metabolism, leading to a relative decrease in fat oxidation compared with carbohydrate or protein oxidation and a relatively greater loss of LBM.[42] The effect of TNF on AIDS patients may depend on its site of production. For example, intracerebral TNF-secreting tumors produced lethal anorexia and weight loss in mice with relative sparing of protein—a model of starvation.[43] TNF-secreting tumors in peripheral muscle tissue resulted in much slower cachexia with a greater loss of protein.[43]

A variety of other potential mechanisms of TNF action have been discussed.[44] Some investigators suggest that the interaction of TNF with other cytokines, such as IL-1, or with other inflammatory mediators may induce anorexia, accelerated protein breakdown, or wasteful energy expenditure.[38,42]

Endocrine Abnormalities

Endocrine dysfunction is another possible etiology of HIV wasting syndrome. Endocrine abnormalities in HIV-infected patients, including changes in gonadal, adrenal, and thyroid function, occur frequently and could lead to weight loss and wasting.[39,44] Low levels of reverse triiodothyronine (rT_3) and a persistence of triiodothyronine (T_3) within the normal range[45] mark HIV infection. This finding is consistent with most severe infections, in which rT_3 rises and T_3 falls. Normal serum T_3 levels may be an inappropriate response to the caloric deprivation of normal illness or result from a cytokine effect, and they might result in continued high energy expenditure leading to weight loss.[45] TNF and IL-1 have been shown to cause an inappropriately normal T_3 and a low rT_3 state in mice and appear to stimulate the enzyme iodothyronine 5'-deiodinase (5'D), which results in increased synthesis of T_3 from T_4 and increased degradation of rT_3.[46] However, other studies suggest that serum T_3 falls appropriately in the presence of AIDS and acute OIs.[44]

Adrenal insufficiency in AIDS has been reported occasionally, often stemming from OIs or the effects of medication.[47] Some patients had a suboptimal cortisol response to the administration of adrenocorticotropic hormone (ACTH) and conceivably could develop clinical adrenal insufficiency during acute infection.[47] The basal cortisol levels are elevated in patients with HIV compared with controls.[48] Elevation in cortisol levels can be a physiological response to severe weight loss as the body attempts to maintain glucose hemostasis in the brain.

Decreased testosterone and dehydroepiandrosterone (DHEA) have been reported in a number of studies of HIV-infected men.[44,49] DHEA and DHEA sulfate (DHEAS) are sterols that are synthesized from cholesterol in humans. DHEAS is water soluble and easily transported by attaching to albumin. It is present in humans at 1000 times the level of DHEA and functions as a inactive reservoir. Because DHEA and DHEAS interconvert, DHEAS often converts to DHEA; however, the conversion of DHEA to DHEAS is much less frequent. DHEA can be converted in tissues to more potent androgens, testosterone, and dihydrotestosterone. It acts as an estrogen as well. DHEA levels and $CD4^+$ T-cell counts decline in HIV-infected people. We showed that DHEA supplementation prevented most of the immune dysfunction, cytokine dysregulation, and loss of nutrients during murine AIDS.[50] Lowered levels of testosterone are correlated with weight loss and decreased survival.[44] In a study of patients with HIV wasting syndrome, free and total testosterone was significantly lower in patients with similar $CD4^+$ T-cell counts but without wasting.[44] Since testosterone is an anabolic hormone, a deficiency could result in decreased LBM and contribute to HIV wasting syndrome.

Steroids and Growth Hormone

If BCM does not increase rapidly despite improved energy intake, anabolic pharmacological approaches may be used to augment nutritional intervention. Because severe loss of BW is directly associated with risk of death and lower survival rates in end-stage AIDS, replacement testosterone therapy should be initiated early.[51]

Recent studies report marked gains in LBM from administration of anabolic steroids. An open study of nandrolone decanoate (100 mg/ml), intramuscularly (IM) administered every 2 weeks for 16 weeks, enrolled 24 patients with HIV infection who had lost 5% to 15% of their usual BW.[52] The study found that nandrolone decanoate resulted in marked increases above baseline in BW, LBM, and quality of life (QOL). Another study spanning 8 weeks with 24 HIV-infected men reported that IM testosterone and oxandrolone (20 mg/day) resulted in considerable increases in LBM, BW, and strength compared with treatment using IM testosterone and a placebo.[53] However, clinical trials providing more data and a larger number of patients are needed in this study before recommendations can be made regarding the inclusion of anabolic steroids in wasting therapy. Another study of oxandrolone (15 mg/day) reported a marked weight increase above baseline compared with placebo-treated patients who lost weight.

Growth hormone (GH) deficiency is postulated to be a possible cause of HIV wasting. AIDS wasting is associated with a GH-resistant state that results in low levels of serum insulin-like growth factor 1 and 2 (IGF-1, IGF-2), IGF-binding protein 3 (IGFBP-3), elevated levels of phosphorylated IGF-binding protein 1 (IGFBP-1), and a reduced ability to form the IGFBP-3 ternary complex.[54] AIDS patients who lost more than 10% of their ideal body mass demonstrated a 50% reduction in serum IGF-1 and a 70% reduction in IGF-2 compared to healthy HIV-negative subjects. The wasting syndrome of rabies infection is found to cause pituitary and hypothalamic dysfunction, resulting in decreased growth hormone production.[55] It is possible that a similar mechanism may occur in AIDS.

Recent studies have shown beneficial effects of GH therapy on LBM, muscle mass, and protein synthesis. A relatively large, double-blind, and placebo-controlled study of recombinant human GH (rhGH) with 178 HIV-infected patients demonstrated that 0.1 mg/kg of rhGH/day induces statistically significant weight gain, accrual of LBM, increased strength, and loss of body fat over 12 weeks of treatment.[56] In a study of six AIDS patients, 0.1 mg/kg of rhGH was shown to induce positive nitrogen balance and a retention of BCM, implicating that adding exogenous rhGH overcomes the acquired GH resistance in these patients.[57] In both studies, GH was well tolerated in AIDS patients. Most adverse effects were mild to moderate and included tissue edema, pain, arthralgia, and myalgia. These adverse symptoms generally responded to a reduction in the dose of rhGH.

The mechanism of action of GH in AIDS is unclear. However, some possibilities have been explored in recent years. GH can induce thymic hyperplasia and the generation of new CD4$^+$ T cells in mice, and IL-7 may be the effector molecule promoting thymopoiesis.[58] In addition, GH potentiates the proliferation and cytokine responses of human antigen-specific CD4$^+$ helper T and CD8$^+$ cytotoxic T-cell clones to their antigens.[59] GH improves the ability of dendritic cells to present a cognate antigen and provide costimulation at a maximal concentration of 10-50 μg/ml.[60]

Regardless of the beneficial effects of GH in AIDS patients, limitations still exist. The cost of GH as a long-term therapeutic reagent is a concern. Therefore researchers have explored the effectiveness of short-term use of GH. A recent study reported that a short-term intervention with rhGH prevents weight loss during acute OIs in patients with AIDS.[61] Another potential concern is the adverse effects of GH therapy, such as mild edema, arthralgia, and possible tumor cell proliferation.[56] Thus after the patient has tried GH therapy, a progress assessment is recommended. In addition, other measures of disease progression, such as CD4$^+$ T-cell count and viral load, should be monitored to ensure that no intervening clinical events have occurred. Continued nutritional support and assessment are also required.

Primary Muscle Disease

HIV wasting syndrome may result from a myopathy. Myopathy may occur as a complication of HIV-1 infection or from its treatment, zidovudine (AZT). No evidence exists to support a direct retroviral etiology. HIV-associated myopathy more likely has an immune-mediated pathogenesis. HIV antigens are localized in macrophages invading muscle, suggesting a role for virus-infected inflammatory cells in muscle degeneration.[62] The lack of significant inflammation in many of the muscle biopsies of individuals who have HIV wasting syndrome may reflect their profound immunological impairment. 5% of patients with HIV wasting syndrome had myopathy by clinical, laboratory (e.g., creatinine kinase and electromyelogram [EMG]), and muscle biopsy criteria.[63] Among these patients, prednisone caused decreases in creatinine kinase and increases in strength.[63] The connection of AZT

and HIV to myopathy and loss of muscle mass requires further evaluation.

Alcohol Abuse

Progression from HIV infection to AIDS took a few months in people consuming large amounts of alcohol instead of the expected 7 to 11 years.[64] Greatly increased alcohol use stimulated HIV replication, suppressed immune defenses, and promoted progression to AIDS.[65] Heavy alcohol use is common among intravenous (IV) drug users. The relative risk of AIDS was 3.8 times higher in heavy alcohol drinkers than in moderate ones.[66] Alcohol abuse was more common among AIDS patients than among HIV-infected drug abusers[66] or uninfected IV drug users. A study involving heavy alcohol drinkers who were HIV-infected showed a 41% increase in CD4$^+$ T cells after cessation of alcohol use,[67] whereas only a 15% increase was seen in uninfected controls who quit drinking. Such changes suggest that the potential direct (i.e., immunotoxic) actions of heavy alcohol use, as well as indirect ones due to undernutrition, by HIV-infected people result in a 30% to 40% decrease in CD4$^+$ T cells over a 4-year period.[67]

We documented the effects of alcohol consumption in murine AIDS.[68,69] Alcohol accentuated the loss of disease resistance due to retrovirus infection even when ethanol consumption had no effect on disease resistance in uninfected mice.[69,70] Thus alcohol acted as a cofactor, which was sufficient for accelerated development of murine AIDS. In our murine AIDS model, alcohol consumption exacerbated cytokine dysregulation,[68] increased immune dysfunction,[71] and further suppressed disease resistance to pathogens common in AIDS patients.[69,70] Although alcohol use in mice who did not have retroviral infection had some effects on cytokine production and immune dysfunction,[72] it was not sufficient to significantly suppress disease resistance to AIDS-associated pathogens.[73] Alcohol use before retroviral infection in mice was sufficient to accelerate development of severe murine retroviral immunosuppression.[74]

Oxidation causes DNA damage to lymphocytes, whereas supplementation with vitamin E, vitamin C, or beta-carotene greatly reduces the DNA damage in lymphocytes of both smokers and nonsmokers.[75] Serum antioxidants (e.g., α-tocopherol, retinol, beta-carotene, glutathione, selenium, zinc) in alcoholics decreased significantly. Since alcohol and retrovirus infection each induce losses in tissue antioxidants, they should promote greater DNA damage and dysfunction in lymphocytes when used together. Reduction of immunostimulatory antioxidants by alcohol abuse is accentuated by retrovirus infection. Micronutrient deficiencies should synergize with HIV immunosuppression to increase immune dysfunction and accelerate progression to AIDS.

MICRONUTRIENT DEFICIENCY AND PROGRESSION TO AIDS

Vitamin A

Progressively decreased serum vitamin A levels in HIV-infected patients are associated with increased M&M. Low levels among pregnant women with HIV are related to low birth weight (LBW), higher maternal and infant mortality, and increased mother-to-child transmission of HIV.[76,77] The biological mechanisms by which vitamin A deficiency could influence mother-to-child transmission of HIV-1 include impairment of immune responses in both mother and infant, abnormal placental and vaginal pathology, and increased HIV viral burden in breast milk and blood. A number of possible causes of low serum vitamin A levels exist, including (1) decreased dietary intake, (2) poor gastrointestinal (GI) absorption, (3) high urinary losses, (4) impaired hepatic protein synthesis, and (5) increased nutritional demands related to chronic infection.[78] Most dietary vitamin A is delivered to the liver and released into the blood to be used by peripheral tissues. The synthesis and release of serum carrier protein and RBP regulate this action. Thus impaired RBP synthesis or release may lead to low serum vitamin A levels despite adequate dietary vitamin A and adequate stores in the liver. However, serum vitamin A levels are also highly correlated with RBP in people who are not infected with HIV, suggesting that this correlation does not indicate impaired hepatic protein synthesis.[79]

HIV-infected patients are most concerned about whether vitamin A supplementation will increase survival and reduce mother-to-child transmission of HIV. HIV-infected patients taking supplemental vitamin A had significantly higher serum vitamin A levels and higher RBP levels than those not taking vitamin A. Moderately high intake of vitamin A slowed progression to AIDS.[80]

Serum beta-carotene concentration is deficient in all HIV-infected persons. The most likely mechanism for the beta-carotene deficiency is related to impairment of free radical (FR) elimination and failure to protect cellular membrane against lipid peroxidation (LP), including damage to CD4$^+$ T cells.[81] Consequently, beta-carotene deficiency, along with other antioxidant deficiencies, may contribute indirectly to the immunological deterioration seen in HIV infection by facilitating CD4$^+$ T-cell apoptosis.

Vitamin B$_6$

Vitamin B$_6$ plays a critical role in nucleic acid and protein metabolism; thus a deficiency significantly alters immune responses.[82] The prevalence of vitamin B$_6$ deficiency in HIV-infected patients ranges from 12% to 52%.[83] Vitamin B$_6$ deficiency also results in the impairment of both cell-mediated and humoral immune responses, including impaired IL-2 production and lymphocyte proliferation in response to mitogens in uninfected animals and people.[84] In HIV-infected persons vitamin B$_6$ causes delayed cutaneous hypersensitivity, depressed cell-mediated immune response, depressed lymphocyte proliferation, decreased CD4$^+$ T-cell counts, and reduced natural killer (NK) cell cytotoxicity.[83,85] Vitamin B$_6$ repletion with coenzyme Q$_{10}$ increases IgG, CD4$^+$ T cells, and the ratio of CD4$^+$/CD8$^+$ lymphocytes in uninfected older people and animals.[86] These increases may be clinically important to accelerate progression to AIDS, suggesting a role for vitamin B$_6$ supplementation in the treatment of nutritional immunodeficiency.

Vitamin B$_{12}$

A significant number of elderly and HIV-positive individuals are at increased risk of vitamin B$_{12}$ deficiency.[87] Decreased serum vitamin B$_{12}$ levels occur in up to 20% of patients with early-stage AIDS.[88] Development of vitamin B$_{12}$ deficiency is associated with a decline in CD4$^+$ T-cell counts and a number of neurological and neuropsychiatric disorders. Neurological damage caused by vitamin B$_{12}$ deficiency may be due to methyl group deficiency as a result of either the patient's inability to synthesize methionine and S-adenosyl-L-methionine (SAM) or the toxicity of homocysteine accumulation.[89] Low serum levels of haptocorrin in HIV-1-positive patients could also lead to the low levels of serum vitamin B_{12} frequently observed in this patient population. In some cases subnormal serum vitamin B_{12} levels adversely contribute to the hematological and neurological dysfunction attributed to HIV.[90] Decreased levels of vitamin B_{12} are also highly prevalent in HIV-infected patients with chronic diarrhea. Low serum vitamin B_{12} concentrations are more closely associated with faster HIV-1 disease progression and a decline in $CD4^+$ T-cell counts than are low vitamin B_6 concentrations.[91] Metabolic and clinical disturbances due to decreased serum vitamin B_{12} levels lowered hemoglobin, leukocytes, and the ratio of $CD4^+/CD8^+$ T-cell counts in HIV-infected patients compared to those in HIV-infected patients with normal serum vitamin B_{12} levels. Thus disease progression to AIDS may be predicted by the change in serum vitamin B_{12} levels and $CD4^+$ T-cell counts and might be slowed by vitamin B_{12} supplementation.

Vitamin E

Plasma concentration of vitamin E is less significantly decreased than that of vitamin A in HIV-infected patients. Vitamin E deficiency is found mostly in patients who have wasting syndrome.[92] Thus low plasma vitamin E levels could be related partly to dietary intake or absorption, suggesting that supplementation may be warranted in HIV-1-infected persons with a vitamin E deficiency. In contrast, circulating vitamin E levels decrease considerably in HIV-positive patients after progression to AIDS.[93] Vitamin E levels are four to five times higher in lymphoid cells than in other cells. Since vitamin E is an antioxidant of cell membranes and plasma lipoproteins, a deficiency of vitamin E is related to the increase of LP. Paradoxically, LP is more significant in asymptomatic HIV-negative patients than in AIDS patients.[94] In early HIV-1 infection, the elevation of plasma IgE levels precedes the decline of $CD4^+$ T-cell counts and is influenced by vitamin E status.[92] Recently HIV-infected people were shown conclusively to lose vitamin E as progression to AIDS occurred.[92] Supplementation with vitamin E slowed this process,[93] and an editorial called for more trials and supplementation of HIV-infected persons.[94] These conclusions are supported by animal model studies. In one animal model, C57BL/6 mice were infected with an LP-BM5 retrovirus causing murine AIDS. Extremely high levels of vitamin E supplementation significantly normalized the levels of IL-2, IL-6,

IL-10, IFN-γ, and TNF-α produced by a splenocyte.[95] Vitamin E supplementation at 15 to 450 times the normal intake for a mouse was not toxic during murine AIDS.[96] However, supplementation restored part of the immune deficits for a time, slowing death.[97] It restored tissue vitamin E and prevented oxidation. When the retrovirally infected mice were treated with a T-cell receptor (TCR) V_β peptide specifically for the retroviral antigen-activated T_H2 cells, their excessive secretion of IL-6 was largely prevented.[98] Maintaining immune function prevented the loss of vitamin E and vitamin A, as well as retrovirus-increase oxidation. Thus immune dysfunction and cytokine dysregulation are critical and necessary for the loss of antioxidants and oxidative damage due to murine retrovirus infection.

Retroviral infection in humans and mice has a profound dysfunctional effect on the regulation of autoantibodies to TCRs.[98] In C57BL/6 mice after murine virus (LP-BM5) infection, injection with human TCR V_β 8.1 CDR1 peptide largely prevented the retrovirus-induced reduction in B- and T-cell proliferation and T_H1 cytokines, including IL-2 and IFN-γ secretion.[99] It also suppressed the excessive T_H2 cytokine (e.g., IL-6 and IL-10) production that was stimulated by retrovirus infection.[100] Retrovirus infection in mice inhibits the release of T_H1 cytokines, stimulates the secretion of T_H2 cytokines, and induces hepatic and cardiac vitamin E deficiency with increased LP. Administration of TCR peptide with doses >100 µg/mouse for 2 to 4 weeks after retrovirus infection maintained production of IL-2 and prevented retrovirus-induced elevated production of IL-6 by splenocytes in vitro. It also ameliorated immune dysfunction and thus prevented increases in tissue LP and vitamin E loss. T-cell immune dysfunction and its prevention by TCR peptide treatment could be important in vitamin E deficiency therapy induced by retrovirus infection.[101] Immune dysfunction during retroviral infection is clearly associated with increased oxidation and loss of antioxidants.

Copper

The serum concentration of copper (Cu) decreases as a result of AZT treatment.[102] The variation is linked to the severity of the disease such as AIDS. However, abnormalities and the effect of supplementation in Cu are still less clearly identified than those in selenium and zinc. Several inhibitory effects of Cu were reported between HIV and its gene products, including HIV-1 integrase, protease, and nucleocapsid protein 7 (Ncp7).[103-105] HIV-1 integrase is required for the integration of a double-stranded DNA copy of the viral DNA genome into a host chromosome and for HIV replication. The enzyme for both integration and disintegration can be inhibited by 1,10-phenanthrolinecuprous complexes at low concentrations (IC$_{50}$ = 1-10 μm, 10-40 μm), although the uncomplexed phenanthrolines are not active below 100 μM.[103] Dialysis experiments and kinetic analyses showed that the inhibition is reversible and that the mode of inhibition by the cuprous complex is noncompetitive with respect to substrate DNA. The protease encoded by HIV-1 is also essential for processing viral polyproteins, which contain the enzymes and structural proteins required for the infectious virus.[104] Cupric chloride in the presence of dithiothreitol (DTT) or ascorbic acid could inhibit the HIV-1 protease. The stable Cu^{1+} (BCDS-Cu^{1+}) is responsible for inhibition of the HIV-1 protease. Inhibition of the HIV-1 protease and of HIV replication by BCDS-Cu^{1+} is dependent on the presence of Cu^{1+}, since bathocuproine disulfonic acid (BCDS) alone is ineffective, indicating that Cu^{1+} is the inhibitory agent. Transcription factor nuclear factor kappa B (NF-κB) regulates the expression of various cellular genes involved in immune responses and viral genes, including HIV.[105] NF-κB is inhibited by binding with protein inhibitor kappa B (I-κB) and by Cu^{2+}, which interferes with the dissociation of the NF-κB-I-κB complex. Cu^{2+} inhibits the release of NF-κB by blocking a signal leading to the phosphorylation of I-κB.

Magnesium

Patients with AIDS have a low serum magnesium (Mg) concentration.[106] Although the serum concentration of Mg normalized after supplementation, the amount of Mg supplementation required to maintain normal serum concentration suggests a persistent intracellular deficiency.[107] Many effects of Mg on HIV are mediated through the stabilization of other enzymes and compounds, including HIV-1 integrase and oltipraz (5-pyrazinyl-4-methyl-1,2-dithiole-3-thione), which is an HIV-1 replication inhibitor.[108] Mg ions, which are metal cofactors, are essentially required for 3'-donor processing activity of HIV-1 integrase in vitro, although the activity can be altered by the

length of nucleotides to which the integrase binds.[109] The relationship between HIV-1 Nef (a myristylated 206-amino-acid protein) and Mg ions was also studied.[110] Nef is normally a predominantly intracellular protein. The release of Nef leads elevated levels of Mg ions at an elevated temperature. However, the importance of Nef in the development of AIDS is unknown. Little evidence shows whether serum levels of Mg and HIV-infected patients have a positive or a negative correlation to each other. The serum concentration of Mg ions in HIV-infected patients was either normal or low without showing statistical significance.[111] Serum Mg values appeared to be independent from the stage of infection.

Manganese

Serum manganese (Mn) concentration was similar in asymptomatic HIV-negative individuals and in healthy controls but was significantly higher in those groups than in AIDS patients.[112] No differences in urinary Mn levels were observed between HIV-infected patients and controls. Researchers have examined the effect of Mn on specific HIV enzymes. HIV integrase protein mediates between two distinct reactions. One is 3'-donor processing activity that includes specific removal of two nucleotides from the 3' ends of the viral DNA. The other is strand transfer reaction that is identified as integration of the viral DNA into target DNA.[113] The integrase requires Mn ions for efficient in vitro activity.[114] In the presence of Mn ions, a stable complex of HIV integrase and viral DNA formed, although some findings suggest that Mg ions are more efficient in stabilizing the complex than Mn ions.[115] Thus the role of Mn ions is to stabilize the bound complexes or to augment DNA affinity of the HIV integrase. Mn ions are also required for ribonuclease H (RNase H) activity, hydrolysis of double-stranded RNA, and HIV-1 reverse transcriptase (RT).[116] RNase H activity depends on the presence of Mn ions rather than Mg ions.

Selenium

Selenium (Se) is an essential biological trace element required for human and animal growth, but higher concentrations have toxic effects.[117] Its deficiency is associated with glutathione peroxidase (GPX) activity, cardiomyopathy, carcinogenesis, and immune dysfunction, including impaired phagocytic function, decreased $CD4^+$ T cells, and AIDS.[118-120] Epidemiological studies indicate a correlation between low plasma Se concentrations and HIV-positive patients, as well as increased risks of AIDS-related pathology.[121] AIDS patients tend to have more severe deficits than those at earlier stages of HIV infection. The Se deficit in AIDS-positive patients may be caused by decreased caloric and protein intake, malabsorption, or various viral and bacterial infections.[122] AIDS patients often experience malabsorption due to intestinal infections related to *Cryptosporidium, Microsporidum, Cytomegalovirus, Mycobacterium avium,* or Kaposi's sarcoma (KS). Malabsorption may even occur without an identified pathogen, and HIV may directly injure the small intestine.[123] Thus poor dietary intake and malabsorption could lead to an Se deficit that has important implications for immune functions in HIV-positive patients.

Low plasma Se concentrations have a negative effect on HIV-positive patients by decreasing plasma cysteine, T-cell glutathione, and plasma vitamin A.[124] They also have an increase in malondialdehyde (MDA), an end product of LP, and reduced homocysteine, a prooxidant substance.[125] An Se deficiency may result in decreased efficacy of GPX, a major antioxidant system. Because FRs are able to stimulate HIV replication and $CD4^+$ T-cell apoptosis, a decreased Se concentration should result in increased oxidative stress, HIV replication, and accelerated $CD4^+$ T-cell death.[126] This concept is supported by selenoproteins discovered in mammalian cells, suggesting Se's essentiality in the body's antioxidant defense and immune system function.[127] GPX activity and reduced glutathione (GSH) values increase after Se supplementation. Because GPX and GSH play an important role in the natural enzymatic defense system by detoxifying hydrogen peroxide (H_2O_2) in water, Se supplementation could be of great interest in protecting cells against oxidative stress. Se deficiency is a mechanism of AIDS-associated congestive cardiomyopathy. In a recent study, a 5-year-old boy with AIDS and cardiomyopathy had a low plasma Se level (29 μg/ml), and his cardiac status improved with Se supplementation.[128] Thus Se causes symptomatic improvements and possibly slows the course of the disease. Since Se inhibits RT activity in RNA virus-infected animals, supplemental Se could also prevent the replication of HIV and retard the development of AIDS in newly HIV-infected subjects.[128] A 100 μg/day Se dosage is sufficient to restore normal plasma concentrations, improve oxidative stress, and decrease $\beta_2$microglobulin, which is a marker of immune activation and a poor prognosis in HIV infection.[126,129] An adequate supply of Se and antioxidant vitamins is also proposed as a measure to reduce the probability of the placental transmission of HIV in pregnancy. However, the potential effects of Se on HIV viral load and the benefit of Se supplementation have not been clearly established. HIV may carry several genes to encode selenoproteins, and one of these proteins may bind with DNA, repressing HIV virus transcription. This mechanism results in turning off the HIV expression, thus slowing the virus proliferation.[128]

Zinc

Zinc (Zn) is one of the most important trace elements for immune function. Congenital or acquired Zn deficiencies are associated with immune dysfunction and increased susceptibility to infectious diseases. A number of immunological abnormalities in HIV-1 infection are observed in both experimental animals and humans with Zn deficiency, which is more severe in stage IV than in stage III of HIV progression.[130] A close correlation between an immune response evaluated by a proliferative response to T-cell mitogens and serum Zn levels was reported in HIV-positive patients.[131] The precise mechanism for Zn-dependent immunodeficiency in T cells is not clear.[132] However, HIV does not replicate in T_H1 cells, which probably contain more Zn, but it replicates preferentially in T_H0 and T_H2 cells because Zn ions inhibit intracellular HIV replication.[133] Researchers have postulated several mechanisms of Zn, and one is probably on lymphocyte proliferation.[134] Zn activates B cells to secrete immunoglobulins and also interacts synergistically with their activators to enhance the activation and differentiation process in vitro.[135] The plasmatic Zn deficiency in AIDS patients also correlates with a decrease in $CD4^+$ T-cell counts, NK cell lytic activity, and thymic hormone activity.[130] Subjects who progressed to AIDS had significantly lower Zn levels than nonprogressors.[136] Supplementation with Zn increased BW stabilization, $CD4^+$ T cells, and the plasma level of active Zn-bound thymulin.[131] Moreover, the frequency of OIs following Zn supplementation was reduced, although its effect was restricted to infections caused by *Pneumocystis carinii* and *Candida*.[130] An increase in the lymphocyte response to mitogens occurs in asymptomatic patients treated by 125 mg of Zn for 3 weeks.[136] Another epidemiological study suggested that the intake of Zn supplements was associated with a lower survival rate (relative hazard [RH] = 1.49, 95% CI 1.02 to 2.18) than that of other micronutrients, such as the B vitamins.[137] In this study, the intakes of most B vitamin supplements were more than five times the recommended dietary allowance. However, the optimal level of Zn intake in HIV-1-infected individuals was not determined.

SUMMARY

Wasting syndrome is one of the early manifestations of the onset of symptomatic AIDS. Because the magnitude of weight loss relates directly to the risk of death, it is critically important to treat HIV-associated wasting to maintain BCM, which is the marker that best characterizes the degree of wasting in patients infected with HIV. Wasting is caused by many factors. Inadequate energy intake can stem from anorexia or malnutrition caused by physical impediments to food ingestion, loss of appetite, and intestinal infections. Cytokine imbalance may also induce wasting. In addition, social behaviors, such as heavy smoking and alcohol and drug abuse, are other influences that induce wasting in HIV-infected patients. Clinical trials therefore should consider all these factors before evaluating the association between wasting and progression to AIDS.

The conclusion from studies of a number of micronutrients in both HIV-infected people and retrovirus-infected animals is that nutritional immunodeficiency develops and promotes progression to AIDS. As an adjunct therapy, micronutrient supplementation has beneficial effects on HIV-infected patients by slowing the progression to AIDS. However, the therapeutic threshold of each supplemental micronutrient needs to be defined.

Recently steroids and GH are gaining recognition in the treatment of AIDS, although some potential side effects are anticipated. GH is not required for normal lymphoid development. However, under certain stressful situations in the treatment of AIDS patients, it stimulates lymphoid proliferation and amplifies other physiological signals to lymphoid expansion. By monitoring an in vivo assessment of immune functions and potential side effects, a large-scale and carefully designed AIDS clinical trial may define a role for GH in the generation of CD4$^+$ T cells and the increase of BW that would provide a better QOL for AIDS patients.

References

1. Pacht ER, Diaz P, Clanton T, et al: Serum vitamin E decreases in HIV-positive subjects over time, *J Lab Clin Med* 130:293-296, 1997.
2. Tang AM, Graham NMH, Semba RD, et al: Association between serum vitamin A and E levels and HIV-1 progression, *AIDS* 11:613-620, 1997.
3. Miguez-Burbano MJ, Shor-Posner G, Fletcher MA, et al: Immunoglobulin E levels in relationship to HIV-1 disease, route of infection, and vitamin E status, *Allergy* 50:157-161, 1995.
4. Watson RR: *Nutrients, foods for AIDS*, ed 1, Boca Raton, Fla, 1997, CRC Press.
5. Melchior JC, Raguin G, Boulier A, et al: Resting energy expenditure in human immunodeficiency virus-infected patients: comparison between patients with and without secondary infections, *Am J Clin Nutr* 57:614-619, 1993.
6. Heijligenberg R, Romijn JA, Westerterp KR, et al: Total energy expenditure in human immunodeficiency virus-infected men and healthy controls, *Metabolism* 46:1324-1326, 1997.
7. Paton NI, Elia M, Jebb SA, et al: Total energy expenditure and physical activity measured with the bicarbonate-urea method in patients with human immunodeficiency virus infection, *Clin Sci* 91:241-245, 1996.
8. Grunfeld C, Pang M, Shimizu L, et al: Resting energy expenditure, caloric intake, and short-term weight change in human immunodeficiency virus infection and acquired immunodeficiency syndrome, *Am J Clin Nutr* 55:455-460, 1992.
9. Melchior JC, Salmon D, Rigaud D, et al: Resting energy expenditure is increased in stable, malnourished HIV-infected patients, *Am J Clin Nutr* 53:437-441, 1991.
10. McCallan DC, Noble C, Baldwin C, et al: Energy expenditure and weight loss in HIV infection, *Int Conf AIDS* 1993.
11. Hellerstein MK, Kahn J, Mudie H, et al: Current approach to the treatment of human immunodeficiency virus-associated weight loss: pathophysiologic considerations and emerging management strategies, *Semin Oncol* 17(6 suppl 9):17-33, 1990.
12. Hommes MJT, Romijn JA, Endert E, et al: Resting energy expenditure and substrate oxidation in human immunodeficiency virus-infected asymptomatic man: HIV affects host metabolism in the early asymptomatic stage, *Am J Clin Nutr* 54:311-315, 1991.
13. Hommes MJT, Romijn JA, Godfried MH, et al: Increased resting energy expenditure in human immunodeficiency virus-infected men, *Metabolism* 39:1186-1190, 1990.

14. Romijn JA, Klein S: One more reason for weight loss in patients with AIDS, *Gastroenterology* 101:861-862, 1991.

15. Kotler DP, Tierney AR, Brenner SK, et al: Preservation of short-term energy balance in clinically stable patients with AIDS, *Am J Clin Nutr* 51:7-13, 1990.

16. Kotler DP, Tierney AR, Wang J, et al: Magnitude of body-cell-mass depletion and the timing of death from wasting in AIDS, *Am J Clin Nutr* 50:444-447, 1989.

17. Weinroth SE, Parenti DM, Simon GL: Wasting syndrome in AIDS: pathophysiologic mechanisms and therapeutic approaches, *Infect Agents Dis* 4:76-94, 1995.

18. Ysseldyke LL: Nutritional complications and incidence of malnutrition among AIDS patients, *J Am Diet Assoc* 91:217-218, 1991.

19. Framm SR, Soave R: Agents of diarrhea, *Med Clin North Am* 81:427-447, 1997.

20. Kapembwa MS, Bridges C, Joseph AEA, et al: Ileal and jejunal absorptive function in patients with AIDS and enterococcidial infection, *J Infect* 21:43-53, 1990.

21. Kapembwa MS, Fleming SC, Griffin GE, et al: Fat absorption and exocrine pancreatic function in human immunodeficiency virus infection, *QJM* 273:49-56, 1990.

22. Zeitz M, Ullrich R, Heise W, et al: Malabsorption is found in early stages of HIV infection and independent of secondary infections, *Proc Int Conf AIDS* 1990.

23. Lim SG, Menzies IS, Lee CA, et al: Small intestinal permeability in HIV-positive patients, *Proc Int Conf AIDS* 1990.

24. Stein TP, Nutinsky C, Condoluci D, et al: Protein and energy substrate metabolism in AIDS patients, *Metabolism* 39:876-881, 1990.

25. Lake-Bakaar G, Quadros E, Beidas S, et al: Gastric secretory failure in patients with acquired immunodeficiency syndrome, *Ann Intern Med* 109:502-504, 1988.

26. Lake-Bakaar G: AIDS gastropathy prevalence and progression: an update, *Gastroenterology* 100:A592, 1991.

27. Russell RM, Krasinski SD, Samloff IM, et al: Folic acid malabsorption in atrophic gastritis: possible compensation by bacterial folate synthesis, *Gastroenterology* 91:1476-1482, 1986.

28. Qin ZH, Krugerkrasagakes S, Kunzendorf U, et al: Expression of TNF by different tumor-cell lines results either in tumor suppression or augmented metastasis, *J Exp Med* 178:355-360, 1993.

29. Vaisman N, Schattner A, Hahn T: Tumor necrosis factor production during starvation, *Am J Med* 87:115-124, 1989.

30. Liang B, Zhang Z, Araghiniknam M, et al: Prevention of retrovirus-induced aberrant cytokine secretion, excessive lipid peroxidation, and tissue vitamin E deficiency by T-cell receptor peptide treatment in C57BL/6 mice, *Proc Soc Exp Biol Med* 14:87-94, 1997.

31. Grunfeld C, Kotler DP: Wasting in acquired immunodeficiency syndrome, *Semin Liver Dis* 12:175-187, 1992.

32. Grunfeld C, Kotler DP, Hamadeh R, et al: Hypertriglyceridemia in acquired immunodeficiency syndrome, *Am J Med* 86:27-31, 1989.

33. Grunfeld C, Kotler DP, Kwan-Shigenaga J, et al: Circulating interferon-α levels and hypertriglyceridemia in acquired immunodeficiency syndrome, *Am J Med* 90:154-162, 1991.

34. Farrar WL, Korner M, Clouse KA: Cytokine regulation of human immunodeficiency virus expression, *Cytokine* 3:531-542, 1991.

35. Hess G, Rossol R: Tumor necrosis factor and interferon as prognostic markers in human immunodeficiency virus infection, *Infection* 19:S93-97, 1991.

36. Godfried MH, Vander-Pall T, Jansen J, et al: Soluble receptors for tumor necrosis factor: a putative measure of disease progression in HIV infection, *AIDS* 7:33-36, 1993.

37. Longo N, Zabay JM, Sempere JM, et al: Altered production of PGE$_2$, IL-1β, and TNF-α by peripheral blood monocytes from HIV-positive individuals at early stages of HIV infection, *J Acquir Immune Defic Syndr Hum Retrovirol* 6:1017-1023, 1993.

38. Grunfeld C, Pang M, Doerrier W, et al: Lipids, lipoproteins, triglyceride clearance, and cytokines in human immunodeficiency virus infection and acquired immune deficiency syndrome, *J Clin Endocrinol Metab* 74:1045-1032, 1991.

39. Jones PD, Shelley L, Wakefield D: Tumor necrosis factor-α in advanced HIV infection in the absence of AIDS-related secondary infections, *J Acquir Immune Defic Syndr Hum Retrovirol* 5:1266-1271, 1992.

40. Chen GJ, Watson RR: Modulation of tumor necrosis factor and gamma interferon production by cocaine and morphine in aging mice infected with LP-BM5, a murine retrovirus, *J Leukoc Biol* 50:349-355, 1991.

41. Dworkin BM, Seaton T, Wormser G: The role of tumor necrosis factor and altered metabolic rate in weight loss in AIDS, *Int Conf AIDS* 6:218-226, 1990.

42. Grunfeld C, Feingold KR: Metabolic disturbances and wasting in acquired immunodeficiency syndrome, *New Engl J Med* 327:329-337, 1992.

43. Tracey KJ, Morgello S, Koplin B, et al: Metabolic effects of cachectin/tumor necrosis factor are modified by site of production, *J Clin Invest* 86:2014-2024, 1990.

44. Coodley GO, Loveless MO, Nelson HD, et al: Endocrine dysfunction in HIV wasting syndrome, *J Acquir Immune Defic Syndr Hum Retrovirol* 7:46-51, 1994.

45. LoPresti JS, Fried JC, Spencer CA, et al: Unique alterations of thyroid hormone indices in acquired immunodeficiency syndrome, *Ann Intern Med* 110:970-975, 1989.

46. Ozawa M, Sato K, Han CD, et al: Effects of tumor necrosis factor-alpha/cachectin on thyroid hormone metabolism in mice, *Endocrinology* 123:1461-1467, 1988.

47. Piedrola G, Casado JL, Lopez E, et al: Clinical features of adrenal insufficiency in patients with acquired immunodeficiency syndrome, *Clin Endocrinol* 45:97-101, 1996.

48. Abbott M, Khoo SH, Wilkins EGL, et al: Adrenocortical deficiency: common in late HIV, *Int Conf AIDS* 1993.

49. Centurelli MA, Abate MA: The role of dehydroepiandrosterone in AIDS, *Ann Pharmacother* 31:639-642, 1997.

50. Araghiniknam M, Liang B, Watson RR, et al: Modulation of immune dysfunction during murine leukemia retrovirus infection of old mice by DHEAS, *Immunology* 90:344-349, 1997.

51. Grinspoon S, Corcoran C, Lee K, et al: Loss of lean body and muscle mass correlates with androgen levels in hypogonadal men with AIDS and wasting, *J Clin Endocrinol* 81:4051-4058, 1996.

52. Gold J, High HA, Li Y, et al: Safety and efficacy of nandrolone decanoate for treatment of wasting in patients with HIV infection, *AIDS* 10:745-752, 1996.

53. Dobs AS: Is there a role for androgenic anabolic steroids in medical practice? *JAMA* 281:1326-1327, 1999.

54. Frost RA, Fuhrer J, Steigbigel R, et al: Wasting in AIDS is associated with multiple defects in the serum insulin-like growth factor system, *Clin Endocrinol* 44:501-514, 1996.

55. Torres-Anjel MJ, Volz D, Torres MJR, et al: Failure to thrive, wasting syndrome, and immunodeficiency in rabies: a hypophyseal/hypothalamic/thymic axis effect of rabies virus, *Rev Infect Dis* 10: S710-725, 1988.

56. Schambelan M, Mulligan K, Grunfeld C, et al: Serostim study group, recombinant human growth hormone in patients with HIV-associated wasting: a randomized, placebo-controlled trial, *Ann Intern Med* 125:873-882, 1996.

57. Mulligan K, Grunfeld C, Hellerstein MK, et al: Anabolic effects of recombinant human growth hormone in patients with wasting associated with human AIDS virus infection, *J Clin Endocrinol Metab* 77:956-962, 1993.

58. Murphy WJ: Role of neuroendocrine hormones in murine T-cell development; growth hormone exerts thymopoietic effects in vivo, *J Immunol* 149:3851-3857, 1992.

59. Tedla N, Dwyer J, Truskett P, et al: Phenotypic and functional characterization of lymphocytes derived from normal and HIV-1-infected human lymph nodes, *Clin Exp Immunol* 117:92-99, 1999.

60. Murphy WJ, Longo DL: Growth hormone as an immunomodulating therapeutic agent, *Immunol Today* 21:211-213, 2000.

61. Abbaticola M, Fisher A: Effects of recombinant human growth hormone and aggressive nutrition support on body weight in HIV infection and concurrent opportunistic infection, Abstract presented at Fourth International Conference on Nutrition and HIV Infection, Cannes, France, 1997.

62. Chad DA, Smith TW, Blumenfeld A, et al: HIV-associated myopathy: immunocytochemical identification of an HIV antigen (gp 41) in muscle macrophages, *Ann Neurol* 28:579-582, 1990.

63. Simpson DM, Bender AN, Farraye J, et al: Human immunodeficiency virus wasting syndrome may represent a treatable myopathy, *Neurology* 40:535-538, 1990.

64. Penkower L, Dew MA, Kingley L, et al: Alcohol consumption as a cofactor in the progression of HIV infection and AIDS, *Alcohol* 12:547-552, 1995.

65. Watson RR, Wang JY, Dehghanpisheh K, et al: T-cell receptor V beta complementarity determining region-1 peptide administration moderates immune dysfunction and cytokine dysregulation induced by murine retrovirus infection, *J Immunol* 155:2282-2291, 1995.

66. Lake-Bakaar G, Grimson R: Alcohol abuse and stage of HIV disease in intravenous drug abusers, *J R Soc Med* 89:389-392, 1996.

67. Pol S, Artu P, Berthelot P, et al: Improvement of the CD4 cell count after alcohol withdrawal in HIV-positive patients, *AIDS* 10:1293-1294, 1996.

68. Wang Y, Huang DS, Watson RR, et al: Ethanol-induced modulation of cytokine production by splenocytes during murine retrovirus infection causing murine AIDS, *Alcohol Clin Exp Res* 17:1035-1039, 1993.

69. Darban H, Watson RR, Darban J, et al: Modification of resistance to *Streptococcus pneumoniae* by dietary ethanol, immunization, and murine retroviral infection, *Alcohol Clin Exp Res* 16:844-851, 1992.

70. Shahbazian M, Huang D, Watson RR, et al: Alcohol and suppression of resistance to *Cryptosporidium parvum* infection during modulation of cytokine production murine-acquired immune deficiency syndrome, *Alcohol Clin Exp Res* 17:539-544, 1993.

71. Watson RR, Odeleye OE, Darban HR, et al: Modification of lymphoid subsets by chronic consumption of alcohol in C57BL/6 mice infected with LP-BM5 murine leukemia virus, *Alcohol* 27:417-424, 1992.

72. Shahbazian M, Stazzone A, Watson RR, et al: Effect of thymosin fraction 5 on immune response of C57BL/6 mice fed ethanol diet and challenged with *Streptococcus pneumoniae*, *Adv Biophys* 86:353-358, 1993.

73. Wang Y, Huang DS, Watson RR, et al: Influence of chronic dietary ethanol on cytokine production by murine splenocytes and thymocytes, *Alcohol Clin Exp Res* 18:64-70, 1994.

74. Wang Y, Watson RR: Chronic ethanol consumption before retrovirus infection alters cytokine production by thymocytes during murine AIDS, *Alcohol* 11:361-365, 1994.

75. Duthie SJ, Ma A, Ross MA, et al: Antioxidant supplementation decreases oxidative DNA damage in human lymphocytes, *Cancer Res* 56:1291-1295, 1995.

76. Semba RD: Overview of the potential role of vitamin A in mother-to-child transmission of HIV-1, *Acta Paediatr* 421:S107-112, 1997.

77. Greenberg BL, Semba RD, Vink PE, et al: Vitamin A deficiency and maternal-infant transmissions of HIV in two metropolitan areas in the United States, *AIDS* 11:325-332, 1997.

78. Hussey GD, Klein M: A randomized, controlled trial of vitamin A in children with severe measles, *New Engl J Med* 323:160-164, 1990.

79. Wolde-Gabriel Z, West CE, Gebru H: Interrelationship between vitamin A, iodine, and iron status in school-children in Shoa Region, central Ethiopia, *Br J Nutr* 70:593-607, 1993.

80. Tang AM, Graham NMH, Kirby AJ: Dietary micronutrient intake and risk of progression to acquired immunodeficiency syndrome (AIDS) in human immunodeficiency virus type 1 (HIV-1)-infected homosexual men, *Am J Epidemiol* 138:938-951, 1993.

81. Rousseau E, Davison AJ, Dunn B: Protection by beta-carotene and related compounds against oxygen mediated cytotoxicity and genotoxicity, *Free Radic Biol Med* 12:407-433, 1992.

82. Chandra RK: *Nutrition, immunity and infection: mechanisms of interactions,* ed 1, New York, 1977, Plenum.

83. Herzlich BC, Schiano TD: Reversal of apparent AIDS dementia-complex following treatment with vitamin B, *J Intern Med* 233:495-497, 1993.

84. Rule SAJ, Hooker M, Costello C, et al: Serum vitamin B_{12} and transcobalamine levels in early HIV disease, *Am J Hematol* 47:167-171, 1994.

85. Grimble RF: Effects of antioxidative vitamins on immune function with clinical applications, *Int J Vitam Nutr Res* 67:312-320, 1997.

86. Trakatellis A, Dimitiadou A, Exindari M, et al: Effect of pyridoxine deficiency on immunological phenomena, *Postgrad Med J* 68:S70-77, 1992.

87. Markle HV: Cobalamin, *Crit Rev Clin Lab Sci* 33:247-356, 1996.

88. Meydani SN, Meydani M, Blumberg JB: Antioxidants and the aging immune response, *Adv Exp Med Biol* 262:57-67, 1990.

89. Herbert V: Vitamin B_{12} deficiency neuropsychiatric damage in AIDS, *Arch Neurol* 50:569-576, 1993.

90. Meydani SN, Meydani M, Verdon CP: Vitamin E supplementation suppresses prostaglandin E2 synthesis and enhances the immune response in aged mice, *Mech Ageing Dev* 34:191-198, 1986.

91. Tang AM, Graham NM, Chandra RK, et al: Low serum vitamin B_{12} concentrations are associated with faster human immunodeficiency virus type-1 disease progression, *J Nutr* 127:345-351, 1997.

92. Coodley GO: Micronutrient concentrations in the HIV wasting syndrome, *AIDS* 7:1595-1600, 1993.

93. Malvy DJM: Relationship of plasma malondialdehyde, vitamin E, and antioxidant micronutrients to human immunodeficiency virus-1 seropositivity, *Clin Chim Acta* 224:89-94, 1994.

94. Favier A: Antioxidant status and lipid peroxidation in patients infected with HIV, *Chem Biol Interact* 91:165-180, 1994.

95. Wang Y, Huang DS, Watson RR, et al: Modulation of immune function and cytokine production by various levels of vitamin E supplementation during murine AIDS, *Immunopharmacology* 29:225-233, 1995.

96. Wang Y, Liang B, Watson RR: Normalization of nutritional status by various levels of vitamin E supplementation during retrovirus infection causing murine AIDS, *Nutr Res* 14:1375-1386, 1994.

97. Wang Y, Huang DS, Watson RR, et al: Nutritional status and immune responses in mice with murine AIDS are normalized by vitamin E supplementation, *J Nutr* 124:2024-2032, 1994.

98. Marchalonis JJ, Lake DF, Watson RR, et al: Autoantibodies against peptide-defined epitopes of T-cell receptors in retrovirally infected humans and mice, *Adv Exp Med Biol* 383:211-222, 1995.

99. Liang B, Ardestani S, Watson RR, et al: T-cell receptor dose and the time of treatment during murine retrovirus infection for maintenance of immune function, *Immunology* 87:198-204, 1996.

100. Watson RR, Wang JY, Dehghanpisheh K, et al: T-cell receptor V beta complementarity-determining region-1 peptide administration moderates immune dysfunction and cytokine dysregulation induced by urine retrovirus infection, *J Immunol* 155:2282-2291, 1995.

101. Liang B, Eskelson C, Watson RR, et al: Vitamin E deficiency and immune dysfunction in retrovirus-infected C57BL/6 mice are prevented by T-cell receptor peptide treatment, *J Nutr* 126:1389-1397, 1996.

102. Baum MK: Aidovudine-associated adverse reactions in a longitudinal study of asymptomatic HIV-1-infected homosexual males, *J Acquir Immune Defic Syndr Hum Retrovirol* 4:1218-1226, 1991.

103. Mazumder A, Gupta M, Perrin DM, et al: Inhibition of human immunodeficiency virus type-1 integrase by a hydrophobic action: the phenanthroline-cuprous complex, *AIDS Res Hum Retroviruses* 11:115-125, 1995.

104. Davis DA, Branca AA, Pallenberg AJ, et al: Inhibition of the human immunodeficiency virus-1 protease and human immunodeficiency virus-1 replication by bathocuproine disulfonic acid Cu^{+1}, *Arch Biochem Biophys* 322:127-134, 1995.

105. Satake H, Suzuki K, Aoki T, et al: Cupricion blocks NF kappa B activation through inhibiting the signal-induced phosphorylation of I kappa B alpha, *Biochem Biophys Res Commun* 216:568-573, 1995.

106. Olree K, Stein-Gocken J: Elevated magnesium and calcium requirements associated with intravenous pentamidine, *Nutr Clin Pract* 9:191-195, 1994.

107. Dubey A, Solomon R: Magnesium, myocardinal ischemia, and arrhythmias: the role of magnesium in myocardial infarction, *Drugs* 37:1-7, 1989.

108. Chavan SJ, Bornmann WG, Prochaska HJ, et al: In-activation of human immunodeficiency virus type-1 reverse transcriptase by oltipraz: evidence for the formation of a stable adduct, *Arch Biochem Biophys* 324:143-152, 1995.

109. Lee SP, Kim HG, Censullo ML, et al: Characterization of Mg^{2+}-dependent 3'-processing activity for human immunodeficiency virus type-1 integrase in vitro: real-time kinetic studies using fluorescence resonance energy transfer, *Biochemistry* 34:10205-10214, 1995.

110. Macreadie IG, Castelli LA, Lucantoni A, et al: Stress- and sequence-dependent release into the culture medium of HIV-1 Nef produced in *Saccharomyces cerevisiae, Gene* 162:239-243, 1995.

111. Bogden JD: Micronutrient status and human immunodeficiency virus (HIV) infection, *Ann N Y Acad Sci* 587:189-195, 1990.

112. Schuhmacher M: Trace elements in patients with HIV-1 infection, *Trace Element Med* 11:130-137, 1994.

113. Vink C, Lutzke RA, Plasterk RH: Formation of a stable complex between the human immunodeficiency virus, integrase protein, and viral DNA, *Nucleic Acids Res* 22:4103-4110, 1994.

114. Engelman A, Craigie R: Efficient magnesium-dependent human immunodeficiency virus type-1 integrase activity, *J Virol* 69:5908-5911, 1995.

115. Huang L, Kim Y, Turch JJ, et al: Structure-specific cleavage of the RNA primer from Okazaki fragments by calf thymus RNase H, *J Biol Chem* 269:25922-25927, 1994.

116. Cirino NM, Cameron CE, Smith JS, et al: Divalent cation modulation of the ribonuclease functions of human immunodeficiency virus reverse transcriptase, *Biochemistry* 34:9936-9943, 1995.

117. Shamberger RJ: Selenium metabolism and function, *Clin Physiol* 4:42-50, 1986.

118. Sappey C, Legrand-Poels S, Best-Belpomme M, et al: Stimulation of glutathione peroxidase activity decreases HIV type-1 activation after oxidative stress, *AIDS Res Hum Retroviruses* 10:1451-1461, 1994.

119. Dworkin BM: Selenium deficiency in HIV infection and AIDS, *Chem Biol Interact* 91:181-186, 1994.

120. Badmaev V, Majeed M, Passwater RA: Selenium: a quest for better understanding, *Altern Ther Health Med* 2:59-62, 65-67, 1996.

121. Cirelli A, Ciardui M, Simone-De C: Serum selenium concentration and disease progress in patients with HIV infection, *Clin Biochem* 24:211-214, 1991.

122. Sammalkorpi K, Valtonen V, Alfthon G, et al: Serum selenium in acute infection, *Infection* 16:222-224, 1988.

123. Ullrich R, Zeitz M, Heise W: Small intestinal structure and function in patients infected with HIV: evidence for HIV-induced enteropathy, *Ann Intern Med* 111:15-21, 1989.

124. Semba RD, Graham NH, Caiffa WT: Increased mortality associated with vitamin A deficiency during HIV type-1 infection, *Arch Intern Med* 153:2153-2154, 1993.

125. Muller F, Svardal A, Ankronst P, et al: Elevated plasma concentration of reduced homocystein in patients with HIV infection, *Am J Clin Nutr* 63:242-248, 1996.

126. Schrauzer GN, Sacher J: Selenium in the maintenance and therapy of HIV-infected patients, *Chem Biol Interact* 91:199-205, 1994.

127. Kavanaugh-McHugh AL, Ruff A, Perlman A: Selenium deficiency and cardiomyopathy in AIDS, *JPEN* 13:347-349, 1991.

128. Taylor EW, Ramanathan CS, Jalluri RK, et al: A basis for new approaches to the chemotherapy of AIDS: novel genes in HIV-1 potentially encode selenoproteins expressed by ribosomal frameshifting and termination suppression, *J Med Chem* 37:2637-2654, 1994.

129. Hori K, Hatfield D, Lee BJ, et al: Selenium supplementation suppresses tumor necrosis factor alpha-induced HIV-1 replication in vitro, *AIDS Res Hum Retroviruses* 13:1325-1332, 1997.

130. Mocchegiani E, Veccia S, Ancarani F, et al: Benefit of oral zinc supplementation as an adjunct to zidovudine (AZT) therapy against opportunistic infections in AIDS, *Int J Immunopharm* 17:719-727, 1995.

131. Baum MK: Zidovudine-associated adverse reactions in a longitudinal study of asymptomatic HIV-1-infected homosexual males, *J Acquir Immune Defic Syndr Hum Retrovirol* 4:1218-1226, 1991.

132. Prasad AS: *Marginal deficiency of zinc and immunological effects, in essential and toxic trace elements in human health and disease,* ed 1, New York, 1993, Wiley-Liss.

133. Sprietsma JE: Zinc-controlled T_H1/T_H2 switch significantly determines development of diseases, *Med Hypotheses* 49:1-14, 1997.

134. Cunningham-Rundles S: Physiological and pharmacological effects of zinc on immune response, *Ann N Y Acad Sci* 587:113-122, 1990.

135. Graham NM: Relationship of copper and zinc levels to HIV-1 seropositivity and progression to AIDS, *J Acquir Immune Defic Syndr Hum Retrovirol* 4:976, 1991.

136. Zazzo JF: Effect of zinc on immune status of zinc-depleted ARC patients, *Clin Nutr* 8:259-267, 1989.

137. Tang AM, Graham NM, Saah AJ: Effects of micronutrient intake on survival in human immunodeficiency virus type-1 infection, *Am J Epidemiol* 143:1244-1256, 1996.

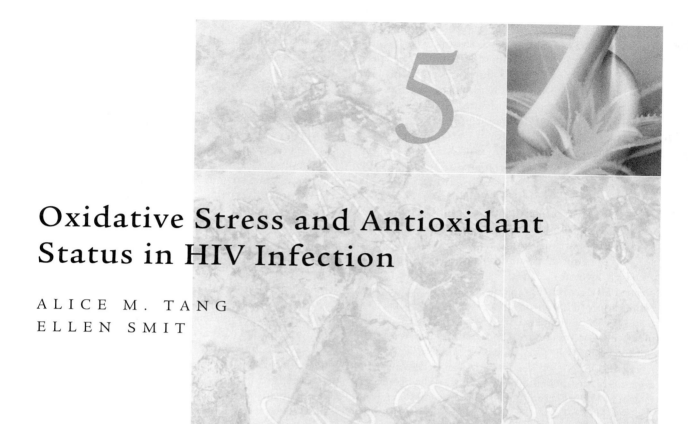

Oxidative Stress and Antioxidant Status in HIV Infection

ALICE M. TANG
ELLEN SMIT

OXIDATIVE STRESS

Oxidative stress is defined as a disturbance in the equilibrium status of prooxidant and antioxidant systems of intact cells.[1] Under normal conditions, cells have intact systems that continuously generate and detoxify oxidants. In the presence of excess oxidative events, the prooxidant systems may overwhelm the antioxidants, leading to oxidative damage of lipids, proteins, carbohydrates, and nucleic acids. Several highly unstable molecular species are involved in oxidative stress. These include (1) reactive radicals of oxygen (e.g., superoxide anion and hydroxyl radicals); (2) reactive nonradical oxygen species (e.g., hydrogen peroxide [H_2O_2] and diatomic oxygen [O_2]); and (3) radicals of carbon, nitrogen, and sulfur. Cellular and plasma antioxidant defenses include (1) enzymes that detoxify oxidants (e.g., superoxide dismutase [SOD], catalase, glutathione peroxidase [GPX], and reductase); (2) glutathione (GSH) and reactive protein sulfhydryls; (3) vitamins C and E; (4) carotenoids; and (5) uric acid.[2,1] The most effective antioxidant to combat the excessive production of reactive oxygen species (ROS) depends on the specific molecules causing the stress and the cellular or extracellular location of the molecular sources.

Mechanisms of Oxidative Stress in HIV Infection

Oxidative stress is hypothesized to contribute to HIV disease progression. However, it is unclear whether the excess ROS produced in HIV infection is a benign side effect of disease progression, or whether it contributes to the pathogenesis of the disease. Prooxidants are normally produced as a result of phagocytic activity and cellular respiration.[3,4] In HIV infection, oxidative stress may be caused by both overproduction of ROS and a simultaneous deficiency of antioxidant defenses.[5] Sources of excess free radical (FR) production in HIV infection include high levels of antigenic stimulation and cytokine activity. Prooxidant activity causes macrophages and monocytes to produce tumor necrosis factor alpha (TNF-α). TNF-α production may lead to further increases in oxidative stress through activation of T-cell respiratory activity and further stimulation of macrophages and neutrophils.[5] Other sources of ROS include the products of lipid peroxidation (LP), immune responses to opportunistic infections (OIs) and cofactors such as concomitant mycoplasma infection.

High levels of oxidative stress may lead to increased HIV replication.[6] Oxygen radicals can induce expression of HIV through activation of a transcription factor, nuclear factor kappa B (NF-κB). When inactive, NF-κB is bound in the cytoplasm to factor inhibitor kappa B (I-κB). When stimulated with a variety of ROS, NF-κB becomes dissociated from I-κB and enters the nucleus, where it binds to the promoter region of the HIV long terminal repeat (LTR) region. This leads to increased transcription of HIV ribonucleic acid (RNA). Furthermore, HIV-infected cells have diminished levels of manganese-SOD (Mn-SOD), which is an antioxidant enzyme, and a decreased ability to evoke this enzyme in response to TNF-α. Downregulation of cellular Mn-SOD by the HIV regulatory protein *tat* leads to an increase in FR production and an increase in HIV viral replication.[7]

Oxidative stress also is linked to T-cell apoptosis, or programmed cell death.[8] H_2O_2 can indirectly kill cells through the oxidation of cell membranes to form lipid hydroperoxides. The toxic forms of lipid hydroperoxides are usually converted to more benign forms through a reaction catalyzed by GPX, an antioxidant enzyme. In experiments using the chronically HIV-infected 8E5 cell line, Sandstrom et al[8] demonstrated a direct relationship between HIV gene expression and impaired GPX activity, which led to lipid hydroperoxide-induced apoptosis.

ANTIOXIDANTS

Several mechanisms of antioxidant depletion that place patients at a higher risk of oxidative stress exist in HIV infection. These include (1) changes in bowel mucosa leading to malabsorption of various nutrients, (2) dysregulation of plasma amino acid levels, which may compromise normal antioxidant defenses, and (3) loss of electron-transport capacity, which leads to an inability to recover reduced forms of GSH, a potent cellular antioxidant.[5] Furthermore, researchers hypothesize that excessive production of FRs directly depletes or uses up available antioxidants.

Several observational studies that measure both indicators of oxidative stress and antioxidant levels in HIV-infected patients show that increased oxidative stress is usually accompanied by a decrease in antioxidant levels. A group of French researchers measured indicators of oxidative stress and several antioxidants (including plasma zinc [Zn] and selenium [Se], red blood cell [RBC] GPX activities, carotenoids, and vitamins C and E) in 43 HIV-positive and 16 HIV-negative subjects.[9,10] Overall they found severe reductions of carotenoids in both asymptomatic HIV-infected patients and AIDS patients. At the same time they found an increase in oxidative stress as measured by plasma hydroperoxides and malondialdehyde (MDA) levels. Another group of researchers[11] measured RBC MDA concentrations, plasma fatty acid (FA) profiles, and plasma levels of vitamins A, E, and Se in 95 HIV-infected patients and 20 HIV-negative controls. The researchers reported significantly lower plasma vitamin A and Se levels in HIV-positive patients compared to those in controls. Higher RBC MDA levels and lower polyunsaturated fatty acid (PUFA) levels provided evidence for increased oxidative stress in this group of patients. Allard et al[12] measured breath-alkane output and LP concentrations as indicators of oxidative stress and found significantly higher levels of LP in HIV-positive patients compared to those in HIV-negative controls. They also found significantly lower concentrations of ascorbic acid, vitamin E, beta-carotene, and Se in the plasma of the HIV-positive patients. In another recent study, lipid hydroperoxide concentrations were significantly elevated, and antioxidant capacity was depleted in 14 HIV-positive patients compared with 14 HIV-negative controls.[13] The researchers reported a slight correlation ($r = 0.41$) between measures of oxidative stress and antioxidant status in the HIV-infected patients, suggesting that depleted antioxidant status is secondary to oxidative stress in patients with HIV.

Revillard et al[14] measured serum MDA levels, as well as serum Se levels, in 63 HIV-positive individuals

(37 with AIDS) and 32 healthy controls. MDA levels were significantly higher in asymptomatic HIV-infected patients than in the controls and were even higher among those with AIDS. However, serum Se levels were not decreased in HIV-infected patients, with or without AIDS. These results, in contrast to the previous studies, suggest that the increase in LP observed in HIV infection is not directly related to a breakdown in Se-dependent GPX activity.

Glutathione

GSH, a low-molecular-weight (LMW) thiol, is the primary soluble antioxidant found in the cytoplasm, nuclei, and mitochondria of all animal cells.[1] GSH protects cells against oxidizing agents that can damage DNA and other cellular components. Intracellular GSH is also important in T-cell function and immune function.[15,16] Studies found decreased levels of GSH in both symptom-free HIV-infected individuals and in AIDS patients. Buhl et al[17] measured concentrations of extracellular GSH in plasma and lung epithelial lining fluid (ELF) of 14 asymptomatic HIV-positive men and 19 healthy HIV-negative controls and found significantly reduced GSH levels in the HIV-positive men compared to those in the controls. Roederer et al[16] demonstrated that peripheral blood mononuclear cells (PBMCs) from HIV-positive individuals had decreased levels of intracellular GSH, which were most pronounced in CD4[+] and CD8[+] T cells. Human CD4[+] and CD8[+] T cells are divided into two subsets: high-GSH and low-GSH T cells. The decreased GSH levels observed in this study were thought to be due to either the loss of high-GSH T cells in these individuals or the conversion of high-GSH T cells to low-GSH T cells. Regardless of the exact mechanism involved, decreased GSH levels place HIV-infected patients at increased risk of disease progression due to the damaging effects of oxidative stress.

Eck et al[18] designed a study to examine plasma thiol levels in HIV-positive individuals and to determine the effects of reduced extracellular cysteine levels on the intracellular GSH concentrations in T cells. They found that plasma thiol concentrations were decreased in HIV-infected individuals (including those who were asymptomatic) and that this decline was accompanied by a decrease in mean intracellular GSH levels. Patients who had been treated with zidovudine (AZT) for 1 year or less showed an increase in their plasma thiol levels, but their intracellular GSH levels remained low. Using cell cultures, the same authors demonstrated that the addition of extracellular cysteine increased the levels of intracellular GSH, and the absence of cysteine led to its decline. Furthermore, the amount of extracellular cysteine correlated positively with the rate of DNA synthesis in mitogenically stimulated T cells.

Aukrust et al[15] measured the ratio between reduced and total intracellular GSH levels from 22 HIV-positive patients and 15 sex- and age-matched healthy controls. They found a significant increase in oxidized GSH and a decrease in the ratio of reduced to total GSH levels in the CD4[+] lymphocytes of HIV-positive patients compared to those of the controls. However, the decreased plasma levels of cysteine found in a previous study[18] were not confirmed by this study. Since only a small fraction of total GSH normally exists in oxidized form, the authors concluded that the marked increase in oxidized GSH levels during HIV infection is a strong indicator of oxidative stress in these cells.

In a more recent study, Marmor et al[19] compared serum thiol levels among 13 HIV-negative and 133 HIV-positive injection drug users (IDUs) from a methadone maintenance program and found that low serum thiol levels were associated with an increased risk of mortality among the HIV-infected IDUs. This association was stronger in persons with AIDS than in those without AIDS. Together these studies show that HIV-infected individuals are more susceptible to a reduction in thiol levels (particularly GSH and cysteine levels) and that this reduction may lead to more rapid disease progression.

Catalase

Catalase, an antioxidant enzyme, is thought to aid in the breakdown of H_2O_2 and superoxide anion. Catalase activity increases during oxidative stress and protects against cell damage. Yano et al[20] showed that catalase activity in RBCs was higher in HIV-positive patients than in healthy controls, whereas the same enzyme activities decreased in mononuclear cells and in granulocytes. Similarly, serum catalase activity was higher in 97 HIV-positive patients than in healthy controls, and the enzyme activity increased progressively with HIV infection.[21] Data from Repetto et al[22], however, showed no significant difference in catalase activity between HIV-positive patients and healthy controls. A slight downward trend of catalase activity was noted with increasing severity of HIV infection and with increasing levels of antiretroviral treatment, indicating that oxidant levels may differ from those in therapy. At the cellular level, Foga et al[23] added catalase and SOD to gp120-induced U937 cells and found that both enzymes decreased the oxidative damage to the cells. Additionally, Leff et al[21] found a reduction in H_2O_2 damage with the addition of catalase but no effect on neutrophil bactericidal activity or mononuclear cell cytotoxicity in cultured cells. The implications of the increase in serum catalase activity observed during HIV infection require further study.

N-Acetylcysteine

N-Acetylcysteine (NAC) is a drug that is used to treat oxidative stress due to overdoses of acetaminophen.[25] It is thought to increase GSH levels and neutralize TNF-α activity.[24] Cysteine is needed for GSH synthesis, and NAC supplementation increases cysteine levels. A study of healthy subjects in vivo showed that T-cell counts were increased by a 4-week oral NAC supplementation in persons with low initial GSH levels, whereas GSH levels decreased. NAC supplementation decreased T-cell counts in those with optimal GSH levels.[26] The researchers concluded that treatment of HIV-positive persons with NAC should be limited to those with low GSH levels and that the levels of GSH may remain suboptimal with NAC treatment.

The effects of NAC in HIV infection have been studied in a few small supplementation trials. De Quay et al[27] gave a one-time NAC supplement to nine HIV-positive patients and six healthy controls and measured NAC levels at baseline and at 2 and 4 hours after supplementation. At baseline, levels of plasma GSH and cysteine were lower in HIV-positive patients than in controls. After supplementation, levels of plasma NAC and cysteine increased after 2 hours but returned to near-baseline levels after 4 hours for both the HIV-positive group and the control group. Levels of plasma GSH did not change after supplementation, but intracellular GSH levels in the HIV-positive group were higher 4 hours after supplementation, as compared to levels at baseline and at 2 hours after supplementation. However, intracellular GSH levels did not normalize with supplementation. Intracellular GSH levels did not change after supplementation in the control group. The researchers concluded that larger and more frequent doses may be needed to maintain increased intracellular GSH levels. In contrast, Clotet et al[25] found that prescribing 3200 mg of NAC per day in combination with AZT treatment versus AZT treatment alone resulted in no benefit of NAC over AZT treatment. In fact, many patients experienced side effects from NAC. The researchers suggested that repeated high-dose NAC supplementation results in poor compliance.

Other studies examined the effects of NAC at the cellular level, and results have been mixed. Cayota et al[28] studied purified CD4+ lymphocytes from 11 HIV-positive patients and 10 healthy controls in vitro, both at baseline and after NAC treatment. At baseline, the researchers observed low intracellular thiol levels in lymphocytes from the HIV-positive group. After NAC treatment, they observed increased thiol levels in a high proportion of the cells from HIV-positive patients. Among those patients whose thiol levels did not change, a high number of cells underwent a programmed cell death. Similarly, Staal et al[29] found that NAC prevents a decrease in thiol levels and blocks activation of NF-κB by using a cell culture that contains the HIV LTR region and is stimulated by phorbol 12-myristate 13-acetate (PMA) and TNF-α. Kalebic et al[30] used U1 cells treated with TNF-α, PMA, or IL-6 to study the effects of NAC. They found that NAC inhibited the level of HIV messenger ribonucleic acid (mRNA) by 90% in those cells stimulated by TNF-α and PMA.

A few studies showed conflicting results. Although Aillet et al[31] showed that NAC inhibited TNF-α or PMA-induced NF-κB activity in U1 cells and suppressed HIV reactivation, they found that NAC did not block chronic active HIV replication. They cautioned that the concentrations used in the study were at near-toxic levels and that at these levels, NAC may compromise immune function. Similarly, Roberts et al[32] found that NAC supplementation (1 mM and 5 mM) increased the antibody-dependent cell-mediated cytotoxicity (ADCC) of neutrophils, using cells from HIV-positive and healthy individuals. However, ADCC decreased at higher levels of NAC, and the researchers felt that the higher level of NAC exceeded levels that could be used in vivo. Jones et al[33] treated murine T cells with NAC and showed that apoptosis decreased when induced by anti-CD3 antibodies, but apoptosis increased when induced by 6-alpha-methylprednisolone. When they repeated the experiment with either a specific GSH inhibitor or the isomer *N*-Acetyl-D-cysteine, the results were similar.

The researchers concluded that the effects of NAC on apoptosis are independent of GSH status.

Chen et al[34] demonstrated a negative effect of NAC. Not only did NAC increase HIV growth in PBMCs in vitro, but it also increased cell-to-cell transmission of HIV at low concentrations.

These studies, both at the cellular level and at the supplementation trial level, indicate mixed results. Researchers should continue to study the usefulness of NAC supplementation. Until stronger evidence for clinical benefits of NAC supplementation exists, physicians should exercise caution when using or prescribing this drug.

Antioxidant Vitamins

The increase in oxidative stress caused by HIV infection increases the body's use of antioxidant vitamins, possibly leading to deficiencies of these nutrients. Vitamin deficiencies, in turn, exacerbate the immune dysfunctions caused by HIV infection, leaving individuals more susceptible to OIs. If left untreated, this cycle will grow worse as the disease progresses.

Vitamin E

Vitamin E is the primary chain reaction–breaking antioxidant in cell membranes.[1] Studies on vitamin E status among HIV-positive individuals showed mixed results. Constans et al[11] found no difference in plasma vitamin E levels among 95 HIV-positive patients compared to those of 20 healthy controls. In contrast, Allard et al[35] showed lower α- and γ-tocopherol levels in 49 HIV-positive patients compared to those of 15 healthy controls. Among HIV-positive participants, vitamin E levels were similar between those who were asymptomatic and those with AIDS. Pacht et al[36] found that, although the mean serum vitamin E level was adequate among 121 HIV-positive individuals, vitamin E deficiency was present in 22% of the study participants. Moreover, they found that serum vitamin E levels decreased after 1 year compared to baseline levels.

The benefits of vitamin E supplementation on retrovirus-induced immune dysfunctions were studied largely using in vitro systems and animal models; fewer studies were done in humans. Suzuki and Packer[37] found that several of the naturally occurring vitamin E derivatives (e.g., vitamin E acetate, α-tocopheryl succinate, and 2,2,5,7,8-pentamethyl-

6-hydroxychromane [PMC]) were successful in inhibiting NF-κB activation in an in vitro system.

In a series of murine AIDS studies, a team of researchers at the University of Arizona in Tucson (including the authors of chapter 4) investigated whether vitamin E supplementation, alone or in combination with other therapies, would be able to modulate cytokine production and restore many of the immune dysfunctions caused by retrovirus infection.[38-41] Although the murine retrovirus (LP-BM5) used in these studies is different from HIV, it shares many of the same characteristics and has a similar pathogenesis. Mice infected with LP-BM5 have inhibited release of IL-2 and IFN-γ (cytokines that promote cell-mediated immunity); increased secretion of IL-4, IL-5, IL-6, and TNF-α (promoters of humoral responses); and decreased hepatic and serum levels of vitamin E. This abnormal cytokine profile is also found in HIV-infected patients. The researchers found that the cytokine and immune dysregulation induced by the retrovirus infection could be reversed with a 15- to 450-fold increase in dietary intake of vitamin E,[40,39] an increased intake of vitamin E plus IFN-γ,[41] or treatment with a T-cell receptor (TCR) peptide.[38]

Two studies in humans support the findings of the previous animal studies. In a 9-year longitudinal study of 310 HIV-positive homosexual men in Baltimore, researchers found that patients in the highest quartile of serum vitamin E levels ($\geq$23.5 mol/L) had a significant decrease in risk of progression to AIDS compared to those in the lower three quartiles combined, after adjusting for several covariates.[42] In addition, a strong correlation existed between the intake of vitamin E supplements (single vitamin or multivitamin) and serum vitamin E levels in the patients, suggesting that oral vitamin E supplements are an effective means of raising vitamin E levels. A randomized clinical trial (RCT) conducted in 40 HIV-positive subjects in Toronto demonstrated that 3 months of supplementation with 800 IU of vitamin E and 1000 mg of vitamin C significantly reduced oxidative stress when compared to a placebo group.[35] In addition, researchers observed a decrease in HIV viral load in the supplemented group but not in the placebo group. These results are consistent with the theories generated by the in vitro and animal studies presented earlier. Taken together, these human and animal studies suggest that not only is vitamin E necessary for proper functioning of the immune system, but therapeutic levels have important immunostimulatory properties.

However, physiological levels of oxidative stress perform critical functions for host defense, and high doses of vitamin E may counteract these benefits. Given this potential, we need to assess whether the evidence is strong enough for vitamin E testing in HIV clinical trials.

Beta-Carotene

Beta-carotene is both an antioxidant and a precursor of vitamin A. It is unclear how beta-carotene contributes to HIV disease progression. As an antioxidant, the role of beta-carotene is much the same as that proposed for vitamin E. Although beta-carotene is the most-studied carotenoid in HIV disease, one study measured individual carotenoids in 35 HIV-positive and 38 healthy individuals.[43] The researchers found that all carotenoids, including lutein, zeaxanthin, cryptoxanthin, lycopene, and beta-carotene, were lower in the HIV-positive patients than in the healthy controls. Sappey et al[10] showed that beta-carotene levels dramatically decreased during early stages of HIV infection, but they did not observe further depletion in later stages of infection. This decrease was attributed to the higher degree of LP in the early stages and a hypothesized decrease in the production of free radicals at later stages due to hyperstimulation of macrophages. Beta-carotene's primary mechanism of action in HIV could be through its conversion to retinol. Since high doses of beta-carotene are associated with few toxic side effects, beta-carotene supplements are safer than vitamin A supplements, which are toxic at high doses.

Early on, the prospect of using beta-carotene as an adjunct therapy to help stimulate the immune response of HIV-positive patients generated much enthusiasm among researchers. However, the results of a few preliminary trials showed remarkably few benefits of beta-carotene supplementation in HIV-infected patients. In 1992 Garewal et al[44] supplemented 11 patients with 60 mg of beta-carotene daily for 4 months and found increases in natural killer (NK) cells and activated lymphocytes after 3 months of treatment. However, the observed increases diminished thereafter. No major changes were seen in $CD4^+$ cell counts. Bianchi-Santamaria et al[45] supplemented 64 AIDS-related complex (ARC) patients with 60 mg of beta-carotene daily in cycles of 20 days per month for nearly 3 years and found improvements in general health and working efficiency, as well as recovery from HIV-related symptoms. However, in the 11 patients who complied with the study protocol, no significant changes in mean $CD4^+$ cell counts were noted over the 24- to 36-month follow-up period. Silverman et al[46] published results from a trial where 11 HIV-positive patients with chronic oral candidiasis were supplemented with 60 to 120 mg of beta-carotene daily for 3 to 7 months. After 6 months, the researchers found no apparent improvements in the control of oral candidiasis or in lymphocyte counts or percentages. Fryburg et al[47] supplemented seven AIDS patients with 60 mg of beta-carotene and a multivitamin daily for 1 month. In the entire group, $CD4^+$ cells increased slightly, but the increase was not statistically significant. In three patients who had baseline $CD4^+$ cell counts >10 cells/L, $CD4^+$ cells increased significantly by approximately 50 cells. Six weeks after the treatment ended, however, the $CD4^+$ cells returned to baseline levels. It is difficult to draw firm conclusions from these trials because they were uncontrolled and included small numbers of patients. Although some of the results may suggest slight improvements in immune response soon after beta-carotene supplementation, the improvements in most of these trials diminished a few months after stopping the treatment.

In 1996 Coodley et al[48] published an extended evaluation of their initial 1993 placebo-controlled trial of beta-carotene. Their initial study[49] showed significant increases in total white blood cell (WBC) counts, $CD4^+$ T-cell counts, and $CD4^+/CD8^+$ ratios after 1 month in those supplemented with beta-carotene compared to those given a placebo. In their extended evaluation, 36 HIV-positive patients were given 180 mg of beta-carotene daily plus a multivitamin supplement, and 36 HIV-positive controls were given a placebo plus a multivitamin. The results showed no significant difference between the two groups with respect to T-cell subsets, NK cells, p24 antigen levels, or body weight (BW) after either 1 month or 3 months of supplementation. The multivitamin supplement given to patients in both arms of the study may have masked the effects of beta-carotene.

In a recent study, Delmas-Beauvieux et al[50] examined the effects of beta-carotene and Se supplementation in HIV-infected patients. They found a slight increase in GPX and a significant increase in GSH status in the beta-carotene supplemented group compared to the placebo group. The Se-supplemented arm of this trial showed greater increases in GPX and GSH, suggesting that Se supplementation is more effective in boosting GPX and GSH levels. Therefore results from these more extensive trials of beta-carotene supplementation have not revealed much of a future role for beta-carotene as an adjunct therapy in HIV infection. However, no studies have yet examined the role of beta-carotene as a precursor of vitamin A. Beta-carotene may still have a role in boosting vitamin A levels in persons who are vitamin A deficient, since it is safer to prescribe high doses of beta-carotene than it is to prescribe high doses of retinol.

Selenium

Selenium acts as part of GPX, which is an antioxidant enzyme. Although Se deficiency is uncommon in the general population, low Se status has been observed among HIV-positive individuals when compared to HIV-negative individuals. Low serum Se levels are associated with anemia, congestive cardiomyopathy, skeletal muscle myopathy, and increased cancer risk. Low Se levels also are associated with a lowered resistance to microbial and viral infections.[51] Moreover, studies show a link between low serum Se levels and low erythrocyte GPX activity, increased activation of NF-κB, and viral transcription.[8,10]

Several studies have examined the association of Se status and HIV disease. One such study by Constans et al[11] involved 95 HIV-positive patients and 20 healthy controls. They found plasma Se levels to be lower in patients who had CD4$^+$ cell counts less than 400 than in controls; however, they observed no differences in serum Se levels between patients with and without OI or with and without wasting. Serum Se levels were positively correlated with serum albumin, CD4$^+$ cell-count, body mass index (BMI), and p24 antigen ($r = 0.41, 0.47, 0.36, 0.60$, respectively). Serum Se was correlated with neither OIs nor antiretroviral drug use.

In a small study of 12 AIDS patients and 27 controls, Dworkin et al[52] found levels of plasma Se, whole blood Se, and RBC Se to be lower among the AIDS patients than the controls. Although serum albumin was normal in both the AIDS patients and the controls, the researchers found a correlation between Se and serum albumin ($r = 0.77$). The correlation between serum albumin and Se in both studies is of interest, since Se is transported in plasma bound to nonalbumin proteins. They also found plasma Se to correlate with hematocrit (Hct), lymphocyte count, and GPX activity ($r = 0.77, 0.53, 0.78$, respectively).

Other studies showed low Se status to be associated with disease progression and mortality. Baum et al[53] studied 125 HIV-positive and 105 HIV-negative drug users for a period of 3.5 years. They found serum Se deficiency to be associated with HIV mortality, independent of CD4$^+$ cell counts (crude relative risk [RR] = 19.9, 95% confidence interval [CI] = 5.52-71.9; adjusted RR = 10.8, 95% CI = 2.37-49.2). In another study of 70 HIV-positive patients, 23% of the patients had high serum Se levels, and 11% had low Se levels.[54] The low Se levels were associated with a lower NK cell activity, whereas high Se levels were associated with lower levels of immunoglobulins (IgG and IgM).

Look et al found that levels of serum Se decreased with disease progression in HIV-positive patients.[55] In a cross-sectional study of 104 HIV-positive individuals and 72 healthy controls, mean serum Se levels were lower in HIV-positive patients who had symptoms (stage II) and in those with AIDS (stage III), compared to the asymptomatic HIV-positive patients (stage I) and the healthy controls. Mean Se levels were lower in stage III than in stage II. After controlling for the presence of hepatitis, the differences remained. Serum Se correlated positively with CD4$^+$ T-cell count ($r = 0.42$) and correlated negatively with TNF receptors ($r = -0.58$), neopterin ($r = -0.5$) and β$_2$microglobulin ($r = -0.4$). The researchers suggested that Se is related more to OIs than to CD4$^+$ T-cell count because the correlations were independent for neopterin and β$_2$microglobulin, whereas CD4$^+$ T-cell count was not an independent factor of Se. They also speculated that a breakdown of erythrocyte GPX activity may exist in end-stage AIDS when serum Se levels fall below a threshold level (approximately 55 µg/L). Look et al concluded that Se deficiency is common among persons with advanced HIV disease and that it may be caused by malnutrition or OIs.

Several small Se supplementation trials showed increased serum Se levels and increased GPX activity with supplementation. Cirelli et al[51] studied 67 HIV-positive patients and 15 healthy controls and found that serum Se levels were similar between the controls and the asymptomatic HIV-positive patients, both of whom had higher serum levels than HIV-positive patients with generalized lymphoadenopathy, ARC, and AIDS. During a second stage of this study, 12 HIV-positive patients received 80 µg Se and 25 mg vitamin E daily for 2 months. Serum Se levels increased after supplementation, whereas no changes were observed in CD4$^+$ T-cell counts, RBC and WBC counts, albumin, hemoglobin, and the erythrocyte sedimentation rate (ESR).

Another supplementation study involved 14 HIV-positive patients who received 100 µg Se daily for 12 months, 13 HIV-positive patients who received 60 mg beta-carotene daily for 12 months, and 18 HIV-positive patients and 26 healthy controls who received no supplement.[50] At baseline, HIV-positive patients had lower plasma Se levels than controls. After Se-supplementation, serum Se levels were higher in the Se-supplemented group than in the beta-carotene or no-supplement groups. Se supplementation resulted in higher GPX activity and GSH status compared to baseline levels. No differences were observed for SOD activity compared to baseline levels. Although beta-carotene supplementation achieved similar results, the differences were fewer.

At the cellular level, Makropoulos et al[56] studied the effects of Se supplementation on NF-κB activation in Se-deprived lymphocytes. They found that Se increased GPX activity and decreased NF-κB activation and that this response was dose-dependent.

Low Se status is related to HIV disease progression. The few supplementation trials suggest that Se supplementation can be beneficial. However, other studies also showed a reduction in immunological function and nonimmunological symptoms, including fatigue and nail and hair changes, with high Se levels. Clinical trials are needed to determine the optimal dose of Se for HIV-positive individuals with low Se levels, as well as for those with normal Se levels.

SUMMARY

Several studies showed lower serum antioxidant levels (mainly vitamins A, C, and E, the carotenoids, Zn, and Se) in HIV-positive populations compared to HIV-negative populations.[9-12,55,58-60] To our knowledge, only one study found a direct, but moderate, link between oxidative stress and antioxidant depletion in HIV-infected patients.[13] Several studies, however, measured both metabolites of oxidative stress and serum levels of antioxidants in the same group of patients. These studies found increased levels of oxidative stress (e.g., MDA levels, breath pentane and ethane output, thiobarbituric acid reactants, and LP levels) and decreased serum levels of antioxidants (e.g., vitamin E, various carotenoids, Se, and Zn) in HIV-positive patients compared to HIV-negative controls.[9,10,12,14,22,59] One limitation of these studies is that they demonstrated increases in mean levels of oxidative stress and decreases in mean levels of antioxidants among the population as a whole. Many of these studies consisted of only a small number of patients.

In recent years the use of antioxidant supplements (particularly vitamin E, beta-carotene, Se, and NAC) as therapeutic agents in various disease states, including cancer and HIV infection, has been popular. However, several researchers have pointed out that ROS and FRs are involved in a number of useful physiological processes and therefore require physicians to be extremely cautious when using or recommending high-dose antioxidant supplementation.[3,4,6,61,62] When generated at low (physiological) levels, ROS perform critical functions in the human body, such as assisting in the bactericidal activity of phagocytes, the synthesis of prostaglandins, and the stimulation of cell proliferation.[61,62] Furthermore, superoxide anion may play a beneficial role in lymphocyte function.[61] Therefore reducing intracellular concentrations of ROS may lead to harmful effects, such as impaired phagocyte microbicidal function, which would render HIV-infected patients more susceptible to OIs. On the other hand, excessive production of FRs may be associated with increased stimulation of HIV replication[6] and apoptosis,[56] which leads to more rapid disease progression. It is important to determine the right balance between too much antioxidant protection and too little antioxidant protection, both of which are likely to be deleterious. Furthermore, in this era of protease inhibitors (PIs), we also need to determine the impact of various treatment regimens on oxidative stress.

References

1. Thomas JA: Oxidative stress, oxidant defense, and dietary constituents. In Shils ME, Olson JA, Shike M, editors: *Modern nutrition in health and disease*, Philadelphia, 1994, Lea & Febiger.
2. Grimble RF: Effect of antioxidative vitamins on immune function with clinical applications, *Int J Vitam Nutr Res* 67:312-320, 1997.
3. Muller F: Reactive oxygen intermediates and human immunodeficiency virus (HIV) infection, *Free Radic Biol Med* 13:651-657, 1992.

4. Schwarz KB: Oxidative stress during viral infection: a review, *Free Radic Biol Med* 21:641-649, 1996.

5. Greenspan HC, Aruoma OI: Oxidative stress and apoptosis in HIV infection: a role for plant-derived metabolites with synergistic antioxidant activity, *Immunol Today* 15:209-213, 1994.

6. Baruchel S, Wainberg MA: The role of oxidative stress in disease progression in individuals infected by the human immunodeficiency virus, *J Leukoc Biol* 52:111-114, 1992.

7. Flores SC, Marecki JC, Harper KP, et al: Tat protein of human immunodeficiency virus type 1 represses expression of manganese superoxide dismutase in HeLa cells, *Proc Natl Acad Sci U S A* 90:7632-7636, 1993.

8. Sandstrom PA, Tebbey PW, Van Cleave S, et al: Lipid hydroperoxides induce apoptosis in T cells displaying a HIV-associated glutathione peroxidase deficiency, *J Biol Chem* 269:798-801, 1994.

9. Favier A, Sappey C, Leclerc P, et al: Antioxidant status and lipid peroxidation in patients infected with HIV, *Chem Biol Interact* 91:165-180, 1994.

10. Sappey C, Leclerc P, Coudray C, et al: Vitamin, trace element and peroxide status in HIV-seropositive patients: asymptomatic patients present a severe beta-carotene deficiency, *Clin Chim Acta* 230:35-42, 1994.

11. Constans J, Peuchant E, Pellegrin JL, et al: Fatty acids and plasma antioxidants in HIV-positive patients: correlation with nutritional and immunological status, *Clin Biochem* 28:421-426, 1995.

12. Allard JP, Aghdassi E, Chau J, et al: Oxidative stress and plasma antioxidant micronutrients in humans with HIV infection, *Am J Clin Nutr* 67:143-147, 1998.

13. McLemore JL, Beeley P, Thorton K, et al: Rapid automated determination of lipid hydroperoxide concentrations and total antioxidant status of serum samples from patients infected with HIV: elevated lipid hydroperoxide concentrations and depleted total antioxidant capacity of serum samples, *Am J Clin Pathol* 109:268-273, 1998.

14. Revillard JP, Vincent CMA, Favier AE, et al: Lipid peroxidation in human immunodeficiency virus infection, *J Acquir Immune Defic Syndr Hum Retrovirol* 5:637-638, 1992.

15. Aukrust P, Svardal AM, Muller F, et al: Increased levels of oxidized glutathione in CD4$^+$ lymphocytes associated with disturbed intracellular redox balance in human immunodeficiency virus type 1 infection, *Blood* 86:258-267, 1995.

16. Roederer M, Staal FJ, Osada H, et al: CD4 and CD8 T cells with high intracellular glutathione levels are selectively lost as the HIV infection progresses, *Int Immunol* 3:933-937, 1991.

17. Buhl R, Holroyd KJ, Mastrangeli A, et al: Systemic glutathione deficiency in symptom-free HIV-seropositive individuals, *Lancet* 2:1294-1298, 1989.

18. Eck H, Gmunder H, Hartmann M, et al: Low concentrations of acid-soluble thiol (cysteine) in the blood plasma of HIV-1-infected patients, *Biol Chem Hoppe-Seyler* 370:101-108, 1989.

19. Marmor M, Alcabes P, Titus S, et al: Low serum thiol levels predict shorter times-to-death among HIV-infected injecting drug users, *AIDS* 11:1389-1393, 1997.

20. Yano S, Colon M, Yano N: An increase of acidic isoform of catalase in red blood cells from HIV(+) population, *Mol Cell Biochem* 165:77-81, 1996.

21. Leff JA, Oppegard MA, Curiel TJ, et al: Progressive increases in serum catalase activity in advancing human immunodeficiency virus infection, *Free Radic Biol Med* 13:143-149, 1992.

22. Repetto M, Reides C, Gomez Carretero ML, et al: Oxidative stress in blood of HIV-infected patients, *Clin Chim Acta* 255:107-117, 1996.

23. Foga I, Nath A, Hasinoff BB, et al: Antioxidants and dipyridamole inhibit HIV-1 gp120 induced free radical-based oxidative damage to human monocytoid cells, *J AIDS Hum Retrovirol* 16:223-229, 1997.

24. Reference deleted in proofs.

25. Clotet B, Gomez M, Ruiz L, et al: Lack of short-term efficacy of N-Acetyl-L-cysteine in human immunodeficiency virus-positive patients with CD4 cell counts <250/mm³, *J Acquir Immune Defic Syndr Hum Retrovirol* 9:98, 1995.

26. Kinscherf R, Fischbach T, Mihm S, et al: Effect of glutathione depletion and oral N-Acetylcysteine treatment on CD4$^+$ and CD8$^+$ cells, *FASEB J* 8:448-451, 1994.

27. de Quay B, Malinverni R, Lauterburg BH: Glutathione depletion in HIV-infected patients: role of cysteine deficiency and effect of oral N-Acetylcysteine, *AIDS* 6:815-819, 1992.

28. Cayota A, Vuillier F, Gonzalez G, et al: In vitro antioxidant treatment recovers proliferative responses of anergic CD4$^+$ lymphocytes from human immunodeficiency virus-infected individuals, *Blood* 87:4746-4753, 1996.

29. Staal FJ, Roederer M, Herzenberg LA: Intracellular thiols regulate activation of nuclear factor kappa B and transcription of human immunodeficiency virus, *Proc Natl Acad Sci U S A* 87:9943-9947, 1990.

30. Kalebic T, Kinter A, Poli G, et al: Suppression of human immunodeficiency virus expression in chronically infected monocytic cells by glutathione, glutathione ester, and N-Acetylcysteine, *Proc Natl Acad Sci U S A* 88:986-990, 1991.

31. Aillet F, Gougerot-Pocidalo MA, Virelizier JL, et al: Appraisal of potential therapeutic index of antioxidants on the basis of their in vitro effects on HIV replication in monocytes and interleukin 2-induced lymphocyte proliferation, *AIDS Res Hum Retroviruses* 10:405-411, 1994.

32. Roberts RL, Aroda VR, Ank BJ: N-Acetylcysteine enhances antibody-dependent cellular cytotoxicity in neutrophils and mononuclear cells from healthy adults and human immunodeficiency virus-infected patients, *J Infect Dis* 172:1492-1502, 1995.

33. Jones DP, Maellaro E, Jiang S, et al: Effects of *N*-Acetyl-L-cysteine on T-cell apoptosis are not mediated by increased cellular glutathione, *Immunol Lett* 45:205-209, 1995.

34. Chen P, Bauer G, Mitchell J, et al: *N*-Acetylcysteine and L-2-oxathiazolidine-4-carboxylic acid enhance contact-dependent growth of HIV in resting peripheral blood mononuclear cells (PBMC) in vitro and increase recovery of HIV from human-PBMC SCID mice, *AIDS* 11:33-41, 1997.

35. Allard JP, Aghdassi E, Narine N, et al: Effects of antioxidant vitamin supplementation in patients with HIV infection, *Nutrition* 13:272, 1997 (abstract).

36. Pacht ER, Diaz P, Clanton T, et al: Serum vitamin E decreases in HIV-seropositive subjects over time, *J Lab Clin Med* 130:293-296, 1997.

37. Suzuki YJ, Packer L: Inhibition of NF-κB activation by vitamin E derivatives, *Biochem Biophys Res Commun* 193(1):277-283, 1993.

38. Liang B, Ardestani S, Chow HH, et al: Vitamin E deficiency and immune dysfunction in retrovirus-infected C57BL/6 mice are prevented by T-cell receptor peptide treatment, *J Nutr* 126:1389-1397, 1996.

39. Wang JY, Liang B, Watson RR: Vitamin E supplementation with interferon-gamma administration retards immune dysfunction during murine retrovirus infection, *J Leukoc Biol* 58:698-703, 1995.

40. Wang Y, Huang DS, Liang B, et al: Nutritional status and immune responses in mice with murine AIDS are normalized by vitamin E supplementation, *J Nutr* 124:2024-2032, 1994.

41. Wang Y, Huang DS, Wood S, et al: Modulation of immune function and cytokine production by various levels of vitamin E supplementation during murine AIDS, *Immunopharmacology* 29:225-233, 1995.

42. Tang AM, Graham NMH, Semba RD, et al: Association between serum vitamin A and E levels and HIV-1 disease progression, *AIDS* 11:613-620, 1997.

43. Lacey CJ, Murphy ME, Sanderson MJ, et al: Antioxidant-micronutrients and HIV infection, *Int J STD AIDS* 7:485-489, 1996.

44. Garewal HS, Ampel NM, Watson RR, et al: A preliminary trial of beta-carotene in subjects infected with the human immunodeficiency virus, *J Nutr* 122(3 suppl):728-732, 1992.

45. Bianchi-Santamaria A, Fedeli S, et al: Short communication: possible activity of beta-carotene in patients with the AIDS related complex: a pilot study, *Med Oncol Tumor Pharmacother* 9:151-153, 1992.

46. Silverman Jr S, Kaugars GE, Gallo J, et al: Clinical and lymphocyte responses to beta-carotene supplementation in 11 HIV-positive patients with chronic oral candidiasis, *Oral Surg Oral Med Oral Pathol* 78:442-447, 1994.

47. Fryburg DA, Mark RJ, Griffith BP, et al: The effect of supplemental beta-carotene on immunologic indices in patients with AIDS: a pilot study, *Yale J Biol Med* 68:19-23, 1995.

48. Coodley GO, Coodley MK, Lusk R, et al: Beta-carotene in HIV infection: an extended evaluation, *AIDS* 10:967-973, 1996.

49. Coodley GO, Nelson HD, Loveless MO, et al: Beta-carotene in HIV infection, *J Acquir Immune Defic Syndr Hum Retrovirol* 6:272-276, 1993.

50. Delmas-Beauvieux MC, Peuchant E, Couchouron A, et al: The enzymatic antioxidant system in blood and glutathione status in human immunodeficiency virus (HIV)-infected patients: effects of supplementation with selenium or beta-carotene, *Am J Clin Nutr* 64:101-107, 1996.

51. Cirelli A, Ciardi M, De Simone C, et al: Serum selenium concentration and disease progress in patients with HIV infection, *Clin Biochem* 24:211-214, 1991.

52. Dworkin BM: Selenium deficiency in HIV infection and acquired immune deficiency syndrome (AIDS), *Chem Biol Interact* 91:181-186, 1994.

53. Baum MK, Shor-Posner G, Lai S, et al: High risk of HIV-related mortality is associated with selenium deficiency, *J Acquir Immune Defic Syndr Hum Retrovirol* 15:370-374, 1997.

54. Mantero-Atienza E, Beach RS, Gavancho MC, et al: Selenium status of HIV-1-infected individuals (letter), *J Parent Enter Nutr* 15(6):693-694, 1991.

55. Look MP, Rockstroh UK, Rao GS, et al: Serum selenium, plasma glutathione (GSH), and erythrocyte glutathione peroxidase (GPX)-levels in asymptomatic versus symptomatic human immunodeficiency virus-1 (HIV-1)-infection, *Eur J Clin Nutr* 51:266-272, 1997.

56. Baier-Bitterlich G, Fuchs D, Wachter H: Chronic immune stimulation, oxidative stress, and apoptosis in HIV infection, *Biochem Pharmacol* 53:755-763, 1997.

57. Reference deleted in proofs.

58. Beach RS, Mantero-Atienza E, Shor-Posner G, et al: Specific nutrient abnormalities in asymptomatic HIV-1 infection, *AIDS* 6:701-708, 1992.

59. Malvy DJM, Richard MJ, Arnaud J, et al: Relationship of plasma malondialdehyde, vitamin E, and antioxidant micronutrients to human immunodeficiency virus-1 seropositivity, *Clin Chim Acta* 224:89-94, 1994.

60. Skurnick JH, Bogden JD, Baker H, et al: Micronutrient profiles in HIV-1-infected heterosexual adults, *J Acquir Immune Defic Syndr Hum Retrovirol* 12:75-83, 1996.

61. Halliwell B, Cross CE: Reactive oxygen species, antioxidants, and acquired immunodeficiency syndrome, *Arch Intern Med* 151:29-31, 1991.

62. Pompella A: Biochemistry and histochemistry of oxidant stress and lipid peroxidation, *Int J Vitam Nutr Res* 67:289-297, 1997.

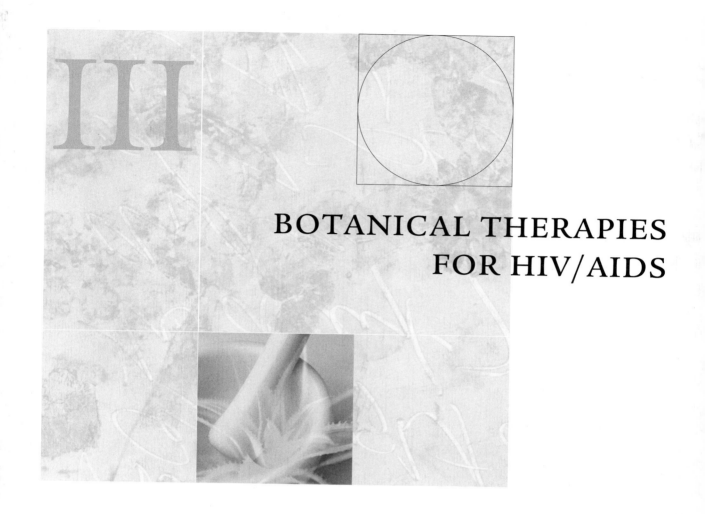

III

BOTANICAL THERAPIES FOR HIV/AIDS

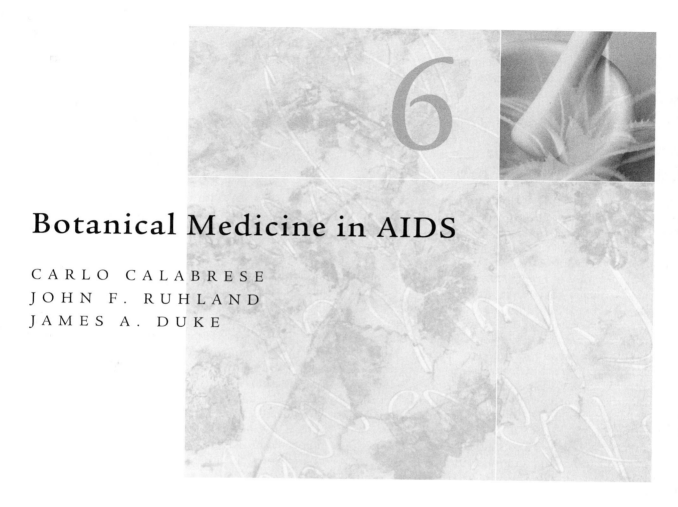

Botanical Medicine in AIDS

CARLO CALABRESE
JOHN F. RUHLAND
JAMES A. DUKE

SCREENING BOTANICALS FOR USE IN AIDS TREATMENT

Both complementary and alternative medicine (CAM) adherents and many conventional biomedical researchers believe that botanical medicines may yield some benefit in the treatment of AIDS. Molecular pharmacologists think that botanicals provide a rich source of specific molecules as lead compounds for drug development. This perspective contrasts with that of herbal practitioners, who believe that useful plant species and preparations are associated with a clinical pathology described in the herbalist's terms. Conscientious members of each group respect the values of the other.

Most herbal practitioners are devoted consumers of traditional scientific literature because herbal therapy is enhanced by studying findings related to the molecular constituents of the *materia medica*. The wise molecular pharmacologist should study traditional herbal remedies to discover which plant species are good to start with and which assays point toward more effective drugs. In the current regulatory and economic environment, however, business interests often discourage pharmacologists from using traditional herbs because funds cannot be committed for FDA-required research without the patent and sales protection provided by novel molecules.

Accordingly, the development of AIDS treatments from botanical products proceeds from one of two sources: (1) semirandom screening for novel molecules or (2) suggestions for clinical testing from traditional clinical use. The result is either drugs that are approved for effectiveness and safety by the FDA or relatively crude herbal extracts or preparations used commercially as dietary supplements. Most traditional herbal preparations are liquid or wet formulations (e.g., tinctures, teas, syrups, oils, ointments, liniments, compresses, and poultices). The modern dietary supplement industry has shifted to solid formulations such as tablets and capsules (e.g., crude dried herbs, dried juices, and, increasingly, extracts dried on an inert powder vehicle).

Botanicals may be used to treat AIDS in one of three ways: (1) by killing or suppressing the virus, (2) by supporting impaired immune function, or (3) by managing opportunistic infections (OIs) and neoplasms. This chapter concentrates on two associated parameters: (1) effect on viral load and (2) lymphocyte populations.

A great deal of research has been done on botanical treatments that can destroy or suppress viral growth. From 1987 to 1992, the National Cancer Institute (NCI) screened 22,000 aqueous and solvent extracts of terrestrial plants and lichens, cultured cyanobacteria, marine invertebrates, and algae. During their primary screen, 18% of these were found to have anti-HIV activity, with the highest percentage among plants, mostly in aqueous extracts.[1] The assay was the inhibition of killing of CD4$^+$ lymphocytes by the HIV-1 RF strain. To narrow down the enormous number of choices, NCI evolved a process to eliminate sulfated polysaccharides and tannins,[2] the most frequent sources of plant-based anti-HIV activity, to focus on novel molecules. After these two chemical classes were eliminated, about 400 NCI-designated active extracts of diverse chemistry remained. Active agents included alkaloids, coumarins, flavonoids, lignans, phenolics, proteins, quinones, phospholipids, and terpenes. Compounds from four of these, including michellamine B from the tropical liana (vine) *Ancistrocladus korupensis* and calanolide A from *Calophyllum lanigerum,* were committed to preclinical drug development by NCI.[3]

Researchers have published numerous papers on anti-HIV activity found in specific plant molecules, chemical classes of natural compounds,[4,5] anti-HIV compounds from particular plant species[6] and plant families,[7] natural products with particular mechanisms of anti-HIV activity,[8] anti-HIV species in regional herbaria,[9-13] and a number of excellent overviews.[3,14-16] They discovered various natural agents that interfered with a number of steps in the HIV life cycle, including (1) virus adsorption to the target cell surface, (2) uncoating of the viral particle, (3) virus-cell fusion, (4) reverse transcription of viral RNA to DNA, (5) integration into the host chromosome, (6) extension of viral latency, (7) RNA transcription before protein production, (8) translation into viral proteins, (9) inhibition of protease that clips viral proteins to the proper length, (10) glycosylation of env proteins, and (11) virion assembly and release.

The NCI screening program does not find prior ethnobotanical use to be valuable in developing lead compounds.[1] Since AIDS is a new clinical entity, the lack of an effective response is common among diverse traditional healer cultures. NCI's screening activity is turning away from cell-based assays and toward enzyme assays, such as protease and reverse transcriptase (RT) inhibition, and is focusing on chemical activities. This indicates a departure from exploring unknown mechanisms that exist in natural products toward making chemical attacks on well-known HIV targets. In contrast, the World Health Organization (WHO), focused on health in numerous underdeveloped countries, has considered ethnobotanical use to be a cost-effective screening method for pharmaceutical candidates.[17] Ethnobotanical use in developed countries provides some evidence of a plant's effectiveness and safety, although it may not be used traditionally for the treatment of AIDS. Beyond those chosen for preclinical development by NCI, plant extracts may exist that could be used as anti-HIV agents on the clinical bases of safety, bioavailability, and effect.

SOME BOTANICAL POSSIBILITIES

The following are a few of the botanical agents that have been considered as possible herbal treatments for AIDS from an herbalist's perspective. They are presented with some supporting in vitro mechanistic evidence. Sometimes a plant species has several mechanisms of action or a benefit that is missed in enzyme-based assays. Each of these species has a long history of safe human use, and safety considerations for some of them are mentioned before the discussion on clinical evidence to follow.

Curcuma Longa

Curcumin, a powerful antioxidant, is the primary active ingredient in the plant, comprising about 4% of the common culinary herb, turmeric. Turmeric is a major ingredient of curry powder. In vitro evidence shows inhibition of HIV integrase[18] and inhibition of HIV-1 long terminal repeat (LTR)-directed transcription[19] at fractional micromolar concentrations, as well as modest inhibition of HIV-1 and -2 proteases.[20] It also inhibits nuclear factor kappa B (NF-κB), which regulates viral transcription.[21] Between 40% to 85% of oral doses may be absorbed from the gastrointestinal (GI) tract,[22] although evidence of substantially lower absorption also exists.[23] Normal doses show little toxicity, although patients have reported GI irritability and other mild side effects.

Glycyrrhiza Glabra

Glycyrrhizin, a licorice root constituent, shows in vitro evidence of inhibition of viral attachment or fusion.[24-26] It may also inhibit protein kinase C (PKC), an activator of NF-κB.[27] Herbalists use it to treat peptic ulcers, hepatitis, and rheumatoid arthritis, and it is also used as an antiviral, an antispasmodic, and a demulcent.[22,28] Between 5% to 10% of the root consists of glycyrrhizin.[29] The root, with a traditional dose of 1 to 4 g/day, provides 50 to 400 mg of glycyrrhizin. In comparison, 400 to 1600 mg of glycyrrhizin was administered intravenously to three HIV-positive hemophiliacs, who demonstrated substantially lowered viral load after 1 month.[24] Long-term use can cause pseudoprimary aldosteronism.[28] It should not be used by patients with a history of hypertension or with renal or cardiac problems.

Hypericum Perforatum

Laboratory evidence shows that constituents of this plant, primarily hypericin, inhibit uncoating,[30-33] fusion,[34] and virion assembly,[31] which is a novel target. Hypericin inhibits viral infectivity factor (vif), an HIV protein that may be essential for viral assembly.[35] It does not show consistent results in clinical research as a single agent. Best known as an antidepressant, *Hypericum* (St. John's wort) is also used traditionally as an antiviral, an antiinflammatory, a sedative, and a hepatoprotective.[22,36,37] It is known to cross the blood-brain barrier. Hypericin can cause phototoxicity. The maximum tolerated oral dose is about 0.05 mg/kg.[38] Some research was performed on its interaction with anti-HIV drugs, with encouraging results.[39] Common

standardized extracts of 0.14% hypericin are available over the counter; higher concentration products are available through AIDS buyers' clubs. A number of sources report anecdotes of improved liver function in HIV patients who also have hepatitis.[40] *Hypericum* is associated with a decrease in serum indinavir sulfate levels in patients taking both drugs.[41]

Hyssopus Officinalis

Crude extracts of the dried leaves of this plant show strong anti-HIV activity as measured by the inhibition of syncytial formation, RT, and the formation of p17 and p24 antigen expression.[42] One constituent, caffeic acid, shows evidence of inhibition of integration of proviral DNA into the host genome.[43] Another constituent, MAR-10, a polysaccharide, also shows strong anti-HIV activity via glycosidase inhibition.[44] Its traditional indications include colds, bronchitis, and anxiety, and it is also used as an antispasmodic and an antiinflammatory at a tincture dose of 1 to 4 ml.[37]

Lentinus Edodes

An extract of the mycelial culture of the *Lentinus edodes* mushroom (LEM) demonstrated inhibition of the HIV antigen expressed from MT-4 cells and inhibition of giant cell formation, as well as inhibition of RT of avian myeloblastosis virus (AMV).[45] Three fractions of LEM inhibited the cytopathic effect of HIV-1 in ATH-8 cells.[46] Its probable effect is during the initial stages of the HIV life cycle. In a clinical study where the mushroom extract was used in combination with didanosine (ddI), it enhanced the action of the antiviral drug.[47] *Lentinus* (shiitake) is the second most popular mushroom in the global market, and it is used medicinally as an immune stimulant, an anti-cancer drug, and an antiviral (AV).[36,37]

Prunella Vulgaris

Prunella extract inhibits interaction between HIV-1 gp120 and immobilized CD4+ receptors.[48,49] An extract of 10 μg/ml was more potent than 4 μg/ml AZT at inhibiting HIV replication and preventing cell-to-cell infection.[50] Traditional Chinese medicinal dosage is 9 to 30 g with a broad antibiotic effect.[51]

Rosmarinus Officinalis

Compounds in rosemary have reported anti-HIV activity. Carnosic acid showed potent HIV-1 protease inhibition in a cell-free assay,[52,53] and carnosol showed action against HIV-1 replication in C8166 cells[54] at concentrations that were not cytotoxic.

Chelidonium Majus

Benzo[c]phenanthridine alkaloids, which are present in traditional phytomedicines, including *Chelidonium* (celandine) and *Sanguinaria canadensis* (bloodroot), inhibit RT from AMV and HIV-1.[55,56]

Spirulina Platensis (Arthrospira Platensis)

Cyanophyta (blue-green algae) are a promising source of anti-HIV pharmaceuticals.[57,58] Aqueous extracts from *Spirulina platensis,* as well as an identified *Spirulina* polysaccharide, reduce syncytial formation and viral production.[59-61] *Spirulina* has a growing market as a human and animal food supplement. A number of reports claim to enhance various immune functions in vitro and in vivo.

Scutellaria Baicalensis

Baicalein, a flavonoid, occurs in many *Scutellaria* species, particularly in *S. baicalensis,* commonly used in Chinese herbal medicine for infectious diseases[62] given at whole root doses of 6 to 15 g.[51] It is also antiinflammatory.[63] Baicalein inhibits HIV-1 RT,[64-66] protease,[67] and attachment.[68] Baicalin also shows reverse transcription inhibition.[62] Furthermore, baicalin may preferentially induce apoptosis in HIV-infected CEM cells over uninfected ones.[69]

The following paragraphs are generally about the list of herbs that precedes them. Although the in vitro anti-HIV research looks promising, it does not take into account bioavailability and half-life, many potential toxicities, nor the activity of metabolites that cause changes in both effectiveness and toxicity. Some common assays, such as syncytial inhibition, overemphasize surface effects in HIV inhibition. Although positive in vitro bioassays are necessary to screen and fractionate lead compounds for pharmaceutical development, botanical mechanisms of action that are irrelevant for a specific bioassay are not identified in these screens. Both the strain of the virus used and the cell system are critical to evaluating agents that may be useful against a prevalent virus or in clinical application. For example, betulinic acid derivatives have IC_{50}s against HIV-1 in the 10 nM range but are inactive against HIV-2,[70] and soulatrolide (a coumarin from *Calophyllum teysmannii* latex) is a potent inhibitor of HIV-1 RT but is inactive against HIV-2 RT.[71] In in vitro research, product variability is critical, and standardization requires attention for replicability. Standardization for clinical research, as exemplified by extracts of the plants discussed earlier and by centuries of herbalist clinical research, may not be molecularly specific, since it is based on agricultural practice, extraction, and administration. Despite the evidence from the research presented earlier on the selected botanical extracts, the NCI screen found little activity in its preparations of *Glycyrrhiza, Hypericum, Lentinus* and none in *Scutellaria, Prunella,* and *Chelidonium. Curcuma* and *Hyssopus* were not tested.[72] Thus large-scale screening programs may have significant limitations due to their inflexibility.

In contrast to the research on AV plant activity, relatively less scientific literature exists on botanicals as potential clinical immune system enhancers in the treatment of AIDS. Although we have known about microbial etiologies in infectious diseases for a century and a half, we have only begun to understand the complex immune system during the last few decades. In fact, much of our knowledge is the result of research precipitated by the AIDS epidemic. In HIV immunology, many researchers focused primarily on finding a vaccine that prevents HIV infection, and some researched therapeutic vaccines to deter cell-to-cell transmission of HIV, but few tried to correct the immune deficiency that allows a variety of infections and neoplasms to arise in AIDS patients. Different compartments of the immune system are stimulated by botanical treatments and may be of help in managing OIs[73] (see Chapters 4 and 20). However, the appropriate therapeutic targets that treat the central immune deficit have not been identified; thus confusion exists over which assays to employ for screening, which is the source of much of the anti-HIV botanical literature. The leading botanical candidates in immune enhancement in AIDS include *Astragalus membranaceus* (huang qi), the ginsengs (*Panax, Eleutherococcus*), mushrooms (maitake, shiitake, *Ganoderma lucidum*) from the East, and *Echinacea* from the West.

THE CLINICAL EVIDENCE

Clinical research has a great advantage over in vitro research in that a holistic response can be evaluated, and the results of unknown therapeutic mechanisms may be detected by positive outcomes. Although animal studies can fill in some of the missing pieces, animal AIDS models do not closely parallel human expression of the disease. In human studies, unpredicted toxicities may also occur, a possibility that calls for caution in designing and entering trials. Thus toxicity testing is the more important use of animal research in drug development. However, herbs that have a long history of safe human use may be entered into human AIDS studies more quickly than newer molecular treatments, especially given the lack of definitive treatments for this life-threatening disease.[17] Clinical AIDS trials with botanicals are not rare; however, most suffer from significant methodological deficits, with few showing substantial benefit as single agents. Nevertheless, worthwhile evidence often exists and, occasionally, a startling outcome. A review of published clinical work with medicinal plants and extracts in the treatment of AIDS reveals some possibilities.

Curcumin

Although it was not tested by the NCI, curcumin is popular among HIV-positive CAM users. A study of 18 HIV-positive patients with $CD4^+$ T-cell counts ranging from 5 to 615 found a significant increase of $CD4^+$ T-cell counts after using curcumin compared with controls. The treatment period was an average of 127 days. The increase occurred primarily during the early stages of treatment.[74] In a second study, curcumin was prescribed to two groups in doses of either 2700 mg/day or 4800 mg/day, based on anecdotal reports of current and historical use. The control was a waiting list. Neither dose had an effect on either $CD4^+$ T-cell count or viral load.[75]

Glycyrrhizin

Between 400 to 1600 mg/day was administered intravenously (IV) to three hemophiliacs with AIDS on six separate occasions lasting 1 month or more. HIV-1 p24 was detected at the beginning of 5 of the 6 courses but was undetectable at the end of 3 of those 5 courses and decreased after the other 2 courses.[24] Another small study of IV treatment with hemophiliacs showed lymphocyte increases in all nine patients, $CD4^+/CD8^+$ ratio increases in six patients, and $CD4^+$ lymphocyte level increases in eight patients.[76] In a third observation of two asymptomatic groups treated for 7 and 4 years, respectively, with daily oral doses of 150-225 mg/day, patients who received glycyrrhizin when their $CD4^+$ T-cell counts were 200 or above maintained counts of at least 200 throughout the treatment. Those with T-cell counts above 500 maintained counts of 500 or above after receiving glycyrrhizin. P24 was not detected throughout the study.[77] Endo[78,79] reported immune enhancements (lymphocytes, $CD4^+$ T-cell counts, $CD4^+/CD8^+$ ratio, and natural killer (NK) cell activity) with glycyrrhizin in six HIV-positive hemophiliacs treated over an 11-year period, and Ikegami[80] reported the same findings in an additional 16 patients treated for 3 to 7 years.

Hypericin

Several studies with plant-derived hypericin show moderate AV effects with relatively low toxicity. In a study of 31 patients treated for a 4-month period, $CD4^+$ T-cell count increased 13% in the 10 patients given hypericin who were not concomitantly on AZT. Although this was not a statistically significant increase, the patients on hypericin and AZT had a significant decrease in $CD4^+$ T cells.[81] In an open pilot study of 18 HIV-positive patients undergoing IV treatment, the majority showed stable or increasing $CD4^+$ T-cell counts. Only two of the 16 compliant patients encountered an OI during the 40 months of observation.[82] In another study, 18 HIV-positive symptomatic patients were treated with plant-derived hypericin (2 ml IV weekly), as well as daily oral *H. perforatum* for 40 months,[83] and were monitored for viral load and p24 antigens. Of the six patients who had positive p24 antigens at baseline, four patients exhibited significant long-term declines in p24 antigen levels; the levels showed no change in the other two patients. Of the 15 patients with a detectable baseline viral load, those with positive p24 antigens showed a decline in viral load from 5.0 to 4.23 log10 copies/ml. Although other patients showed an increase in viral load (without reported deterioration in clinical condition), the investigators considered the treatment nontoxic and continued clinical trials. Conversely, a study using synthetic hypericin found no AV results and dose-limiting phototoxic reactions.[84] Another study with synthetic hypericin also showed no AV effects after 12 weeks.[85] Finally, a third study of synthetic hypericin with four arms (0.25 or 0.5 mg/kg of body weight [BW] twice weekly, or 0.25 mg/kg 3 times weekly, or oral hypericin 0.5 mg/kg daily) in a total of 30 patients had 16 of them discontinue early due to toxicity.[86] Viral load and CD4+ T-cell counts did not change significantly. These contrasting results raise the hypothesis that plant-derived hypericin and crude *H. perforatum* have profiles of both effect and toxicity that differ markedly from those of synthetic hypericin.

SPV-30: Boxwood Extract
(*Buxus Sempervirens*)

In a well-designed 30-week study of 145 asymptomatic patients with CD4+ T-cell counts of 250 to 500 treated with two different doses (990 and 1980 mg/day) of SPV-30 versus a placebo, patients who received a 990 mg dose had fewer dropouts due to therapeutic failure and fewer increases in viral load. This was the lower of the two doses; at the higher dose, outcomes were similar to placebo.[87] An earlier phase I trial showed a rise in CD4+ T-cell counts, which did not appear in the controlled trial. In a follow-up community-organized US observational study, subjects who were not on antiretroviral drug therapy had a median fall of viral load of 35% after 6 months.

Chelidonium Majus

Two case study reports show that an IV-administered semisynthetic compound of alkaloids called Ukrain was associated with reducing the size and coloration of Kaposi's sarcoma (KS) lesions. No new lesions appeared during the 30-day interval after the beginning of treatment. There was an increase in total leukocytes, as well as in T-cell and T-suppressor counts in both patients, and an increase in helper T cells in one patient.[88] Clinical results with a combination of *Chelidonium* and *Sanguinaria* have been few.[89]

Andrographis Paniculata

An approach with the terpenes from this plant is described in a separate chapter (see Chapter 7). The preparation showed an indication of CD4+ lymphocyte protection in 13 HIV-positive patients not taking antiretrovirals, but dosing and toxicity questions remain.[90]

Momordica Charantia (Bitter Melon)

After a constituent, MAP-30, showed promising in vitro results, a community-based study provided a preliminary report that a decoction of bitter melon, administered orally or rectally, normalized the CD4+/CD8+ ratio with a concomitant improvement in the sense of well-being based on data from four patients with AIDS and two who were HIV-positive.[91]

Trichosanthin (Compound Q; GLQ233; *Tricosanthes Kirilowii*)

Trichosanthin has an interesting history in the AIDS epidemic. This extracted protein is a ribosomal inhibitor; in vitro it blocked HIV replication in lymphocytes and macrophages. Byers[92] in the United Kingdom reported that in a study of 51 patients with advanced disease, three injections of trichosanthin showed increased CD4+ T-cell counts and decreased serum p24 antigen levels, with one patient converting to antigen-negative. There were significant side effects—usually a flu-like syndrome but also possibly related dementia. In a second study of 112 HIV-positive patients with CD4+ T-cell counts less than 500 who were also on AZT or ddI but failing those drugs, there was a modest increase in CD4+ T-cell counts, but p24 antigen levels did not change.[93] A study of 61 HIV-positive patients found that Compound Q "stabilized and improved" the condition of all the patients. White blood cell (WBC) counts tripled, but CD4+ lymphocytes and the CD4+/CD8+ ratio did not increase.[94] In a study of 20 patients, eight patients showed a decrease in the size of their lymph nodes after the first treatment; eight patients had increased energy and improved appetites, and they experienced an overall weight gain,[95] but the concerns on side effects continued in this and other studies. In a phase I study of nine men, there was no disease progression, and the therapy was tolerated without significant toxicity for at least 6 months in four patients who agreed to take high doses of trichosanthin.[96] Further studies at the University of California–San Francisco published in 1994 showed moderate and sometimes equivocal results.[96a] Side effects continued to be an issue. There have been no further clinical trials with trichosanthin in the treatment of AIDS.

Viscum Album (Iscador, Mistletoe)

A study of 12 symptomatic patients with an injectable preparation found that, if beginning CD4[+] T-cell counts were above 200, the median increase in CD4[+] T cells was 35%, with all patients increasing above baseline. The patients were followed for 6 years and sustained the benefit.[97] In a second study of 40 self-injecting patients with CD4[+] T-cell counts greater than 200, 77% had an increase in CD4[+] T cells of at least 20%, lowered $\beta_2$microglobulin by about one-third, and two of eight patients who were HIV p24 antigen-positive became antigen-negative.[98] The investigators in these studies continued to report similar findings in a further phase I study.[99]

Aloe Vera, *Aloe Barbadensis* (Acemannan)

In a 1987 study by McDaniel in which 53 patients were treated for 3 months with Acemannan (ACE-M), a polysaccharide from *A. barbadensis,* statistical improvement was found in clinical and laboratory parameters. In 1990 McDaniel refined his criteria and on follow-up in 1993, suggested that the long-term survival of participants in the earlier study was related to ACE-M.[99a,99b] In a randomized controlled trial (RCT) versus a placebo, although the rate of decline in CD4[+] lymphocytes favored ACE-M, there was no difference after 48 weeks and no significant effect on p24 viral antigens.[100] In another blinded RCT of 63 patients on AZT or ddI with CD4+ T-cell counts between 50 to 300/mm³, no effect was found on either CD4+ T-cell counts or viral load.[101]

Lentinus Edodes (Shiitake)

Lentinan, a β1-3 glucan and an active ingredient of shiitake, showed a modest increase in CD4[+] T cells in an open trial with an IV preparation in 15 HIV-positive hemophiliacs[102] and significantly increased the CD4[+] T-cell count with ddI in a controlled study of 107 patients whose baseline CD4[+] T-cell count was between 200 to 500 cells/mm³.[47] In a follow-up, changes were considered provocative but insignificant in trends toward immunological benefit, although the medication was generally tolerated.[103]

Combinations of Chinese Herbs

Herbs from the traditional Chinese *materia medica* are commonly used in combinations based on individual prescriptions. However, despite the disparity with the usual practices of traditional Chinese medicine, a number of combinations have been applied to AIDS and evaluated in clinical study as though the combination was a standardized drug with a disease indication for persons with the Western diagnosis.

After a successful trial in a simian model of HIV infection that showed superior results to AZT,[104] a combination called ZY-1 was tried in 51 Tanzanian patients. Most symptoms were alleviated, and immune function improved in 14 patients and was stable in 16 patients. One patient, whose immune function was high, seroreverted.[105] When patients were treated with any of several combinations, Lu had eight cases of seroreversion. False-positive baseline tests for most of these were ruled out.[106] Chief components of the remedies were *A. membranaceus, Glycyrrhiza uralensis, Cordyceps sinensis,* and *S. baicalensis.*

Another Chinese formula called the "Spring of Life" (SOL) was administered in a controlled trial versus a placebo for 3 months to HIV-positive persons with a follow-up after 20 months. Twenty-five of the 27 herb-treated cases had positive results with a decrease of symptoms and increases in total lymphocytes, CD4[+] T cells, and CD8[+] lymphocytes.[107] SOL inhibits HIV-1, HIV-2, and many bacteria in vitro and shows no toxic effect at usual doses in acute and chronic toxicity tests. Results reported later on 56 cases were inconclusive.[108]

Young and Sinclair[109] treated 391 persons for 12 weeks with individualized acupuncture and a standardized herbal formula. Two hundred eighty-six patients completed the study (172 asymptomatic, 39 with ARC, and 75 with AIDS). They reported a statistically significant decrease of clinical and subjective symptoms.

Forty HIV-positive children between ages 2 to 6 were treated with the herbal combinations Chan Bai San (CBS) and Astol and were compared to 80 chemically treated children in a 3- to 5-year study.[110] The authors reported that nine of the herb-treated children became asymptomatic, whereas only one of the children in the comparison group did so. Morphometric measurements were better with herbs, CD4[+] lymphocytes increased, infections were reduced, and mortality was reduced by one-third.

XQ-9302, a combination of 20 herbs, was reported to be associated with an increase in CD4[+] lymphocytes and a one log decrease in viral load.[111]

At the Highbridge Woodycrest Center, a nursing facility in south Bronx, New York, a Chinese herbal formula was given in capsules to 103 patients for a period of 3 to 24 months. Goh reported an increase in CD4+ lymphocytes with a concomitant amelioration of symptoms compared to patients who did not take the herbs.[112]

In controlled trials, Chinese herb combinations have not fared as well. Burack et al[113] evaluated a combination of 31 herbs (28 pills/day) sold as two mixtures (Enhance and Clear Heat) against a placebo. Although there were no statistically significant differences, life satisfaction improved and symptoms lessened with the herbs. In a second blinded RCT against a placebo in 68 patients, another combination of 35 Chinese herbs also showed no marked differences between the test subjects and the controls.[114]

African Traditional Herbal Treatments

African traditional treatments are typically combinations. In a case series of an inexpensive herbal treatment, clinicians found the herbs to be effective during the early stages of AIDS. Among 112 patients who completed the treatment, 13 patients who began the treatment during advanced stages of AIDS died; four others were reported to have seroreverted.[115]

In a study of chronic diarrhea, chronic wasting, and herpes zoster (HZ) in 414 test and 136 control HIV-positive patients, 327 (79%) test and 99 (73%) control patients were followed for up to 36 weeks. HZ patients healed at the same rate whether under herbal ($n = 35$) or acyclovir ($n = 45$) treatment. At the end of the follow-up, however, 11% of herbally treated HZ patients versus 44% of HZ controls reported postherpetic neuralgia ($p < 0.005$). Among 187 patients with chronic diarrhea, 144 (77%) responded totally or partially to herbal treatment in contrast to 15 out of 35 controls (43%, $p < 0.005$).[116] Homsy continued his work in HZ and repeated his findings on HZ in a similar observational study.[117]

Other herbs recently studied in Africa include *Punica granatum* (pomegranate) for AIDS diarrhea and a compound called ELS. A home herbal pharmacy for which local women are encouraged to plant medicinal gardens is part of a public health project in the Rakai District in Uganda.[117a]

Ayurvedic Herbal Combinations

Minimal evidence exists on several combinations of Ayurvedic herbs prescribed according to different schools of thought. Bora et al[118] reported the results of the use of an Ayurvedic formula in 14 persons, who showed a slight increase in CD4+ lymphocytes and a decrease in $\beta_2$microglobulin after 12 weeks. Kothandaraman[119] claimed that five patients were cured from a group of 500 male and female HIV-positive persons treated by Siddha medicine. Singh et al[120] reported an average weight gain of 1.68 kg with improved subjective and functional measures after individualized treatment with nutrition, lifestyle change, and Rasayana therapy (mixtures of herbs and fruits). A comparison of an Ayurvedic approach and triple antiretroviral therapy (ART) was done in a very small group. HIV-1 viral load fell dramatically among the drug-treated patients, whereas the patients in the Ayurvedic group showed no change in viral load but gained more weight than the drug-treated group.[121]

Other Combinations

Caprani et al[122] reported the results of a study on a combination of three Brazilian herbs, named CHAM3, which was prescribed to 12 HIV-positive persons for a 9-month period. Nine patients took it as a single therapy; three maintained conventional therapy. All patients showed a significant improvement of laboratory findings (median CD4+ T-cell level rose from 204 to 460 mm³), and there were no adverse side effects.

ACA (also called Perthon), a Westernized combination of a southeast Asian herbal tradition of eleven herbs, including *Boswellia carteri* resin, Sumatra benzoin, *Curcuma zedoaria*, cinnamon, and cloves, attained investigational new drug (IND) status from the FDA in 1994 on the basis of preliminary data collected in Australia. Fifteen HIV-positive patients treated for up to 2 years showed significant improvements in weight and CD4+/CD8+ ratio.[123]

Among herbs that have been used frequently in Western countries to treat HIV, a combination was developed based on the partial efficacy of individual constituents in other studies, including curcumin, bitter melon, glycyrrhizin, and freeze-dried leaves of boxwood (*B. sempervirens*), known as SPV-30.[124] Eight patients used the combination for approximately 8 weeks; 3 of the 8 patients had viral load reductions from baseline of one log or greater; 2 remained stable or saw less than a one log reduction; and 2 had viral load increases. An eighth individual initially saw a >one log reduction over 1 month but then experienced a dramatic increase.

ISSUES OF SAFETY AND EFFICACY

Herbal practitioners proclaim their *materia medica* to be safe. In general, their relative safety in comparison to pharmaceutical drugs is the same as the results indicated by botanical studies. This is the rule except when a molecule is extracted, purified, or synthesized and applied unalloyed. Safety is more assured when plants are used in their traditional contexts by practitioners who know their effects. Nevertheless, safety issues are of primary concern, and it is important to collect toxicity data as well as efficacy data.

Medicinal plant AIDS research, even when it does not isolate active molecular species, needs to increase the consideration of compound variability so that the benefits detected can be replicated and transferred to other settings. This may mean measures from the assurance of proper species identification to the stabilization of agricultural, collection, and manufacturing practice, assuring the stability of herbal products, and standardizing for the concentration of one or more constituents in a preparation. Standardization by bioassay helps by accounting to some degree for the range of interactions among molecular constituents. Bioassay standardization, in addition to the long-practiced chemical standardization, is emerging as a manufacturing innovation. Its increased use benefits researchers, botanical practitioners, and patients.

Although most single herbs have not been fully researched, combination treatments often achieve more significant results. Studies initiated by herbal practitioners rather than herb-based pharmaceutical companies indicate that combination botanical treatment is the rule rather than the exception in medical practice. The ubiquitous employment of combination treatments must be considered if ethnobotanical use is considered valuable. At a higher level of complexity, medical systems that provide prescriptions for individuals in their own terms rather than on a Western disease diagnosis need evaluation. Adequate study on this basis has not been done even for Ayurvedic and Chinese medicine. Combination treatments with Western rationales such as naturopathy are unexplored, with rare exceptions.[125]

One arena of combination treatments drawing a great deal of attention is the interaction of frequently used botanicals with pharmaceutical drugs and, particularly, with antiretroviral drugs taken by HIV-positive patients. The prime example is *H. perforatum's* effect on the serum concentration of indinavir sulfate in both healthy volunteers and HIV-positive patients, in which indinavir serum's concentrations decreased from 20% to 50%.[126] The mechanism is either the induction of the cytochrome P3A4 or the alteration of p-glycoprotein by *H. perforatum.* The concern is the possibility of antiretroviral treatment failure or the emergence of viral resistance. However, other botanicals, as well as many common foods and numerous drugs, also affect the relevant metabolic systems. On the other hand, a few studies demonstrate benefit to combinations of pharmaceutical drugs and botanicals.[47]

Clinicians who wish to use botanicals in AIDS treatments should try the indicated traditionally used botanicals rationally and carefully, whether with or without conventional treatment. Clinicians should consider safety first and effectiveness second. Many medical practitioners are using botanicals or herbs in the treatment of AIDS and are willing to share their experiences. If clinicians decide to use botanicals, reporting the results in a public forum would be valuable for others. Patients should try indicated botanicals that have a history of safe human use, should monitor symptoms and laboratory tests carefully, and should work with a responsible and responsive professional. Whether botanical treatments work or not, both the clinician and the patient should let others know about the results.

References

1. Cragg GM, Boyd MR, Cardellina JH II, et al: Ethnobotany and drug discovery: the experience of the US National Cancer Institute, *Ciba Found Symp* 185:178-196, 1994.
2. Cardellina JHD, Munro MH, Fuller RW, et al: A chemical screening strategy for the dereplication and prioritization of HIV-inhibitory aqueous natural products extracts, *J Nat Prod* 56(7):1123-1129, 1993.
3. Vlietinck AJ, De Bruyne T, Apers S, et al: Plant-derived leading compounds for chemotherapy of human immunodeficiency virus (HIV) infection, *Planta Med* 64(2):97-109, 1998.
4. Gnabre JN, Brady JN, Clanton DJ, et al: Inhibition of human immunodeficiency virus type 1 transcription and replication by DNA sequence-selective plant lignans, *Proc Natl Acad Sci U S A* 92(24):11239-11243, 1995.

5. Ben KL, Zheng YT: Antihuman immunodeficiency virus type-1 activities of proteins from 17 species of plants, *Int Conf AIDS* 12:782 (abstract no. 41203), 1998.

6. Kalvatchev Z, Walder R, Garzaro D: Anti-HIV activity of extracts from *Calendula officinalis* flowers, *Biomed Pharmacother* 51(4):176-180, 1997.

7. Yamasaki K, Nakano M, Kawahata T, et al: Anti-HIV-1 activity of herbs in *Labiatae, Biol Pharm Bull* 21(8):829-833, 1998.

8. Ng TB, Huang B, Fong WP, et al: Antihuman immunodeficiency virus (anti-HIV) natural products with special emphasis on HIV reverse transcriptase inhibitors, *Life Sci* 61(10):933-949, 1997.

9. Abdel-Malek S, Bastien JW, Mahler WF, et al: Drug leads from the Kallawaya herbalists of Bolivia: 1. Background, rationale, protocol, and anti-HIV activity, *J Ethnopharmacol* 50(3):157-166, 1996.

10. Chang RS, Yeung HW: Inhibition of growth of human immunodeficiency virus in vitro by crude extracts of Chinese medicinal herbs, *Antiviral Res* 9:163-176, 1988.

11. Collins RA, Ng TB, Fong WP, et al: A comparison of human immunodeficiency virus type-1 inhibition by partially purified aqueous extracts of Chinese medicinal herbs, *Life Sci* 60(23):PL345-351, 1997.

12. el-Mekkawy S, Meselhy MR, Kusumoto IT, et al: Inhibitory effects of Egyptian folk medicines on human immunodeficiency virus (HIV) reverse transcriptase, *Chem Pharm Bull (Tokyo)* 43(4):641-648, 1995.

13. Walder R, Kalvatchev Z, Garzaro D, et al: Natural products from the tropical rain forest of Venezuela as inhibitors of HIV-1 replication, *Acta Cient Venez* 46(2):110-114, 1995.

14. Bianchi A, Adamoli R, Durante A, et al: The clinical research on medicinal plants used in HIV infection: a bibliographic search, *Int Conf AIDS* 12:852 (abstract no. 42393), 1998.

15. Chang RY, Kong XB: Meta-survey of plant and herb material as a treatment for HIV, *Int Conf AIDS* 11(1):22, 1996.

16. Houghton PJ: Compounds with anti-HIV activity from plants, *Trans R Soc Trop Med Hyg* 90(6):601-604, 1996.

17. World Health Organization (WHO): In vitro screening of traditional medicines for anti-HIV activity: memorandum from a WHO meeting, *Bull World Health Organ* 67(6):613-618, 1989.

18. Mazumder A, Raghavan K, Weinstein J, et al: Inhibition of human immunodeficiency virus type-1 integrase by curcumin, *Biochem Pharmacol* 49(8):1165-1170, 1995.

19. Li CJ, Zhang LJ, Dezube BJ, et al: Three inhibitors of type 1 human immunodeficiency virus long terminal repeat-directed gene expression and virus replication, *Proc Natl Acad Sci U S A* 90(5):1839-1842, 1993.

20. Sui Z, Salto R, Li J, et al: Inhibition of the HIV-1 and HIV-2 proteases by curcumin and curcumin boron complexes, *Bioorg Med Chem* 1(6):415-422, 1993.

21. Singh S, Aggarwal BB: Activation of transcription factor NF kappa-B is suppressed by curcumin, *J Biol Chem* 270(42):2495-5000, 1995.

22. Pizzorno J, Murray M, editors: *Textbook of natural medicine,* Seattle, 1993, Bastyr University Publications.

23. Ammon HP, Wahl MA: Pharmacology of *Curcuma longa, Planta Med* 57(1):1-7, 1991.

24. Hattori T, Kematsu S: Preliminary evidence for inhibitory effects of glycyrrhizin on HIV replication in patients with AIDS, *Antiviral Res* 11(5-6):255-261, 1989.

25. Ito M, Nakashima H, Baba M, et al: Inhibitory effect of glycyrrhizin on the in vitro infectivity and cytopathic activity of the human immunodeficiency virus [HIV (HTLV-III/LAV)], *Antiviral Res* 7(3):127-137, 1987.

26. Tochikura TS, Nakashima H, Ohashi Y, et al: Inhibition (in vitro) of replication and of the cytopathic effect of human immunodeficiency virus by an extract of the culture medium of *Lentinus edodes* mycelia, *Med Microbiol Immunol (Berl)* 177(5):235-244, 1988.

27. Ito M, Nakashima H, Baba M, et al: Inhibitory effect of glycyrrhizin on the in vitro infectivity and cytopathic activity of the human immunodeficiency virus [HIV (HTLV-III/LAV)], *Antiviral Res* 7(3):127-137, 1987.

28. Wichtl M: *Herbal drugs and phytopharmaceuticals,* Boca Raton, Fla, 1994, Medpharm Scientific Publishers.

29. Willard T: *Textbook of advanced herbology,* Calgary, Canada, 1992, Wild Rose College of Natural Healing.

30. Degar S, Prince AM, Pascual D, et al: Inactivation of the human immunodeficiency virus by hypericin: evidence for photochemical alterations of p24 and a block in uncoating, *AIDS Res Hum Retroviruses* 8(11):1929-1936, 1992.

31. Lavie G, Valentine F, Levin B, et al: Studies of the mechanisms of action of the antiretroviral agents hypericin and pseudohypericin, *Proc Natl Acad Sci U S A* 86(15):5963-5967, 1989.

32. Meruelo D, Lavie G, Lavie D: Therapeutic agents with dramatic antiretroviral activity and little toxicity at effective doses: aromatic polycyclic diones hypericin and pseudohypericin, *Proc Natl Acad Sci U S A* 85(14):5230-5234, 1988.

33. Schinazi RF, Chu CK, Babu JR, et al: Anthraquinones as a new class of antiviral agents against human immunodeficiency virus, *Antiviral Res* 13(5):265-272, 1990.

34. Lenard J, Rabson A, Vanderoef R: Photodynamic inactivation of infectivity of human immunodeficiency virus and other enveloped viruses using hypericin and rose bengal: inhibition of fusion and syncytia formation, *Proc Natl Acad Sci U S A* 90(1):158-162, 1993.

35. Yang X, Goncalves J, Gabuzda D: Phosphorylation of Vif and its role in HIV-1 replication, *J Biol Chem* 271(17):10121-10129, 1996.

36. Brinker FJ, Alstat E: *Eclectic dispensatory of botanical therapeutics,* Sandy, Ore, 1995, Eclectic Medical Publications.

37. Hoffman D: *Therapeutic herbalism: a correspondance course in phytotherapy,* Seattle, 1996, Bastyr University Publications.

38. Pitisuttithum P, Migasena S, Sunjtharasamai P: Hypericin: safety and antiretroviral activity in Thai HIV-positive volunteers, *Int Conf AIDS* 11(1):285, 1996.

39. Foster BC, Bayne MA, et al: Preclinical in vitro toxicological evaluation of hypericin and zidovudine on human leukocytes, *Int Conf AIDS* 8(2):B185, 1992.

40. James J: *AIDS Treat News* 146, 1992.

41. Piscitelli SC, Burstein AH, Chaitt D, et al: Indinavir concentrations and St John's wort, *Lancet* 355(9203):547-548, 2000.

42. Kreis W, Kaplan MH, Freeman J, et al: Inhibition of HIV replication by *Hyssop officinalis* extracts, *Antiviral Res* 14(6):323-337, 1990.

43. Fesen MR, Kohn KW, Leteurtre F, et al: Inhibitors of human immunodeficiency virus integrase, *Proc Natl Acad Sci U S A* 90(6):2399-2403, 1993.

44. Gollapudi S, Sharma HA, Aggarwal S, et al: Isolation of a previously unidentified polysaccharide (MAR-10) from *Hyssop officinalis* that exhibits strong activity against human immunodeficiency virus type 1, *Biochem Biophys Res Commun* 210(1):145-151, 1995.

45. Tochikura TS, Nakashima H, Yamamoto N: Antiviral agents with activity against human retroviruses, *J Acquir Immune Defic Syndr Hum Retrovirol* 2(5):441-447, 1989.

46. Suzuki H, Okubo A, Yamazaki S, et al: Inhibition of the infectivity and cytopathic effect of human immunodeficiency virus by water-soluble lignin in an extract of the culture medium of *Lentinus edodes* mycelia (LEM), *Biochem Biophys Res Commun* 160(1):367-373, 1989.

47. Gordon M, Guralnik M, Kaneko Y, et al: A phase II controlled study of a combination of the immune modulator, lentinan, with didanosine (ddI) in HIV patients with CD4 cells of 200-500/mm³, *J Med* 26(5-6):193-207, 1995.

48. Collins, RA, Ng TB, Fong WP, et al: A comparision of human immunodeficiency virus type 1 inhibition by partially purified aqueous extracts of Chinese medicinal herbs. *Life Sci* 60(23):PL345-351, 1997.

49. Tabba HD, Chang RS, Smith KM: Isolation, purification, and partial characterization of prunellin, an anti-HIV component from aqueous extracts of *Prunella vulgaris, Antiviral Res* 11(5-6):263-273, 1989.

50. Yao XJ, Wainberg MA, Parniak MA: Mechanism of inhibition of HIV-1 infection in vitro by purified extract of *Prunella vulgaris, Virology* 187(1):56-62, 1992.

51. Bensky FJ, Gamble A, Kapchuk T, editors: *Chinese herbal medicine,* rev ed, Seattle, 1993, Eastland Press.

52. Paris A, Strukelj B, Renko M, et al: Inhibitory effect of carnosic acid on HIV-1 protease in cell-free assays, *J Nat Prod* 56(8):1426-1430, 1993.

53. Pukl M, Umek A, Paris A: Inhibitory effect of carnosolic acid on HIV-1 protease, *Planta Med* 58(suppl 1): A632, 1992.

54. Aruoma OI, Halliwell B, Aeschbach R, et al: Antioxidant and prooxidant properties of active rosemary constituents: carnosol and carnosic acid, *Xenobiotica* 22(2):257-268, 1992.

55. Kakiuchi N, Hattori M, Ishii H, et al: Effect of benzo[c]phenanthridine alkaloids on reverse transcriptase and their binding property to nucleic acids, *Planta Med* 53(1):22-27, 1987.

56. Tan G, Pezzuto JM, Kinghorn AD: Screening of natural products as HIV-1 and HIV-2 reverse transcriptase inhibitors. In *Natural products as antiviral agents,* New York, 1992, Plenum Press.

57. Gustafson KR, Cardellina JHD, Fuller RW, et al: AIDS-antiviral sulfolipids from cyanobacteria (blue-green algae), *J Natl Cancer Inst* 81(16):1254-1258, 1989.

58. Lau AF, Siedlecki J, Anleitner J, et al: Inhibition of reverse transcriptase activity by extracts of cultured blue-green algae *(cyanophyta), Planta Med* 59(2):148-151, 1993.

59. Ayehunie S, Belay A, Hu Y, et al: Inhibition of HIV-1 replication by an aqueous extract of *Spirulina platensis (Arthospira platensis), Intl Assoc Applied Algology, Book of Abstracts* 22, 1996.

60. Hayashi K, Hayashi T, Kojima I: A natural sulfated polysaccharide, calcium spirulan, isolated from *Spirulina platensis:* in vitro and ex vivo evaluation of anti-herpes simplex virus and anti-human immunodeficiency virus activities, *AIDS Res Hum Retroviruses* 12(15):1463-1471, 1996.

61. Hayashi T, Hayashi K, Maeda M, et al: Calcium spirulan, an inhibitor of enveloped virus replication, from a blue-green alga *Spirulina platensis, J Nat Prod* 59(1):83-87, 1996.

62. Li BQ, Fu T, Yan YD, et al: Inhibition of HIV infection by baicalin—a flavonoid compound purified from Chinese herbal medicine, *Cell Mol Biol Res* 39(2):119-124, 1993.

63. Harbone J, Baxter H: *Phytochemical dictionary: a handbook of bioactive compounds from plants,* Bristol, Pa, 1993, Taylor & Francis.

64. Ono K, Nakane H: Mechanisms of inhibition of various cellular DNA and RNA polymerases by several flavonoids, *J Biochem (Tokyo)* 108(4):609-613, 1990.

65. Ono K, Nakane H, Fukushima M, et al: Inhibition of reverse transcriptase activity by a flavonoid compound, 5,6,7-trihydroxyflavone, *Biochem Biophys Res Commun* 160(3):982-987, 1989.

66. Ono K, Nakane H, Fukushima M, et al: Differential inhibitory effects of various flavonoids on the activities of reverse transcriptase and cellular DNA and RNA polymerases, *Eur J Biochem* 90(3):469-476, 1990.

67. Brinkworth RI, Stoermer MJ, Fairlie DP: Flavones are inhibitors of HIV-1 proteinase, *Biochem Biophys Res Commun* 188(2):631-637, 1992.

68. Mahmood N, Pizza C, Aquino R, et al: Inhibition of HIV infection by flavonoids, *Antiviral Res* 22(2-3):189-199, 1993.

69. Wu X, Akatsu H, Okada H: Apoptosis of HIV-infected cells following treatment with Sho-Saiko-to and its components, *Jpn J Med Sci Biol* 48(2):79-87, 1995.

70. Mayaux JF, Bousseau A, Pauwells R, et al: Triterpene derivatives that block entry of human immunodeficiency virus type 1 into cells, *Proc Natl Acad Sci U S A* 91(9): 3564-3568, 1994.

71. Pengsuparp, T, Serit M, Hughes SH, et al: Specific inhibition of human immunodeficiency virus type 1 reverse transcriptase mediated by soulatrolide: a coumarin isolated from the latex of *Calophyllum teysmannii, J Nat Prod* 59(9): 839-842, 1996.

72. Stringner, SY: Personal communication, April 9, 1998.

73. Wong CK, Leung KN, Fung KP, et al: Immunomodulatory and antitumour polysaccharides from medicinal plants, *J Int Med Res* 22:299-312, 1994.

74. Copeland R et al: Curcumin therapy in HIV-infected patients initially increase CD4 and CD8 cell counts, *Int Conf AIDS* 10(2):216, 1994.

75. Elion RA, Cohen C: Complementary medicine and HIV infection, *Comp Alt Ther Prim Care* 24(4):9, 1997.

76. Mori K, Sakai H, Suzuki S, et al: Effects of glycyrrhizin (SNMC: stronger neo-minophagen C) in hemophilia patients with HIV-1 infection, *Tohoku J Exp Med* 162(2):183-193, 1990.

77. Kinoshita S, Tsujino G, Yoshioka K, et al: Evaluation of long-term oral administration of glycyrrhizin in asymptomatic HIV-1 carrier, *Int Conf AIDS* 10(1):222, 1994.

78. Endo Y: The immunotherapy for AIDS with glycyrrhizin and/or neurotropin, *Int Conf AIDS* 9(1):492 (abstract no. P.O.B28.2143), 1993.

79. Endo Y: The immunoactivetherapy for patients with positive HIV using glycyrrhizin, *Int Conf AIDS* 10(1):218, 1994.

80. Ikegami N, Akatani K, et al: Prophylactic effect of long-term oral administration of glycyrrhizin on AIDS development of asymptomatic patients, *Int Conf AIDS* 9(1):234 (abstract no. PO.A25.0596), 1993.

81. Cooper WC, James J: An observational study of the safety and efficacy of hypericin in HIV-positive subjects, *Int Conf AIDS* 6(2):369, 1990.

82. Steinbeck-Klose A, Wernet P: Successful long-term treatment over 40 months of HIV-patients with intravenous hypericin, *Int Conf AIDS* 9(1):470, 1993.

83. Vonsover A, Steinbeck KA, Rudich C, et al: HIV-1 virus load in the serum of AIDS patients undergoing long term therapy with hypericin, *Int Conf AIDS* 11(1):120 (abstract no. Mo.B.1377), 1996.

84. Mcauliffe V, Gulick R, Hochster H, et al: A phase I dose escalation study of synthetic hypericin in HIV-infected patients (ACTG 150), *Natl Conf Hum Retroviruses Relat Infect* (1st), Dec 12-16, 159, 1993.

85. Furner V, Bek M, Gold J: A Phase I/II unblinded dose ranging study of hypericin in HIV-positive subjects, *Int Conf AIDS* 7(2):199, 1991.

86. Gulick RM, McAuliffe V, et al: Phase I studies of hypericin, the active compound in St. John's wort, as an antiretroviral agent in HIV-infected adults, AIDS Clinical Trials Group Protocols 150 and 258, *Ann Intern Med* 130(6):510-514, 1999.

87. Durant J, Chantre P, Gonzalez G, et al: Efficacy and safety of *Buxus sempervirens* L. preparations (SPV30) in HIV-infected asymptomatic patients: a multicentre, randomized, double-blind, placebo-controlled trial, *Phytomedicine* 5(1):1-10, 1998.

88. Voltchek IV, Liepins A, Nowicky JW, et al: Potential therapeutic efficacy of Ukrain (NSC 631570) in AIDS patients with Kaposi's sarcoma, *Drugs Exp Clin Res* 22(3-5):283-286, 1996.

89. D'Adamo P: *Chelidonium and Sanguinaria* alkaloids as anti-HIV therapy, *J Naturopathic Med* 3(1):31-34, 1992.

90. Calabrese C, Berman S, Babish J, et al: A phase I trial of andrographolide in HIV-positive patients and normal volunteers, *Phytother Res* 14(5):333-338, 2000.

91. Zhang Q, Khanyile C: Primary report on the use of Chinese herbal extract of *Momordica charantia* (bitter melon) in HIV-infected patients, *Int Conf AIDS* 8(3):148, 1992.

92. Byers VS, Levin AS, Waites LA, et al: A phase I/II study of trichosanthin treatment of HIV disease, *AIDS* 4:1189-1196, 1990.

93. Byers VS, Levin AS, Waites L, et al: A phase II study of the effect of trichosanthin treatment in combination with zidovudine in HIV disease, *Int Conf AIDS* 7(2):224, 1991.

94. Zhang QC: Compound Q in the treatment of AIDS: observation of self-administered AIDS treatment with injections of trichosanthin, *Int J Orient Med* 16(2):107-113, 1991.

95. Mayer RA, Sergios PA, Coonan K, et al: Trichosanthin treatment of HIV-induced immune dysregulation, *Eur J Clin Invest* 22(2):113-122, 1992.

96. Kahn JO, Arri C, Gorelick KJ, et al: Safety of high dose GLQ223 in ARC: phase IC study report, *Int Conf AIDS* 9(1):72, 1993.

96a. Byers VS, Levin AS, Malvino A, et al: A phase II study of effect of addition of trichosanthin to zidovudine in patients with HIV disease and failing antiretroviral agents, *AIDS Res Hum Retroviruses* 10(4):413-420, 1994.

97. Gorter R, Khwaja T, Linder M: Anti-HIV and immunomodulating activities of *Viscum album* (mistletoe), *Int Conf AIDS* 8(3):84, 1992.

98. Gorter R, Stoss M, el Arif N, et al: Immune modulating and anti-HIV activities of *Viscum album* (Iscador), *Int Conf AIDS* 9(1):496, 1993.

99. Gorter RW, van Wely M, Reif M, et al: Tolerability of an extract of European mistletoe among immuno-compromised and healthy individuals, *Altern Ther Health Med* 5(6):37-44, 47-48, 1999.

99a. McDaniel HR, Carpenter R, Kemp M, et al: HIV-1-infected patients respond favorably to oral Acemannan (ACE-M), *Int Conf AIDS* 6(3):209, 1990.

99b. McDaniel HR, Rosenberg LJ, McAnalley BH: CD4 and CD8 lymphocyte levels in Acemannan (ACE-M)-treated HIV-1-infected long-term survivors, *Int Conf AIDS* 9(1):498, 1993.

100. Singer J, Gill J, Arseneau R, et al: A randomized placebo-controlled trial of oral Acemannan as an adjunctive to antiretroviral therapy in advanced HIV disease, *Int Conf AIDS* 9(1):494 (abstract no. PO-B28-2153), 1993.

101. Montaner JS, Gill J, Singer J, et al: Double-blind placebo-controlled pilot trial of Acemannan in advanced HIV disease, *J Acquir Immune Defic Syndr Hum Retrovirol* 12(2):153-157, 1996.

102. Shirahata A, Mori K, Kishida K, et al: The usefulness of LEM (the extract of cultured *Lentinus edodes* mycelia) in HIV-infected hemophiliacs, *Int Conf AIDS* 6(2):372, 1990.

103. Gordon M, Bihari B, Goosby E, et al: A placebo-controlled trial of the immune modulator, lentinan, in HIV-positive patients: a phase I/II trial, *J Med* 29(5-6):305-330, 1998.

104. Fen GC, Xiaoxian W, Yaozeng L, et al: Experimental research on traditional Chinese medicinal herbs: ZY-I recipe for AIDS treatment, *Int Conf AIDS* 11(2):58, 1996.

105. Lu W, Gu YH, Wang J, et al: Clinical observation on ZY-1 in treating 52 HIV-infected patients, *Int Conf AIDS* 11(2):271, 1996.

106. Lu Weibo et al: A report on 8 seronegative converted HIV/AIDS patients with traditional Chinese medicine, *Chin Med J* 108(8):634-637, 1995.

107. Li YK, Li M, Wang K: Treat AIDS and ARC with Chinese traditional medicine "the spring of life": 27 case report, *Int Conf AIDS* 11(2):90, 1996.

108. Li M, Li Y, Kun W, et al: Treat AIDS-related multiple organs lesions (ARMOL) with Chinese traditional medicine "extract spring of life"—a report of 56 cases, *Int Conf AIDS* 12:1012 (abstract no. 60062), 1998.

109. Young MG, Sinclair TM: Proposed model of a traditional Chinese medicine treatment and research program for HIV/AIDS, *Int Conf AIDS* 11(2):271, 1996.

110. Michio T, Matusa R: Morphometrical and clinical improvement with natural remedies in infantile AIDS, *Int Conf AIDS* 11(2):270, 1996.

111. Kang LY, Pan XZ, Yang WX, et al: A study on Chinese herbal formula XQ-9302 treatment for AIDS patients, *Int Conf AIDS* 12:1004 (abstract no. 60010), 1998.

112. Goh M: Herb tea #1 treatment for AIDS patients in an AIDS nursing facility, *Int Conf AIDS* 10(2):218 (abstract no. PB0884), 1994.

113. Burack JH, Cohen MR, Hahn JA, et al: Pilot randomized controlled trial of Chinese herbal treatment for HIV-associated symptoms, *J Acquir Immune Defic Syndr Hum Retrovirol* 12(4):386-393, 1996.

114. Weber R, Loy M, Christen L, et al: Treatment of HIV-infected persons with Chinese herbs: a randomized, placebo-controlled trial, *Int Conf AIDS* 12:850 (abstract no. 42381), 1998.

115. Chileshe J: Treating AIDS-related symptoms using traditional medicine, *Int Conf AIDS* 11(2):424, 1996.

116. Homsy J, Kabatesi D, Mubiru F, et al: Herbal medicine shows potential effectiveness in PWAs with chronic diarrhea and h. zoster in Kampala, Uganda, *Int Conf AIDS* 10(2):218, 1994.

117. Homsy J, Katabira E, Kabatesi D, et al: Evaluating herbal medicine for the management of herpes zoster in human immunodeficiency virus-infected patients in Kampala, Uganda, *J Altern Complement Med* 5(6):553-565, 1999.

117a. Ssenyonga M, Brehony E: Herbal medicine—its use in treating some symptoms of AIDS, *Int Conf AIDS* 9(1):75, 1993.

118. Bora PC, Bokil A, Hira S, et al: Efficacy of Ayurvedic formulation among HIV-infected persons, *Int Conf AIDS* 11(2):269, 1996.

119. Kothandaraman R: Prevention of HIV/AIDS diseases through Siddha medicines, *Int Conf AIDS* 12:305 (abstract no. 22213), 1998.

120. Singh H, Bora P, Hira SK, et al: Comprehensive management of HIV disease—Ayurvedic approach, *Int Conf AIDS* 12:851 (abstract no. 42386), 1998.

121. Samuel M, Paramehwari S, Raja D, et al: Immunological and virological analysis of a triple combination pilot study and traditional drugs in HIV-1-infected patients in south India, *Int Conf AIDS* 12:853 (abstract no. 42395), 1998.

122. Caprani A, Miramor B, Avicenne J, et al: Drastic increase of CD4 cell counts by CHAM3 therapy in HIV-infected patients, *Int Conf AIDS* 11(2):269, 1996.

123. Bielory L: Advanced Plant Pharmaceuticals, Inc, New York, Personal communication, 2000.

124. Carter GM, Onstott M, Bingham F: Case reports of potential combination therapy using botanical substances, selected on the basis of their antiviral activity, *Int Conf AIDS* 12:851 (abstract no. 42388), 1998.

125. Standish LJ, Guiltinan J, McMahon E, et al: One year open trial of naturopathic treatment of HIV infection class IV-A in men, *J Naturopathic Med* 3:42-64, 1992.

126. Piscitelli SC: Use of complementary medicines by patients with HIV: full sail into uncharted waters, *Medscape HIV/AIDS* 6(3), 2000.

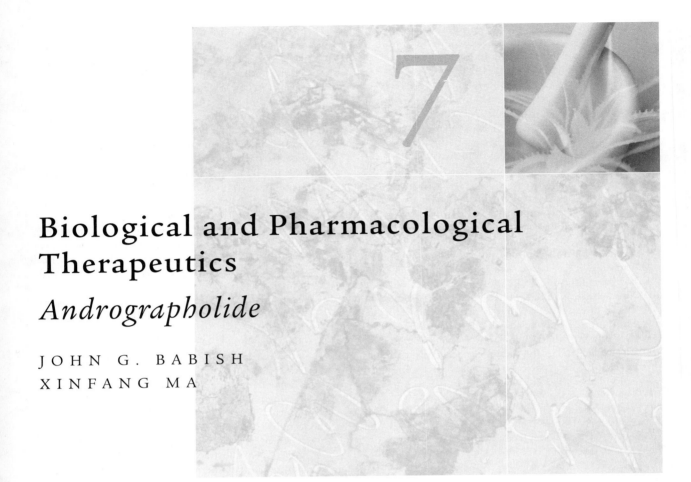

Biological and Pharmacological Therapeutics
Andrographolide

JOHN G. BABISH

XINFANG MA

ABSTRACT

*A*ndrographolide is a diterpene lactone and the main constituent of the traditional Chinese and Indian medicinal herb, *Andrographis paniculata*. Known primarily for its usefulness as a tonic and as a treatment of common viral infections, *A. paniculata* was suggested as a way to control HIV-1 infections in developing nations. When tested under laboratory conditions, andrographolide affects several facets of HIV-1 infection. These include (1) inhibition of HIV-1 cell-to-cell transmission, (2) inhibition of viral replication in peripheral blood mononuclear cells (PBMCs), and (3) inhibition of CD4+ T-cell death. An open-label, phase I clinical trial in 13 HIV-1-positive patients indicated that the patients displayed increased CD4+ T-cell counts after 6 weeks of andrographolide administration. At the molecular level, andrographolide acts as a kinase inhibitor and downregulates the expression of the cell cycle–related enzymes cyclin B and cyclin-dependent kinase 1 (CDK-1) in either cancer cells or HIV-1 infected cells. By combining andrographolide with natural compounds that target other molecular sites necessary for viral reproduction, the prospect of formulating a safe and cost-effective "natural cocktail" to control HIV-1 infections is promising. Such attributes project a possible role for andrographolide in the future management of HIV/AIDS. Since AIDS is becoming less life-threatening, the search for cost-effective medicines that can improve health and enhance the quality of life (QOL) is becoming increasingly important.

TRADITIONAL USES OF *A. PANICULATA*

The herb, *A. paniculata,* is widely used in Chinese, Thai, and Indian forms of traditional medicine. Medicinal blends of the herb generally consist of the leaves from the aerial part of the plant. In traditional Chinese medicine (TCM), *A. paniculata* is described as "bitter and cold," is related to the functions of the digestive, cardiovascular, and urinary systems, and is considered effective as an antipyretic, a detoxicant, and an anti-inflammatory agent.[1,2] In China the ground herb is known as *Chuanxinlian,* and other formulations include (1) *Chunlianqiaolio,* (2) *Yiqianxi,* (3) *Ganhelian,* (4) *Kudanchao,* and (5) *Zhanshejian.*[3] Numerous concoctions of *A. paniculata* exist in Ayurvedic medicine, and both the fresh and dried leaves, as well as the juice extracted from the shrub, are listed in the *Indian Pharmacopoeia.*[4] In Thai folklore, a preparation consisting of the leaves of *A. paniculata* is known as *Fah Talai Joan.*[5]

Typical uses of *A. paniculata* in indigenous medical systems include (1) the treatment of upper respiratory (URI) infections, (2) fever, (3) pharyngolaryngitis, (4) tonsillitis, (5) pneumonia, (6) tuberculosis, (7) herpes, (8) cough with thick sputum, (9) diarrhea, (10) bacterial dysentery, (11) ulcer, and (12) snakebite.[3,5-10] In India and other Southeast Asian countries, the herb is used as a stomachic, an antipyretic, and an antihelmintic. Diseases for which the herb is often prescribed include dysentery, enteritis, and diabetes.[5] Despite its extensive uses in traditional Oriental medicine, however, modern research on its composition, efficacy, effectiveness, mechanisms of action, and other potential clinical applications spans only the last two decades.[2]

PHARMACOLOGICALLY ACTIVE COMPONENTS OF *A. PANICULATA*

The main active chemical constituent of *A. paniculata* is the diterpene lactone andrographolide, a colorless, crystalline substance with a very bitter taste (Figure 7-1). Balmain and Connolly[11] reported

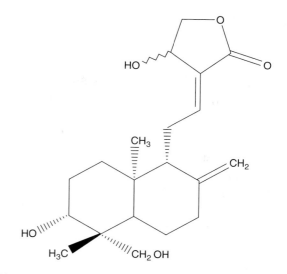

Figure 7-1 Structure of andrographolide [1R-1α [E(S*)],4a§,5α,6α,8aα]]-3-[2-[Decahydro-6-hydroxy-5-(hydroxymethyl)-5,8a-dimethyl-2-methylene-1-naph-thaleneyl]ethylidene]dihydro-4-hydroxy-2(3H)-furanon).

the isolation and identification of three diterpene lactone constituents from *A. paniculata*. They were termed *andrographolides A* (deoxyandrographolide), *B* (andrographolide), and *C* (neoandrographolide), of which *B* was the major component. Other predominant diterpene lactones identified in the herb include (1) deoxyandrographolide-19-β-D-glucoside, (2) homoandrographolide, (3) andrographan, (4) andrographon, and (5) andrographosterin. Minor diterpene lactones isolated from the whole plant include (1) 14-deoxy-11-oxoandrographolide, (2) 14-deoxy-11, (3) 12-didehydroandrographlide (andrographolide *D*), (4) andrographiside, and (5) 19-glucosyl-deoxyandrographolide.[3,12] In addition, stigmasterol was isolated from the hexane fraction of *A. paniculata.*[7]

The content of diterpene lactones in the leaves and stems of *A. paniculata* varies by season and growing region. Within a region, the highest yield of andrographolide is found before the plant blooms, and at this time the amount of andrographolide ranges from 1% to 2% of the dry weight of the leaf. For this reason, harvesting is done in the early fall. The plant grows well and is cultivated in China, India, Thailand, Sri Lanka, Indonesia, and other parts of Southeastern Asia.[2,3,13]

General Pharmacology of *A. Paniculata* and Diterpene Lactones

A. paniculata is frequently prescribed with other herbs or drugs for a variety of diseases. This was especially true in Asian countries with little exposure to Western medicines or during periods of political isolation in China, such as the Cultural Revolution. Most published studies of such combinations of herbal treatments claimed efficacy. Diseases reported to be effectively treated solely by the herb include (1) Japanese B encephalitis, (2) cervical erosion, (3) pelvic infection,[1] (4) otitis media purulenta,[14] (5) cutaneous gangrene in infants,[15] (6) vaginitis,[16] (7) leprosy,[17] (8) herpes,[18,19] (9) chicken pox and mumps,[19] (10) neurodermatitis, (11) eczema, and (12) burns.[20]

Although the range of uses for *A. paniculata* and andrographolide is impressive, the most common modern application of the herb is for the treatment of infectious diseases. Reports in scientific literature describe the successful treatment of bacterial dysentery, as well as throat and respiratory infections. However, neither *A. paniculata* nor its diterpene lactones convincingly demonstrated direct antimicrobial activity. Other applications of *A. paniculata* that are supported by clinical and laboratory research include hepatoprotection and immune stimulation.

Hepatoprotection

When *A. paniculata* products were administered before administration of the toxic agent, they showed certain protective effects against hepatotoxicity in rats induced by CCl_4 (800 mg/kg), D-semilactomine, or acetaminophen. Hepatoprotection was measured by the reduced serum concentrations of the liver-associated enzymes serum glutamate pyruvate transaminase (SGPT), serum glutamate oxaloacetate transaminase (SGOT), and alkaline phosphatase (AP) and by decreased damage to hepatocytes.[21,22] *A. paniculata* also protected against CCl_4-induced hepatic microsomal lipid peroxidation (LP),[23] and *Plasmodium berghei*-infected hepatic damage.[24] Administration of andrographolide, andrographiside, or neoandrographolide at 100 mg/kg/day for 7 days caused an elevation of cellular antioxidant defenses and a reduction in LP, resulting from a cytotoxic dose of CCl_4. In these studies, the protective effects of the glycoside forms of the diterpene lactones were greater than hepatoprotection by andrographolide.[25]

In two similar studies, administering several diterpene lactones from *A. paniculata* intraperitoneally to mice at 100 mg/kg for 3 consecutive days resulted in a significant reduction in malondialdehyde (MDA) formation and reduced glutathione (GSH) depletion and enzyme leakage after a dose of CCl_4.[26,27] As in the previous study, the diterpene lactones containing glycoside residues afforded greater hepatoprotection. Andrographolide demonstrated significant hepatoprotective activity only when administered 4 hours before the CCl_4 dose, and administration of the same 5 mg/kg/day dose over a 15-day period did not provide protection against CCl_4 hepatotoxicity.[23]

All diterpene lactones from *A. paniculata* are potent stimulators of gallbladder function. Intragastric administration of several analogs of andrographolide to rats or guinea pigs significantly increased bile flow and also induced qualitative changes in the physical properties of bile.[21,28] Andrographolide produced a significant dose-dependent (1.5 to 12 mg/kg) choleretic effect (4.8% to 73%). Furthermore, the acetaminophen-induced decrease in the volume and content of bile was prevented by andrographolide pretreatment[21]; in this study, andrographolide was more potent than silymarin, a clinically useful, natural hepatoprotective agent.

Immune Responses

A decoction of the herb *A. paniculata* increased the ability of leukocytes to engulf *Staphylococcus aureus*.[3] Animal studies indicated that the diterpene lactones from the herb increased the level of murine serum lysozyme and the phagocytic activity of phagocytes and neutrocytes.[1] Oral administration of the decoction was reported to boost the skin reaction to tuberculotoxin in cancer patients as well as in healthy individuals, suggesting that *A. paniculata* has immune stimulating effects.[29] Continual administration of sulfonated andrographolide to rabbits or mice improved the phagocytic ability of peripheral phagocytes against *Pneumonococcus* or *S. aureus*.[1]

Although diterpene lactones stimulate the immune system, they can be immunosuppressive at high doses. Murine blood clearance tests revealed that andrographolide, at a dose of 2 g/kg or higher, significantly prolonged the time needed for clearing charcoal particles from venous blood pool.[30] In vitro experiments also indicated that sulfonated andrographolide and several closely related water-soluble derivatives inhibited the incorporation of high concentrations of ^3H-thymidine to lymphocytes.[1]

Antiinfective Activity

Acute bacterial dysentery and diarrhea. Acute bacterial diarrhea was treated with a dosage regimen totaling 500 mg andrographolide per person, divided over three dosing periods per day for 6 days (2.5 to 3.0 mg/kg tid), and combined with initial rehydration therapy. This regimen cured 66 out of 80 individuals (82.5%). Seven additional patients responded favorably to the treatment, whereas only seven patients (8.8%) showed no response. The results of the treatment were confirmed by laboratory tests of stool samples.[1] In another reported study, *A. paniculata* was used to treat 1611 cases of bacterial dysentery and 955 cases of diarrhea[31]; overall effectiveness was reported to be 91%.

Although it was assumed that andrographolide and *A. paniculata* were effective against bacterial dysentery and diarrhea because they were antibacterial, studies could not confirm the antibacterial activity of either *A. paniculata* or its products. Researchers designed a clinical study to examine the antibacterial activity of *A. paniculata* in the treatment of both acute diarrhea and URT infections. They did not see any antimicrobial activity in either direct in vitro assays of the herb or in the serum of human volunteers given four different doses of the herb.[32]

In the first experiment, a direct assay of antibacterial activity of *A. paniculata* powder was performed using single isolates of *Salmonella, Shigella, Escherichia coli,* group A *streptococci,* and *S. aureus*. No antibacterial activity was detected, even at the highest concentrations of *A. paniculata*. A second study was designed to detect bactericidal activity in the serum of 10 healthy volunteers who each received a single oral dose of 1, 2, 3, or 6 g *A. paniculata*. Serum antibacterial activity was undetectable using five strains of each of the previously indicated pathogens. The researchers concluded that *A. paniculata* possessed no antimicrobial activity.

In vitro studies confirmed the lack of antibacterial activity of deoxyandrographolide, andrographolide, neoandrographolide, dehydroandrographolide, and their water-soluble derivatives from *A. paniculata*.[29,31,33] However, andrographolides exhibited excellent antidiarrheal activity against enterotoxin-induced diarrhea in animal models.[10,34] Therefore it is reasonable to infer that the antibacterial and antidiarrheal activities of *A. paniculata* or its products are not a function of direct antimicrobial activity. Rather, the apparent antiinfective efficacy of andrographolides may be due to observed immunostimulatory properties of diterpene lactones (see the section on immune responses).

Throat and respiratory tract infections. Researchers reported successful treatment of the pain and fever associated with tonsillitis with *A. paniculata*.[5] A randomized, double-blind study treated 152 adult patients with either acetaminophen or a dose of either 3 or 6 g *A. paniculata* per day for 7 days. Three days after administration of the drugs, the efficacy of acetaminophen and the higher dose of *A. paniculata* were significantly better than the lower dose of the herb in terms of the relief of fever and sore throat. No differences among the three groups were seen on the seventh day.

In two controlled, double-blind studies, Kan Jang, an *A. paniculata* product developed in Sweden, demonstrated effectiveness for the treatment of common colds when compared with placebo controls. Patients in the *A. paniculata*-treatment group experienced much shorter periods of sick leave and less severe symptoms.[2]

Infective hepatitis and jaundice. Both the hepatoprotective and antiviral effects of *A. paniculata* are demonstrated in clinical research on the efficacy of *A. paniculata* products for the treatment of viral infections of the liver. In a study reported from India, 20 cases of infective hepatitis (hepatitis A), representing both males and females, were treated over a 24-day period with a decoction of *A. paniculata* (Kalmegh) equivalent to 40 g of Kalmegh. All 20 patients exhibited normal urine and conjunctivae color. Ninety percent of the patients regained their appetite, and 83% exhibited relief from general depression. Overall, 80% of the patients were considered to be cured, and 20% were relieved of symptoms, based on biochemical and symptomatic variables.[35] A similar efficacy rate of 83% was reported on the use of *A. paniculata* for the treatment of 112 cases of hepatitis in China.[31]

Human immunodeficiency virus type 1. Researchers have reported[36-38] that extracts of heat clearing and detoxifying medicinal herbs inhibit human immunodeficiency virus-1 (HIV-1) replication; *A. paniculata* was one herb reported to have an inhibitory effect on HIV-1 replication. Additional in vitro studies of the anti-HIV-1 activity of *A. paniculata* assessed the ability of the plant extract to inhibit cell-to-cell transmission of the HIV-1 virus, using the cervical epithelial cell line ME180.[39] These experiments showed that a methanol extract of *A. paniculata* containing approximately 20% andrographolide was positive for the inhibition of viral spreading, with a median inhibitory

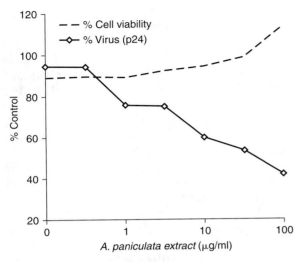

Figure 7-2 Inhibition of HIV-1 cell-to-cell transmission by a methanol extract of the herb *A. paniculata.* Data represent mean inhibition of three replicates. A 95% methanol extract of *A. paniculata* was prepared by Soxhlet's apparatus extraction of 100 g of finely ground leaves; two successive 24-hour extractions were combined, and the methanol was removed under vacuum. Testing of the inhibition of HIV-1 cell-to-cell transmission by the extract was performed using the cervical epithelial cell line ME180. Cells were plated in the interior wells of a 96-well flat-bottom microtiter plate at a density of 5×10^3 cells per well and incubated overnight. Chronically infected H9 cells (H9-SK1) were treated with 200 μg/ml mitomycin C (Sigma, St. Louis, Mo.) in complete medium for 1 hour, washed extensively, and resuspended at 4×10^5 cells per ml. The concentration of mitomycin C used resulted in the killing of the chronically infected cells within 48 hours of treatment, allowing sufficient time for cell-to-cell transmission of the virus to the ME180 cells, while assuring that the virus endpoint quantification would not include a contribution from the chronically infected cells. The *A. paniculata* extract and chronically infected cells (2×10^4 cells) were added to each well containing ME180 cells and incubated for 6 hours. After co-cultivation, the monolayer was washed extensively, and a fresh medium was added. Medium was removed, and fresh medium was added at 24 and 48 hours after infection to remove dead lymphocytes. Virus transmission was monitored by the presence of p24 in the cellular supernatant fractions at 6 days after infection. Toxicity was evaluated simultaneously using the yellow dye 3-(4,5-dimethyl-2-thiazolyl)-2,5-diphenyl-2H-tetrazolium bromide.[86]

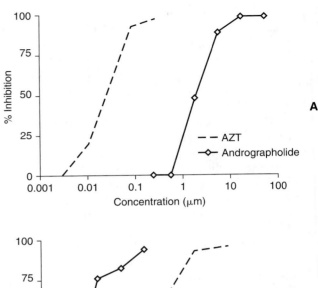

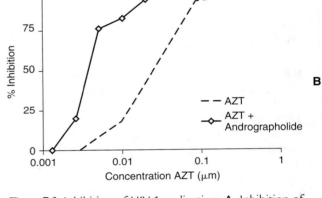

Figure 7-3 Inhibition of HIV-1 replication. **A,** Inhibition of replication of a low passage clinical HIV-1 viral isolate by AZT (positive control) and andrographolide. **B,** Demonstration of antiviral (AV) synergy over six doses of AZT with a constant 0.2 μm andrographolide concentration. Values presented represent the means of two experiments performed in duplicate as described.[84] Experiments performed with AZT and andrographolide demonstrated that the mixture of the two compounds exhibited synergistic AV activity; the IC_{50} for AZT was reduced twentyfold in the presence of 0.2 μm andrographolide.

concentration (IC_{50}) of 17 μg/ml based on p24 quantification (Figure 7-2). Inhibition of HIV transmission by the extract of *A. paniculata* was not due to overt toxicity of the ME180 cells, since the cells remained viable at the highest doses tested (100 μg extract/ml).

Andrographolide treatment of PBMCs infected with HIV virus in vitro significantly inhibited viral replication. The IC_{50} of HIV replication by andrographolide was 2 μm (Figure 7-3, *A*), whereas in the same assay system the IC_{50} of zidovudine (AZT) was 0.08 µm. In addition, andrographolide was not cytotoxic to the PBMCs. However, at doses greater than 10 µm, ^3H-thymidine incorporation was inhibited by andrographolide. Experiments performed with AZT and andrographolide demonstrated that the mixture of the two compounds exhibited synergistic antiviral (AV) activity; the IC_{50} for AZT was reduced 20-fold in the presence of 0.2 µm andrographolide (Figure 7-3, B).

An analog of andrographolide, dehydroandrographolide succinic acid monoester (DASM), was reported to inhibit HIV-1 in vitro.[40] DASM was nontoxic to H9 cells at a dose of 50 to 200 µg/ml and was inhibitory to the HIV-1(IIIB) strain at concentrations ranging from 1.6 to 3.1 µg/ml; the therapeutic ratio was approximately fiftyfold. In human PBMCs, the medium toxic concentration (TC_{50}) and the median effective concentration (EC_{50}) were between 200 to 400 µg/ml and between 0.8 to 2.0 µg/ml, respectively. Furthermore, DASM partially interfered with HIV-induced cell fusion and with the binding of HIV to the H9 cell at subtoxic concentrations.

In addition to transmission and replication, another important aspect of HIV infection and AIDS progression is T-cell depletion. Loss of T cells in AIDS is attributed to virus-infected $CD4^+$ T cells interacting with uninfected $CD4^+$ T cells. Cytopathic signaling generated via viral gp120/41-binding to CD4 receptors results in (1) G_2/M-phase cell cycle arrest, (2) the formation of syncytia, and (3) T-cell death.[41-45] This biological response was modeled using T-cell lines that properly process and express the HIV-1 envelope glycoprotein.[41] Using this model system, researchers discovered that andrographolide also blocked syncytia formation and subsequent T-cell killing (Figure 7-4) with an IC_{50} value of approximately 2 µm.[39]

Clinical trial. An open-label, phase I clinical trial in 13 male and female HIV-1-positive patients was recently reported.[46] The HIV-1-positive patients entered the study with $CD4^+$ T-cell counts between 200 and 703 cells/mm³. All persons received 5 mg andrographolide/kg tid for 3 weeks, followed by 3 weeks of 10 mg andrographolide/kg tid and a final 3 weeks of 20 mg andrographolide/kg tid.

Twelve of the 13 patients reported at least one adverse event during the study. The most common events reported were (1) headache, (2) fatigue, (3) rash, (4) loose stools or diarrhea, (5) itchy hands and feet, and (6) a bitter or metallic taste in the mouth. One patient displayed a severe allergic hypersensitivity during the second dosing period that required treatment with epinephrine and prednisone. Three of the five HIV-negative patients reported at least one adverse event, and one of the control subjects dropped from the trial due to a body rash. Such reactions were previously reported for injections of andrographolide or *A. paniculata* products. The reporting frequency of adverse events was greater during the first 3 weeks of the study, when the patients were receiving the lower 5 mg/kg dose, than it was during the second 3 weeks, when the dose was doubled. The adverse events that persisted through the second dosing period were altered taste sensation, diarrhea, and puritis. Due to the adverse events reported, including an anaphylactic reaction in one patient, a dose escalation planned at 6 weeks was replaced with a 3-week observational period.

During the first 3 weeks of the study, andrographolide administration was accompanied by a median increase of 62% in viral load (0.42 log units; $p < 0.05$). Two individuals demonstrated decreases of 77% in viral load (0.64 log units), whereas the viral load in seven persons increased by more than 50% (0.3 log units). One of the viral load increases was greater than 2 log units (99%). At the end of week 6, which represented the termination of the 10 mg/kg dosage, median viral loads had decreased by 74% (0.59 log units) from week 3 results. Twelve of the 13 patients experienced decreases in viral load; eight of these decreases were greater than 50% (0.3 log units). The viral load of one patient decreased by approximately 90% (1 log unit) during this time period. During the 3-week andrographolide withdrawal period, viral loads increased to prestudy values. Overall, the change in plasma HIV RNA levels from baseline was not statistically significant at either dose.

$CD4^+$ T-cell counts did not follow the same negative trend that was seen for viral load during the first 3-week period (Figure 7-5). A median increase in $CD4^+$ T cells of 6.8% was noted, representing an increase of 25 cells/mm³. In patients with $CD4^+$ T-cell counts less than 300, the observed increase was 26%, or 66 cells/mm³. By week 6, $CD4^+$ T cells exhibited a median increase of 105 cells/mm³, or 29% from baseline ($p < 0.05$). Three individuals experienced $CD4^+$ T-cell count increases of 47% or greater (>200 cells/mm³). No changes from baseline were noted in CD8 cells during any of the sampling periods. After the cessation of andrographolide administration, median

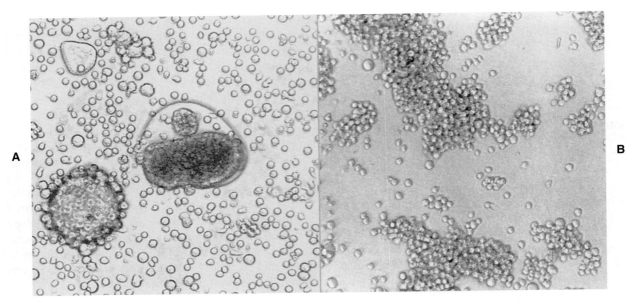

Figure 7-4 Inhibition of HIV-1 envelope glycoprotein-mediated cytopathicity. Photograph of HIV-1 envelope-mediated syncytia formation **A,** as seen under ×10 magnification. Cells were cultured as described.[41] **B,** Cells treated with 10 μm andrographolide at time of co-culture. The cell lines used in the assay protocol include the following: HIV-env 2-2 (gp160 expression, noncytopathic); HIV-env 2-8 (gp120/41 expression, cytopathic); Jurkat CD4+ T-cell line (clone E6-1), and SupT1 cell line. Cell lines were cultured in Roswell Park Memorial Institute (RPMI) medium (Gibco, Grand Island, N.Y.) and supplemented with 1% L-glutamine (Sigma, St. Louis, Mo.), 2% penicillin, 2% streptomycin, and 10% FBS-HI (Intergen, Purchase, N.Y.). The Jurkat CD4+ T-cell line (E6-1) was obtained from American Type Culture Collection (Bethesda, Md.). All other cell lines were gifts of the National Institutes of Health (NIH). The HIV-env 2-2 or HIV-env 2-8 cells were plated with both CD4+ T-cell lines (1 × 10^3 cells per cell line in 16 μl of media) in a 96-well tissue culture plate, with 50 μl of media containing varying andrographolide concentrations. The final volume was approximately 100 μl. Plates were gently shaken to ensure adequate mixing of the assay components. Cells were then co-cultured at 5% CO_2, 37° C, and 95% humidity. Syncytia were visually counted in ×10 microscope fields after 20 to 24 hours of co-culture. Assessments of cell viability were performed by both visual observation and trypan blue dye exclusion.

CD4+ T-cell counts dropped 46% but were still elevated from the median prestudy baseline values by 57 cell/mm^3 ($p < 0.05$).

Contrasting andrographolide clinical results with other therapies. Although the initial clinical results of andrographolide in HIV-1-positive patients are promising, it is difficult to judge the potential role of this natural product in HIV-1 management. The reasons for this are (1) HIV-1 therapy is complex and (2) this study was short and represented a rather small number of subjects. One way of estimating the therapeutic potential of andrographolide, however, is to compare the CD4+ T-cell responses elicited with andrographolide administration to those of HIV-1 therapeutics in clinical studies of similar size and duration.

Figure 7-6 compares the median increases in CD4+ T-cell count for andrographolide and ateviridine,[47] didanosine (ddI),[48] indinavir,[49] nevirapine,[50] ritonavir,[51] saquinavir,[52] and AZT.[53] The studies were similar to the andrographolide clinical trial in that they had a relatively short duration and used only a single test agent (monotherapy). The doses used in these trials were difficult to match, but they are both above and below the doses of andrographolide administered in

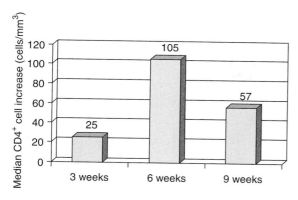

Figure 7-5 CD4+ T-cell count for 13 HIV-1-positive persons receiving 5 mg andrographolide/kg tid for 3 weeks, followed by 3 weeks of 10 mg andrographolide/kg tid and no test material during the final 3 weeks. Subjects were recruited from the Bastyr University Integrated Care Clinic (ICC) and the general population of Seattle, Washington. The HIV-1-positive patients entered the study with CD4+ T-cell counts between 200 and 703 cells/mm³ and were not currently receiving any antiretroviral therapy. During the first 3-week period, a median increase in CD4+ T cells of 6.8% was noted, representing an increase of 25 cells/mm³. In patients with CD4+ T-cell counts less than 300, the observed increase was 26%, or 66 cells/mm³. By week 6, CD4+ T cells exhibited a median increase of 105 cells/mm³, or 29% from baseline ($p < 0.05$). Three individuals experienced CD4+ T-cell increases of 47% or greater (>200 cells/mm³). No changes from baseline were noted in CD8 cells during any of the sampling periods. After cessation of andrographolide administration, median CD4+ T-cell counts dropped 46% but were still elevated from prestudy median baseline values by 57 cell/mm³ ($p < 0.05$).

the previous trial. After eliminating the nonperforming drugs ateviridine and nevirapine, the median increase in CD4+ T-cell counts was 83 cells/mm³. This compares favorably with the 110 cell/mm³ increase in CD4+ T-cell counts exhibited by andrographolide.

Mechanism of Action

At present, researchers' knowledge of how andrographolide functions in the myriad of its demonstrated pharmacologic effects is incomplete. However, the results of the research of the last 2 years indicate that the biochemical role of andrographolide in HIV-1

is as a kinase inhibitor. In other words, it interferes with the phosphorylation of proteins, specifically, enzymes involved in signal transduction pathways that are necessary for cell cycle progression and programmed cell death. This conclusion is based on results obtained with signal transduction pathways that are relevant to the physiological effects of andrographolide in normal, transformed, and HIV-1-infected cells.

Cell Cycle Arrest

In normally dividing MCF-7 human breast cancer cells, andrographolide (5 to 10 µm) causes the cells to arrest during G_1 within 48 to 72 hours. Continued exposure to concentrations causing cell cycle inhibition leads to death in nearly all cell types. At lower concentrations (1 to 2 µm) and in different T-cell types, such as the HL60 leukemia cell, andrographolide induces a G_2/M block and apoptosis. This information provides a clue as to where to begin the search for the cellular site of action of andrographolide. An examination of the signal transduction pathways involved in cell division could provide an understanding of the mechanism of action of andrographolide in both cancer and AIDS.

To describe the effect of andrographolide on signal transduction pathways involved in abnormal cell division, it is necessary to first examine the interaction between andrographolide and tyrosine phosphorylation pathways. In normal cells, tyrosylphosphoproteins represent an extremely small percentage of the total protein-linked phosphate, about 0.1%. Transformed cells have several-fold higher levels of phosphotyrosine in their proteins than normal cells.[54] Incubation of MCF-7 cells with andrographolide at concentrations between 5 to 10 µm results in the complete elimination of 4 tyrosylphosphoproteins at 85, 45, and 33 kd within 24 hours. One of these proteins, the 33 kd protein, was identified as the cell cycle control kinase CDK-1.[39] This effect is specific in that many other tyrosylphosphoproteins are not affected, even at higher concentrations of andrographolide.

Down-regulation of Cyclin B and CDK-1

MCF-7 breast cancer cells incubated with 10 µm andrographolide exhibit a rapid down-regulation of both cyclin B (Figure 7-7) and CDK-1 (Figure 7-8). As noted by the decrease in the size of the thicker, upper band in Figure 7-7, andrographolide inhibited the phosphorylation of cyclin B relative to untreated cells within the

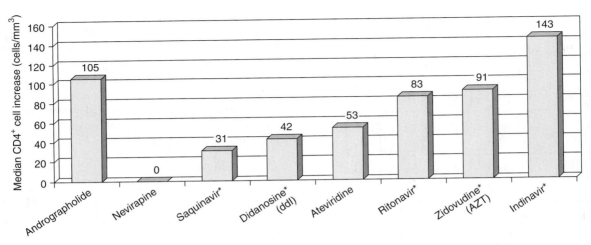

Figure 7-6 Contrasts in increases in CD4+ T-cells for eight compounds. Data for each compound were abstracted from the following publications: ateviridine,[47] ddI,[48] indinavir,[49] nevirapine,[50] ritonavir,[51] saquinavir,[52] and AZT.[53] The studies were similar to the andrographolide trial in that they were of relatively short duration (~12 weeks) and used a single test agent (monotherapy). *Indicates a US FDA-approved AIDS therapeutic.

first 24 hours of treatment. After 48 hours of postexposure, total phosphorylated cyclin B expression decreased more than 50% compared to that of controls. In a similar fashion but delayed in time, CDK-1 phosphorylation decreased relative to controls, with the maximal response occurring 48 hours after treatment (Figure 7-8).

Other recent studies indicate that andrographolide exhibits dose-responsive inhibition of c-Mos, mitogen-activated protein kinase (MAPK), and the apototic proteins c-Myc, p53, Bcl-2, Bcl-xL, and Bax.[39] In these studies, the inhibition of the apototic proteins correlated with both the inhibition of syncytium formation by the HIV-1 protein gp120/41 and cell death.

Signal Transduction Pathways Shared in HIV-1 Infection and Cancer

It is interesting that the effects of andrographolide on both cancer cells and HIV-infected cells follow similar dose-response profiles. This implies that andrographolide affects signal transduction pathways that are critical for cancer cell division, as well as HIV-1 replication. In this regard, one putative target for andrographolide is the CDK-1/cyclin B complex, also known as the maturation promoting factor or the M-phase promoting factor (MPF).[55,56] These proteins belong to a family of cell division control enzymes that serve to con-

trol and coordinate the molecular events of cell division in all eukaryotic cells.[57] In resting cells, neither CDK-1 nor cyclin B are expressed. As the cell prepares to divide, CDK-1 concentrations increase through G_1 and the G_1/S transition, reaching maximal levels in the S, G_1, and M phases.[58] CDK-1 functions as a serine/threonine kinase. Its catalytic activity is regulated primarily through posttranslational modifications, including cycles of phosphorylation and dephosphorylation,[59] interactions with the cyclins, such as cyclin B,[59,60] and intracellular compartment translocation.[60]

Overexpression of CDK-1 and cyclin B is reported for many cancer types.[61-66] Also, the formation of syncytia by the interaction of HIV-infected and noninfected T cells, as well as HIV-1 replication, are accompanied by overexpression of cyclin B, hyperphosphorylation of CDK-1, and induced expression of c-Mos.[42,44,45,67] Therefore andrographolide may inhibit HIV-1 cytopathicity and replication by limiting the formation of the CDK-1/cyclin B complex necessary for the establishment of the G_2/M block.

The pathways involved in this proposed action of andrographolide are presented schematically in Figure 7-9. As mentioned earlier, andrographolide inhibits the activation of cyclin B through a signaling pathway that may involve c-Mos. By inhibiting the phosphorylation of cyclin B, the formation of the active CDK-1/cyclin B complex is prevented. The steps

MCF-7 lysate with α-cyclin B antibody

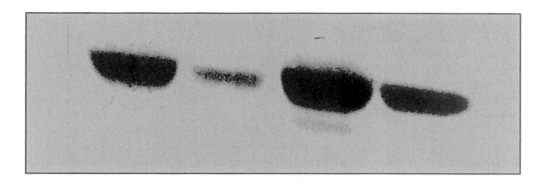

Control   5 μg/ml   Control   5 μg/ml

48 hr   24 hr

Figure 7-7. The down-regulation of cyclin B by 10 μm andrographolide in MCF-7 human breast cancer cells at 24 and 48 hours of exposure. The human breast adenocarcinoma cell line MCF-7 was cultured at 370° C in a 5% CO_2 balanced air environment. Cells were subcultured by centrifuging (1000X g for 3 minutes) and suspending in 100 ml of fresh media to a cell density of 5.0 × 10^5 cell/ml. After exposure to 10 μm andrographolide, cells were harvested at 24 and 48 hours by centrifugation and washed three times in PBS (phosphate-buffered saline) at 40° C and lysed in 20 mm Tris buffer (pH 8.0) with 137 mm NaCl, 10% glycerol, 1% Nonidet P-40, 1 mm phenyl-methylsulfonyl fluoride (PMSF), 0.15 units/ml of aprotonin, and 1 mm sodium orthovanadate at 40° C for 20 minutes. Sodium dodecylsulfate-polyacrimide gel electrophoresis (SDS-PAGE) was carried out as described,[85] using 7.5% to 10% polyacrylamide gels with the modification that MCF-7 cell lysates (100 μg protein/lane) were subjected to heat treatment (100° C) for 8 minutes. The immunoblotting was carried out as described[87]; however, a MilliBlot-SDE electroblot apparatus (Millipore, Bedford, Mass.) was used to transfer proteins from polyacrylamide gels to an Immobilon membrane filter (Millipore, Bedford, Mass.). Complete transfers were accomplished between 25 to 30 minutes at 500 mA. Membrane filters were blocked by incubating in Tris buffer saline (TBS) (50 mm Tris, 150 mm NaCl, pH 7.5) containing 5% commercial nonfat dry milk for 30 minutes at room temperature and incubated for 2 hours with 5 μg/ml antibody in TBS with Tween 20 (TBST) (0.05% Tween 20 in TBS). Molecular weights of immunostained proteins were estimated by adding molecular weight standards to reference lanes and by staining the membrane filters with Amido black 10 B. To visualize the antibody reactions, the membranes were incubated for 2 hours at room temperature with alkaline phosphatase-conjugated antirabbit IgG diluted 1:1000 in TBST and developed for 15 minutes. Both the concentration and phosphorylation status of cyclin B were reduced at 24 and 48 hours after dosing in MCF-7 whole cell lysates exposed to 10 μm andrographolide. However, unlike CDK-1, it was the nonphosphorylated form (lower band) of cyclin B that was more demonstrably affected during the 24-hour time period.

MCF-7 lysate with α-p34 cdc2 antibody

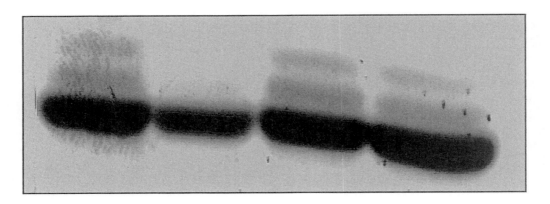

Control   5 μg/ml   **Control   5 μg/ml**

48 hr   **24 hr**

Figure 7-8 The down-regulation of CDK-1 (p34 cdc2) by 10 μm andrographolide in MCF-7 human breast cancer cells at 24 and 48 hours of exposure. The human breast adenocarcinoma cell line MCF-7 was cultured at 370° C in a 5% CO_2 balanced air environment. Cells were subcultured by centrifuging (1000X g for 3 minutes) and suspending in 100 ml of fresh media to a cell density of 5.0×10^5 cell/ml. After exposure to 10 μm andrographolide, cells were harvested at 24 and 48 hours by centrifugation and washed three times in PBS (phosphate-buffered saline) at 40° C and lysed in 20 mm Tris buffer (pH 8.0) with 137 mm NaCl, 10% glycerol, 1% Nonidet P-40, 1 mm phenylmethylsulfonyl fluoride, 0.15 units/ml of aprotonin, and 1 mm sodium orthovanadate at 40° C for 20 minutes. Sodium dodecylsulfate-polyacrimide gel electrophoresis (SDS-PAGE) was carried out as described,[85] using 7.5% to 10% polyacrylamide gels with the modification that MCF-7 cell lysates (100 μg protein/lane) were subjected to heat treatment (100° C) for 8 minutes. The immunoblotting was carried out as described[87]; however, a MilliBlot-SDE electroblot apparatus (Millipore, Bedford, Mass.) was used to transfer proteins from polyacrylamide gels to an Immobilon membrane filter (Millipore, Bedford, Mass.). Complete transfers were accomplished between 25 to 30 minutes at 500 mA. Membrane filters were blocked by incubating in TBS (50 mm Tris, 150 mm NaCl, pH 7.5) containing 5% commercial nonfat dry milk for 30 minutes at room temperature and were incubated for 2 hours with 5 μg/ml antibody in TBST (0.05% Tween 20 in TBS). Molecular weights of immunostained proteins were estimated by adding molecular weight standards to reference lanes and by staining the membrane filters with Amido black 10 B. To visualize the antibody reactions, the membranes were incubated for 2 hours at room temperature with alkaline phosphatase-conjugated antirabbit IgG diluted 1:1000 in TBST and developed for 15 minutes. Both the concentration and phosphorylation status of CDK-1 were reduced at 24 and 48 hours after dosing in whole cell lysates exposed to 10 μm andrographolide. Control samples exhibited three staining bands with the anti-CDK-1 antibody. The lowest band represents the nonphosphorylated form, whereas the two upper bands represent increasing phosphorylation status. Within 24 hours, a decrease in the extent of phosphorylation of CDK-1 can be readily observed as a loss in the staining intensity of the hyperphosphorylated band compared to that of the controls. At 48 hours, both upper bands representing phosphoprotein had nearly disappeared, and a decrease was noted in the major staining band as well.

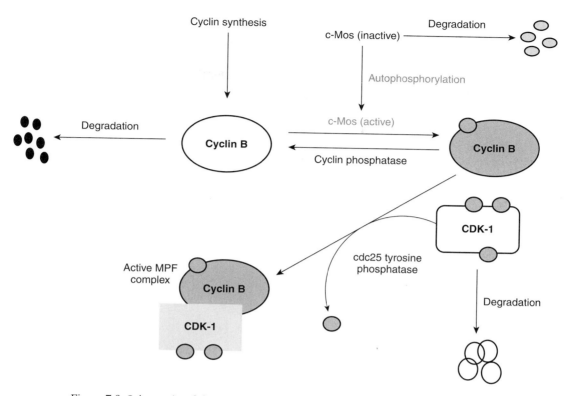

Figure 7-9 Schematic of the proposed mechanism of action of andrographolide.

necessary for the formation of an enzymatically active CDK-1/cyclin B complex include (1) activation of cdc25 tyrosine phosphatase by cyclin B, (2) removal of a phosphate from a tyrosine residue of CDK-1 by cdc25, and (3) the interaction of phosphorylated cyclin B with dephosphorylated CDK-1.[68] Blocking the formation of the active CDK-1/cyclin B complex through the inhibition of cyclin B phosphorylation by andrographolide thereby suppresses HIV-1 replication, syncytia formation, and infectivity.

Synergy with Other Natural Products for AIDS Treatment

Since researchers now recognize that the control and management of HIV-1 can only be achieved through multiple drug therapy,[69] this chapter includes speculation about a possible role for andrographolide in a multiple drug regimen. Searching the scientific literature for other natural products with AV effects leads to some possibilities, which are examined in the next section.

Combinations with Natural Plant Products

The bioflavonoid quercetin is a naturally occurring, antiviral compound that possesses the ability to inhibit a wide variety of tyrosine kinases.[70-72] Specifically, quercetin inhibits the binding of HIV-1 gp120 to CD4 receptors,[73] HIV-1 integrase,[74] and Moloney murine leukemia virus reverse transcriptase (MMLV-RT).[75] In vitro median inhibitory concentrations for quercetin against MMLV-RT were reported to be 0.06 μm. Figure 7-10 depicts these results in comparison with other bioflavanoids tested. The glucoside form of quercetin also inhibits HIV-1 RT.[76] The speculation that quercetin, in combination with andrographolide, is a potent inhibitor of HIV-1 replication is supported by the observations that quercetin (1) is active at molecular sites distinct from those affected by andrographolide and (2) demonstrates synergy with other compounds in viral systems.[77-79]

The triterpenic compound oleanolic acid is similar to andrographolide with respect to the range of its pharmacological effects.[80] Many of these effects, such

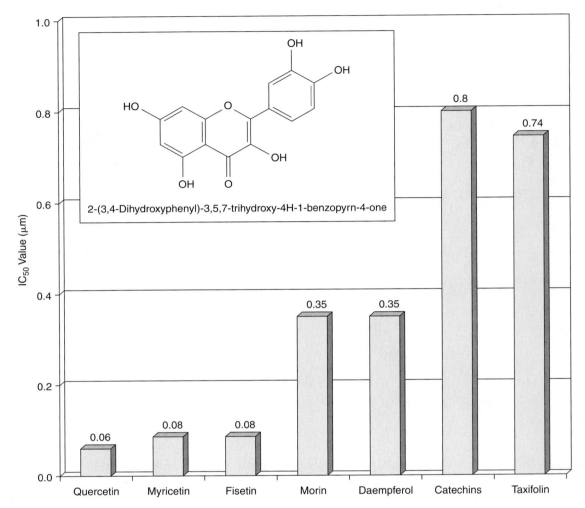

Figure 7-10 Median inhibitory concentrations of seven flavonoids on Moloney murine leukemia virus reverse transcriptase activity (MMLV-RT).[75] Structure presented in graph is that of quercetin, the most active of the flavonoids tested.

as hepatoprotective effects, immune stimulating effects, AV effects, and antineoplastic effects, overlap those of andrographolide. In addition to these biological activities, oleanolic acid is described in the scientific literature as a potentially excellent inhibitor of HIV-1 protease dimerization.[81]

The active protease of HIV-1 is formed of two identical half-molecules that contribute to the formation of one active site. This dimerization process is a critical step in the formation of the active protease and is sensitive to inhibition by certain triterpenes and peptides. The triterpene oleanolic acid fits the molecular criteria for a nonpeptide pharmacophore capable of intercalating between the monomers and preventing the formation of an active dimer.[81] With a calculated median inhibitory constant of 1 m, oleanolic acid projects greater AV activity than any of the other natural triterpenes modeled (Figure 7-11). Assuming that oleanolic acid targets molecular sites that differ from those of andrographolide and quercetin, it could function in concert with andrographolide and quercetin in an anti-HIV natural cocktail.

This combination of natural products has several distinct advantages. First, the molecular targets in-

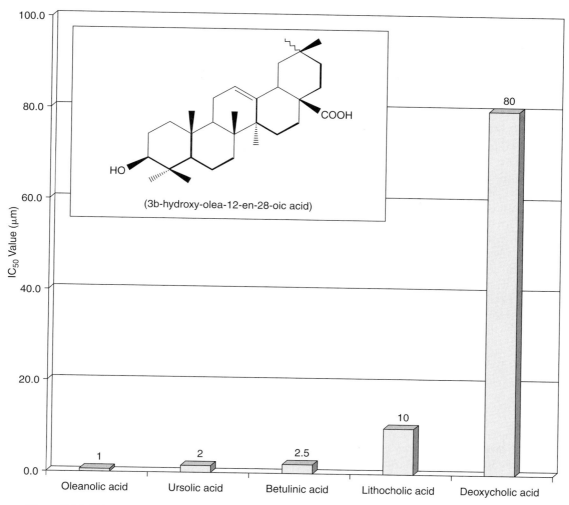

Figure 7-11 Triterpenes as potential dimerization inhibitors of HIV-1 protease, presented with median inhibitory concentrations of five triterpenes.[81] Structure presented in graph is that of oleanolic acid, estimated to be the most active of the series.

clude both HIV-1 RT and integrase, which are unique to the virus, and a cellular enzyme that is necessary for viral infectivity and replication. Such a group of sites dramatically decreases the probability of viral resistance to the drug regimen. Second, since they have demonstrated synergy with AZT and other drug combinations, they may be useful in current combinations. Third, in addition to its anti-HIV activity, either andrographolide or oleanolic acid may be useful as an hepatoprotectant. Similarly, quercetin's and oleanolic acid's functions as antioxidants may also be useful against drug toxicities and as immunostimulants.

APPLICATIONS

Those persons in whom current drug therapies have either failed or elicited toxicity could use either this combination or a similar one. It is estimated that multidrug therapy for AIDS fails between 40% to 60% of the time.[82] Additionally, the low cost of such a cocktail would enable it to be used in developing countries where the impact of AIDS is greatest and the cost of triple combination therapy is prohibitive.[83] Specifically, research on the in vitro effectiveness of combinations of active natural products on HIV-1 replication and infectivity, coupled with historical data on human toxicity, could define a botanical cocktail with high AV activity and a wide margin of safety.

SUMMARY

Although further research is needed to establish the role of andrographolide in the management of HIV-1, certain consistent, reproducible effects of andrographolide can be summarized. Andrographolide (1) arrests the growth of cancer cells at low concentrations; (2) inhibits HIV-1 cell-to-cell transmission, replication, and syncytia formation; (3) stimulates immune function; (4) increases the effectiveness of AZT; (5) protects against chemically induced liver damage; (6) maintains pharmacological activity with oral administration; and (7) possesses a wide margin of safety. Such characteristics project a possible role for andrographolide in the future management of HIV/AIDS. Since AIDS is becoming less life-threatening, the search for medicines that can improve health and enhance the quality of life (QOL) is becoming increasingly important.

References

1. Yin J, Guo L: *Contemporary traditional Chinese medicine,* Beijing, 1993, Xie Yuan.
2. Sandberg F: *Swedish herbal institute: Andrographis herba Chuanxinlian,* Austin, Tex, 1994, American Botanical Council.
3. Huang TK: *Handbook of compositions and pharmacology of traditional Chinese medicine,* Beijing, 1994, China Medical and Technology Press.
4. Bhat VS, Nanavati DD: *A. paniculata* (Kalmegh), *Indian Drugs* 15:187-190, 1978.
5. Thamlikitkul V, Dechatiwongse T, Theerapong S, et al: Efficacy of *Andrographis paniculata* Nees for pharyngotonsillitis in adults, *J Med Assoc Thai* 74:437-442, 1991.
6. Huang KC: *The pharmacology of Chinese herbs,* Boca Raton, Fla., 1993, CRC Press.
7. Siripong P, Kongkathip B, Preechanukool K, et al: Cytotoxic diterpenoid constituents from *Andrographis paniculata* Nees leaves, *J Sci Soc Thai* 18(4):187-194, 1992.
8. Nadkarni AK: *Indian materia medica, vol 1,* Panvel, India, 1976, Dhootpapeshwar Prakashan, Ltd.
9. Madav S, Tripathi HC, Tandan SK, et al: Analgesic, antipyretic, and antiulcerogenic effects of andrographolide, *Indian J Pharm Sci* 57:121-125, 1995.
10. Gupta S, Choudhry MA, Yadava JNS, et al: Antidiarrheal activity of diterpenes of *Andrographis* (Kalmegh) against *Escherichia coli* enterotoxin in in vivo models, *Int J Crude Drug Res* 28:273-283, 1990.
11. Balmain A, Connolly JD: Isolation and identification of three diterpene constituents from *Andrographis paniculata, J Chem Soc Pekin Trans* I:1247-1251, 1973.
12. Matsuda T, Kuroyanagi M, Sugiyama S, et al: Cell differentiation-inducing diterpenes from *Andrographis paniculata* Nees, *Chem Pharm Bull (Tokyo)* 42:1216-1225, 1994.
13. Taludar PB, Datta AK: Quantitative estimation of andrographolide by TLC, *Indian J Applied Chem* 32:25-32, 1969.
14. Anonymous: Baoan County Hospital of Guangdong: effects of *Andrographis paniculata* on intestinal function in typhoid fever patients, *New Med* 5:29-30, 1972.
15. Qi WC: Investigation of 45 cases of infant cutaneous gangrene treated by Yi-Jian-Xi cream, *Trad Chinese Med Fujian* 4:32, 1965.
16. Anonymous: Lingtang Town Hospital of Gaoyou County: treating vaginitis using *Andrographis paniculata, Jiangshu Med* 6:45-46, 1975c.
17. Anonymous: No. 31 Field Hospital of the Peoples' Liberation Army: a summary of the clinical effects of *Andrographis paniculata* and andrographolide on 112 leprosy cases, *J Protect Cure Derm Dis* 2:158-164, 1975b.
18. Huang QZ: Treating herpes using *Andrographis paniculata* products, *Guangxi Health* 5:43, 1974.
19. Hang QZ: Treating herpes, chicken pox, mumps, and neurodermatitis using *Andrographis paniculata* products, *Barefoot Doctor Guangxi* 9:21, 1978.
20. Anonymous: Cooperative Clinic of Zuoqiao, Sanca, Douchang, Jiangxi: treating burns using pumpkin pulp plus *Andrographis paniculata* powder, *J Barefoot Doctor* 4:11, 1975a.
21. Visen PK, Shukla B, Patnaik GK, et al: Andrographolide protects rat hepatocytes against paracetamol-induced damage, *J Ethnopharmacol* 40:131-136, 1993.
22. Handa SS, Sharma A: Hepatoprotective activity of andrographolide against galactosamine and paracetamol intoxication in rats, *Indian J Med Res* 92:284-292, 1990.
23. Choudhury BR, Poddar MK: Andrographolide and Kalmegh *(Andrographis paniculata)* extract: in vivo and in vitro effect on hepatic lipid peroxidation, *Methods Find Exp Clin Pharmacol* 6:481-485, 1984.
24. Chander R, Srivastava V, Tandon JS, et al: Antihepatotoxic activity of diterpenes of *Andrographis paniculata* (Kalmegh) against plasmodium berghei-induced hepatic damage in mastomys natalensis, *Int J Pharmacog* 33:135-138, 1995.
25. Koul IB, Kapil A: Effect of diterpenes from *Andrographis paniculata* on antioxidant defense system and lipid peroxidation, *Indian J Pharmacol* 26:296-300, 1994.
26. Kapil A, Koul IB, Banerjee SK, et al: Antihepatotoxic effects of major diterpenoid constituents of *Andrographis paniculata, Biochem Pharmacol* 46:182-185, 1993.
27. Darmograi VN, Krivenchuk PE, Litvinenko VI: Flavonoids of *Gypsophila paniculata* L., *Farmatsiia* 18:30-32, 1969.

28. Chaudhuri SK: Influence of *Andrographis paniculata* (Kalmegh) on bile flow and hexabarbitone sleeping in experimental animals, *Indian J Exp Biol* 16:830-832, 1978.

29. Anonymous: Traditional Chinese Herbal Medicine Group of the Second People's Hospital of Hangzhou City, *Newsletter Sci Technol* (Med Health section) 4:36, 1978.

30. Ou ZN: Effect of andrographolide on the clearance of carbon particles from mouse venous blood, *Acad J First Med College People's Lib Army* 8(1):37, 1988.

31. Deng WL: Outline of current clinical and pharmacological research on *Andrographis paniculata in* China, *Newsletter Chinese Herb Med* 10:27-31, 1978b.

32. Leelarasamee A, Trakulsomboon S, Sittisomwong N: Undetectable antibacterial activity of *Andrographis paniculata* (Burma) wall, ex ness, *J Med Assoc Thai* 3:299-304, 1990.

33. Deng WL: Preliminary studies on the pharmacology of the *Andrographis* product dihydroandrographolide sodium succinate, *Newsletter Chinese Herb Med* 8:26-28, 1978a.

34. Gupta S, Yadava JNS, Tandon JS: Antisecretory (antidiarrhoeal) activity of Indian medicinal plants against *Escherichia coli* enterotoxin-induced secretion in rabbit and guinea pig ileal loop models, *Int J Pharmacog* 31(3):198-204, 1993.

35. Chaturvedi GN, Tomar GS, Tiwari SK, et al: Three clinical studies on Kalmegh *(Andrographis paniculata)* in infective hepatitis, *J Int Institute Ayurveda* 2:208-211, 1983.

36. Weibo Lu: Prospect for study on treatment of AIDS with traditional Chinese medicine, *J Tradit Chinese Med* 15(1):3-9, 1995.

37. Otake T, Mori H, Morimoto M, et al: Screening of Indonesian plant extracts for antihuman immunodeficiency virus type 1 (HIV-1) activity, *Phytother Res* 9(1): 6-10, 1995.

38. Wu B: Recent development of studies on traditional Chinese medicine in prophylaxis and treatment of AIDS, *J Tradit Chinese Med* 12:10-20, 1992.

39. Ma X, Rininger J, Chigurupati P, et al: Biochemical pathways of inhibiting human immunodeficiency virus 1 replication and cytopathicity by andrographolide, *Am Soc Microbiol* T12:538, 1997 (abstract).

40. Chang RS, Ding L, Gai QC, et al: Dehydroandrographolide succinic acid monoester as an inhibitor against the human immunodeficiency virus, *Proc Soc Exp Biol Med* 197:59-66, 1991.

41. Tani Y, Tian H, Lane HC, et al: 1993 Normal T-cell receptor-mediated signaling in T-cell lines stably expressing HIV-1 envelope glycoproteins, *J Immunol* 151:7337-7348, 1993.

42. Cohen DI, Tani Y, Tian H, et al: Participation of tyrosine phosphorylation in the cytopathic effect of human immunodeficiency virus 1, *Science* 256:542-545, 1992.

43. Tani Y, Donoghue E, Sharpe S, et al: Enhanced in vitro human immunodeficiency virus type 1 replication in B cells expressing surface antibody to the TM Env protein, *J Virol* 68:1942-1950, 1994.

44. Kolesnitchenko V, King L, Riva A, et al: A major human immunodeficiency virus type 1-initiated killing pathway distinct from apoptosis, *J Virol* 71:9753-9763, 1997.

45. Tian H, Lempicki R, King L, et al: HIV envelope-directed signaling aberrancies and cell death of CD4$^+$ T cells in the absence of TCR co-stimulation, *Int Immunol* 8:65-74, 1996.

46. Calabrese C, Berman SH, Babish JG et al: A phase I trial of andrographolide in HIV-positive patients and normal volunteers, *Phytother Res* 14(5):333-338, 2000.

47. Mieke A, Been-Tiktak B, Williams I, et al: Safety, tolerance, and efficacy of atevirdine in asymptomatic human immunodeficiency virus-infected individuals, *Antimicrob Agents Chemother* 40:2664-2668, 1996.

48. Ragni MV, Amato DA, LoFaro ML, et al: Randomized study of didanosine monotherapy and combination therapy with zidovudine in hemophilic and non-hemophilic subjects with asymptomatic human immunodeficiency virus-1 infection, AIDS Clinical Trial Groups, *Blood* 85(9):2337-2346, 1995.

49. Stein DS, Fish DG, Bilello JA, et al: A 24-week open-label phase I/II evaluation of the HIV protease inhibitor MK-639 (indinavir), *AIDS* 10(5):485-492, 1996.

50. deJong MD, Vella S, Carr A, et al: High-dose nevirapine in previously untreated human immunodeficiency virus type 1-infected persons does not result in sustained suppression of viral replication, *J Infect Dis* 175(4):966-970, 1997.

51. Markowitz M, Sagg M, Powderly WG, et al: A preliminary study of ritonavir, an inhibitor of HIV-1 protease, to treat HIV-1 infection, *New Engl J Med* 333(23):1534-1539, 1995.

52. Schapiro JM, Winters MA, Stewart F, et al: The effect of high-dose saquinavir on viral load and CD4$^+$ T-cell counts in HIV-infected patients, *Ann Intern Med* 124(12): 1039-1050, 1996.

53. Brun-Vezinet F, Boucher C, Loveday C, et al: HIV-1 viral load, phenotype, and resistance in a subset of drug-naive participants from the Delta trial, The National Virology Groups, Delta Virology Working Group and Coordinating Committee, *Lancet* 350(9083):983-990, 1997.

54. Hunter T: A thousand and one protein kinases, *Cell* 50:823-829, 1987.

55. O'Connor PM, Ferris DK, White GA, et al: Relationships between cdc2 kinase, DNA cross-linking, and cell cycle perturbations induced by nitrogen mustard, *Cell Growth Differ* 3:43-52, 1992.

56. Pines J, Hunter T: Human cyclins A and B1 are differentially located in the cell and undergo cell cycle-dependent nuclear transport, *J Cell Biol* 115:1-17, 1991.

57. Draetta G: Cell cycle control in eukaryotes: molecular mechanisms of cdc2 activation, *Trends Biochem Sci* 15:378-383, 1990.

58. Loyer P, Glaise D, Cariou S, et al: Expression and activation of CDKs (1 and 2) and cyclins in the cell cycle progression during liver regeneration, *J Biol Chem* 269:2491-2500, 1994.

59. Krek W, Nigg EA: Differential phosphorylation of vertebrate p34 cdc2 kinase at the G_1/S and G_2/M transitions of the cell cycle: identification of major phosphorylation sites, *EMBO J* 10:305-316, 1991.

60. Booher R, Beach D: Interaction between cdc13$^+$ and cdc2$^+$ in the control of mitosis in fission yeast: dissociation of the G_1 and G_2 roles of the cdc2$^+$ protein kinase, *EMBO J* 6:3441-3447, 1987.

61. Rice RH, Steinmann KE, deGraffenried LA, et al: Elevation of cell cycle control proteins during spontaneous immortalization of human keratinocytes, *Mol Biol Cell* 4:185-194, 1993.

62. Steinmann KE, Pei XF, Stoppler H, et al: Elevated expression and activity of mitotic regulatory proteins in human papillomavirus-immortalized keratinocytes, *Oncogene* 9:387-394, 1994.

63. Oshima J, Steinmann KE, Campisi J, et al: Modulation of cell growth, p34 cdc2, and cyclin A levels by SV-40 large T-antigen, *Oncogene* 8:2987-2993, 1993.

64. Yasui W, Ayhan A, Kitadai Y, et al: Increased expression of p34 cdc2 and its kinase activity in human gastric and colonic carcinomas, *Int J Cancer* 53:36-41, 1993.

65. Keyomarsi K, Pardee AB: Redundant cyclin overexpression and gene amplification in breast cancer cells, *Proc Natl Acad Sci U S A* 90:1112-1116, 1993.

66. Kamb A: Cell cycle regulators and cancer, *Trends Genet* 11:136-140, 1995.

67. Kolesnitchenko V, Wahl LM, Tian H, et al: Human immunodeficiency virus 1 envelope-initiated G_2-phase programmed cell death, *Proc Natl Acad Sci U S A* 92:11889-11893, 1995.

68. Galaktionov K, Beach D: Specific activation of cdc25 tyrosine phosphatases by B-type cyclins: evidence for multiple roles of mitotic cyclins, *Cell* 67:1181-1194, 1991.

69. Doran CM: New approaches to using antiretroviral therapy for the management of HIV infections. *Ann Pharmacother* 31:228-236, 1997.

70. Daikoku T, Shibata S, Goshima F, et al: Purification and characterization of the protein kinase encoded by the UL13 gene of herpes simplex virus type 2, *Virology* 235:82-93, 1997.

71. Angeletti PC, Engler JA: Tyrosine kinase-dependent release of an adenovirus preterminal protein complex from the nuclear matrix, *J Virol* 70:3060-3067, 1996.

72. Formica JV, Regelson W: Review of the biology of quercetin and related bioflavonoids, *Food Chem Toxicol* 33:1061-1080, 1995.

73. Mahmood N, Piacente S, Pizza C, et al: The anti-HIV activity and mechanisms of action of pure compounds isolated from *Rosa damascena*, *Biochem Biophys Res Commun* 229:73-79, 1996.

74. Fesen MR, Kohn KW, Leteurtre F, et al: Inhibitors of human immunodeficiency virus integrase, *Proc Natl Acad Sci U S A* 90:2399-2403, 1993.

75. Chu SC, Hsieh YS, Lin JY: Inhibitory effects of flavonoids on Moloney murine leukemia virus reverse transcriptase activity, *J Nat Prod* 55:179-183, 1992.

76. el-Mekkawy S, Meselhy MR, Kusumoto IT, et al: Inhibitory effects of Egyptian folk medicines on human immunodeficiency virus (HIV) reverse transcriptase, *Chem Pharm Bull (Tokyo)* 43:641-648, 1995.

77. Ohnishi E, Bannai H: Quercetin potentiates TNF-induced antiviral activity, *Antiviral Res* 22:327-331, 1993.

78. Amoros M, Simoes CM, Girre L, et al: Synergistic effect of flavones and flavonols against herpes simplex virus type 1 in cell culture: comparison with the antiviral activity of propolis, *J Nat Prod* 55:1732-1740, 1992.

79. Mucsi I, Gyulai Z, Beladi I: Combined effects of flavonoids and acyclovir against herpesviruses in cell cultures, *Acta Microbiol Hung* 39:137-147, 1992.

80. Liu J: Pharmacology of oleanolic acid and ursolic acid, *J Ethnopharmacol* 49:57-68, 1995.

81. Quere L, Wenger T, Schramm HJ: Triterpenes as potential dimerization inhibitors of HIV-1 protease, *Biochem Biophys Res Commun* 227:484-488, 1996.

82. Puzzanghera J: AIDS drugs fail many, Knight-Ridder Newspapers, Sept 30, 1997.

83. Anonymous: World's AIDS—the worst is still to come (news), *Science* 278(5344):1715, 1997.

84. Buckheit RW Jr, Fliakas-Boltz V, Decker WD, et al: Biological and biochemical anti-HIV activity of the benzothiadiazine class of nonnucleoside reverse transcriptase inhibitors, *Antiviral Res* 25:43-56, 1994.

85. Laemmli UK, Favre M: Maturation of the head of bacteriophage T4: I. DNA packaging events, *J Mol Biol* 80:575-599, 1973.

86. Mossman T: Rapid colorimetric assay for cellular growth and survival: applications to proliferation and cytotoxicity assays, *J Immunol Methods* 65:55-63, 1983.

87. Towbin H, Staehelin T, Gordon J: Electrophoretic transfer of proteins from polyacrylamide gels to nitrocellulose sheets: procedure and some applications, *Proc Natl Acad Sci U S A* 76:4350-4354, 1979.

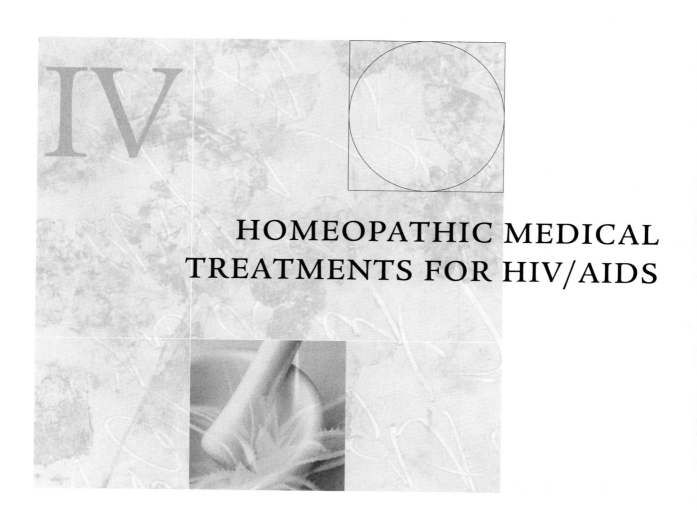

HOMEOPATHIC MEDICAL
TREATMENTS FOR HIV/AIDS

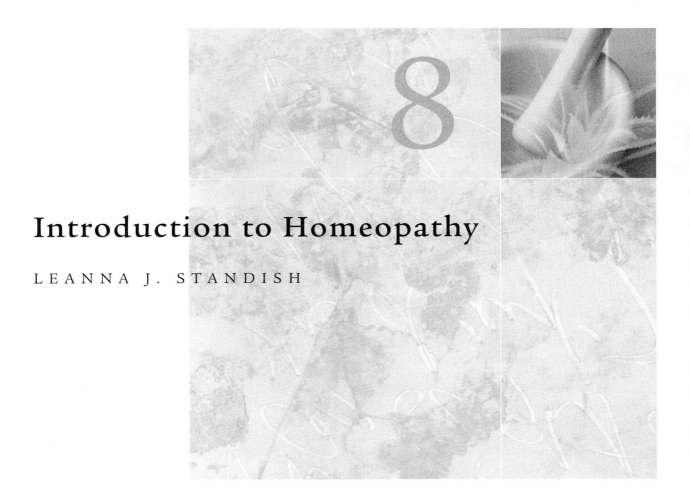

Introduction to Homeopathy

LEANNA J. STANDISH

Homeopathy is perhaps the most controversial area of alternative medicine. To most scientists trained in the dominant paradigm of molecular medicine, its tenets seem counterintuitive, even irrational. The notion that minute concentrations of medicines administered to human biological systems can exert therapeutic biological and clinical effects emerged from the medical discipline of homeopathy more than 180 years ago. The history of homeopathy began in Germany in 1810 with the publication of Samuel Hahnemann's *Organon of The Medical Art.*[1]

Homeopathy is defined as a system of medical practice that treats a disease with minute concentrations of medicines that, if administered at higher doses to a healthy person, would produce symptoms of that disease. That is, if a high concentration of a substance causes a medical problem, the homeopathic law of similars predicts that the same substance will effectively treat that problem when prescribed in exceedingly small concentrations.

Homeopathic medicine continues to be practiced widely in both Europe and India. Homeopathy played a major role in North American medicine at the turn of the twentieth century and for the next few decades. It fell out of wide professional use in the United States during the middle to late twentieth century. Currently both scientific and clinical interest in and practice of homeopathic medicine in the United States has undergone a resurgence. All known schools of homeopathy agree on two basic principles: the law of similars, also known as the "similar principle," and the principle of dilution and potentiation.

The law of similars predicts that a substance that causes disease symptoms in healthy patients will reverse those same symptoms in patients who have that disease. The principle of dilution and potentiation predicts that the molecular activity of the diluted substance is maintained and potentiated with repeated agitated serial dilution.[2] Ultrahigh dilutions (UHDs) are traditionally prepared by using either a decimal system (1:10 dilutions), referred to as "X," or a centesimal system (1:100 dilutions), referred to as "C." Commonly used centesimal dilutions (or "potencies" in homeopathic terminology) are 6 C, 9 C, 12 C, 30 C, 200 C, and 1 M ("M" refers to a 1:100 serial dilution performed 1000 times). At each step, the dilution is agitated by a method called succussion (shaking or vortexing). Substances serially diluted by succussion to 12 C (10^{-24} M) and beyond the reciprocal of Avogadro's constant are diluted to such an extent that the chances of a single molecule being present are extremely small. The biological effects of such potentiated UHDs are theorized to occur even at this metamolecular level.[2] The law of similars and the law of dilution and potentiation are clinically derived concepts that are currently being studied to evaluate their validity in the similar but divergent fields of homeopathy and UHD biology.

The basic tenets of homeopathy find support in one of the earliest empirically derived laws of pharmacology, known as the Arndt-Schultz law. Formulated by Arndt in 1888 and restated by Hueppe a few years later, the law states that "for every substance, small doses stimulate, moderate doses inhibit, large doses kill." The existence of inverse effects on a changing dose has long been described in pharmacology, in which such terms as hormesis and the Arndt-Schultz law are used to identify positive, stimulatory effects of either low doses of inhibitors or toxins or low doses of radiation.[2] These concepts predict that the dose-response curve for some biologically active substances is nonlinear and complex.

Some preliminary data from immunological experiments suggest that the dose-response curve for some substances is oscillatory and perhaps even sinusoidal (Figure 8-1). The law of dilution and potentiation states that serial agitated dilutions potentiate the activity of the molecule that is diluted. Together the Arndt-Schultz law and the law of dilution and potentiation suggest the testable hypothesis that the action of some biologically active substances can best be described as a complex and perhaps repeating oscillatory curve that extends into the metamolecular range (dilutions beyond 12 C or 10^{-24} M). This theoretical concept is illustrated in Figure 8-1.

Modern molecular and pharmacological medicine rests on the biochemical tenet that substances exert their effects on living systems through a direct molec-

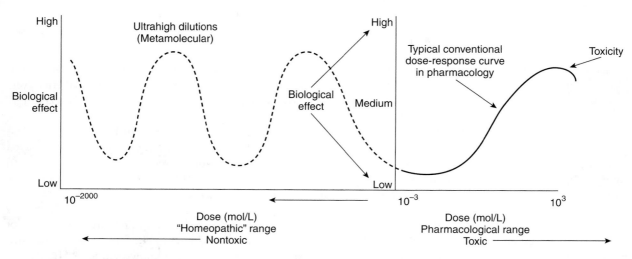

Repeating sinusoidal curve more fully describes the relationship between dose and response

Figure 8-1 Theoretical dose-response curve from the work of Arndt-Schultz and the tenets of homeopathy.

ular interaction with cells. Receptor-ligand interactions have been the focus of most pharmaceutical developments for the past 50 years. Thus most clinical and basic pharmacological research is limited to concentrations of molecular species that are mostly in the 10^{-3} to 10^3 M range. Outside of the homeopathic scientific community, few researchers have studied the effects of compounds beyond Avogadro's constant of 10^{-24} M (12 C in homeopathic terminology), since the probability of the existence of even a single molecule in such a diluted preparation is extremely small. Dose-response curves in the narrow dose range used in most pharmacological studies are typically sigmoidal, or S-shaped. The possibility exists that the pharmacological sigmoid curve describing dose response is only a small section, or a dose window, of a much larger curve, one that is sinusoidal (perhaps even repetitively so) with a possibly unique frequency modulation for each substance.

ULTRAHIGH DILUTIONAL BIOLOGY IS DIFFERENT FROM HOMEOPATHY

The fields of homeopathy and UHD biology differ. Homeopathy focuses on the law of similars, whereas UHD biology focuses on the law of dilution and potentiation. Homeopathy may be considered to be a special case of UHD biology. Scientific evidence for the homeopathic similiar principle is still provisional and uncertain.[3] To date, the law of similars remains a clinically derived concept that is not proven to be a scientific law.

DOSE-RESPONSE CURVES FOR SOME BIOLOGICALLY ACTIVE MOLECULES ARE COMPLEX AND NONLINEAR

The developments of modern molecular and pharmacological medicine occurred independently of homeopathic theory and practice until the 1990s. One of the first published modern studies that supported both the concept of oscillatory, sinusoidal dose-response action and the theory that repetitive, serial agitated dilutions alter the biological effects of a compound came from the work of a French immunologist, Jacques Benveniste. In a highly controversial pa-

per published in the June 1988 issue of *Nature*, Benveniste and his colleagues presented data showing that highly diluted antihuman IgE antibodies at concentrations ranging from 10^{-2} to 10^{-120} M caused oscillatory peaks in histamine release from basophils in vitro (Figure 8-2). These findings were reproduced by Benveniste in 1991[4,5] and by other research groups.[6] The 1991 replication studies by Benveniste[7,8] used additional control dilutions of either antihuman IgG antiserum or distilled water and demonstrated that UHDs of various substances have effects that differ from those of water. These results were replicated by the original research team, as well as by other investigators.[6-9] Independent investigators in other labs made three attempts to replicate this study. Two research teams failed to replicate the results,[10,11] whereas a recently published multicenter study involving four independent labs succeeded in replicating the original results.[12]

Studies that tested the effects of UHD substances at serial dilutions on specific in vitro and in vivo experimental models suggest the existence of complex dose-response relationships, with both stimulatory and inhibitory effects occurring at different UHD doses, or potencies. Such studies suggest the existence

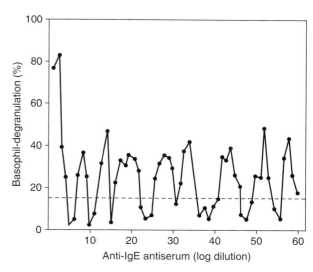

Figure 8-2 Actual data generated by high dilutions of anti-IgE antiserum, which causes basophil degranulation. Note that the scale shows log dilutions and captures the oscillatory dose-response curve. (From Davenas E, Beauvais F, Amara J, et al: Human basophil degranulation triggered by very dilute antiserum against IgE, *Nature* 333:816-818, 1988.)

of complex and nonlinear dose-response curves over a wide concentration range, from toxic pharmacological levels at the high dose end to UHD metamolecular levels at the low dose end, which are many log units lower in concentration compared to the pharmacological doses typically studied in biomedical research. Researchers reported UHD effects that are both similar to and opposite of (inverse) those seen at pharmacological doses. Both similar and inverse effects were observed in a wide diversity of endogenous substances, homeopathic remedies, and UHD substances that are considered toxic at high doses.[13-24] For example, thyroxin has either stimulatory or inhibitory effects on the development of frogs, depending on the dilution applied.[19,20] Dose-response effects were historically associated with the narrow range of dilutions usually investigated in hormesis studies, which were still within the molecular range of pharmacological, physiological, and lower doses.[25-28] However, recent studies report that measurable biological effects also occur with solutions diluted to 10^{-23} M (the reciprocal of Avogadro's number)[13-24] and beyond.[21,22,29,30] These data refute the assumption held by some homeopaths that all UHD doses have the opposite, or inverse, effects as pharmacological doses of the same substance.

EVIDENCE FOR UHD EFFECTS

A small but growing body of scientific literature provides evidence for UHD effects across a diverse range of models. Evidence for UHD and homeopathic phenomena has emerged from five fields: (1) toxicology, (2) pharmacology, (3) endocrinology, (4) immunology, and (5) human clinical trials of homeopathic medicine. This evidence is summarized below.

Toxicology

A number of studies that demonstrate protection from toxic agents have been published, using either low (10^{-2} M) or very low (10^{-24} M) doses of identical or similar agents. Examples of such studies are summarized below.

- Cadmium and cisplatin have marked effects on kidney tubules when administered in pharmacological doses. The pretreatment of kidney cell cultures with very low doses (10^{-16} M) of cadmium and cisplatin had a protective effect against the

toxicity caused by medium to high doses (10^{-5} to 10^{-6} M) of these substances.[31]

- In a rodent nephrotoxicity model, rats treated with either 9 C or 15 C dilutions of mercury were significantly protected against the nephrotoxicity of both medium and high doses (5 to 6 mg/kg) of mercury,[32,33] as evidenced by reduced mortality.
- Phosphorus is hepatotoxic at high doses. Homeopathically prepared phosphorus administered at doses of 30 C (10^{-60} M) inhibited fibrosis in the liver caused by chronic administration of CCl_4 in rats.[34]
- A toxicology metanalysis of 105 publications indicated that "four of five outcomes meeting quality and comparability criteria for metanalysis showed positive effects for [UHD] preparations."[35]

Pharmacology

Serially agitated UHDs of pharmacological agents induced effects in both tissue culture and ex vivo and in vivo biological systems. Contrary to homeopathic theory, the effects are not always opposite to those induced by pharmacological doses. Selected studies are summarized below.

- Cytostatic agents (e.g., vincristine, methotrexate, fluorouracil) at relatively high concentrations (100 mg to 10 ng/ml) inhibited lymphoblastic transformation and granulocyte phagocytosis, whereas very low concentrations (10 pg to 10 fg/ml) stimulated them. Intermediate doses were ineffective.[36-39]
- An experimental model of carcinogenesis in rats was used to test the effect of highly diluted carcinogens and tumor promoters on the development of carcinomas caused by high doses of the same agents.[40] A large percentage of rats who received dietary 2-aminoacetylfluorene (0.03% for 21 days) and phenobarbitol (0.05% for 12 months) developed hepatocellular carcinomas after 9 to 20 months. The treatment of these animals with either 9 C of 2-aminoacetylfluorene or 9 C of phenobarbitol added to their drinking water significantly reduced and delayed the development of liver tumors compared to the control group, which received only the serially agitated solvent.
- Benveniste and colleagues[41,42] studied the effects of high dilutions of histamine on an isolated perfused guinea pig heart. The coronary flow increased with the infusion of very high dilutions of

histamine (above 30 X), which normally occurs with low pharmacological doses. The vasodilatory activity of histamine in very high dilutions was destroyed by either heat treatment at 70° C for 30 minutes or by exposing these dilutions of histamine to a magnetic field of 50 Hz for 15 minutes.

- Pharmacological doses of β-agonists, such as isoproterenol, salbutamol, and tulobuterol, caused relaxation of the tracheobronchial muscles. Callens et al[43] showed that extremely low concentrations (from 10^{-20} to 10^{-36} M in potentiated decimal dilutions) of these agents induced measurable relaxation of basal tone in isolated guinea pig trachea.

- Alloxan 9 C partly inhibited the diabetogenic effect of 40 mg/kg alloxan in mice.[44]

- High dilutions of bee venom *(Apis mellifica)* are used in homeopathy to treat edema, erythema, and itching. High dilutions (from 7 to 9 C) had a protective effect on x-ray-induced erythema in the albino guinea pig.[9,45,46]

- Conventional hematological journals reported a paradoxical effect of acetylsalicylic acid (aspirin). In healthy volunteers, homeopathic dilutions of aspirin (2 ml of a 5 C solution corresponding to 0.000000002 mg by sublingual administration) caused a statistically significant reduction in bleeding time when compared to distilled water. Since pharmacological doses (from 50 to 500 mg) of aspirin cause an increase in bleeding time, the findings of this study support the law of similars and suggest a complex nonlinear dose-response curve.[47]

Endocrinology

- Immune function can be reinstituted by the homeopathically prepared hormone bursin in chicks who received bursectomies as embryos. An in ovo administration of UHDs of bursin (10^{-30} to 10^{-40} g/ml), theoretically no longer containing any molecules of the original substance, restore the immune response as measured by antibody production in adult chickens in response to an antigen bovine thyroglobulin.[14]

- Physiological doses of thyroxine stimulated metamorphosis and activity in frogs. UHD thyroxine (30 C) also induced metamorphosis and activity. However, depending on the dosing schedule, UHD thyroxine can also induce inhibitory effects. Investigators found stimulatory effects when doses were repeated every 8 hours and inhibitory effects when doses were repeated every 48 hours.[14]

- The nonlinearity of UHD dose-response curves is supported by another study of the effect of UHD thyroxine on frogs.[19] Researchers compared UHD thyroxine (30 X) to a control (30 X diluted water) and showed that this potency of UHD thyroxine inhibited climbing activity, which is the opposite effect of physiological doses of thyroxine. The results of these two studies on frogs[19,20,30] suggested that the direction of the response, whether inhibitory or stimulatory, varies according to the UHD dilution.

Immunology

- In chicks who received bursectomies as embryos, UHDs of the peptide hormone bursin (5×10^{-27} g) induced the recovery of normal antigen-induced melatonin response and normal melatonin circadian rhythms.[22,23] Mice who were pretreated with a potent immunogen, keyhole limpet hemocyanin (KLH), at UHDs of 4 C, 5 C, 6 C, 7 C, and 15 C adminstered either orally or parenterally showed an increase in both IgM and IgG response.[48] The greatest response occurred with a UHD of 15 C. These researchers suggested that UHDs of an antigen transfers modulatory signals to the immune system.

- Jonas and Dillner[29] showed in a well-controlled study that oral administration of UHDs (e.g., 3 C, 7 C, 14 C, 30 C, 200 C, 1000 C) of tissue from *Francisella tularensis*-infected mice induced protection against an infectious challenge by the same organism. The results suggested that UHD tularemia increases immune response to tularemia infection in mice.

- A decrease of the cellular immune response against mastocytoma murine cells was induced when mice were treated with UHD thymulin ranging from 10^{-3} to 10^{-11} ng. The most effective inhibitory dose was a 9 C dilution.[17,18]

- Highly diluted thymulin (9 C) modified the humoral response in Swiss mice and amplified seasonal variations of the humoral response.[49,50]

- Homeopathically prepared *Phytolacca decandra* (poke root) has been used as a treatment for lymphadenopathy for many years. Pharmacological concentrations of *P. decandra* contain a glycoprotein with mitogenic activity that can induce lymphoblastic transformation of B cells in culture. In resting lymphocytes, 5 C, 7 C, and 15 C dilutions of *P. decandra* had no mitogenic effect, but in lymphocytes stimulated with pharmacological doses of phytohemagglutinin (PHA), these UHDs exerted a 28% to 73% inhibitory effect on mitosis.[51]

- Researchers have studied the effects of high dilutions of silica on the production of platelet-activating factor (PAF) by peritoneal murine macrophages.[52] High dilutions of silica at 9 C (corresponding to 1.66×10^{-19} M) were added to the mice's drinking water. Macrophages extracted from the mice thus treated had a 30% to 60% greater capacity to respond to yeast extracts compared to macrophages extracted from untreated mice. Lower dilutions of 5 C were less effective.

- Three doses of interferon-alpha,beta (IFN-α,β), ranging from 10^3 IU/ml, 1.6 IU, and 1.6×10^{-10} IU (approximately 9 C) modulated phorbol 12-myristate 13-acetate (PMA)-induced activation of peritoneal macrophages in vitro, as measured by changes in chemiluminescence.[53,54]

- UHD IFN-α,β (2×10^{-10} IU/0.2 ml, approximately equivalent to 9 C), administered intraperitoneally, stimulated humoral and allospecific T-cell responses in mice significantly more than saline control. Higher concentrations (but still pharmacologically low doses) of 2 IU/0.2 ml were without effect.[13]

- Serial agitated UHDs of tumor necrosis factor-alpha (TFN-α) (at 100 X from 100 mg/ml starting concentration) significantly elevated H_2O_2 production of neuroblastoma cells compared to a vehicle control.[55]

- UHDs of IL-2 (4 C and 9 C) showed stimulatory immunomodulating effects on specific humoral immune response in mice when treatment occurred for the primary response (stimulating effect). When the dilutions were injected after repeated immunizations (secondary response), a decrease in antibody levels occurred.[13,14]

STATISTICAL ISSUES IN UHD AND HOMEOPATHIC BIOLOGY

Although the studies cited in the previous paragraphs report intriguing data, researchers must be cautious in concluding that the data show some biological effects of UHDs. The proper statistical analysis is imperative to avoid the risk of a type I error (i.e., rejecting the null hypothesis that UHD preparations have no biological effect when the null hypothesis is actually true). The risk of such an error increases with repeated tests in a single experiment that evaluates the effect of numerous dilutions of a particular substance on small groups of tissue culture plates or experimental animals. Researchers must consider carefully whether the results they observe for some dilutions are simply the result of the random variation that necessarily comes with multiple comparisons. The field of UHD biology will advance when the proper statistical issues are considered and when independent labs replicate the results for specific dilutions.

EVIDENCE FROM PUBLISHED, CONTROLLED, HUMAN CLINICAL TRIALS OF HOMEOPATHY

Although many published clinical trials of homeopathic preparations are of low methodological quality, a small but significant body of well-designed controlled clinical trials reporting positive evidence of the efficacy of homeopathic treatment in a number of conditions exists. Kleijnen et al[56] conducted a meta-analysis and review of 107 clinical trials in homeopathy. They used the same rigorous assessment criteria that are used in conventional clinical drug trials. On the basis of these criteria, 22 publications were judged to be of good quality. Fifteen of these reported positive results in favor of a homeopathic effect. Out of the 107 trials whose results could be interpreted, 81 yielded positive results, whereas the remainder showed no significant differences between homeopathic drugs and placebo.

Other metanalyses by Linde et al[57-59] and by Reilly et al[60,61] also make a strong case for homeopathy. However, Walach[62] cautioned the scientific community with several caveats. He pointed out that, although Linde's metanalysis showed a significant odds ratio of 2.45 for all placebo-controlled clinical trials, this odds ratio dropped to 1.66 with a confidence interval between 1.33 and 2.08 for the 26 studies that were considered methodologically sound. If recently published studies that showed clear negative results were included,[63-65] the odds ratio would drop to insignificance. Walach[62] also pointed out that little evidence exists for the efficacy of homeopathy from independent replications. He suggested that "homeopathy depends on the presence of complementary states of mind," i.e., a nonlocal, noncausal synchronistic relationship between patient and physician. Clearly more well-designed, placebo-controlled, randomized clinical trials (RCTs) of homeopathy are required to increase the certainty that homeopathic medicines have clinical effects independent of placebo, beliefs, or intention on the part of either patient or physician. More trials are needed to determine the effect size and replicability of clinical homeopathy.

SUMMARY OF IN VITRO, ANIMAL, AND HUMAN CLINICAL RESEARCH IN ULTRAHIGH DILUTIONAL BIOLOGY

Taken together, these in vitro, ex vivo, and in vivo animal and human studies in a diversity of systems, including (1) toxicology, (2) pharmacology, (3) endocrinology, (4) immunology, and (5) human clinical trials of homeopathy, suggest the possibility that UHD or homeopathically prepared substances can exert measurable effects in vitro, ex vivo, and in vivo in several biological systems. Some studies also suggest the testable hypothesis that the dose-response relationship of UHD potencies is complex and nonlinear. Some dose-response relationships may even be oscillatory or sinusoidal. The scientific literature indicates that some potencies of UHD substances may have effects that are either similar or inverse to those induced by physiological doses. Although the field of high dilutional pharmacologicals and biologicals is relatively new, some new evidence exists that supports the following hypotheses:

1. The dose-response curve for some biologically active substances is complex, often paradoxical, and nonlinear.
2. High metamolecular dilutions of toxic chemicals can, under several experimental conditions, inhibit the toxic biological effects of the same molecule administered at high material doses.
3. High metamolecular dilutions of several cytokines, hormones, neurotransmitters, drugs, and immunomodulatory compounds can, under several experimental conditions, influence immune cells in culture, organs maintained in physiological isolation, and whole organisms.
4. A small set of human clinical studies exists that

suggests that high dilutional compounds can exert measurable clinical effects.

A CONSERVATIVE STANCE IS WARRANTED

Although the preliminary existing data suggest the possibility that homeopathic medicines and UHDs have biological activity, the field is still in the early stages of scientific validation. A systematic review or metanalysis for in vitro and in vivo effects of UHD biologicals and pharmacologicals has yet to be published. Both the risk of a type I statistical error and a publication bias in favor of positive results exist in homeopathy, which should be considered when assessing the evidence for biological activity of UHDs. A significant publication bias in homeopathic literature may exist, causing negative results to be less likely to be either submitted for publication or published. Negative results are less likely to be published because, for many scientific reviewers, homeopathy and UHD biology are accused by some scientists as lacking a plausible mechanism of action, and therefore publishing negative results is not of scientific interest.

At this time cautious researchers believe that the scientific literature contains some intriguing findings studying the biological and clinical activity of homeopathically prepared substances in extremely low concentrations. These preliminary studies encourage the scientific community to continue studying homeopathic medicine. In the meantime, several plausible hypotheses attempt to explain the mechanism of activity of such substances, the verity of which is still provisional.

MECHANISTIC HYPOTHESES

Both the claims made by homeopaths and the data from in vitro experiments, animal studies, and clinical trials call for an explanatory mechanism of action. At the very least, the homeopathic scientific community should posit hypothetical mechanisms of action to explain the complex, nonlinear effects of homeopathic doses, from the pharmacological range to the UHD and metamolecular range. Most researchers discussing this topic suggest that the mode of action is biophysical instead of biochemical. Many UHD researchers currently agree that both receptor dynamics and the sensitivity of receptors to specific molecular and electromagnetic signals play a role in UHD effects.

Several hypothetical mechanisms have been proposed to explain the effects of UHD compounds on biological systems. These explanatory mechanisms are summarized in Bellavite and Signorini's book *Homeopathy: A Frontier in Medical Science*.[2] These proposed mechanisms include:

- Priming effects of low doses on receptors
- Stimulation of antiidiotype immune responses
- Potentiation or desensitization of cell activity by receptor dynamics
- Retention of molecular and electromagnetic solute information by the cluster structure of water
- Retention of electron cloud patterns created by molecular solute in vicinal water
- Coherence and resonance effects on membrane-bound and intracellular receptors
- Holographic retention of information in the high frequency domain
- Fractal effects of iterative biological processes
- Decrease in biological chaos by repetition of small signals

Insufficient basic scientific research exists that allows differentiation among these various proposed mechanisms of action. In the meantime, most homeopathic research has focused on demonstrating that homeopathic preparations of various substances can exert biological and clinical effects. Further demonstrations of the in vitro and in vivo activity of nonmaterial homeopathic doses may inspire basic mechanistic research.

HOMEOPATHY AND AIDS

Many HIV-positive patients seek the care of lay homeopaths and licensed physicians who also practice homeopathy (e.g., MDs, NDs, and DOs). The Bastyr University AIDS Research Center's observational study of 1666 HIV-positive men and women indicates that, nationwide, approximately 9% of HIV-infected individuals who use complementary and alternative medicine (CAM) were treated by a homeopathic prescriber. In India homeopathy is more widely used and is used to treat the growing HIV-positive population. To our knowledge, only two papers that report on the clinical effects of constitutional homeopathic medicine in HIV-positive patients have been published in a

peer-reviewed journal. Rastogi and his colleagues in India conducted both studies. Rastogi et al[66] studied 129 asymptomatic HIV-positive patients in India who were treated with homeopathic medicines (with potencies from 30 C to 1 M), based on each individual's constitutional characteristics. They reported that 12 patients became enzyme-linked immunosorbent assay (ELISA)-negative after 3 to 16 months. In 1999 Rastogi et al[67] published a controlled trial comparing the effect of individualized homeopathic medicines with placebo in 100 HIV-positive patients between the ages of 17 and 50 (71% men) who were randomized to receive either a single homeopathic remedy or a placebo. The group receiving verum showed statistically significant increases in $CD4^+$ T cells after 6 months.

Within the broad area of homeopathy and AIDS, two avenues of research currently present themselves. The first avenue is the investigation of the efficacy of classical constitutional homeopathy in the treatment of HIV/AIDS. The second, more recent direction is the application of homeopathic principles to molecular biology. Some devoted advocates of homeopathy, patients and practitioners alike, claim that constitutional homeopathic medicine not only can help HIV-positive patients but also can cure AIDS. These claims demand scientific evidence. The homeopathic *materia medica* consists of over 1000 homeopathic substances that are "proven" to induce symptoms in healthy people but that can be used to treat sick people who have those same symptoms. It is still unknown whether expert constitutional homeopathic prescriptions can increase immune status, lower viral activity, ameliorate HIV-related symptoms, or improve the patient's quality of life (QOL).

Another application of homeopathic theory is the desensitization of antibiotic drugs. Bissuel et al[68] used homeopathically prepared trimethoprim-sulfamethoxazole (TMP-SMX, Bactrim, Septra, Cotrim) to desensitize HIV-positive patients to an antibiotic used to prevent *Pneumocystis carinii* pneumonia. Many HIV-positive patients who begin TMP-SMX therapy developed hypersensitivity reactions that manifested as a skin rash. Bissuel's small study suggested that oral administration of UHD TMP-SMX may prevent such reactions.

Administration of homeopathic nosodes is another area of homeopathic medicine that deserves investigation. Nosodes are serially agitated UHDs of antigenic material taken from diseased tissues that are usually administered either orally or sublingually. Homeopathic physicians in India sometimes use homeopathically prepared HIV concentrated in the buffy coat of centrifuged blood samples to treat HIV/AIDS. The use of nosodes has a long history within homeopathic medicine, and some of the key homeopathic constitutional medicines (polycrests) are nosodes. For example, the polycrest remedies *Medorrhinum, Syphlinum,* and *Tuberculinum* are made from gonorrheal-, syphilitic-, and tubercular-infected tissue, respectively. Many naturopathic physicians in Europe and the United States prescribe homeopathically prepared viral nosodes for the treatment of HIV co-factor viruses, such as hepatitis, human papilloma virus (HPV), Epstein-Barr virus (EBV), and cytomegalovirus (CMV). To our knowledge, none of these nosodes have been clinically evaluated in controlled clinical trials in HIV disease. Sufficient in vitro and animal data from other UHD research suggest that this approach is worthy of systematic study.

Novel applications of homeopathic theory to molecular medicine are in their infancy. The most comprehensive research in this area to date is by Brewitt and her colleagues (see Chapter 9). In an early study, Brewitt and Standish[15] evaluated the clinical, hematological, and immunological effects of growth factors (GFs) and cytokines administered in extremely high oral doses in a small controlled study with HIV-positive patients. Four GFs and cytokines with known or suspected immunomodulatory actions were evaluated at extremely low concentrations and administered orally in a randomized, double-blind, placebo-controlled trial to 24 HIV-positive adults with baseline CD4 cell counts between 125 and 500. The GFs and cytokines tested included (1) platelet-derived growth factor BB (PDGF-BB), (2) insulin-like growth factor-1 (IGF-1), (3) transforming growth factor-beta-1 (TGF-β1), and (4) granulocyte-macrophage colony-stimulating factor (GM-CSF) at dilutions of 10^{-60}, 10^{-400}, and 10^{-2000} M. Each dose was well beyond Avogadro's number. Statistically significant improvements were detected in the treatment group for CD4 cells, CD8 cells, erythrocyte sedimentation rate (ESR), weight gain, platelets, and viral load. Patients receiving GFs and cytokines had reduced occurrences of opportunistic infections (OIs), increased platelet counts in thrombocytopenic patients, lower viral load (0.3 log unit), increased weight, and stabilized CD4 and CD8 cell counts.[15]

The new field of UHD cytokines and GFs stems from the integration of homeopathic theory with modern molecular biology. This line of research raises the question of whether it is possible to influence immunological, virological, and clinical outcomes using GFs and cytokine peptides in UHDs that are selected based on the law of similars. It also raises the question whether other cytokines, such as IL-2, can be useful at UHDs. IL-2 shows immunological efficacy in HIV-positive patients at pharmacological doses, but the common adverse reactions (e.g., myalgia, fever, and flu-like symptoms) limit its medical usefulness.

Chapter 9 describes 3 years of clinical studies of HIV-positive patients receiving oral doses of homeopathically prepared GFs and cytokines. The rationale for this research is based both on the law of similars and the law of dilution and potentiation. GFs and cytokines that induce down-regulation of immune function and increased HIV activity at pharmacological doses were selected based on the law of similars. These GFs and cytokines were then potentiated using standard homeopathic serial dilution methods at extremely low concentrations. Dilutions beyond 12 C have a miniscule chance of even a single molecule being present in the orally administered fluid. The results of the three studies presented by Brewitt and her colleagues provide preliminary evidence that UHDs of GFs and cytokines may exert biological activity. Their work suggests a whole new field of promising clinical and basic research.

References

1. Brewster O'Reilly W: *Organon of the medical art by Dr. Samuel Hahnemann (1842),* Redmond, Wash, 1996, Birdcage Books.
2. Bellavite P, Signorini A: *Homeopathy: a frontier in medical science,* Berkeley, Calif., 1995, North Atlantic Books.
3. Bellavite P, Andrioli G, Lussignoli S, et al: A scientific reappraisal of the "principle of similarity," *Med Hypotheses* 49:203, 1997.
4. Benveniste J: Defense of diluted water, *Nature* 353:787, 1991a (letter).
5. Benveniste J: Commentary, *Homint R D Newsletter* 2:3, 1991b.
6. Sainte-Laudy J, Belon P: Inhibition of human basophil activation by high dilutions of histamine, *Agent Actions* 38:C245, 1993.
7. Benveniste J, Davenas E, Ducot B, et al: L'agitation de solutions hautement diluees n'induit pas d'activite biologique specifique, *C R Acad Sci III* 312:461, 1991.
8. Benveniste J, Davenas E, Ducot B, et al: Basophil achromasia by dilute ligand: a reappraisal, *FASEB J* 5:A3706, 1991.

9. Poitevin B, Davenas E, Benveniste J: In vitro immunological degranulation of human basophils is modulated by lung histamine and *Apis mellifica, Br J Clin Pharmacol* 25:439, 1998.

10. Hirst SJ, Hayes NA, Burridge J, et al: Human basophil degranulation is not triggered by very dilute antiserum against human IgE, *Nature* 366:525, 1993.

11. Ovelgonne JH, Bol AW, Hop WC, et al: Mechanical agitation of very dilute antiserum against IgE has no effect on basophil staining properties, *Experientia* 48:504, 1992.

12. Belon P, Clumps J, Ennis M, et al: Inhibition of human basophil degranulation by successive histamine dilutions: results of a European multicenter trial, *Inflamm Res* 48(suppl 1):S17, 1999.

13. Daurat V, Dorfman P, Bastide M: Immunomodulatory activity of low doses of interferon alpha,beta in mice, *Biomed Pharmacother* 42:197-206, 1988.

14. Bastide M: Immunological examples on ultrahigh dilution research. In Endler PC, Schulte J, editors: *Ultra high dilution: physiology and physics,* Dordrecht, the Netherlands, 1994, Kluwer Academic Publishers.

15. Brewitt B, Standish LJ: High dilution growth factors/cytokines: positive immunological, hematological, and clinical effects in HIV/AIDS patients, *Eleventh Int Conf AIDS* Abstract TH 4108, 1996.

16. Bastide M, Lagache, A: A communication process: a new paradigm applied to high-dilution effects on the living body, *Altern Ther Health Med* 3:35, 1997.

17. Bastide M, Daurat V, Doucet-Jaboeuf M, et al: Immunomodulatory activity of very low doses of thymulin in mice, *Int J Immunother* 3:191, 1987.

18. Bastide M, Doucet-Jaboeuf M, Daurat V: Activity and chronopharmacology of very low doses of physiological immune inducers, *Immunol Today* 6:234-235, 1985.

19. Endler PC, Pongratz W, Kastberger G, et al: The effect of highly diluted agitated thyroxine on the climbing activity of frogs, *Vet Hum Toxicol* 36:56, 1994.

20. Endler PC, Pongratz W, Smith CW, et al: Nonmolecular information transfer from thyroxine to frogs with regard to homeopathic toxicology, *Vet Hum Toxicol* 37:(3)259-260, 1995.

21. Davenas E, Beauvais F, Amara J, et al: Human basophil degranulation triggered by very dilute antiserum against IgE, *Nature* 333:816-818, 1988.

22. Youbicier-Simo BJ, Boudard F, Mekaouche M, et al: A role for bursa fabricii and bursin in the ontogeny of the pineal biosynthetic activity in the chicken, *J Pineal Res* 21:35, 1996.

23. Youbicier-Simo BJ, Boudard F, Cabaner C, et al: Biological effects of continuous exposure of embryos and young chickens to electromagnetic fields emitted by video display units, *Bioelectromagnetics* 18:514, 1997.

24. Brewitt B: Homeopathic growth factors: understanding like cures like from the scientific and medical literature, *Altern Ther Health Med* 3:92, 1997 (letter, comment).

25. Calabrese EJ, Baldwin LA: Hormesis as a biological hypothesis, *Environ Health Perspect* 106(suppl 1):357, 1998.

26. Calabrese EJ, Baldwin LA: Chemical hormesis: its historical foundations as a biological hypothesis, *Toxicol Pathol* 27:195, 1999.

27. Calabrese EJ, Baldwin LA: The marginalization of hormesis, *Toxicol Pathol* 27:187, 1999.

28. Eskinazi D: Homeopathy re-revisited: is homeopathy compatible with biomedical observations? *Arch Intern Med* 159:1981, 1999.

29. Jonas WB, Dillner DK: Protection of mice from tularemia infection with ultralow serial agitated dilutions prepared from *Francisella tularensis*-infected tissue, *J Sci Exploration,* 2000 (in press).

30. Endler PC, Pongratz W, van Wijk R, et al: A zoological example on UHD research: energetic coupling between the dilution and the organism in a model of *Amphibia.* In Endler PC, Schulte J, editors: *Ultra high dilution: physiology and physics,* Dordrecht, the Netherlands, 1994, Kluwer Academic Publishers.

31. Delbancut A, Dorfman P, Cambar J: Protective effect of very low concentrations of heavy metals (cadmium and cisplatin) against cytotoxic doses of these metals on renal tubular cell cultures, *Br Homeopath J,* 82:123, 1993.

32. Cambar J, Desmoulieres A, Cal JC, et al: Mise en evidence de l'effet protecteur de dilutions homeopathiques de Mercuris corrosivus vis-à-vis de la mortalite au chlorure mercurique chez la souris, *Ann Hom Fr* 25(5):160, 1983.

33. Guillemain J, Cal JC, Desmoulieres A, et al: Effet protecteur de dilutions homeopathiques de metaux nephrotoxiques vis-à-vis d'une intoxication mercurielle, *Cah Biotherapie* 81(suppl):27, 1984.

34. Palmerini CA, Codini M, Floridi A, et al: The use of phosphorus 30 CH in the experimental treatment of hepatic fibrosis in rats. In Bornoroni C, editor: *Omeomed 92,* Bologna, Italy, 1993, Editrice Compositori.

35. Linde K, Jonas WB, Melchart D, et al: Critical review and metanalysis of serial agitated dilutions in experimental toxicology, *Hum Exp Toxicol* 13:481, 1994.

36. Wagner H: Neue Untersuchungen uber die immunostimilierende Wirkung einiger pflanzlicher Homoopathica, *Biologische Medizin* 2:399, 1985.

37. Wagner H: Studi immunologici in vitro e in vivo con farmaci vegetali a bassi dosaggi, *Riv Ital Omotossicol* 6(3):13, 1988.

38. Wagner H, Kreher B, Juric K: In vitro stimulation of human granulocytes and lymphocytes by pico- and femtogram quantities of cytostatic agents, *Arzneimittelforschung Drug Res* 38:273, 1988.

39. Wagner H, Kreher B: Cytotoxic agents as immunomodulators, Proceedings of the third meeting of the International Group on Very Low Dose Effects, Atelier Alpha Bleu, Paris, 1989.

40. De Gerlache J, Lans M: Modulation of experimental rat liver carcinogenesis by ultra low doses of the carcinogens. In Doutrempuich C, editor: *Ultra low doses,* London, 1991, Taylor & Francis, Inc.

41. Hadji L, Arnoux B, Benveniste J: Effect of dilute histamine on coronary flow of isolated guinea pig heart, *FASEB J* 5:A1583, 1991.

42. Benveniste, J: Further biological effects induced by ultra high dilutions: inhibition by a magnetic field. In Endler PC, Shulte J, editors: *Ultra high dilution: physiology and physics,* Dordrecht, the Netherlands, 1994, Kluwer Academic Publishers.

43. Callens E, Debiane H, Santais MC, et al: Effects of highly diluted β_2-adrenergic agonists on isolated guinea pig trachea, *Br Homeopath J* 82:123, 1993.

44. Cier A, Boiron J, Vingert C, et al: Sur le traitement de diabete experimental par des dilutions infinitesimales d'alloxane, *Ann Hom Fr* 8:137, 1966.

45. Bastide P, Aubin B, Baronnet S: Etude pharmacologique d'une preparation d'*Apis mellifica* (7CH) vis-à-vis de l'erytheme aux rayons UV chez le cobayes albinos, *Ann Hom Fr* 17(3):289, 1975.

46. Bildet J, Guyot M, Bonini F, et al: Demonstrating the effects of *Apis mellifica* and Apium virus dilutions on erythema induced by UV radiation on guinea pigs, *Berlin J Res Homeopathy* 1:28, 1990.

47. Doutrempuich C, de Seze O, Anne MC, et al: Platelet aggregation on whole blood after administration of ultralow dosage acetylsalicylic acid in healthy volunteers, *Thromb Res* 47:373-377, 1987.

48. Weisman Z, Topper R, Oberbaum M, et al: Immunomodulation of specific immune response to KHL by high dilution of antigen. In *GIRI Meeting,* Paris, 1992.

49. Doucet-Jaboeuf M, Pelegri A, Cot MC, et al: Seasonal variations in the humoral immune response in mice following administration of thymic hormones, *Ann Rev Chronopharmacol* 1, 1985.

50. Doucet-Jaboeuf M, Guillemain J, Piechaczyk M, et al: Limit-dose evaluation of serum thymic factor activity, *C R Seances Acad Sci III* 295:283, 1982.

51. Colas H, Aubin M, Picard PH, et al: Inhibition du test de transformation lymphoblastique (TTL) a la phytohemagglutinine (PHA) par phytolacca americana en dilution homeoapthiques, *Ann Hom Fr* 17(6):629, 1975.

52. Davenas E, Poitevin B, Beneviste J: Effect on mouse peritoneal macrophages of orally administered very high dilutions of silica, *Eur J Pharmacol* 135:313, 1987.

53. Carriere V, Bastide M: Influence of mouse age on PMA-induced chemiluminescence of peritoneal cells incubated with alpha, beta interferon, *Int J Immunother* 6:211, 1990.

54. Carriere V, Dorfman P, Bastide M: Evaluation of various factors influencing the action of mouse alpha, beta interferon on the chemoluminescence of mouse peritoneal macrophages, *Int J Immunopharmacol* 10:9, 1988.

55. Carmine TC: Effects of high potencies of tumour necrosis alpha on H_2O_2 production in cultured neuroblastoma cells by enhanced luminol-dependent chemiluminescence (ECL), *Br Homeopath J* 86:66, 1997.

56. Kleijnen J, Knipschild P, ter Riet G: Clinical trials of homeopathy, *Br Med J* 302:316, 1991.

57. Linde K, Clausius N, Ramirez G, et al: Are the clinical effects of homeopathy placebo effects? A metanalysis of placebo-controlled trials, *Lancet* 350:834, 1997.

58. Linde K, Melchart D: Randomized controlled trials of individualized homeopathy: a state-of-the-art review, *J Altern Complement Med* 4:371, 1998.

59. Linde K, Scholz M, Ramirez G, et al: Impact of study quality on outcome in placebo-controlled trials of homeopathy, *J Clin Epidemiol* 52:631, 1999.

60. Reilly DT, Taylor MA, McSharry C, et al: Is homeopathy a placebo response? Controlled trial of homeopathic potency, with pollen in hay fever as a model, *Lancet* Oct 18;2(8512):881-886, 1986.

61. Reilly D, Taylor MA, Beattie NG, et al: Is evidence for homeopathy reproducible? *Lancet* 344(8937):1601-1606, 1994.

62. Walach H: Magic of signs: a nonlocal interpretation of homeopathy, *Br Homeopath J* 89(3):127-140, 2000.

63. Walach H: Does a highly diluted homeopathic drug act as a placebo in healthy volunteers? Experimental study of belladonna 30 C in double-blind crossover design: a pilot study, *J Psychosom Res* 37(8):851-860, 1993.

64. Whitmarsh TE, Coleston-Shields DM, Steiner TJ: Double-blind randomized placebo-controlled study of homeopathy prophylaxis of migraine, *Cephalagia* 17(5):600-604, 1997.

65. Friese KH, Feuchter U, Moeller H: Homeopathic treatment of adenoid vegetations: results of a prospective, randomized, double-blind study, *HNO* 45(8):618-624, 1997.

66. Rastogi DP, Singh VP, Dey SK: Evaluation of homeopathic therapy in 129 asymptomatic HIV carriers, *Br Homeopath J* 82:4, 1993.

67. Rastogi DP, Singh VP, Singh V, et al: Homeopathy in HIV infection: a trial report of double-blind placebo controlled study, *Br Homeopathy* 88(2):49-57, 1999.

68. Bissuel F, Cotte L, Crapanne JB, et al: Trimethoprim-sulfamethoxazole rechallenge in 20 previously allergic HIV-infected patients after homeopathic, *AIDS* 9(4):407-408, 1995.

9

Homeopathic Growth Factors as Treatment for HIV
Recovery of Homeostasis and Functional Immune System

BARBARA BREWITT

MICHAEL TRAUB

CARL HANGEE-BAUER

LYN PATRICK

LEANNA J. STANDISH

SETTING THE STAGE FOR POSSIBILITY

Look Again—Another Perspective

Conventional medical wisdom has largely avoided the immune system in its quest for human immunodeficiency virus (HIV) treatments, instead favoring designer drugs targeted to every part of HIV's outer coat or enzymatic mechanism. However, human survival depends on the immune system. Our bodies protect themselves from the daily barrage of changing pathogens via complex adaptive immune mechanisms that recognize "self" versus "nonself" elements. When these mechanisms break down, our bodies suffer from diseases such as HIV. It therefore makes sense that the treatment of immune system diseases is best addressed by bolstering the immune system—a goal that can be accomplished because of recent developments in human growth factors (GFs).

Cellular immunity, which is unique to vertebrates, specifically recognizes "self" as it evolves, while also being flexible and capable of specifically attacking "nonself" invaders or pathogens. These adaptive mechanisms are grounded in a cell-to-cell communication network that bridges the immune and neuroendocrine systems.[1-3] This integration of physical, emotional, and hormonal sensations creates an adaptive cellular immune response, which produces billions of T lymphocytes that specifically attack newly recognized foreign pathogens.

Misinterpretation of Clinical Effects of Growth Factors

Cell-to-cell communication occurs via signaling molecules such as GFs, cytokines, neuropeptides, neurotransmitters, and some hormones. GFs are multifunctional, small polypeptides that regulate and effectively coordinate immune communication, enabling the immune system to work as a cohesive whole.[4,5] Because of their crucial role in maintaining a healthy immune system, pharmacological doses of GFs were tested in clinical studies during the early 1990s for treatment of HIV disease. However, clinical and other in vitro studies on high-dose GFs evoked unwanted and unpredictable effects, such as increased HIV replication, suppression of lymphocyte proliferation, lymph node swelling, and inhibition of macrophage function.

These side effects caused many researchers to largely abandon a GF treatment approach in favor of other strategies aimed at killing HIV.[6-10] They did not recognize that these abnormally high concentrations of growth were the reason for the adverse effects. Actually, the side effects supported the theory of the homeopathic law of similars and justified their medical use at low homeopathic concentrations. Conventional researchers chose to directly attack HIV viral mechanisms, whereas homeopathic medical researchers chose to support the body's immune system.

Dr. Samuel Hahnemann's law of similars states, "If a substance can cause symptoms or unwanted side effects at high concentrations, the same substance may effectively treat the symptoms when prepared homeopathically."[11] His writings also clarify the theory that the more powerful the substance, the more dilute it must be for therapeutic effectiveness.[12] His years of clinical observation taught him a guiding principle of pharmacology, namely, that "a drug directly affects the body, and then the body reacts to the drug, producing either healing or adverse symptoms." A toxic concentration of a drug evokes the first symptoms of toxicity in the organ or organs where the drug action is most efficacious.

Currently, conventional treatment largely consists of antiviral (AV) drugs designed to inhibit replication of HIV. However, these new drugs are not designed to renew, repair, or mimic cellular communication, which is the cornerstone of immune system health. HIV replication patterns are nonlinear and complex, and treatment with highly active antiretroviral therapy (HAART) has not effectively stopped viral replica-

tion.[13,14] Unfortunately, 78% of people taking HAART are resistant to one form or another of these drugs, and 27% are resistant to all HAART drugs.[15] About 12% of these patients are infected with a strain of HIV that has mutated in a region for which current drug-resistant tests can not account, suggesting that up to 90% of people taking HAART experience drug resistance due to HIV viral mutations. Another 40% of people on HAART suffer from unwanted side effects, such as insulin resistance and hyperglycemia.[16] People who either live in underdeveloped countries or lack economic resources find that the cost of HAART therapy is out of reach and that the therapy has unwanted, unacceptable side effects.

GFs, which were used and rejected at pharmacological concentrations in the 1990s, can be practical, safe, and economically feasible when used homeopathically. Homeopathic GFs (hoGFs) represent one frontier of medical practice, which is rooted in fundamental healing principles that integrate the mental, emotional, and spiritual living truths within the physical body.[17] Medical practitioners have a responsibility to research and identify potentially effective healing approaches that awaken the body's innate and adaptive ability to survive, thrive, and defend itself as an integrated whole without causing adverse side effects. This can now be accomplished because of advances in new homeopathic human GF products.

The Immune System Must Destroy HIV

Contrary to almost all research reports and after more than 15 years of research into the cause and potential cure for AIDS, the message remains the same: the human immune system must destroy HIV.[18,19] Researchers from the National Institutes of Health (NIH) report that even the most sophisticated of today's antiretroviral (ART) AIDS drugs may never completely cure HIV-infected individuals. After conventional drug therapy causes HIV levels to drop initially, the virion's outer coat mutates and becomes drug-resistant. HIV sequesters itself deep into the lymphatic vessels and lymph nodes, the exclusive home territory of the immune system, where the virus is largely protected from drug access. At this point HIV viral load becomes stable at some level, whether at 100,000 RNA copies/ml or at undetectable levels, but the virus is still present. Whatever the patient's contributing factors to viral load stability, including age, gender, lifestyle, and nutritional status may be, the task of final elimination and management of the viral invasion is ultimately up to the immune system. Thus the popular concept that HAART eliminates high turnover rates of HIV is giving way to new attempts to restore immune function and reestablish homeostasis.[20-22]

The Immune System Relies on Cell-to-Cell Communication

The immune system, like HIV, is highly dynamic, mobile, and adaptive. The one thing that HIV particles lack in comparison to immune cells is cell-to-cell communication, which is the Achilles' heel of all viruses. HIV particles act like single soldiers attacking a cohesive armory of immune cells. Cell-to-cell communication may be the key to successfully overcoming HIV infection.

Macrophages play a central role in the complex, nonlinear communication dynamics underlying immune responses. The immune system's homeostasis depends on cell-to-cell signaling feedback loops.[23] Circulating monocytes and tissue macrophages, strategically located in prominent organs, stimulate adaptive immune responses by secreting GFs and presenting (exposing) foreign antigens to CD4[+] T-cell surfaces.[24-26] GF signals and antigen presentation stimulate clonal expansion of highly targeted CD4[+] T cells to aggressively search for and destroy foreign invaders. GFs are biologically active polypeptide proteins that stimulate cell proliferation, modulate cell growth, alter gene expression, and sustain healthy homeostasis by supporting complex intercellular and intersystemic communications.[5,27,28] After the initial activation, T cells secrete other types of GFs, such as interleukins (ILs) and cytokines, to coordinate the immune response against foreign antigens.

When given proper GF signals and correct nutritional support for repair, the immune system is capable of restoring billions of CD4[+] T cells on a bimonthly basis[21,22] while also repairing and rebuilding tissue. GFs are the body's guides to complete healing through their ability to orchestrate healing processes, repair damaged DNA segments, and increase the uptake of nutrients. Researchers can take advantage of these healing abilities in the battle against HIV.

HIV Breaks Down Cell-to-Cell Communication in the Immune System

Macrophages, the immune system's front-line defenders, and CD4[+] T cells are primary targets for HIV infection.[29] One of the first aberrations to occur during HIV infection is the abnormal production of GFs by macrophages.[30-32] HIV particles sabotage macrophages to secrete GFs that increase virion replication.[30,33-38] Once a macrophage becomes infected, its presentation of antigen to CD4[+] T cells perpetuates continual infection.

HIV is cytotoxic to T cells and its precursors.[39-41] Binding the HIV-gp120 surface to the CD4[+] T-cell surface stimulates cell signals that evoke inappropriate activities, such as premature programmed cell death (apoptosis), unresponsiveness to antigen presentation (anergy), or reactivity against self-antigen (autoimmunity).[29,42] Because HIV has a rapid bimonthly replication, 25% of CD4[+] T cells within the lymph nodes are infected during the early stages of the infection process.[21,22,43] This constant immune reactivity depletes other CD4[+] T-cell–dependent immune response cells, such as CD8[+] T-cells, natural killer (NK) cells, and B cells.[39]

As HIV disease continues, immune dysfunction deepens, resulting in the destruction of lymph node and lymph vessel architecture.[44] At this point a person becomes susceptible to opportunistic infections (OIs) by bacteria, other viruses, and fungi. Protection of tissue integrity throughout the body, whether lean body mass (LBM) or lymph node histology, correlates with long-term survival.[45,46] Unfortunately, the widespread use of HAART has not reduced incidences of wasting.[47-48b]

Under What Conditions Can the Immune System Effectively Overcome HIV?

A monumental struggle takes place between CD4[+] T-cell killing of HIV and HIV replication dynamics in an infected person's body.[21,22,44,49,50] The struggle can be represented as two periodic, oscillating forces opposing one another; i.e., when CD4[+] T cells are high, more HIV is destroyed, and when HIV replication is high, more CD4[+] T cells undergo infection and cell death.

The randomness or irregularity of immune response activities that becomes unpredictable over time in HIV infection fits exactly with the definition of chaos. Chaos theory proposes that turbulence results when two forces constantly oppose each other within the same physiological system.[51,52] Over time, this turbulence progresses and reaches a transition point, whereby chaos appears. Chaos drives one of the two opposing forces to collapse. The most effective way to rescue the favored force from entering into this destructive chaos is to introduce a periodic attractor.[53] A periodic attractor is another force that parallels and stabilizes a favored force. The periodic attractor provides support for feedback control mechanisms. The feedback stabilizes the favored force and drives the unwanted force to an undesired bifurcation point and inevitable collapse. In the scenario between HIV and immune cells, this means reinforcing the replication dynamics of CD4$^+$ T cells and displacing the dynamics of HIV. GFs are ideal candidates to serve as periodic attractors, since GFs control every aspect of the immune system: (1) immune responsiveness, (2) wound healing, (3) tissue repair, and (4) cell growth under healthy or infected conditions.

The concepts of homeostasis, self-defense, and self-recovery are fundamental principles of homeopathy as articulated by the law of similars.[17,54,55] The restoration of cellular immunity and the reestablishment of homeostasis are central issues in HIV disease; thus a homeopathic GF (hoGF) approach seems logical as a viable, nontoxic, affordable, and effective way to provide an HIV-infected person with a periodic attractor. HoGFs are predicted to improve immune system function (see Chapter 16).[17,56]

The clinical practices of homeopathy have shown effectiveness for the last 200 years and have been proven efficacious by many statistical studies.[57-59] For example, Dr. Madeleine Bastide's research group in France proved the nonlinear, dose-related effectiveness of homeopathic epidermal GF in stimulating and inhibiting cell proliferation in vitro.[60] IGF-1 at homeopathic concentrations inhibits HIV-1 replication in cultured cells.[61] Randomized, double-blind, placebo-controlled clinical studies at three different test sites also demonstrated that homeopathic recombinant human growth hormone (rhGH) provided physiological and psychological benefits similar to injectable rhGH while simultaneously eliminating symptoms that match those resembling common side effects of

pharmacological rhGH.[62] Using hoGFs thus offers an opportunity to gain therapeutic benefits while avoiding adverse side effects.

Two approaches can be used to identify which GFs might act as periodic attractors in a clinical setting: (1) the Hahemannian method of symptom appraisal and (2) analyses of common molecular and genetic regulatory sites shared by both HIV and GFs. The first method involves carefully applying the law of similars to symptoms of HIV infection and GFs. Table 9-1 presents the major organs and early symptoms of HIV infection with the known adverse side effects of pharmacological doses of some GFs. The symptom picture is created by high concentrations of four GFs: (1) insulin-like GF-1 (IGF-1), (2) platelet-derived GF (PDGF), (3) transforming GF-beta (TGF-β), and (4) granulocyte-macrophage colony-stimulating factor (GM-CSF). These GFs closely matched early presenting symptoms of HIV infection, thus making them potential candidates for clinical study.

Table 9-2 provides additional information from studies in vivo and in vitro regarding the adverse side effects of these four GFs on the immune system when used at higher-than-normal physiological concentrations. The reports of adverse side effects on immune responsiveness strengthened the rationale for selecting these specific GFs for homeopathic treatment of HIV. High concentrations of these GFs suppress and inhibit both lymphocyte and macrophage proliferation and stimulate HIV replication.

The second method for selecting these GFs was their well-characterized molecular and genetic activities. IGF-1, PDGF, TGF-β, and HIV compete for the same G protein signaling processes, now identified as requisite coreceptors for HIV infection of human cells.[63,64] G proteins are the first site of information transfer from the cell membrane surface to its DNA. At the genetic level, these GFs use the same genetic transcription AP-1 site that HIV also targets: a regulatory area that controls what gene is expressed into viable proteins.[65-67] This is the key decision point that determines whether HIV viral proteins or needed human proteins will be synthesized. It is during the early G$_1$ phase of the cell cycle that critical decisions are made regarding cell fate, such as cell proliferation, cell differentiation, or cell death. Also during this phase, HIV manipulates cell cycle dynamics to up-regulate HIV expression and replication, while concurrently displacing feedback communications necessary for

TABLE 9-1

Target Organs and Early HIV Symptoms Compared to GF Adverse Side Effects

Tissues most frequently infected by HIV	Primary (bold) and early symptoms of HIV infection (Schacker et al, 1996; Griffin et al, 1998)	GF	Adverse side effects
Bone marrow	Malaise	GM-CSF TGF-β	Malaise, bone pain, presyncope (Cinti et al, 1999), osteoblast hyperplasia (Terrell et al, 1993)
Central nervous system	Fatigue, fever, painful nerves, myalgias, arthralgias, shingles, herpes, short-term memory loss	GM-CSF IGF-1	Fever (Cinti et al, 1999) Myalgias, arthralgias (Nguyen et al, 1998)
Colon	Diarrhea, anal herpes, anal sores	TGF-β	Inflammation, gastritis, and general inflammation (Terrell et al, 1993)
Gastrointestinal tract	Mild weight loss, abdominal pain, yeast infections	TGF-β	Mild weight loss, gastritis (Terrell et al, 1993)
Liver	Night sweats, headaches	IGF-1 TGF-β	Headaches (Nguyen et al, 1998), liver weight loss, hepatocyte cell death, high liver enzymes, increased hematocrit, and high bilirubin (Terrell et al, 1993)
Lean body mass (LBM)	Loss of LBM	IGF-1	Loss of LBM (Lee et al, 1996)
Lungs	Weight loss, pharyngitis	TGF-β	Weight loss, inflammation (Terrell et al, 1993)
Lymph nodes	Swollen lymph nodes	PDGF	Swollen lymph nodes (Bunone et al, 2000)
Skin	Skin rashes, skin ulcers, herpes	PDGF	Erythematous rash (Smiell 1998)
Spleen	Swollen lymph nodes	PDGF	Swollen lymph nodes (Bunone et al, 2000)
Thymus	Swollen lymph nodes	PDGF	Swollen lymph nodes (Bunone et al, 2000)
Adrenals	Fatigue	IGF-1	Fatigue (Nguyen et al, 1998)

TABLE 9-2

Homeopathic GFs Meet the Law of Similars and May Effectively Treat HIV

Adverse response	Type of study	Tissue function	GF
Suppress T and B cell proliferation	In vitro	Cellular immunity, CD4$^+$ T cells	IGF-1 (Hunt & Eardley, 1986)
Suppress Thy-1, 2+ cells from entering spleen	In vivo	Spleen	IGF-1 (Bergerot et al, 1996)
Increased inflammation	In vivo	Cellular immunity	IGF-1 (Higgins, 1997)
Enlarged lymph nodes	In vivo	Lymph nodes	PDGF (Poli et al, 1994)
Nonadherence of cells to lymph nodes	In vitro	Lymph nodes	TGF-β (Poli et al, 1994)
Inhibit CD4$^+$ T-cell secretion of IL-2		CD4$^+$ T cells	TGF-β (Kehrl et al, 1991; Matsushima et al, 1993)
Inhibit CD8$^+$ T-cell activity		CD8$^+$ T cells	TGF-β (Kehrl et al, 1991; Matsushima et al, 1993)
Suppress macrophage function	In vitro	Macrophage function	TGF-β (Poli et al, 1994)
Pulmonary fibrosis	In vivo	Lung	PDGF (Yi et al, 1996)
Higher-than-normal expression	In vivo	HIV-infected persons	TGF-β (Kekow et al, 1990)
Higher-than-normal expression	In vivo	HIV-infected persons	GM-CSF (Perno et al, 1996; Poli et al, 1994)
Stimulate HIV replication	Clinical	HIV-infected persons	GM-CSF (Perno et al, 1996; Poli et al, 1994; Poli et al, 1991; Scadden, 1990)
Stimulate HIV replication	In vitro	No cell growth control	TGF-β (Poli et al, 1994; Poli et al, 1991; Scadden, 1990)
Abnormal increase in receptors	In vitro	No cell growth control	IGF-1 (Lal et al, 1993)
Abnormal production of PDGF	In vitro	No cell growth control	PDGF (Goustin et al, 1990)
Chills and nausea	Clinical	Cellular immunity	TGF-β and GM-CSF (Poli et al, 1991; Scadden, 1990)

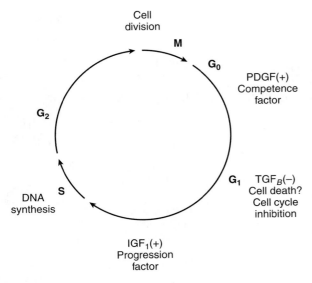

Figure 9-1 Diagram of cell cycle. The classically under-stood phases of the cell cycle include (1) resting G_0, (2) active G_1, (3) DNA synthesis S, (4) synthesis of proteins necessary for cell division G_2, and (5) cell division M. Growth factor PDGF acts as a competence factor to drive the cell from G_0 through G_1 via positive (+) feed-back. After cells become competent in G_1, they reach another time lag that prevents their progression from G_1 to S phase, where DNA synthesis occurs. IGF-1 acts as a progression factor that enables cells to enter S phase via positive feedback. PDGF often couples with progression factors, such as IGF-1, to assure that cells complete all phases of DNA synthesis and reach the stage of mitosis. TGF-β plays two important regulatory roles in the cell cycle. First, TGF-β provides negative feedback to cells, such as T-cells, to inhibit cell growth. Second, TGF-β induces programmed cell death (apoptosis) when appropriate. During the G_1 phase of the cell cycle, major decisions are made regarding cell division, cell differenti-ation, and cell death. (Data from Moses et al, *CIBA Found Sympos,* 157:66-80, 1991; Pimentel, *Handbook of growth factors: vol. 1: general basic aspects,* Ann Arbor, Mich., 1994, CRC Press; Pledger et al, *Proc Natl Acad Sci USA* 74(10):4481-4485, 1977; Pledger et al, *Proc Natl Acad Sci U S A* 75(6):2839-2843, 1978; Schimpff et al, *Acta Endocrinol (Copenh)* 102(1):21-26, 1983; Stiles et al, *Proc Natl Acad Sci U S A* 76:1279-1284, 1979.)

healthy cell function. Figure 9-1 schematically repre-sents the roles of PDGF, IGF-1, and TGF-β in regulat-ing cell fate.

In our investigation, we selected homeopathic IGF-1, PDGF, TGF-β1, and GM-CSF to clinically eval-uate therapeutic efficacy. Preliminary clinical studies on HIV-positive patients receiving subtle-energy elec-tromagnetic signals simulating hoGFs demonstrated appropriate GF potencies to raise $CD4^+$ and $CD8^+$ T-cell counts (see Chapter 16). Homeopathic poten-cies* selected for clinical testing were (1) 1 M IGF-1, (2) 30 C and 1 M PDGF-BB, (3) 30 C and 1 M TGF-β1, and (4) 200 C GM-CSF. Treatment efficacy was deter-mined by measurements of $CD4^+$ and $CD8^+$ T cells, HIV viral load, total body weight (BW), LBM, and gen-eral inflammation, as determined by the erythrocyte sedimentation rate (ESR). Four clinical studies were conducted: two double-blind, placebo-controlled studies and two follow-up studies over a 2½-year pe-riod as shown in Table 9-3.

We tested the homeopathic law of similars with re-gard to these specific GFs that act like periodic attrac-tors to restore immune function in 85 HIV-positive participants. The average length of HIV infection was between 7 to 20 years in 75% of patients and between 1 to 6 years in the remainder of patients. The median period of time between HIV infection and the onset of clinical symptoms of AIDS was 10 to 12 years in West-ern countries.[39,68]

Replication of Results in Different Eras of Antiretroviral Therapy

Patient and study designs are described in Table 9-3. There were enough similarities in terms of years of in-fection and preference for natural therapies for com-parisons between studies. In Studies A, C, and D, 80% of the participants were naïve to ART, whereas only 25% of Study B participants were naïve to ART.

Regardless of treatment or placebo in Study A, a high correlation existed between immune cells that nor-mally have tightly controlled feedback loops between them; i.e., $CD4^+$ and $CD8^+$ T cells (correlation coeffi-cients of 0.7 or greater, $p < 0.001$). However, in Study B, where ART therapy was three times more common

---

*Homeopathic potencies are equivalent to very low concentrations of drugs, such that 30 C = 10^{-60} molar, 200 C = 10^{-400} molar, and 1 M = 10^{-2000} molar (also called 1000 C).

TABLE 9-3

Study Designs and Patient Population Enrollment Criteria

	Study A	Study B	Study C	Study D
Year	1995	Began 1997	1995-199	1996-1997
Numbers	$n = 21$	$n = 55$	$n = 27$	$n = 26$
Type	Double-blind placebo*	Double-blind placebo	Open label	Open label
Study Length	16 weeks	8 weeks	36 weeks	52 weeks
Exclusion	Antiretroviral or corticoid steroid or weight/LBM therapy	Antiretroviral or corticoid steroid or weight/LBM therapy	Antiretroviral or corticoid steroid or weight/LBM therapy	
Inclusion	CD4$^+$ T cells 130-570 cells/μl and only natural medicines		Enrolled in study A† + 9 newly enrolled	Follow-up on study A and C subjects
Location	Seattle	Seven multisite study†	Seattle	Seattle
Treatment	Nat.‡ + GFs‡ No antiretrovirals	Nat. + GFs No antiretrovirals	Nat. + GFs No antiretrovirals	GFs or natural or antiretrovirals
Test Purpose	Original hypothesis	Test replication	Evaluate stability of immune system	Follow-up and evaluate survival

GF, Growth factor; *LBM,* lean body mass; *Nat.,* natural therapy.

*A replication test of the Seattle study was conducted in the following multisite study design enrolling 55 persons during 1997 at each of seven different locations (1) Portland, (2) Kailua-Kona, (3) Tucson, (4) New York, (5) San Francisco, (6) Los Angeles, and (7) San Diego for a 2-month, double-blind, placebo-controlled trial (Study B).

†All eligible persons from Study A who were available enrolled in Study C. One person from the treatment group had committed suicide, and two persons from the placebo group had developed OIs and began ART, thus becoming ineligible for the study.

‡Because calcium is a significant second messenger for GF signaling and calcium levels were on the low side of normal range at study entry, all patients in Study A were asked to take either 1000 mg calcium citrate or calcium chelated to an amino acid moiety each evening.

before study enrollment, this correlation between CD4[+] and CD8[+] T cells was not observed. This lack of correlation in Study B raised questions about the reproducibility of Study A findings and the possibility that ART therapy may disrupt tightly regulated cell-to-cell communication between CD4[+] and CD8[+] T cells within the body. However, other researchers found a high correlation between changes in CD4[+] T-cell counts and CD8[+] T-cell counts in HIV-positive individuals.[69]

Treatment with hoGFs stabilized CD4[+] T-cell counts when placebo and hoGF treatment groups were matched for sex and baseline CD4[+] T-cell counts (Figure 9-2). These hoGF treatment findings were replicated through multisite testing 2 years later. Long-term stability in CD4[+] T-cell counts was maintained in the original hoGF group ($n = 10$) over a 12-month period (see Figure 16-3). CD4[+] T-cell count is an important and accepted indicator of HIV disease progression.[20,70] Because of rapid immune system dynamics, a treatment effect is observable within 14 days.[70] For example, the placebo groups in both Studies A and B had a downward trend, losing approximately -85 CD4[+] T cells/μl. These losses of CD4[+] T cells indicated disease progression. A good indicator for hoGF treatment efficacy was the increase of $+16$ CD4[+] T-cell counts/μl after the placebo group crossed over to hoGF treatment. The replication of findings in the treatment group and their stark difference from CD4[+] T-cell losses in the placebo group suggested that hoGFs represent a periodic attractor capable of rescuing disease-related declines in CD4[+] T-cells.

Under conditions where HIV-positive men are not using antiretroviral or chemotherapeutic agents, losses of -51 CD4[+] T cells/μl in 6 months are expected.[71] HIV disease progression also averaged losses of -85 to -100 CD4[+] T cells/μl/year compared to -6 CD4[+] T cells/μl/year losses in HIV-positive long-term

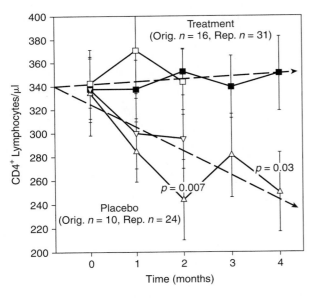

Figure 9-2 CD4 T-cell counts in Studies A and B. Treatment groups (□, ■) show stability in both the 4-month single-site study ($n = 16$) and the multisite 2-month study ($n = 31$). Placebo groups show downward trends (△) for single-site Study A and (▽) for multisite Study B. T-test statistical significance between groups in the single-site study is shown at the appropriate time period. Standard error bars are shown. Linear regressions are shown by dashed lines with arrows.

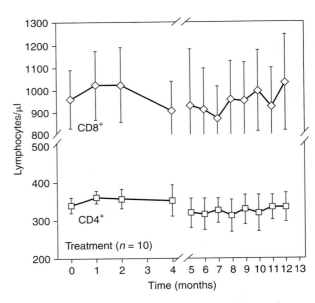

Figure 9-3 CD4[+] (□) and CD8[+] ◇ T-cell counts in the original Study A treatment group ($n = 10$) followed throughout Studies A and C. Standard error bars are shown. Breaks along the X-axis denote a short interim where patients were off treatment.

nonprogressors or −7 CD4+ T cells/μl/yr in healthy controls undergoing normal aging.[72] The patients taking hoGFs were aligned with the categories of HIV-positive, long-term nonprogressors and healthy persons. Only 5% of the population of HIV-positive individuals are nonprogressors; thus it was unlikely that everyone in the hoGF treatment groups were long-term nonprogressors at the time of study entry.[45,73] The more reasonable conclusion was that hoGFs acted as periodic attractors.

CD8+ T-cell counts also stabilized in hoGFs (Figure 9-3). There were no statistical differences noted in total white blood immune cell (WBC) counts between the treatment and placebo groups suggesting that the hoGF effect was specific to cells, specifically restoring these cells to the immune system. CD4+ and CD8+ immune cells worked together in a coordinated attack on HIV.[74] The high correlation between these two cell types in patients who were naïve to ART and the stability of these two cell types gained in patients administering hoGF suggests that restoration of homeostasis occurred in the treatment groups.

LONG-TERM FOLLOW-UP

We lost contact with the study subjects for 9 months after the beginning of the HAART era with widespread use of protease inhibitors (PIs). To understand how hoGFs compared with AV therapies, we initiated Study D. At entry into Study D, three new subgroups of patients had formed voluntarily, as shown in Table 9-3, mixing persons from the previous Study A placebo group into the hoGF group. Because of this heterogeneous grouping and the passage of time, baseline CD4+ T-cell counts were lower at entry into Study D. The three groups were followed quarterly over the course of the next year.

The trends of CD4+ T-cell counts between hoGF, AV, and natural therapies (NAT) differed over time (Figure 9-4). Average CD4+ T-cell counts increased by +23 cells/μl in persons on hoGF treatment. In contrast, persons on AV had a downward trend of −29 CD4+ T cells/μl. There was also a downward trend of −41 CD4+ T cells/μl in the people on NAT without GFs. These findings again support the theory that hoGFs act over the long term as periodic attractors to strengthen the immune system, enabling expansion of the CD4+ immune cell pool. On the other hand, nei-

ther AV nor NAT therapies successfully strengthened the immune system. At the end of Study D, CD4+ T-cell counts of patients using hoGFs were not statistically different than those of patients using AV therapy (see Figure 9-4).

If the immune system is strengthened by hoGF treatment, then it would be expected that OIs, (responsible for most HIV-related morbidity and mortality) would be reduced. This was the case. No hospitalizations or OIs occurred in the hoGF group in Studies A, C, and D. However, as might be predicted, losses in CD4+ T-cell counts in the NAT group were coupled with 40% of hospitalizations by the third quarter of Study D due to OIs and other disease-related infections. Twenty-five percent of the AV group also were hospitalized for the same reasons. OIs of 20% and 17% occurred in the placebo groups of Studies A and B, respectively. Similarly, we experienced one case of an OI, herpes zoster, after 1 month of hoGF treatment (3% incidence) in Study B. This led us to believe that hoGF treatment may not prevent an OI from progressing once it has begun, but it may prevent an OI from taking hold by stimulating appropriate protective immune responses.

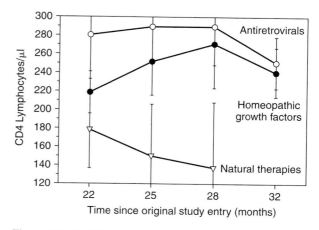

Figure 9-4 CD4 T-cell counts in Study D in subgroups of patients using antiretrovirals (open circles), homeopathic GFs (filled circles), and natural therapies (▽). Time is shown as months since entry in Study A. A high percentage of the patients in the natural treatment group were hospitalized and had OIs, thus they were no longer able to participate.

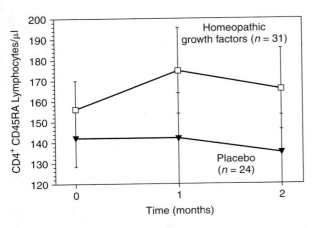

Figure 9-5 CD4⁺-CD45⁺RA T-cells in treatment (□) and placebo (▼) groups. Standard error bars are shown.

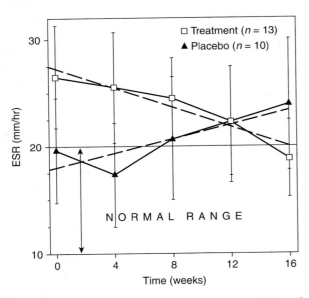

Figure 9-6 ESR values in Study A with treatment (□) and placebo (▲) groups matched for numbers of women to prevent distorted values between groups. Normal ESR values with women are 20 mm/hr or below. Standard error bars are shown.

Naïve cells, which are subsets of CD4⁺ and CD8⁺ T cells, may best characterize functional immunity and are relatively resistant to productive HIV infection.[75] Naïve cells with the CD45RA⁺ antigenic marker can be fully primed to kill their target, even HIV. We studied naïve CD4⁺ T cells to evaluate func-

tional immunity. The hoGF treatment group increased approximately +19 naïve cells/μl within the first month, which leveled out to +10 cells/μl by the second month (Figure 9-5). In contrast, the placebo group had a downward trend of −7 naïve cells/μl throughout the study. An average increase of +19 naïve cells/μl within the first month of hoGF treatment was significant. ART did not show similar short-term increases.[14] Triple combination ART took more than 36 months to raise the CD45RA⁺ population by 50 cells/μl.[14] Once activated, naïve cells returned home to the peripheral lymphatic tissue out of the blood stream to provide cell mediated immunity. The decrease in naïve cell counts during the second month of GF treatment may reflect homing events. Increases in naïve cells in patients using hoGFs supported the conclusion that cell-mediated immunity was strengthened and became more functional than before their use.

FUNCTIONAL IMMUNITY REDUCES INFLAMMATION AND INCREASES IDEAL WEIGHT AND LEAN MASS

A functional immune system would additionally protect tissue integrity, prevent inflammation, and prevent infection. We used ESR measures to determine general inflammation and infection in the body (Figure 9-6). Before widespread evaluation of HIV viral load, research showed that ESR values, in addition to CD4⁺ T-cell counts and $\beta_2$microglobulin, were beneficial in assessing the stage of HIV.[76] Patients randomized to hoGF treatment at Study A entry had higher-than-normal levels of ESR. Treatment reduced these levels to normal levels 4 months later ($p < 0.02$). In contrast, the placebo group's ESR trends rose from normal to higher-than-normal during the same time period. Long-term follow-up showed that patients who remained on hoGF remained in the normal ESR range for 2½ years. In contrast, the AV and NAT groups, who had above normal ESR levels at Study D entry, remained out of normal range for a majority of the time (Figure 9-7). Again, this finding suggested that a unique functional cellular immunity was operating with hoGFs that reduced the stress of the immune system by reducing inflammation and infection in the body, in contrast to the immunity operating with AV or NAT therapies.

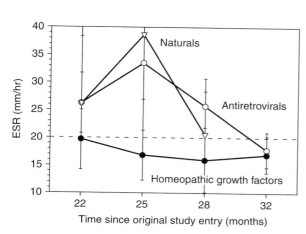

Figure 9-7 ESR values in Study D for each of the three subgroups are shown: (1) antiretroviral (open circle), (2) homeopathic GFs (filled circles), and (3) natural therapies (▽). The dotted line denotes the normal ESR range. Standard error bars are shown.

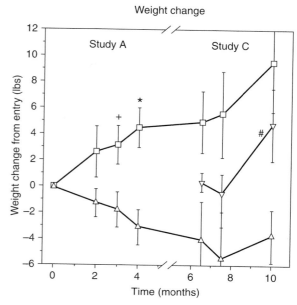

Figure 9-8 Total BW change during Study A and Study C. The treatment in Study A was divided into two groups and consisted of an originally enrolled group (□) and a group that enrolled later during Study C (▽). The Study A placebo group (△) is also shown. Symbols denote statistical differences as shown along the X-axis. Standard error bars are shown. The break in the line denotes when Study A placebo crossed over to treatment, the original Study A treatment continued treatment, and the newly enrolled Study C group began therapy. The symbol # denotes a significance of $p = 0.01$ from the previous month. The symbol * denotes a significance of $p = 0.0004$ versus placebo. The symbol + denotes a significance of $p = 0.009$ versus placebo.

Deterioration in cellular immunity and tissue integrity contributes to early symptoms of lost LBM, weight loss, and cell death.[32,77,78] During the early stages of the HIV epidemic, a direct correlation existed between weight loss, disease progression, and death.[79,80] The same GFs secreted by macrophages to activate CD4[+] T cells also stimulated cell growth, cell repair, and anabolic processes. Loss of cell signaling leads to loss of cell mass and LBM, even in otherwise asymptomatic HIV-infected individuals.[46,77] Given this correlation, it would be expected that any therapy that supported anabolic processes would also necessarily increase cell-to-cell communication.

Incidences of wasting are increasing at an alarming rate, despite primary HIV ART, which has reduced incidences of bacterial infections and other disease complications.[47,48,81] Weight loss is characterized by intermittent periods of acute weight loss interspersed with periods of recovery.[77] Today, with widespread use of AV therapy and increased incidences of lipodystrophy, hyperlipidemia, and hyperglycemia, researchers find that BW is not as good an indicator of disease progression as

are measures of LBM.[82] Specifically, when LBM is reduced to 65% of the ideal BW, life can no longer be supported.[77] Measurements of LBM are even better predictors of long-term survival than CD4[+] T-cell counts.[46]

Homeopathic GFs were selected for their ability to increase cell-to-cell communication and for their known positive effects on cell growth. Before the widespread use of AV/PI therapy, such as the time of Studies A and C, total weight loss was a major concern during HIV infection. There was statistically significant net weight gain on GF treatment in Study A ($+2.84 \pm 1.65$ lbs), and this finding was reproduced in new patients in Study C (Figure 9-8). However, the placebo group in Study A, who were taking

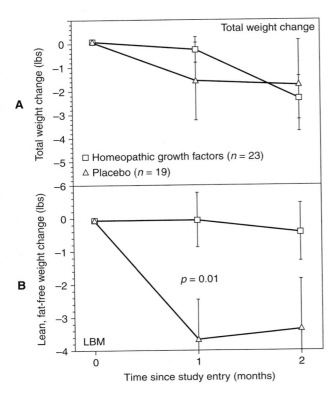

Figure 9-9 Total weight change and LBM change in Study B. **A,** Total weight change in the treatment (□) and placebo (△) groups was not initially different (see Table 9-2). **B,** Statistically significant differences in LBM change ($p = 0.01$) occurred between groups after 1 month of treatment with homeopathic GFs. Standard error bars are shown.

only natural supplements, lost -3.39 ± 1.10 lbs ($p < 0.01$). When patients on placebo crossed over to treatment in Study C, their BWs increased an average of $+0.18 \pm 0.11$ lbs/month. There was continued weight gain of $+9.64 \pm 3.80$ lbs in the treatment group of Study A that was followed for the next 8 months. These findings of weight gain supported a preliminary conclusion that hoGFs increased cell-to-cell communication necessary for anabolic growth.

Once practices of HAART became popular, particularly during the time of Study B, incidences of lipodystrophy rose, and most HIV-infected patients became overweight. In Study B, between 75% to 80% of patients had been on a AV/PI protocol before entering the study. Both the hoGF treatment and placebo groups lost weight, -2.3 ± 0.9 lbs and -1.8 ± 1.8 lbs, respectively, during the 2-month study (Figure 9-9, *A*). Persons in Study A were largely naïve to AV therapy compared to persons in Study B, a majority of whom had used AV therapies. The confounding issue of lipodystrophy required another form of BW analysis (i.e., ideal BW and LBM).

We analyzed the percentage of people in both study groups A and B who were below, within, and above their ideal weight (Table 9-4). We found that 20% and 17% of the patients in the less-than-ideal BW categories at Studies A and B entry, respectively, moved into the ideal BW category by the time they exited the study. No one in the placebo groups experienced any changes in ideal BW. In Study A, we found no change in the percentage of people who were overweight either before or after treatment. In contrast, Study B showed a significant change in the percentage of people who moved from the overweight category to the underweight category. At the start of Study B, 69% of patients were in the overweight category, a figure that decreased to 17% after treatment. Some of these people (26%) became underweight, whereas 8% of the people who were underweight transitioned to their ideal BW. Another 29% of the overweight group entered the ideal BW group. Although the placebo had no effect on weight change, hoGF treatment stimulated changes leading to ideal BW.

However, BW alone is an unreliable measure of cellular and tissue health. Study B also measured LBM

TABLE 9-4

Analyses of Ideal Body Weight

Study assignment	Below ideal BW at entry % of group	Below ideal BW at finish % of group	Within ideal BW at entry % of group	Within ideal BW at finish % of group	Above ideal BW at entry % of group	Above ideal BW at finish % of group
Treatment A	30	10	**0**	20	70	70
Treatment B	18	52	**13**	30	69	17
Placebo A	33	33	0	0	67	67
Placebo B	15	15	0	0	85	85

via bioelectric impedance analysis (BIA).[83,84] LBM statistically differed between the hoGF treatment group and the placebo group within the first month (Figure 9-9, *B; p* = 0.01). The placebo group lost an average of -3.6 ± 1.3 lean lbs within the first month and -3.3 ± 1.6 lbs by the second month. The treatment group had no LBM loss during either the first month ($+0.04 \pm 0.8$ lbs) or the second month (-0.33 ± 0.89 lbs). LBM distinctly indicated that cellular immunity was supported with hoGF compared to placebo. The statistical significance of weight gain in Study A ($p = 0.001$) and maintenance of LBM in Study B ($p = 0.01$) support the conclusion that hoGFs sustained cell mediated immunity during HIV infection compared to placebo.

If hoGF treatment acted as a periodic attractor and strengthened the immune system, then in theory, HIV viral load would decrease. The hoGF treatment may weaken HIV replication dynamics. We evaluated HIV viral load because it indicates the speed of disease progression. HIV viral load tests were not available until the last 2 months of Study A and thereafter. Viral loads decreased on hoGF treatment in all studies, ranging from an average 0.3 log decrease to a 0.7 log decrease, depending on how high the viral load was at entry and how long the patient was on hoGFs (Figure 9-10). Downward trends in viral loads were reproducible in the various studies and were similar, paralleling general downward trends. Higher viral loads dropped dramatically within a 4-month period, since those patients increased the dosage frequency of hoGF to four times/day.

In contrast, the placebo group's viral load moved upward (Figure 9-10, *A*), until they crossed over to hoGF treatment (data not shown). The upward trend in viral load was reproducible. We noted that in Study B, both the placebo and hoGF treatment groups began with similar viral loads. However, within 8 weeks of the study, the outcomes were very different, with the hoGF treatment group having statistically lower viral load levels than the placebo group ($p < 0.05$). Throughout our studies, those patients using either placebo or NAT therapies experienced increased viral loads.

In our long-term follow-up of Study D, people using AV therapy showed signs of either viral resistance or viral mutation (Figure 9-10, *B*), which is an expected common occurrence using this conventional AV treatment strategy.[85] This resistance was not observable in either long-term follow-up of people using hoGFs in Study C and Study D (Figures 9-10, *A* and *B*). Although absolute numbers of HIV-RNA copies/ml were not different between hoGF and AV treatments, there were signs of viral resistance in AV. HoGFs probably acted as periodic attractors to simultaneously strengthen the immune system while weakening HIV, which fits the chaos theory.

SIGNIFICANCE AND SUMMARY

Cell-to-cell communication is unique to multicellular organisms and humans. It is not found in HIV virions. Thus the human immune system has an advantage in its battle against single-soldier-virion particles. The immune system fights foreign invaders by using well-orchestrated and integrated immune response networks that operate effectively via cell-to-cell feedback loops. In this way, immune cells work together in a coordinated effort that involves cell-to-cell communication. It is no surprise that HIV's first disruption in the body involves a breakdown of GF cellular communication networks that would normally facilitate

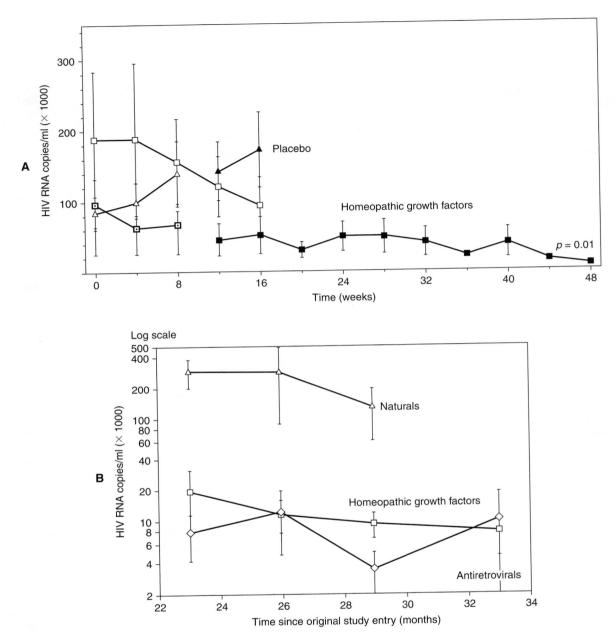

Figure 9-10 HIV viral loads in Studies A, B, C, and D. **A,** Viral loads of Study A treatment group (■) were taken only during weeks 12 and 16 and then every 4 weeks throughout Study C, i.e., weeks 20 through 48. Study C newly enrolled treatment group (□) is shown between weeks 0 and 16 and had high viral loads at entry of approximately 200,000 RNA copies/ml. Study B treatment group (◨) is shown between weeks 0 and 8 at approximately 100,000 RNA copies/ml. The Study A placebo group (▲) had viral loads measured during weeks 12 and 16, whereas the Study B place-bo group (△) had viral loads measured between weeks 0 and 8 at about 90,000 RNA copies/ml. Standard error bars are shown. Note that groups on treatment have downward trends in all cases, whereas placebo groups have upward trends. **B,** Viral loads of Study D. The natural therapies group (△) show 1 log-higher viral loads than the homeopathic GF group (□) and the antiretroviral group (◇). No statistical difference in viral load exists between homeopathic GFs and anti-retrovirals. Standard error bars are shown.

immune cell-to-cell signaling, the cornerstones for immune strength and renewal.[86]

In general, HIV replication dynamics and CD4+ immune cell replication dynamics are complete opposites and become increasingly complex over time. Generally, when high numbers of CD4+ T cells exist, low HIV viral load also exists, and vice versa; when high numbers of viable HIV virions exist, greater infection and low CD4+ T-cell counts exist as well. As cell death increases and the periodic transitions between HIV replication and CD4+ T-cell replication become more frequent, turbulence occurs within the body. This situation becomes more complex and chaotic over time. This chaos leads to an inevitable collapse of one of the two opposing forces. Conditions similar to this periodic and chaotic activity have been modeled for B-cell (humoral) immunity and antibody production using chaos theory.[87]

We applied chaos theory to cellular immunity and HIV infection to gain insight and derive new medical approaches for treating HIV-positive patients. Within chaos theory there exists the concept of a periodic attractor that supports the normal replication dynamics of the CD4+ T cells in an inherently complex system that involves feedback loops. In chaos theory, the periodic attractor creates greater stability (and hence rescues) CD4+ immune cells. As one force is stabilized, the other force (i.e., HIV replication cycles) should be directed toward an undesired transition (bifurcation) that leads toward destructive chaos and collapse. We proposed that a periodic attractor could be identified to strengthen the immune system and hence, according to chaos theory, drive HIV to a predicted weakened end.

The concepts of homeostasis, self-defense, and self-recovery are fundamental principles of homeopathy, as articulated by the law of similars.[54,55] The restoration of cellular immunity and the reestablishment of homeostasis are central issues in healing from HIV disease; thus we integrated the concepts of periodic attractors, homeopathy, and GF biotechnology to strengthen cellular immunity. Using the homeopathic law of similars, we chose four hoGFs (IGF-1, PDGF, TGF-β1, and GM-CSF) to provide positive support of immune system feedback loops, to stabilize CD4+ T-cell dynamics, and to slow HIV disease progression.

We enrolled more than 85 HIV-positive persons from eight different cities and conducted two randomized, double-blinded, placebo-controlled studies

and two follow-up studies over 2½ years. In three of the studies, the persons enrolled were using only self-selected natural medicines, and we added either hoGFs or placebo to the study design. In the final study, we conducted follow-up comparison studies on these persons using hoGFs, ARTs, or only their favorite self-selected natural medicines.

The studies showed that hoGFs stabilized immune responsiveness and protected tissue integrity. On average, no CD4+ T cells were lost in the hoGF treatment groups in either of the double-blinded, placebo-controlled studies. There were increases in naïve cell counts, which is a good indicator of cellular immunity. There was maintenance of LBM and the achievement of ideal BW. Likewise, in both of the open label follow-up studies, little-to-no disease progression was observed in the persons using hoGFs. At entry of Study D, 21 months postentry, individuals using hoGFs generally increased their CD4+ T-cell counts. There were no hospitalizations, no OIs, and no measures of general inflammation or general infection in the tests we ran. These people were not experiencing wasting. Their HIV viral loads trended steadily downward. People using hoGFs over the course of 2½ years had HIV viral loads equal to that of people using AV therapy without any sign of viral resistance. No toxic or adverse events occurred with people using hoGFs at these potencies. HoGF treatment significantly slowed disease progression.

In contrast, patients who used only NATs of their choice or placebo with their NATs experienced HIV-disease progression. In long-term follow-up of persons using only NATs, viral loads reached 1.5 log higher than entry. There were reproducible losses of CD4+ T cells and reproducible rises in HIV viral loads. We also measured losses of naïve cells, losses of LBMs, 40% hospitalizations, and OIs. There were upward trends in general inflammation and infection similar to those reported previously in HIV-positive individuals using only NATs.[88]

The major natural therapies chosen by the patients consisted largely of spiritual practices, vitamin C, vitamin B$_{12}$, garlic, zinc, unspecified Chinese herbs, acupuncture, and beta-carotene. Our studies point to a genuine need for systematic analyses of NATs and their combinations with and without hoGFs. An enhanced therapeutic effect may be established between hoGFs and the correct combination of other natural medicines. The use of alternative therapies with and without supplemental ART by HIV-positive persons

25. Raines EW, Rosenfeld ME, Ross R: The roles of macrophages. In Fuster V, Ross R, Topol EJ, editors: *Atherosclerosis and coronary artery disease,* Philadelphia, 1996, Lippincott-Raven Publishers.

26. Raines EW, Ross R: Macrophage-derived GFs. In Zembala M, Anderson GL, editors: *Human monocytes,* New York, 1989, Academic Press.

27. Pimentel E: *Handbook of GFs: vol. 1: general basic aspects,* Ann Arbor, Mich., 1994, CRC Press.

28. Bradshaw RA, Rubin JS: Polypeptide GFs: some structural and mechanistic considerations, *JSS* 14:183-199, 1980.

29. Fauci AS, Schnittman SM, Poli G, et al: Immunopathogenic mechanisms in human immunodeficiency virus (HIV) infection, *Ann Intern Med* 114(8):678-693, 1991.

30. Valdez H, Lederman MM: Cytokines and cytokine therapies in HIV infection, *AIDS Clin Rev* 187-228, 1997-1998.

31. Fauci AS, Pantaleo G, Stanley S, et al: Immunopathogenic mechanisms of HIV infections, *Ann Intern Med* 124:654-663, 1996.

32. Perno CF, Balestra E, Aquaro S, et al: Potent inhibition of human immunodeficiency virus and herpes simplex type 1 by 9-(2-phosphonoylmethoxyethyl) adenine in primary macrophages is determined by drug metabolism, nucelotide pools, and cytokines, *Mol Pharmacol* 50(2):359-366, 1996.

33. Sharma UK, Song H, Casella SJ, et al: Failure of insulin-like GF type 1 to suppress HIV type 1 in adult or umbilical cord mononuclear blood cells, *AIDS Res Hum Retroviruses* 13(1):105-110, 1997.

34. Li JM, Shen Z, Hu PP, et al: Transforming GF beta stimulates the human immunodeficiency virus 1 enhancer and requires NF-kappa-β activity, *Mol Cell Biol* 18(1):110-121, 1998.

35. Lipman MC, Johnson MA, Poulter LW: Functionally relevant changes occur in HIV-infected individuals' alveolar macrophages before the onset of respiratory diseases, *AIDS* 11(6):765-772, 1997.

36. Graziani A, Galimi F, Medico E, et al: The HIV-1 nef protein interface with phosphatidylinositol 3-kinase activation, *J Biol Chem* 271(12):6590-6593, 1996.

37. Bailer RT, Lazo A, Ng-Bautista CL, et al: Comparison of constitutive cytokine release in high and low histological grade AIDS-related Kaposi's sarcoma cell strains and in sera from HIV-positive/KS+ and HIV-positive/KS− patients, *J Interferon Cytokine Res* 15(5):473-483, 1995.

38. De SK, Marsh JW: HIV-1 nef inhibits a common activation pathway in NIH-3T3 cells, *J Biol Chem* 269(9):6656-6660, 1994.

39. Pantaleo G, Graziosi C, Fauci AS: The immunopathogenesis of human immunodeficiency virus infection, *N Engl J Med* 328(5):327-335, 1993a.

40. Stanley SK, Kessler SW, Justement JS, et al: CD34+ bone marrow cells are infected with HIV in a subset of seropositive individuals, *J Immunol* 149(2):689-697, 1992.

41. Schnittman SM, Denning SM, Greenhouse JJ, et al: Evidence for susceptibility of intrathymic T-cell precursors and their progeny carrying T-cell antigen receptor phenotypes TCR alpha beta+ and TCR gamma delta+ to immunodeficiency virus infection: a mechanism for CD4+ (T4) lymphocyte depletion, *Proc Natl Acad Sci U S A* 87(17):7727-7731, 1990.

42. Laurent-Crawford AG, Krust B, Muller S, et al: The cytopathic effect of HIV is associated with apoptosis, *Virology* 185(2):829-839, 1991.

43. Embretson J, Zapancic M, Ribus JL, et al: Massive covert infection of helper T cells and macrophages by HIV during the incubation period of AIDS, *Nature* 362(6418):359-362, 1993.

44. Pantaleo G, Graziosi C, Demarest JF, et al: HIV infection is active and progressive in lymphoid tissue during the clinically latent stage of disease, *Nature* 362(6418):355-358, 1993b.

45. Pantaleo G, Menzo S, Vaccarezzo M, et al: Studies in subjects with long-term nonprogressive human immunodeficiency virus infection, *N Engl J Med* 332:209-216, 1995.

46. Ott M, Lembcke B, Fischer H, et al: Early changes of body composition in human immunodeficiency virus-infected patients: tetrapolar body impedance analysis indicates significant malnutrition, *Am J Clin Nutr* 57:15-19, 1993.

47. Kotler D: Management of nutritional alterations and issues concerning quality of life, *J Acquir Immune Defic Syndr Hum Retrovirol* 16(suppl 1):51-52, 1997

48. Schambelan M, Mulligan K, Grunfeld C, et al: Recombinant human growth hormone in patients with HIV-associated wasting: a randomized placebo-controlled trial, Serostim Study Group, *Ann Intern Med* 125(1):932-934, 1996.

48a. Rietschel P, Corcoran C, Stanley T, et al: Prevalence of hypogonadism among men with weight loss related to human immunodeficiency virus infection who were receiving highly active antiretroviral therapy, *Clin Infect Dis* 31(5):1240-1244, 2000.

48b. Wanke Ca, Silva M, Knox TA, et al: Weight loss and wasting remain common complications in individuals infected with human immunodeficiency virus in the era of highly active antiretroviral therapy, *Clin Infect Dis* 31(3):803-805, 2000.

49. Pantaleo G, Demarest JF, Soudeyns H, et al: Major expansion of CD8+ T cells with a predominant V beta usage during the primary immune response to HIV, *Nature* 370(6489):463-467, 1994.

50. Daar ES, Moudgil T, Meyer RD, et al: Transient high levels of viremia in patients with primary human immunodeficiency virus type-1 infection, *N Engl J Med* 324(14):961-964, 1991.

51. Glass L, Mackey MC: *From clocks to chaos: the rhythms of life,* Princeton, N.J., 1988, Princeton University Press.

52. Gleick J: *Chaos: making a new science,* New York, 1988, Penguin Books.

53. Liebovitch LS: *Fractals and chaos: simplified for the life sciences,* New York, 1998, Oxford University Press.

54. VanWyk R, Wiegant FAC: The similia principle as a therapeutic strategy: a research program on stimulation of self-defense in disordered mammalian cells, *Altern Ther Health Med* 3(2):33-38,1997.

55. Jacobs J, Moskowitz R: Homeopathy. In Micozzi MS, editor: *Fundamentals of complementary and alternative medicine,* New York, 1996, Churchill Livingstone.

56. Brewitt B, Standish LJ: High dilution GFs/cytokines: positive immunological, hematological, and clinical effects in HIV/AIDS patients, *Eleventh Intl Conf AIDS,* Vancouver, BC, Canada, July 7-12, 1996, pp 270-271.

57. Linde K, Clausius N, Ramirez G, et al: Are the clinical effects of homeopathy placebo effects? a metanalysis of placebo controlled trials, *Lancet* 350:834-843, 1997.

58. Reilly D, Taylor MA, Beattie NGM, et al: Is evidence for homeopathy reproducible? *Lancet* 344:1601-1606, 1994.

59. Kleijnen J, Knipschild P, ter Riet G: Clinical trials of homeopathy, *BMJ* 302:316-323, 1991.

60. Fougeray S, Moubry K, Vallot N, et al: Effect of high dilutions of epidermal GF (EGF) on in vitro proliferation of keratinocyte and fibroblast cell lines, *Br Homeopath J* 82(2):124-125, 1993.

61. Germinario RJ, DeSantis T, Wainberg MA: Insulin-like GF 1 and insulin inhibit HIV type-1 replication in cultured cells, *AIDS Res Hum Retroviruses* 11(5):555-561, 1995.

62. Brewitt B, Hughes J, Welsh EA, et al: Homeopathic human growth hormone for physiologic and psychologic health: three double-blind, placebo-controlled studies, *Alternative Complementary Therapies* 5(6):373-385, 1999.

63. Feng Y, Broder CC, Kennedy PE, et al: HIV-1 entry cofactor: functional DNA cloning of a seven-transmembrane, G protein-coupled receptor, *Science* 272:872-877, 1996.

64. Alkhatib G, Combadiere C, Broder CC, et al: CC CKR5: A rantes, MIP-1α, MIP-1β receptor as a fusion cofactor for macrophage-trophic HIV-1, *Science* 272:1955-1958, 1996.

65. Biggs TE, Cooke SJ, Barton CH, et al: Induction of activator protein-1 (AP-1) in macrophages by human immunodeficiency virus type-1 nef is a cell-type-specific response that requires both hck and MAPK signaling events, *J Mol Biol* 290(1):21-35, 1999.

66. Gibellini D, Re MC, Bassini A, et al: HIV-1 gp120 induces the activation of both c-fos and c-jun immediate-early genes in HEL megakaryocytic cells, *Br J Haematol* 104(1):81-86, 1999.

67. Bulanova EG, Budagyan VM, Yarilin AA, et al: Expression of protooncogenes during lymphocyte activation by GFs, *Biochemistry (Mosc)* 62(9):1021-1025, 1997.

68. Hessol NA, Koblin BA, van Griesven GJ, et al: Progression of human immunodeficiency virus type 1 (HIV-1) among homosexual men in hepatitis B vaccine trial cohorts in Amsterdam, New York, and San Francisco, 1978-1991, *Am J Epidemiol* 139(11):1077-1087, 1994.

69. Burgisser P, Hammann C, Kaufmann D, et al: Expression of CD28 and CD38 by CD8+ T cells in HIV infection correlates with viral load and CD4+ T-cell number at baseline and during treatment, Twelfth World AIDS Conference, Geneva, June 28-July 3, 1998, Abstract #31170.

70. Daar E: AIDS update 1998, Primary Care Essentials CMEA Conference, San Francisco, May 15-19, 1998.

71. Baum MK: Micronutrient deficiencies in HIV infection populations, Update on wasting, metabolism, and altered body shape in HIV/AIDS symposium, Preconference to Twelfth World AIDS Conference, Geneva, June 28, 1998, Tufts University School of Medicine.

72. Buchbinder SP, Katz MH, Hessol NA, et al: Long-term HIV-1 infection without immunological progression, *AIDS* 8:1123-1128, 1994.

73. Cao Y, Qin L, Zhang L, et al: Virilogical and immunological characterization of long-term survivors of human immunodeficiency virus type-1 infection, *N Engl J Med* 332(4):201-208, 1995.

74. Levy J: *HIV and the pathogenesis of AIDS,* Washington, DC, 1993, ASM Press.

75. Ginaldi L, DeMartinis M, D'Ostillio A, et al: Activated naïve and memory CD4+ and CD8+ subsets in different stages of HIV infection, *Pathobiology* 65:91-99, 1997.

76. Schwardtlander B, Bek B, Skarabis H, et al: Improvement of the predictive values of CD4+ lymphocyte count by β2microglobulin, immunoglobulin A, and erythrocyte sedimentation rate, The Multicenter Cohort Study Group, *AIDS* 7:813-821, 1993.

77. Griffin GE, Paton NI, Cofrancesco Jr J, et al: Nutrition and quality of life in HIV infection: the role of growth hormone in HIV-associated wasting, Update on AIDS wasting and lipodystrophy: one-day seminar, Twelfth World AIDS Conference, Geneva, June 28, 1998.

78. Vingerhoets J, Dohlsten M, Penne G, et al: Superantigen activation of CD4+ and CD8+ T cells from HIV-infected subjects: role of co-stimulatory molecules and antigen-presenting cells (APC), *Clin Exp Immunol* 111(1):12-19, 1998.

79. Kotler DP, Tierney AR, Wang J, et al: Magnitude of body cell mass depletion and the timing of death from wasting in AIDS, *Am J Clin Nutr* 50(3):444-447, 1989.

80. Kotler DP, Wang J, Pierson RJ: Body composition studies in patients with the acquired human immunodeficiency syndrome, *Am J Clin Nutr* 42:1255-1265, 1985.

81. Carr A, Samaras K, Chisholm DJ, et al: Pathogenesis of HIV-1-protease inhibitor-associated peripheral lipodystrophy, hyperlipidaemia, and insulin resistance, *Lancet* 351:1881-1883, 1998.

82. Horn T, Pieribone T: The wasting report: current issues in research and treatment of HIV-associated wasting and malnutrition, *Eleventh Intl Conf Aids,* Vancouver, BC, Canada, July 7-12, 1996.

83. Girandola RN, Contarsy S: The validity of bioelectrical impedance to predict human body composition, Olympic Scientific Congress, New Horizons of Human Movement, Seoul, Korea, September 10, 1988.

84. Jodoin RR, Trott SG, Shizgal HM, Determination of whole body composition from whole body electrical impedance, *Surg Forum* 39:50-52, 1988.

85. Cohen J: The daunting challenge of keeping HIV suppressed, *Science* 277:32-33, 1997.

86. Montaner LJ: Cytokine HIV regulation in macrophages and lymphocytes and in AIDS pathogenesis: from in vitro to in vivo, *Res Immunol* 145:575-577, 1994.

87. Zhang L-B, Du C-Y, Qi A-S: Complex behaviours of AB model describing idiotypic network, *Bull Math Biol* 56(2)323-336, 1994.

88. Standish L, Guiltinan J, McMahon E, et al: One-year open trial of naturopathic treatment of HIV infection class IV-A in men, *J Naturopath Med* 3(1):42-64, 1992.

89. Anderson W, O'Connor BB, MacGregor RR, et al: Patient use and assessment of conventional and alternative therapies for HIV infection and AIDS, *AIDS* 7(4):561-566, 1993.

90. Ullman R, Reichenberg-Ullman J, *The patient's guide to homeopathic medicine*, Edmonds, Wash, 1995, Picnic Point Press.

91. Pert CB, Ruff MR, Weber RJ, et al: Neuropeptides and their receptors: a psychosomatic network, *J Immunol* 135:(suppl 2):820s-826s, 1985.

Suggested Reading

Raines EW, Ross R: Multiple GFs are associated with lesions of atherosclerosis: specificity or redundancy? *Bioessays* 18(4):271-282, 1995.

References for Table 9-1

Bunone G, Uggeri M, Mondelline P, et al: RET receptor expression in thyroid follicular epithelial cell derived tumors, *Cancer Res* 60(11):2845-2849, 2000.

Cinti S, Coffey M, Sullivan A, et al: Killing of mycobacterium avian by neutrophils and monocytes from AIDS patients treated with recombinant granulocyte-macrophage colony-stimulating factor, *J Infect Dis* 180(1):229-233, 1999.

Lee PD, Pivarnik JM, Bukar JG, et al: A randomized placebo-controlled trial of combined insulin-like GF 1 and low dose growth hormone therapy for wasting associated with human immunodeficiency virus infection, *J Clin Endocrinol Metab* 81(8):2968-2975, 1996.

Nguyen BY, Clerici M, Venzon DJ, et al: Pilot study of the immunological effects of recombinant human growth hormone and recombinant insulin-like GF in HIV-infected patients, *AIDS* 12(8):895-904, 1998.

Smiell JM: Clinical safety of becaplermin (rhPDGF-BB) gel, Becaplermin Studies Group, *Am J Surg* 176(suppl 2A):68S-73S, 1998.

Terrell TG, Working PK, Chow CP, et al: Pathology of recombinant human transforming GF-B1 in rats and rabbits, *Int Rev Exp Pathol* 34B:43-67, 1993.

References for Table 9-2

Bergerot I, Fabien N, Thivolet C: Effects of insulin-like GF-1 and insulin on effector T cells generating autoimmune diabetes, *Diabetes Metab* 22:235-239, 1996.

Goustin AS, Galanopoulos T, Kalyanaraman V, et al: Coexpression of the genes for platelet-derived GF and its receptor in human T-cell lines infected with HTLV-1, *Growth Factors,* 2:189-195, 1990.

Higgins C: Erythrocyte sedimentation tests as aid to diagnosis, *Nurs Times* 93(6):60-61, 1997.

Hunt P, Eardley DD: Suppressive effects of insulin and insulin-like GF-1 (IGF-1) on immune responses, *J Immunol* 136(11):3994-3999, 1986.

Kehrl JH, Taylor A, Kim S-J, et al: Transforming GF-B is a potent negative regulator of human cells, *Ann N Y Acad Sci* 628:345-353, 1991.

Kekow J, Wachsman W, McCutchan JA, et al: Transforming GF-B and noncytopathic mechanisms of immunodeficiency in human immunodeficiency virus infection, *Proc Natl Acad Sci U S A* 87:8321-8325, 1990.

Lal RB, Rudolph DL, Folks TM, et al: Over-expression of insulin-like GF receptor type 1 in T-cell lines infected with human T-lymphotropic virus types I and II, *Leuk Res* 17:31-35, 1993.

Matsushima K, Sone S, Onozaki K, et al: Meeting report of the international symposium of molecular cell biology of macrophages '92, *Cytokine* 5(2):91-94, 1993.

Perno CF, Balestra E, Aquaro S, et al: Potent inhibition of human immunodeficiency virus and herpes simplex type 1 by 9-(2-phosphonoylmethoxyethyl) adenine in primary macrophages is determined by drug metabolism, nucleotide pools, and cytokines, *Mol Pharmacol* 50(2):359-366, 1996.

Poli G, Kinter AL, Justement JS, et al: Transforming GF-B suppresses human immunodeficiency virus expression and replication in infected cells of the monocyte/macrophage lineage, *J Exp Med* 173:589-597, 1991.

Poli G, Kinter AL, Vicenzi E, et al: Cytokine regulation of acute and chronic HIV infection in vitro: from cell lines to primary mononuclear cells, *Res Immunol* 145:578-582, 1994.

Scadden DT: Granulocyte macrophage colony-stimulating factor (GM-CSF) in AIDS. In *Hematopoietic GFs in transfusion medicine,* New York, 1990, Wiley-Liss.

Yi ES, Lee H, Sin S, et al: Platelet-derived GF causes pulmonary cell proliferation and collagen deposition in vivo, *Am J Pathol* 149(2):539-548, 1996.

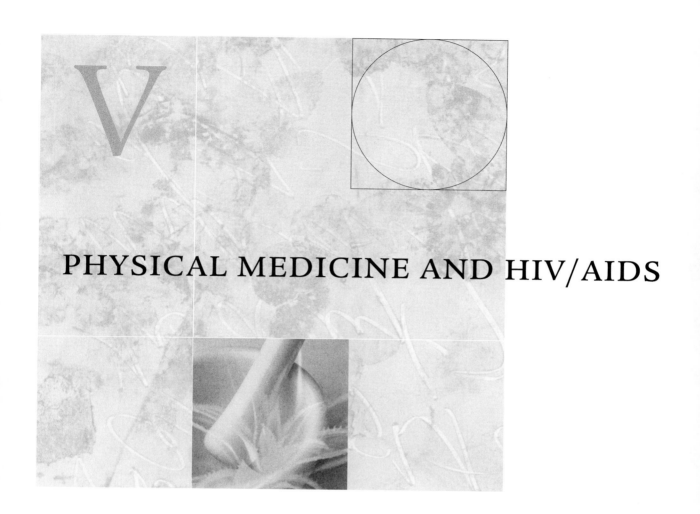

PHYSICAL MEDICINE AND HIV/AIDS

Introduction to Physical Medicine

MARY LOU GALANTINO

The positive effects of exercise, massage, therapeutic touch, and manual therapies on the immune system securely place both alternative therapies and psychoneuroimmunology (PNI) in the domain of interventions for people living with chronic diseases.[1,2] Psychoneuroimmunology shows that healing is facilitated not only by an alternative approach but by the therapeutic presence and holistic nature of the interaction between patient and practitioner.[3] The characteristics of a medical practitioner who acts as a therapeutic agent with his or her patients reflect the philosophy of holism.[4] This section presents various treatment modalities from a physical medicine perspective. At the forefront, however, is patient/practitioner interaction.

The chronic nature of HIV disease warrants various interventions to ease the side effects of medica-

tion. A nonpharmacological approach to pain management is discussed in Chapter 11. Electroacupuncture provides a modality for the management of HIV-related peripheral neuropathy. Small electrical stimulation units can be issued to manage pain at home. This requires a basic working knowledge of the location of acupuncture points for the application of electrical stimulation. Chapter 11 presents data on two different types of electrical currents for the treatment of HIV-related peripheral neuropathy syndrome.

Beyond mechanistic pain management is the use of manual therapies. Massage for newborns and adults is explored in Chapter 12. A review of the data on massage and its alteration of the immune system provides evidence of the healing power of touch. Functional outcome measurements further the support of

149

massage as a useful method for the management of chronic HIV disease.

Chapter 13 expands on additional manual therapy techniques for people living with HIV disease. CranioSacral Therapy (CST), myofascial release (MFR), and lymphatic drainage technique are just a few of the interventions discussed. Few studies have been conducted on these manual therapies; however, their high rates of use are noteworthy.[5]

Movement is crucial to vibrant living. A sedentary nature leads to statis. Extensive research has been conducted in the area of exercise and its beneficial effects on the immune system. Chapter 14 explores the immunoenhancing qualities of aerobic exercise. The prevention of HIV wasting syndrome and lipodystrophy can be augmented through exercise that involves progressive resistance. Various movement therapies, such as Tai Chi, can also improve flexibility and balance, which are important for agile living. This chapter provides the reader with guidelines for embarking on movement interventions.

References

1. Galantino ML, McCormack GL: Pain management. In Galantino ML: *Clinical assessment and treatment of HIV: rehabilitation of a chronic illness*, Thorofare, N.J., 1992, Slack, Inc.
2. LaPerriere A, Antoni M, Fletcher MA, et al: Exercise and health maintenance in HIV. In Galantino ML: *Clinical assessment and treatment of HIV: rehabilitation of a chronic illness*, Thorofare, N.J., 1992, Slack, Inc.
3. Davis CM: Psychoneuroimmunology: the bridge to the coexistence of two paradigms. In Davis CM: *Complementary therapies in rehabilitation*, Thorofare, N.J., 1997, Slack, Inc.
4. Davis CM: *Patient practitioner interaction: an experiential manual for developing the art of health care,* ed 2, Thorofare, N.J., 1994, Slack, Inc.
5. Standish LJ, Greene KB, Bain S, et al: Alternative medicine use in HIV-positive men and women: demographics, utilization patterns, and health status, *AIDS Care* 13(2):197-208, 2001.

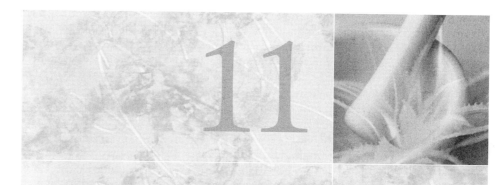

Neuromuscular Manifestations of HIV and Electroacupuncture

MARY LOU GALANTINO
SUNDAY T. EKE-OKORO

Human immunodeficiency virus (HIV) infection has many neuromuscular complications, including loss of lean muscle tissue, involuntary weight loss or wasting, peripheral neuropathies (PNs), and myopathies.[1] AIDS wasting may be caused by reduced food intake, malabsorption of food, increased energy expenditure, hormonal abnormalities, and psychosocial problems.[2,3] Furthermore, loss of body cell mass (BCM) or lipodystrophy may be complications of long-term highly active antiretroviral therapy (HAART).

Peripheral muscle wasting and myopathy have a detrimental effect on muscle performance and physical functioning. Patients with AIDS are already more likely to depend on others for assistance with activities of daily living (ADLs),[4] have a decreased quality of life (QOL), and experience pain. However, the relationship between muscle wasting, pain, and physical functioning requires further research.

Although myopathy is a frequently reported complication of HIV infection, it is not clearly defined in the scientific literature. Previous researchers have discussed other complications, including (1) muscle wasting and weakness,[5] (2) muscle aching or cramps, (3) elevated creatine phosphokinase (CPK) levels,[6] and (4) changes in muscle biopsy or electromyography (EMG).[7] Myopathy is mistakenly diagnosed as myalgia in as many as 24% of people infected with HIV.[6] The cause of myopathy in HIV-positive persons is frequently attributed to the effect of zidovine (AZT).[8] However, Simpson et al have demonstrated in several studies that myopathy may be a consequence of HIV infection rather than AZT.[1,6,7]

Testosterone deficiency in patients with AIDS-related wasting is correlated with both decreased lean body mass (LBM) and poor performance on tests measuring physical functioning, such as a 6-minute walking test and a sit-to-stand test.[9,10] Researchers have established that hormone replacement therapy (HRT) effectively increases body weight (BW),[11] increases LBM, and improves strength.[12] Berger et al[5] found that oxandralone was helpful in increasing BW; subjective improvements in appetite, strength, and physical activity were also noted in patients with AIDS-wasting myopathy. These patients experienced unexplained weight loss and demonstrated proximal muscle weakness but had no other evidence of myopathy.

Exercise may improve strength in HIV-AIDS patients.[13-15] However, any pain must be managed before beginning weight-bearing exercises. Chapter 15 further discusses the benefits of therapeutic exercise and provides alternative strategies for enhancing strength and well-being.

Another frequent neuromuscular complication of HIV infection is distal symmetrical PN (DSPN). This is the most common form of neuropathy in HIV infection, and it includes frequent complaints of numbness, burning, and paresthesias in the feet. These symptoms are typically symmetrical and are often so severe that patients experience contact hypersensitivity and gait disturbances. Neuropathy in the upper extremities and distal weakness may occur during later stages of DSPN. Neurological examination shows a loss of sensory pain and temperature in a stocking/glove distribution, increased vibratory thresholds, and diminished ankle reflexes compared to knee reflexes.[16] Patients with AIDS frequently have concurrent central nervous system (CNS) disorders and neuropathy, which are characterized by hyperactive knee reflexes and depressed ankle reflexes.

The incidence of DSPN increases with advancing immunosuppression, parallel with decreasing $CD4^+$ T-cell counts.[17] Thirty-five percent of patients with AIDS may present with electrophysiological or clinical abnormalities.[18] Furthermore, pathological evidence of DSPN is present in almost all patients who die of AIDS.[19] Researchers have proposed various theories regarding the mechanism of DSPN. Formerly researchers thought that DSPN was caused by direct HIV invasion of the nervous system[20]; most investigators now feel that this is not the case.[21] A "dying-back" neuropathy affecting all fiber types, with prominent macrophage infiltration of the peripheral nerve, has been described.[19] Cytokines, tumor necrosis factor (TNF), and interleukin-1 (IL-1) have been identified in the peripheral nerves of AIDS patients.[22]

BALANCE AND POSTURAL MECHANISMS

The neurological manifestations of HIV disease are numerous, and they involve the central, peripheral, and autonomic nervous systems.[23-25] Polyneuropathy due to AZT (AZT-polyneuropathy) and cytomegalovirus (CMV), which is a common pathogen in AIDS (inflammatory polyneuropathy), may manifest as generalized asymmetric demyelination and chronic denervation of muscles.[26] The demyelination and denervation of nerves that supply postural muscles may weaken these muscles and result in balance problems (e.g., distal pain, paresthesia, or numbness). Also, aside from muscle demyelination and denervation, the pathological process that includes macrophage infiltration of neural structures could spread and affect the vestibular neural complex of the inner ear, which is very important in the maintenance of both static and dynamic balance. Our clinical experience shows that sensory changes are common in the lower limbs of neuropathic HIV/AIDS patients. The balance problems of these patients are connected to a lack of adequate proprioception from the legs while standing, and diminished sensory information makes gait control more difficult.

As in myopathy, DSPN weakens the neuromuscular system and limits functional activities. These effects on the neuromuscular system manifest as disturbances of postural control. Appropriate posture is the starting position for any functional activity. However, compromise of the postural pattern is so characteristic of DSPN that it is a diagnostic for HIV-1 infection.[27] The neurological abnormality resulting from PN in HIV/AIDS patients produces postural disturbances,[28] which may take various forms that exacerbate the severity of the neuropathy[29] and compromise functional activity at various levels. In other words, as the condition of HIV/AIDS patients deteriorates, balance deficits may increase.

According to Husstedt et al,[30] PN in HIV disease progresses much more rapidly than that associated with diabetes or hereditary polyneuropathies. Also, as HIV progresses, DSPN increases, resulting in depression of certain motor functions, such as gait and manual dexterity. Demyelination causes the condition to grow worse.[30] Therefore HIV neuropathy should be treated as soon as it is diagnosed to avoid complications.

The balance problems of HIV-1 infection were studied in a group of 50 patients whose conditions were complicated by neuropathy.[31] The researchers recorded the patients' postural performance by using a postural platform and found an increase of pathological sway path values and gait ataxia. They suggested that the patients' balance problems were caused by reduced somatosensory feedback and the probable involvement of central motor and sensory systems. They also felt that monitoring the balance problems could provide information on the neurological course of HIV/AIDS.

Somatosensory feedback from the lower limbs of neuropathic patients is therefore important in triggering centrally organized postural synergies.[32] Postural imbalance, aside from being an early sign of CNS penetration of HIV, could indicate how the disease progresses.[31] The balance problems of HIV/AIDS patients are generally connected to neuropathic or myopathic conditions that develop either through the original viral infection or as a result of antiretroviral therapy (ART). Neuropathy ultimately leads to postural imbalance, which adversely affects any ADLs that require standing and walking.

Our research group has identified PN and its complications as the cause of functional derangement in HIV/AIDS patients. For instance, a patient who experiences balance derangement resulting from PN may not function effectively in ADLs. Functional limitations cause people to leave the workplace, which is true for persons with HIV/AIDS-related PN. Pain is the limiting factor in the ability to return to work. Any intervention that reduces functional limitations should be applied.

HIV/AIDS patients with neuropathy face balance problems resulting from deranged proprioceptive and kinesthetic systems. In fact, they may become concomitantly weakened, and the nervous system may become incapable of integrating balance signals. Patients may lose their balance while performing more demanding ADLs, such as walking. Therefore researchers need to study balance in HIV/AIDS patients to formulate a precise rehabilitation approach based on the underlying neurophysiological deficit.

PAIN

Pain is another factor closely related to the neuropathy of HIV/AIDS patients. Most AIDS patients require various pain treatment interventions. Painful DSPN is the most common PN complaint in patients with HIV-1 infection.[33] PN is also one of the most common types of pain reported by HIV-infected men.[34] PNs occur in as many as 40% to 60% of patients with HIV disease—the most common of which is DSPN. This manifests itself in hyperesthesia, sensory ataxia, weakness, and hypoactive deep tendon reflexes of the ankle. When neuropathy results in painful distal paresthesia, imbalances in stance and gait may result from compensatory measures aimed at relieving pain in dynamic standing activities. Postural compensations may further exacerbate musculoskeletal, cervical, thoracic, or low back pain.

Pain management is a critical part of the overall care of individuals with HIV disease. Pain is the second most common reason for the hospitalization of AIDS patients.[35] A study of 72 AIDS patients found that 97% experienced pain that was related to their disease process.[36] Newshan and Wainapel, who surveyed 100 patients with AIDS-associated pain, showed that the two reported pain types were abdominal and neuropathic pain. In a longitudinal study of HIV-infected men, Singer et al[34] found that painful PN was one of the most common types of pain.

PHARMACOLOGICAL THERAPY

HIV Disease

HIV disease has been treated mostly by a combination of antiretroviral agents, some of which are protease inhibitors (PIs). Using ART in combination with PIs increases the survival of patients with CMV retinitis.[37] Nucleoside analogs (e.g., AZT, didanosine (ddI), zalcitabine (ddC), lamivudine (3TC), stavudine (d4T), and ziagen), nonnucleoside analogs (e.g., viramune, rescriptor, and sustiva), and PIs (e.g., fortovase, crixivan, norvir, viracept, agenerase) are potent pharmacological agents that have improved the QOL of HIV-infected persons. PIs produce a substantial decrease in plasma viral load,[38] and the triple drug regimen given as an initial therapy in HIV-infected individuals also significantly reduces viral load.[39] Although medication has helped increase life expectancy in

HIV-infected individuals, the drugs have difficult side effects. The following antiretroviral drugs are connected with various pathologies: (1) prolonged AZT therapy causes myopathy,[40,41] (2) ddI causes pancreatitis and PN,[42] and (3) ddC is both neuropathogenic[43] and cardiomyopathic.[44] Chemotherapeutic agents can also cause PN.

Neuropathic Pain

Common drugs used to treat HIV-related neuropathic pain are grouped into opioid and nonopioid substances. Nonopioid drugs, such as aspirin and acetaminophen, are used for mild to moderate pain, whereas opioid drugs (e.g., codeine, oxycodone, and hydrocodone) are used for persistent, severe pain. Opioid substances are very effective analgesics, but they may have serious side effects. Adjuvant analgesics also include tricyclic antidepressants (e.g., amitriptyline, desipramine, and doxepin) and anticonvulsants (e.g., Neurontin).[45]

NONPHARMACOLOGICAL APPROACHES TO THE TREATMENT OF PN

Acupuncture

DSPN exhibits painful paresthesia that may be resistant to pharmacological treatment.[23] Our clinical experience shows that conventional transcutaneous electrical stimulation (TENS) may exacerbate peripheral pain in HIV/AIDS patients. Conventional TENS is based on the gate-control theory, and it can be placed percutaneously over the painful area or over specific nerve roots of the lumbar spine to augment the pain distally. Because of the painful hypersensitivity common in DSPN, researchers decided to evaluate the effects of alternative modalities, such as electroacupuncture.

The use of acupuncture is growing in popularity in most Western countries,[46] and the effectiveness of electroacupuncture as a modality for pain treatment is shown by a significant decrease in visual analog scale scores.[47] The therapeutic effects of acupuncture have been the subject of several Chinese investigations for many years.[48-52] Acupuncture encourages the production of endorphins, which reduce pain, promote sleep, and regulate body systems. AIDS patients who experience pain, coughing, weight loss, or gland inflammation respond well to acupuncture.[53]

In a study by Shlay et al,[54] acupuncture and amitriptyline were compared to evaluate the effectiveness of pain reduction in HIV-related PN. They found that, after 14 weeks of treatment, patients in all treatment groups reported some pain relief, but neither active treatment was more effective than the placebo in relieving neuropathic pain. However, with the increasing acceptance of acupuncture as an effective modality for pain treatment, its scope of research has widened considerably, and further research is required to evaluate its efficacy in various neuromuscular manifestations of HIV disease.

Acupuncture is used to complement drug therapy in some patients.[55] The intensive research efforts on other therapeutic effects of acupuncture have produced encouraging results.[56-59] These results indicate reduction of pain and spasticity, improvement of motor function, better balance, and improved gait; they therefore have a neurophysiological basis and require a neurophysiological interpretation. Among individuals with HIV/AIDS, the therapeutic effects of acupuncture are expected to improve the functions of the affected neuromuscular system. One of the possible mechanisms by which acupuncture affects motor function is stimulation of the release of endogenous opioids.[60]

Changing the amplitude of end plate potential thus facilitates events at the neuromuscular junctions. Peripheral factors contribute to the potentiation of a reflex (e.g., the H-reflex) and may affect the afferents and the neuromuscular junction.[61]

Stimulation of the sensory system results in integrative actions at the spinal cord level, where acupuncture may facilitate the stretch reflex arc through both gamma and alpha motor neurons. Facilitation may depend upon the intensity and timing of the stimuli used to activate muscle afferents.[62]

MICROCURRENT AND MICROCURRENT ACUPUNCTURE

A combination of several features distinguishes microcurrent from other electrotherapy modalities. (1) Microcurrent uses a monophasic, or direct current

(DC) rectangular waveform. The polarity of microcurrent may either stay constant or shift during treatment, but it is maintained at 1 polarity for at least 1 second before shifting. (2) Microcurrent uses a 50% duty cycle. As a result, the total current delivered is independent of the frequency of stimulation; the current flows for one half of the total treatment time. Frequency and pulse width (or pulse duration) have a fixed relationship. (3) Microcurrent produces low maximum current values, which are typically in the 300 to 600 µA (0.3 to 0.6 mA) range. By comparison, TENS devices use maximum currents, which are over 50 times greater (in the 50 to 100 mA range). (4) Microcurrent has a broad frequency range, from 0.3 Hz to 1000 Hz. In comparison, TENS devices typically have frequencies from 1 to 120 Hz.[63] Researchers have described the differences between microcurrent and TENS and have recommended microcurrent application in PN.[64] In this chapter, microcurrent acupuncture refers to the application of microcurrent electrodes at specific acupuncture points for a therapeutic purpose. The method of application uses electrodes and is noninvasive.

Microcurrent Effects on Pain

A 1991 review of the outpatient records of HIV/AIDS patients at an HIV clinic based in Houston found that 80% of patient referrals were for pain management. Thirty-seven percent of those referrals presented with painful PNs.[65] In 1998 a review of an HIV pain management program at an early intervention clinic in Voorhees, New Jersey revealed that 54% of the patients suffering from pain had a diagnosis of PN.[66] Lerner and Kirsch[67] evaluated the effects of microcurrent stimulation on 201 patients with chronic neuromusculoskeletal back pain. The patients' perception of pain was evaluated using several pain-rating scales for 2 weeks before treatment was initiated to establish a baseline pain level. A prototype of a low voltage stimulator with stimulus capabilities similar to those of low-volt microcurrent stimulation delivered a biphasic microcurrent of variable frequency. Patients were treated with either actual or placebo stimulation along painful areas of the back or extremities at points previously identified as having low skin impedance. Each point was stimulated twice for a period of 6 seconds. Patients received treatment 3 times/week

for 2 weeks. Pain levels were assessed by the patients hourly during waking hours and were recorded on a graph. Results indicated that patients in both the placebo and stimulation groups experienced transient pain relief.

Our research group treated 15 patients with a diagnosis of DSPN. All patients were evaluated to rule out any preexisting acute CNS disorder or other competing pathologies. Two patients were eliminated because of additional pathologies. In addition to the evaluation, gait efficiency was measured by counting the number of steps taken in a distance of 20 feet. Patients were also asked to rank their pain on a scale of 0 to 10.

Patients were randomly assigned to experimental and control groups. There were a total of seven patients in the experimental group and six in the control group. All patients read the study protocol and signed a consent form before the study. Two physical therapists collected data and administered the treatment. Both therapists clinically evaluated the patients by using the ranking scale and counting the number of steps.

A chi-square was used to analyze the data; the step frequency of the control group was compared to the step frequency of the experimental group. The study claimed that both groups would walk 20 feet with an equal step frequency. The level of significance was set at $p < 0.05$. The change score between the pretests and posttests for ranking pain on a scale of 0 to 10 and the number of steps taken in 20 feet was used for the chi-square. The experimental group exhibited a significant difference for both pain reduction and improved gait. The control group demonstrated no significant difference for either pain or gait from pretest to posttest. A follow-up Mann-Whitney test was performed. The change score for improved gait approached significance at $z = 1.8970$ and $p = 0.0578$ for the experimental group. The change score for pain using the Mann-Whitney test failed to reach significance, with $z = 1.1967$ and $p = 0.2314$ for each group.

The conclusions drawn from this study were limited by several factors. Two therapists were involved in the data collection. No intratests or intertests of reliability were performed. However, both therapists were trained before the data collection. Despite these limitations, the study provided the first prospective work performed on the effectiveness of treatment modalities in individuals with HIV disease experiencing painful DSPN.

SUPRATHRESHOLD CURRENT ELECTROACUPUNCTURE

Noninvasive Electroacupuncture and the Use of the H-wave Stimulator

In our trial of an alternative treatment, we used suprathreshold electroacupuncture derived from the H-wave therapeutic unit (Electronic Waveform Lab, Inc., Cardiff, Calif.) on seven patients. We identified acupuncture points on which noninvasive electrodes were placed, and the suprathreshold current passed for 20 minutes/day for 30 days. The four acupuncture points (Figure 11-1) were selected on the basis of their use in a previous study. They were originally selected in consultation with experienced acupuncturists. However, the study was designed for home stimulation, and patients would have to apply the electrodes themselves; we had to eliminate the L5-S1 electrode position because patients could not accurately apply the electrodes to their backs without visual guidance. This point was replaced with Liv3, which was one of the alternative points recommended in our preliminary study. The chosen acupuncture points were readily accessible to the patients during the application of electrodes, and they corresponded to acupuncture points used in the treatment of lower extremity pain. The noninvasive method avoided use of needles and allowed home stimulation. Patients were assessed both before and after the intervention with the Medical Outcomes Study (MOS)-HIV, a 30-item instrument questionnaire that measures QOL. Tibial H-reflex (Hoffmann reflex) was similarly recorded from the right calf muscle to measure the integrity of the nervous system. H-reflex is a well-known monosynaptic reflex used for clinical assessment of the neuromuscular system. Its parameters include the latency of the reflex (H-latency) and the amplitude (H-amplitude). The direct muscle response obtained during the elicitation of the H-reflex is known as the M-response, and its latency is known as the M-latency. These parameters are used during clinical assessment of the neuromuscular system. Aside from a possible effect on pain, electroacupuncture may produce other neurophysiological effects. To explore these effects, the H-reflex was monitored before and after the intervention. The H-reflex has been used as a CNS model to test the effects of chemical and nonchemical agents on the nervous system.[61] The H-reflex is a postural re-

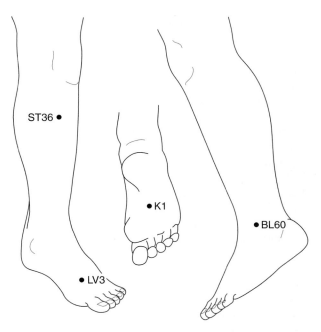

Figure 11-1 Acupuncture points used for electroacupuncture. (From Galantino et al, Electroacupuncture and peripheral neuropathy, *J Altern Complement Med* 5(2):135-142, 1999.)

flex and has also been used to determine S1 radiculopathy[68] and neuropathy.[69,70]

The patients' conditions improved spontaneously. They felt much better and reported having increased physical strength. The outcomes on the MOS-HIV 30-item instrument and H-reflex, which used multivariate analysis of variance (MANOVA) and paired *t*-test, showed significant overall improvement in functional activities when preintervention and postintervention assessments were compared. It is not easy to explain how electroacupuncture produced these results. Since an elaborate experimental design is necessary to explore the process of electroacupuncture effects, we only suggested processes based on well-known neurophysiological principles. For example, increases in H_{max} and M-amplitudes of the H-reflex suggest that electroacupuncture produces an excitatory effect on the neuromuscular system. This effect may be seen in membrane potential (possibly through the influence of ionic transport) and improvement in body fluid circulation. At the peripheral level, acupuncture modulates receptor sensitivity via sympathetic innervation.[71]

Acupuncture also facilitates physiological reflexes in response to the patient's internal or external environment[72] and as a type of sensory stimulation. Patients treated with acupuncture improved significantly in both mobility and balance.[73] Stroke patients who were given sensory stimulation recovered faster than controls.[74] In her review of sensory stimulation, Johansson[73] suggested that acupuncture improves the plasticity of the brain, resulting in an improvement in the patient's condition.

M-latency decreased after the intervention, whereas H-latency was not affected. M-latency does not involve a circuitry such as the reflex arc of the H-reflex. Its decrease may be related to an improvement in the status of the patient's musculocutaneous tissue through electroacupuncture. Such an influence on the neuromuscular system may be connected to improved blood supply to the neuromuscular tissues. Blood vessels are innervated by sensory nerve fibers that contain vasodilator neuropeptides, and electroacupuncture may increase blood flow in musculocutaneous surgical flaps of rats by releasing vasodilatory substances from sensory neurons, inhibiting sympathetic vasoconstriction, or a combination of both.[75]

We also examined the relationship between H-latency and the duration of HIV/AIDS. The H-latency (measured in ms) of a normal person is approximately equal to one sixth of that person's height, and H-reflex latency increases with height.[61] By using the one-sixth height formula, an estimate of the H-reflex latency of a normal person who is 6 feet tall (183 cm) equals 30.48 ms. The expected latency value for an HIV/AIDS patient was therefore calculated as one sixth of his or her height (as corrected for height) and compared with the recorded value from the patient's calf. A comparison of expected (predicted) and recorded values showed that the recorded value was prolonged in relation to the expected value. The conclusion was that H-latency is prolonged as the duration of HIV/AIDS increases. The increase in H-latency is similar to the decrease of nerve conduction velocity in HIV patients.[76,77]

Pain level was reduced after intervention. Electroacupuncture may have caused this effect through a release of endogenous opioids that are essential in the induction of functional changes of different organ systems; endorphins exert effects by binding to opioid receptors.[71] Acupuncture therefore causes a release of the body's own CNS endorphins and enkephalins, which can inhibit either pain or pain transmission. According to Thomas, Collins, and Strauss,[78] acupuncture modulates sympathetic nervous system responses,

which play an integral part in somatic pain. They suggested that sympathetic activation produces vasodilation mediated by prostaglandin release in experimental arthritis, and they concluded that the most significant effect of acupuncture is the reduction of sympathetic activity with an increase in cutaneous temperature. They treated 20 outpatients with acupuncture, and they obtained pain relief and reduced sympathetic activity (increased skin temperature with a mean change of $0.55°$ C) with a significant difference in temperature before and after treatment ($p < 0.01$).

Further research is needed to evaluate the efficacy of various nonpharmacological approaches to the management of DSPN. This study indicates that other types of PN should be investigated through electroacupuncture. The limitations of the study include a lack of diagnostic tests that can discern the etiology of changes in PN. For example, EMG, muscle, and nerve biopsies could provide more information regarding PN and its treatment. Additional limitations include the number of patients in the study and patient subjective reports. Greater control of electroacupuncture could be attained through stimulation at various clinic locations. However, home electroacupuncture stimulation may be efficient and easy to use in light of cost-effective pain management.

This trial study of an alternative treatment for HIV/AIDS-related PN shows that electroacupuncture can ameliorate the complications of HIV-related PN syndrome. Similar studies could also be expedited to evaluate the efficacy of electroacupuncture for pain associated with HIV myopathy. Future studies should give more insight into the process by which electroacupuncture produces its effects on neuromuscular manifestations in patients with HIV/AIDS.

References

1. Wulff EA, Simpson DM: Neuromuscular complications of the par human immunodeficiency virus type 1 infection, *Semin Neurol* 19:157-164, 1999.
2. Abbaticola MM: A team approach to the treatment of AIDS wasting, *J Assoc Nurses AIDS Care* 11:45-56, 2000.
3. Corcoran C, Grinspoon S: Drug therapy: Treatments for wasting in patients with acquired immunodeficiency syndrome, *New Engl J Med* 340:1740-1750, 1999.
4. Stanton DL, Wu AW, Moore RD, et al: Functional status of persons with HIV infection in an ambulatory setting, *J Acquir Immune Defic Syndr Hum Retrovirol* 7:1050-1056, 1994.

5. Berger JR, Pall L, Hall CD, et al: Oxandrolone in AIDS-wasting myopathy, *AIDS* 10:1657-1662, 1996.

6. Simpson DM, Katzenstein DA, Hughes MD, et al: AIDS Clinical Trials Group 175/801 Study Team, Neuromuscular function in HIV infection: analysis of a placebo-controlled combination antiretroviral trial, *AIDS* 12:2425-2432, 1998.

7. Simpson DM, Citak KA, Godfrey E, et al: Myopathies associated with human immunodeficiency virus and zidovine: can their effects be distinguished? *Neurology* 43:971-976, 1993.

8. Casademont J, Barrientos A, Grau JM, et al: The effect of zidovine on skeletal muscle mtDNA in HIV-1-infected patients with mild or no muscle dysfunction, *Brain* 119:1357-1364, 1996.

9. Grinspoon S, Corcoran C, Lee K, et al: Loss of lean body and muscle mass correlates with androgen levels in hypogonadal men with acquired immune deficiency syndrome and wasting, *J Clin Endocrinol Metab* 81(11):4051-4058, 1996.

10. Grinspoon S, Corcoran C, Rosenthal D, et al: Quantitative assessment of cross-sectional muscle area, functional status, and muscle strength in men with acquired immune deficiency syndrome and wasting syndrome, *J Clin Endocrinol Metab* 84:201-206, 1999.

11. Mulligan K, Grunfeld C, Hellerstein M, et al: Anabolic effects of recombinant human growth hormone in patients with wasting associated with human immunodeficiency virus infection, *J Clin Endocrinol Metab* 77:956-962, 1993.

12. Sattler F, Jaque SV, Schroeder ET, et al: Effects of pharmacological doses of nandrolone decanoate and progressive resistance training in immunodeficient patients infected with human immunodeficiency virus, *J Clin Endocrinol Metab* 84:1268-1276, 1999.

13. Roubenoff R, McDermott A, Weiss L, et al: Short-term progressive resistance training increases strength and lean body mass in adults infected with human immunodeficiency virus, *AIDS* 13:231-239, 1999a.

14. Roubenoff R, Weiss L, McDermott A, et al: A pilot study of exercise training to reduce trunk fat in adults with HIV-associated fat redistribution, *AIDS* 13:1373-1375, 1999b.

15. Spence D, Galantino ML, Mossberg K, et al: Progressive resistance exercise: effect on muscle function and anthropometry of a select AIDS population, *Arch Phys Med Rehabil* 71:644-648, 1990.

16. Simpson DM, Tagliati M: Neurological manifestation of HIV infection, *Ann Intern Med* 121:769-785, 1994.

17. Simpson DM, Tagliati M, Grinell J, et al: Electrophysiological findings in HIV infection: association with distal symmetrical polyneuropathy and CD4 level, *Muscle Nerve* 17:1113, 1994 (abstract).

18. So YT, Holtzman DM, Abrams DI, et al: Peripheral neuropathy associated with acquired immunodeficiency syndrome: prevalence and clinical features based on a population-based survey, *Arch Neurol* 45:945-948, 1988.

19. Griffin JW, Crawford TO, Tyor WR, et al: Predominantly sensory neuropathy in AIDS: distal axonal degeneration and unmyelinated fiber loss, *Neurology* 41(suppl 1):374, 1991.

20. Ho DD, Rota TR, Schooley RT, et al: Isolation of HTLV-III from cerebrospinal fluid and neural tissues of patients with neurological syndromes related to acquired immune deficiency syndrome, *N Engl J Med* 313:1493-1497, 1985.

21. Simpson DM, Olney RK: Peripheral neuropathies associated with human immunodeficiency virus infection. In Dyck PJ, editor: *Peripheral neuropathy,* Philadelphia, 1994, WB Saunders.

22. Griffin JW, Wesselingh S, Oaklander AL, et al: mRNA fingerprinting of cytokines and growth factors: a new means of characterizing nerve biopsies, *Neurology* 43(suppl 2):A232, 1993 (abstract).

23. Scherer P: How HIV attacks the peripheral nervous system, *Am J Nurs* 90(5):66-70, 1990.

24. Berger J: Neurological complications of HIV disease, *PAAC Notes* 1992:236-240, 1992.

25. Vinter H, Andres K: *Neuropathology of AIDS,* Boca Raton, Fla, 1990, CRC Press.

26. Morgello S, Simpson DM: Multifocal cytomegalovirus demyelinative polyneuropathy associated with AIDS, *Muscle Nerve* 17:176-182, 1994.

27. Petiot P, Vighetto A, Charles N, et al: Isolated postural tremor revealing HIV-1 infection, *J Neurol* 240(8):507-508, 1993.

28. Arendt G, Maecker HP, Purramann J, et al: Control of posture in patients with neurologically asymptomatic HIV infection and patients with beginning HIV-1-related encephalopathy, *Arch Neurol* 51(12):1232-1235, 1994.

29. Boucher P, Teasdale N, Courtemanche R, et al: Postural stability in diabetic polyneuropathy, *Diabetes Care* 18(5):638-645, 1995.

30. Husstedt I, Grotemeyer K, Heiner B, et al: Progression of distal-symmetrical polyneuropathy in HIV infection: a prospective study, *AIDS* 7(8):1069-1073, 1993.

31. Trenkwalder C, Straube A, Paulus W, et al: Postural imbalance: an early sign in HIV-1-infected patients, *Eur Arch Psychiatry Clin Neurosci* 241:267-272, 1992.

32. Inglis JT, Fay B, Horak FB, et al: The importance of somatosensory information triggering and scaling automatic postural responses in humans, *Brain Res* 101:159-164, 1994.

33. Bradley WG, Verma A: Painful vasculitic neuropathy in HIV-1 infection: relief of pain with prednisone therapy, *Neurology* 47(6):1446-1451, 1996.

34. Singer E, Zorilla C, Fahy-Chandon B, et al: Painful symptom reported by ambulatory HIV-infected men in a longitudinal study, *Pain* (54):15-19, 1993.

35. Lewis M, Warfield C: Management of pain in AIDS, *Hosp Pract (Off Ed)* Oct 30, 51-54, 1990.

36. Newshan G, Wainapel S: Pain characteristics and their management in persons with AIDS, *J Assoc Nurses AIDS Care* 4(2):53-59, 1993.

37. Walsh JC, Jones CD, Barnes EA, et al: Increasing survival in AIDS patients with cytomegalovirus retinitis treated with combination antiretroviral therapy including HIV protease inhibitors, *AIDS* 12:613-618, 1998.

38. Rhone SA, Hogg RS, Yip B, et al: The antiviral effect of ritonavir and saquinavir in combination amongst HIV-infected adults: results from a community-based study, *AIDS* 12:619-624, 1998.

39. Hogg RS, Rhone SA, Yip B, et al: Antiviral effect of double and triple drug combinations amongst HIV-infected adults: lessons from the implementation of viral load-driven antiretroviral therapy, *AIDS* 12:279-284, 1998.

40. Chalmers AC, Greco CM, Miller RG: Prognosis in AZT myopathy, *Neurology* 41:1181-1184, 1991.

41. Manji H, Harrison MJ, Round RH, et al: Muscle disease, HIV, and zidovudine: the spectrum of muscle disease in HIV-infected individuals treated with zidovudine, *J Neurol* 240(8):479-488, 1993.

42. Lambert JS, Seidlin M, Reichman RC, et al: 2,3-dideoxy-inosine (ddI) in patients with acquired immune deficiency syndrome or AIDS-related complex, *N Engl J Med* 322:1333-1340, 1990.

43. Merigan TC, Skowron G: ddC Study Group of the AIDS Clinical Trials Group of the National Institute for Allergy and Infectious Diseases: safety and tolerance of dideoxycytidine as a single agent, *Am J Med* 99(suppl 5B):11S-15S, 1990.

44. Herskowitz A, Willoughby SB, Baughman KL, et al: Cardiomyopathy associated with antiretroviral therapy in patients with human immunodeficiency virus infection: a report of 6 cases, *Ann Intern Med* 116:311-313, 1992.

45. Breitbart W, McDonald M: Pharmacologic pain management in HIV/AIDS, *J Int Assoc Physicians AIDS Care* 21(7):17-26, 1996.

46. Senior K: Acupuncture: can it take pain away? *Mol Med Today* 2(4):150-153, 1996.

47. Kumar A, Tandon OP, Bhattacharya A, et al: Somatosensory evoked potential changes following electroacupuncture therapy in chronic pain patients, *Anaesthesia* 50(5):411-414, 1995.

48. Yuan F, Ymeng C, Qimeiz: CT Scanning and therapeutic effects of acupuncture on 108 cases of hemiplegia due to apoplexy, *Int J Clin Acupunct* 1(1):1-6, 1990.

49. Chen CH, Chou P, Hu HH, et al: Further analysis of a pilot study for planning an extensive clinical trial in traditional medicine: with an example of acupuncture treatment for stroke, *Am J Chin Med* 22(2):127-136, 1991.

50. Raoqi K: Treatment of apoplectic hemiplegia with scalp needling, using withdrawing-replenishing method plus physical exercise: a clinical observation, *Int J Clin Acupunct* 3(2):175-178, 1992.

51. Hu HH, Chung C, L'edu T, et al: A randomized controlled trial on the treatment for acute partial ischemic stroke with acupuncture, *Neuroepidemiology* 12:106-113, 1993.

52. Yukang W, Gao X, Guilan L, et al: Treatment of apoplectic hemiplegia with scalp acupuncture in relation to CT findings, *J Tradit Chin Med* 13(3):182-184, 1993.

53. Sommers B: Chinese medicine and acupuncture in the treatment of AIDS, *Sidahora* Oct/Nov, 37-38, 1995.

54. Shlay JC, Chaloner K, Max MB, et al: Acupuncture and amitriptyline for pain due to HIV-related peripheral neuropathy, *JAMA* 280:1590, 1998.

55. Huson C: Acupuncture and traditional Oriental medicine in the treatment of HIV and AIDS, *STEP Perspect* 8(1):2-3, 1996.

56. Xiaoshan D: Clinical observation on acupuncture treatment of 200 cases of hemiplegia, *Int J Clin Acupunct* 1(3):229-233, 1990.

57. Shoukang L: Acupuncture therapy for apoplectic hemiplegia, *Int J Acupunct* 2(4):333-335, 1992.

58. Chen A: Effective acupuncture therapy for stroke and cerebrovascular diseases, part I, *Am J Acupunct* 21(2):105-122, 1993.

59. Naeser MA, Alexander MP, Stiassy-Elder D, et al: Laser acupuncture in the treatment of paralysis in stroke patients: a CT scan lesion site study, *Am J Acupunct* 23(1):13-28, 1995.

60. Hans JS, Terenius L: Neurochemical basis of acupuncture analgesia, *Annu Rev Pharmacol Toxicol* 22:193-220, 1982.

61. Eke-Okoro ST: The H-reflex studied in the presence of alcohol, aspirin, caffeine, force, and fatigue, *Electromyogr Clin Neurophysiol* 22:579-589, 1982.

62. Jankowska E, Perfilieva EU, Ridell JS: How effective is integration of information from muscle afferents in spinal pathways? *Neuroreport* 7(14):2337-2340, 1996.

63. Carley PJ, Wainapel SF: Electrotherapy for acceleration of wound healing: low intensity direct current, *Arch Phys Med Rehabil* 66:443-446, 1985.

64. McReynolds MA: Rehabilitation management of the lower extremity in HIV disease, *J Am Podiatr Med Assoc* 85(7):392-402, 1995.

65. McReynolds MA, Galantino ML (unpublished).

66. Galantino ML, Jermyn RT: Comprehensive pain management for HIV disease: strategies for the rehabilitation team. A case study, Abstract presented at the National APTA Conference, Seattle, 1999.

67. Lerner FN, Kirsch DL: Microstimulation and placebo effect in short-term treatment of the chronic back pain patient, *ACA J Chiropractic* 15:101-106, 1981.

68. Braddom RL, Johnson EW: Standardization of the H-reflex and diagnostic use in radiculopathy, *Arch Phys Med Rehabil* 55:161-166, 1974.

69. Chandran AP, Singal KK, Mahajan SK, et al: H-reflex latency and sensory conduction in the assessment of neuropathy in patients of chronic obstructive lung disease, *Electromyogr Clin Neurophysiol* 31(2):99-107, 1991.

70. Ciompi ML, Marini D, Siciliano G, et al: Cryoglob-ulinemic peripheral neuropathy: neurophysiologic evaluation in 22 patients, *Biomed Pharmacother* 50(8): 329-336, 1996.

71. Andersson S: The functional background in acupuncture effects, *Scand J Rehabil Med Suppl* 29:31-60, 1993.

72. Yao T: Acupuncture and somatic nerve stimulation: mechanism underlying effects on cardiovascular and renal activities, *Scand J Rehabil Med Suppl* 29:7-18, 1993.

73. Johansson BB: Has sensory stimulation a role in stroke rehabilitation? *Scand J Rehabil Med Suppl* 29:87-96, 1993.

74. Johansson K, Lindgren I, Winder H, et al: Can sensory stimulation improve the functional outcome in stroke patients? *Neurology* 43:2189-2192, 1993.

75. Jansen G, Lundberg T, Kjartansson J, et al: Acupuncture and sensory neuropeptides increase cutaneous blood flow in rats, *Neurosci Lett* 97:305-309, 1989.

76. Lange DJ, Britton CB, Younger DS, et al: The neuromuscular manifestations of human immunodeficiency virus infections, *Arch Neurol* 45:1084-1088, 1988.

77. Husstedt I, Grotemeyer K, Busch H, et al: Early detection of distal symmetrical polyneuropathy during HIV infection by paired stimulation of sural nerve, *Electroencephalogr Clin Neurophysiol* 93:169-174, 1994.

78. Thomas D, Collins S, Strauss S: Somatic sympathetic vasomotor changes documented by medical thermographic imaging during acupuncture analgesia, *Clin Rheumatol* 11(1):55-59, 1992.

HIV-Exposed Newborns and Massage Therapy Effects on the HIV-Exposed Newborn and Adult

TIFFANY FIELD

Heterosexual contact and intravenous (IV) drug use continue to contribute to human immunodeficiency virus type 1 (HIV-1) infection among women of childbearing age.[1] In his review of North American and European surveys, Andiman[1] notes that between 0.1% to 0.3% of women of childbearing age are infected with HIV. The use of antiretroviral therapy (ART) by HIV-positive mothers markedly reduced the risk of vertical HIV-1 transmission.[1] Recent advances in diagnostic urology led to the definitive identification of infants who were infected with HIV by approximately 3 to 4 months of age.

In a review by Campbell,[2] mother-to-child transmission of HIV (vertical transmission) was the main cause of pediatric HIV worldwide. The rate of vertical transmission was approximately 15% to 20%, although the rate was significantly lower in less-developed coun-

tries (30%). According to this review, approximately 40% of HIV-positive children developed AIDS within the first 4 years of life. Associated conditions were common among these children and frequently took the form of developmental delays, neurological symptoms, specific cognitive difficulties, and behavioral problems.

In a comparative study on the first year of growth in HIV-infected and uninfected infants, 102 infants were diagnosed with HIV status, and 21.5% were infected with HIV.[3] From 2 to 4 months of age, the averages of the weights and heights of the HIV-infected infants were lower than those of the uninfected infants. Abnormal clinical signs were found in most HIV-infected infants by the time they were between 9 to 12 months old. In a related study,[4] somatic growth and the relationship between nutritional status and

161

mortality were explored in HIV-infected infants. The mean weight-for-age and length-for-age curves of the HIV-positive children were significantly lower than those of the HIV-negative controls and seroreverters. Fifty-four percent of the HIV-positive infants died before their second birthday, compared with 1.6% and 5.6% mortality in HIV-negative infants and seroreverters. A study by Culnane et al[5] suggests that even uninfected children born to HIV-infected women showed growth delays. At the age of 18 months, the growth of uninfected children born to HIV-infected women, whether or not they were exposed to zidovudine (AZT) in utero, remained significantly below the growth of infants born to healthy HIV-negative women.

One problem with seroreverters is that it takes approximately 4 to 6 months to determine whether an infant has HIV disease. Thus the HIV-positive mothers were uncertain about the HIV status of their infants and their own HIV disease while forming a mother-child relationship.[6] This uncertainty invariably affects the interactions between the mothers and infants, which in turn may contribute to growth and developmental delays, as has been noted in many other high-risk infant populations. An example of this problem is given in a study by Byrne,[7] in which she observed a sample of HIV-exposed infants on the Nursing Child Assessment Satellite Training (NCAST) Feeding Scale during one feeding session. The mothers and infants demonstrated significant weaknesses in their interaction, especially a deficiency in the contingency of their behavior. This suggests that even those infants who do not become HIV-positive are significantly handicapped during the early months of their lives.

Since very little is known about the effects of HIV exposure on newborns, this chapter reviews studies that we have conducted on these effects. We also review our data on alleviating these effects with massage therapy and altering immune function in HIV-positive adults after massage therapy.

Researchers know very little about the neonatal outcome of infants who are exposed to HIV but do not necessarily become HIV-positive. We recently conducted a study to determine the effects of HIV exposure on newborn behavior. The sample comprised 48 full-term infants and their HIV-positive and HIV-negative mothers. The women had a low socioeconomic status (SES) (based on the Hollingshead Index of Social Position [ISP]), and 86% were single women. Their ethnic distribution was 11% Caucasian, 11% Hispanic, and 78% African American. The Brazelton Neo-natal Behavior Assessment Scale (NBAS) was administered to each infant within 48 hours after birth. The infant's performance was summarized according to seven factors: (1) habituation, (2) orientation, (3) motor behavior, (4) range of state, (5) regulation of state, (6) autonomic stability, and (7) abnormal reflexes.[8]

Table 12-1 shows that the mothers of the HIV-exposed infants were older, had been pregnant more often, and had more obstetrical complications.

Although the groups differed on obstetrical complication scores, which were entered into the data analysis as a covariate, the HIV-exposure and non-HIV-exposure groups did not differ on birth measures, including gestational age (GA), length, and head circumference (HC). However, despite the similarity between the groups on the standard birth measures, the HIV-exposed infant group showed inferior performance on the orienting items and had more deviant reflexes (Table 12-2).

Despite the fact that only 22% to 39% of infants born to HIV-positive mothers will become HIV-positive themselves,[9] exposure to HIV appears to disadvantage the infants from birth. Their mothers experienced more obstetrical complications, and the infants had inferior orienting scores and a greater number of abnormal reflexes on the Brazelton NBAS. These effects could possibly be explained by other maternal factors, such as potential drug abuse that was not detected by urine screens or poor maternal nutrition, resulting in intrauterine growth deprivation that was not detected by the ponderal index (PI; a weight/height index that indicates growth retardation). HIV exposure may indirectly affect the infants by compromising the mother's capacity to support intrauterine development. The direct effects of HIV exposure are not the only ones that place the fetus at risk. As far as we could determine, the women had similar demographic and health characteristics besides HIV status (e.g., prenatal medical care and drug abuse). Three factors not related to HIV status that were different between the two groups could have contributed to differential fetal development; namely, mothers (1) who were older, (2) who had higher rates of pregnancy, and (3) who had more obstetrical complications. Statistically covarying the effects of obstetrical complications may not have been adequate.

Although HIV-exposed newborns had inferior orienting and reflex factor scores, most of the Brazelton NBAS measures between the two groups were the same. This was surprising, since all of these factors de-

TABLE 12-1

Means for Demographics and Birth Measures*

| Variables | Groups | | f† |
	HIV ($n = 24$)	Non-HIV ($n = 24$)	
Mother's age	25.9 (4.9)	18.6 (3.7)	13.082
Mother's gravida	3.2 (0.5)	1.6 (0.2)	12.932
OCS	90.2 (19.2)	105.7 (20.1)	6.19‡
GA	38.7 (4.3)	38.1 (4.1)	0.69
Birth weight	3039.7 (1861)	3112.4 (1828)	1.72
Length	49.5 (8.7)	49.6 (7.3)	0.78
HC	33.2 (4.7)	33.4 (4.5)	0.65

GA, Gestational age; HC, head circumference; OCS, Obstetric Complications Scale.
*Standard deviations in parentheses.
†$df = 1, 46$.
‡$p = 0.01$.

TABLE 12-2

Means for Brazelton Scale Scores*

| Variables | Groups | | f† |
	HIV ($n = 24$)	Non-HIV ($n = 24$)	
Brazelton NBAS scores			
Habituation	6.2 (0.6)	5.9 (0.5)	1.47
Orientation	4.6 (0.8)	5.5 (0.9)	5.17‡
Motor	4.4 (0.7)	4.7 (0.7)	0.63
Range of state	3.4 (0.5)	3.7 (0.5)	0.71
Regulation of state	5.2 (0.8)	5.0 (0.8)	0.59
Autonomic stability	5.8 (0.7)	5.8 (0.7)	0.00
Reflexes	3.0 (0.4)	1.4 (0.2)	9.24§

NBAS, Neonatal Behavior Assessment Scale.
*Standard deviations in parentheses.
†$df = 1, 46$.
‡$p = 0.05$.
§$p = 0.005$.

pend upon similar functional systems. However, the infants' suboptimal performance on the orientation and abnormal reflexes may be related to adequate performance on other factors. The suboptimal orientation ratings may stem from these infants' higher stimulation thresholds, which require more stimulation to become oriented to stimuli. This same characteristic contributes to high thresholds for irritability and disorganized behavior, which could explain the infants' adequate performance on the range of state, regulation of state, and autonomic stability factors. Their

high reflex scores were related to hypertonicity, which, because of good muscle tone and lack of flaccid motor behavior, may have paradoxically contributed to their adequate motor scores.

Inferior performance on these Brazelton NBAS factors may be precursors of the developmental problems in later infancy noted in this population. For example, the greater number of abnormal reflexes (mainly hypertonicity) may be a precursor of the later hypertonicity and hyperflexia documented by several investigators.[10-12] Similarly, the newborn problem of orienting to visual and auditory stimuli may be a precursor of the visual-spatial delays noted in later development.[11]

These data suggest that future studies are needed to assess more subtle perceptual and cognitive functions in HIV-exposed newborns, such as habituation and conditioning studies. Further longitudinal studies are needed to track the developmental trajectory of these functions from the newborn period to later infancy to determine whether deficits persist even in HIV-exposed infants who do not become HIV-positive. At least two recent studies converge to suggest that development proceeds normally in HIV-exposed infants who are not infected,[13] particularly in the absence of confounding drug exposure effects.[14] Finally, early interventions are needed to reduce these early differences.

MASSAGE THERAPY TO ALTER EFFECTS OF HIV EXPOSURE IN NEONATES

In our study on Brazelton NBAS performance of HIV-exposed newborns, deficits were noted in Brazelton NBAS performance of perinatal HIV-exposed versus unexposed infants.[15] However, in a study on older children, developmental delays were reported for the HIV-infected children but not for the uninfected but exposed children.[16] Thus the data on children who were only exposed to HIV were mixed. Nonetheless, because the exposed newborns showed inferior neonatal performance in the Scafidi and Field[15] study, and at least 30% of a sample of exposed infants are expected to be at risk for developmental delays caused by infection, we investigated the effects of massage therapy with a sample of perinatally HIV-exposed newborns.

Several investigators have examined the effects of tactile/kinesthetic stimulation on the behavior and development of neonates[17-21] but not on newborns of HIV-positive mothers. In general, tactile/kinesthetic stimulation has facilitated infant growth and development. In a metanalytic study, Ottenbacher et al[22] estimated that 72% of the infants receiving tactile stimulation did better than the unstimulated control infants. In several studies conducted by our group, positive effects associated with touch included (1) increased weight gain, (2) more optimal sleep/wake states, (3) better performance on the Brazelton NBAS, (4) decreased stress behavior, and (5) increased norepinephrine and epinephrine levels.[23-25] We designed the

HIV massage therapy study to determine whether tactile/kinesthetic stimulation could facilitate weight gain, improve cognitive and developmental performance, and reduce stress behaviors in infants born to HIV-positive mothers.

The sample comprised 28 singleton neonates who were identified as HIV-exposed and were randomly assigned to the treatment (massage therapy) or control groups at a mean age of 24 hours. The two groups did not differ on any birth parameters, and the women all had a low level of education ($M = 10.5$ years) and a low SES ($M = 4.5$ on the Hollingshead ISP). Their ethnic distribution was 67% African American and 33% Hispanic.

The infants in the massage therapy group were massaged for three 15-minute periods for 3 consecutive hours each day for a 10-day period. The first stimulation session began approximately 30 minutes after the noon feeding, the second session began approximately 45 minutes after completion of the first session, and the third session began approximately 45 minutes after completion of the second session. The 15-minute stimulation session was comprised of three standardized 5-minute phases. The first and third phases involved tactile stimulation, and the middle phase involved kinesthetic stimulation.

The infant was placed in a prone position during the tactile phase. The research associate providing the stimulation firmly stroked the infant with the flats of the fingers of both hands. Some pressure was applied to avoid a tickling sensation. The stroking continued over each region of the infant's body for five 1-minute segments in the following sequence: (1) six strokes from the top of the infant's head, down the side of the face to the neck, and back up to the top of the head (each of the strokes lasted 10 seconds); (2) six 10-second strokes from the back of the neck, across the shoulders, and back to the neck; (3) six 10-second strokes from the upper back, down to the waist, and back to the upper back. For this segment the stimulator's hands were placed on each side of the spine with the flats of the fingers on the back; (4) six 10-second strokes from the thigh, down to the ankle, and back to the thigh. Both legs were done simultaneously; (5) six 10-second strokes from the shoulder, to the wrist, and back to the shoulder on both arms simultaneously.

For the kinesthetic phase, the infant was placed in a supine position with the head turned to the infant's preferred side. The middle phase also comprised five

1-minute segments. Each segment consisted of six passive flexion/extension movements lasting approximately 10 seconds apiece. Each 1-minute segment involved a different extremity and was performed in the following sequence: (1) right arm, (2) left arm, (3) right leg, (4) left leg, and (5) both legs simultaneously. For each segment, the stimulator gently contained the long bone of the limb, avoiding the soles of the feet and the palms of the hands to avoid eliciting a reflex response. The infant was then turned to a prone position for the final phase of tactile stimulation, which is the same as that described for the first phase of stimulation. The stimulator warmed his or her hands before touching the infant and remained silent throughout the procedure.

The massage therapy group had more optimal score changes on several Brazelton NBAS clusters. These included habituation, motor, range of state, and autonomic stability scores. The massage therapy group also received better scores on excitability and stress behaviors. Finally, the massage therapy group averaged a significantly greater increase in weight gain (Table 12-3).

The results of this study are probably not surprising, since improved performance on the Brazelton NBAS and greater weight gain were noted after 2 weeks of massage therapy in other studies.[23-25] However, although the infants in this study had a shorter gestation period and a smaller birth weight than

TABLE 12-3

Means (and Standard Deviations in Parentheses) for Brazelton NBAS Scores and Daily Weight Gain

Brazelton NBAS score	Massage		Control		
	Day 1	Day 10	Day 1	Day 10	p
Habituation†	6.9‡	6.8	6.2	4.6	0.01
	(0.6)[a]	(0.4)[a]	(0.5)[a]	(0.5)[b]	
Orientation†	3.6	4.5	3.8	4.4	NS
	(0.2)[a]	(0.3)[a]	(0.4)[a]	(0.5)[a]	
Motor†	4.3	5.2	3.8	4.5	0.001
	(0.5)[a]	(0.5)[b]	(0.4)[a]	(0.4)[a]	
Range of state†	3.5	4.3	3.2	3.6	0.05*
	(0.3)[a]	(0.4)[b]	(0.5)[a]	(0.3)[a]	
Regulation of state†	4.7	4.0	5.4	4.5	NS
	(0.4)[a]	(0.6)[a]	(0.6)[a]	(0.7)[a]	
Autonomic stability†	5.8	6.2	6.0	5.0	0.003
	(0.5)[a]	(0.7)[b]	(0.8)[a]	(0.5)[a]	
Reflexes	3.3	2.2	3.2	2.7	NS
	(0.2)[a]	(0.3)[a]	(0.4)[a]	(0.2)[a]	
Excitability	2.5	1.5	1.8	3.2	0.01
	(0.2)[a]	(0.4)[b]	(0.3)[b]	(0.4)[a]	
Depression	3.5	3.0	4.8	2.9	NS
	(0.5)[a]	(0.4)[a]	(0.5)[a]	(0.4)[a]	
Stress behaviors	2.4	1.8	1.8	3.6	0.004
	(0.2)[a]	(0.2)[b]	(0.4)[b]	(0.5)[a]	
Daily weight gain§	22.5	33.4	20.2	26.3	0.01
	(2.4)[a]	(4.3)[b]	(3.7)[a]	(3.9)[a]	

NBAS, Neonatal Behavior Assessment Scale; *NS*, not specified.
*Using the more conservative Bonferroni correction factor, the range-of-state factor would not be significant.
†Higher score is optimal.
‡Superscripts (a, b) indicate significant differences between columns.
§Day 1 means the first day of the study, although it was, on average, the infants' third day after birth.

normal babies, which is not unusual for HIV-exposed infants, they had a longer gestation period and a larger birth weight than the infants of the previous massage studies. Therefore the significant weight gain after extra stimulation was more surprising.

Many of the Brazelton NBAS score differences were accounted for by the improvement of the massage therapy group and by the stasis or decline of the control group. These trends were very different than those noted in our earlier massage therapy studies on massaged preterm infants, who simply improved more than the control group preemies. The preterm control groups did not stay the same or decline but improved in their performance, as would be expected with development. Exposure to HIV may contribute to developmental delays and failure to thrive as early as the newborn period in the absence of compensatory treatment provided by extra stimulation. These effects possibly resulted from other risk conditions, such as maternal drug use or intrauterine growth deprivation. Nonetheless, the surprising finding was the unusual number of inferior scores received by the HIV-exposed control infants on several Brazelton NBAS dimensions, suggesting a generalized, pervasive influence of HIV exposure on newborn behaviors. The early appearance of developmental delay and failure to thrive in the control group is somewhat surprising, since supposedly only 22% to 39% of these infants reputedly were HIV-positive.[9,26,27]

On the positive side, deterioration in HIV-exposed newborns apparently can be attenuated by the use of massage therapy. The underlying stimulation-weight gain and stimulation-improved performance mechanisms are not clear. The weight gain may relate to increased vagal activity after massage, which in turn facilitates the release of food absorption hormones, such as insulin, as noted in a study we conducted on preterm neonates exposed to cocaine.[28] Improved performance on the Brazelton NBAS could also relate to increased vagal activity, since infants with higher performance scores typically have higher vagal activity.[29] Future studies could examine vagal activity, as well as several other variables, including sleep/wake behavior and immune function changes, after massage therapy was adminstered to HIV-exposed infants. In addition, follow-up studies are needed to assess the duration of the positive effects after the massage therapy.

MASSAGE THERAPY ENHANCES IMMUNE FUNCTION IN ADULTS

Unfortunately, we had difficulty getting immune measures from newborns, but we were able to do so in a study on HIV-positive men.[30] The effects of massage therapy on the neuroendocrine system have been noted in several studies. In a study on children and adolescents who were hospitalized for depression, five massage therapy sessions led to decreases in urinary norepinephrine and cortisol levels.[31] In a more recent study, researchers noted decreases in urinary norepinephrine and cortisol levels in depressed adolescent mothers after massage therapy.[32] Decreased cortisol levels seemingly lead to improved immune function.

Although the scientific literature does not include articles on the impact of massage on traditional immune measures, the data from relaxation studies may be relevant, since massage is a type of relaxation. Progressive muscle relaxation is associated with significant increases in natural killer (NK) cell activity, decreases in herpes simplex virus (HSV) antibody titers in geriatric adults,[33] and higher helper T-cell percentages in medical students undergoing exams who practiced relaxation more frequently.[34] In combination with stress management techniques, relaxation training is also associated with increases in NK cell cytotoxicity (NKCC) and NK cell numbers in melanoma patients (and a small decrease in the percentage of helper T cells 6 months after the end of the intervention).[35] Finally, in an HIV-positive sample, patients who practiced relaxation more frequently had better immune functioning 1 year after receiving news of HIV-positive status and had slower disease progression 2 years after this news.[36,37]

In our HIV massage study,[38] changes in anxiety levels, relaxation, and endocrine function were also assessed as possible mechanisms by which immune alteration could occur (see Antoni et al[39] for a review of potential mechanisms). Twenty-three HIV-positive and 10 HIV-negative men were recruited for the study. After attrition, 20 HIV-positive and nine HIV-negative men completed the month-long massage protocol. We recruited gay men who had no AIDS-defining symptoms. We also tried to recruit subjects who had not taken antiretrovirals. Men who were on ART had to have used ART for at least 3 months without anticipating any drug regimen changes during the study. We excluded drug abusers, men who drank more than one unit of alcohol a day, men who smoked more than one pack of cigarettes a day, men who were on antidepressant medications or other medications that might affect the immune system, such as steroids, antihistamines, or β blockers, and men with any chronic illness other than HIV.

The sample comprised well-educated (two thirds were college graduates), middle SES gay men who had an average age of 33.2. $CD4^+$ T-cell counts were predominantly above 500. Most of the patients were asymptomatic. Five of the 23 HIV-positive patients were HIV-symptomatic before the study (one had thrush and shingles, one had shingles, one had thrush and night sweats, one had diarrhea and night sweats, and one had night sweats alone). Only two of the patients were on antiretrovirals (both were on AZT).

The study was conducted in two cohorts. The first cohort (10 HIV-positive and 10 HIV-negative men), received 1 month of daily (Monday through Friday) 45-minute massages. Biological measures (e.g., blood draws and 24-hour urine collections) and psychological questionnaires were obtained before the first massage and at the end of the month, as described later. The first cohort contained both HIV-positive and HIV-negative men in case the massages had different effects on each of the two groups. (The two groups in this cohort did not experience significantly different effects.) Because our preliminary results from this cohort were promising (trends were only significant on one-tailed tests), and in order to increase power, a second cohort of 13 HIV-positive men underwent the month-long massage period (we continued accepting subjects until 20 HIV-positive men had completed the month-long regimen). In addition, we added a control period for this second cohort, which lasted for a month (the same time period as the massage group), during which no massages took place. For one half of the second cohort sample, the control period preceded the massage period (separated by 1 month); for the other half, the order was reversed. A within-subject design was chosen for the second cohort (rather than a randomized between-subject design) because it maximized power (especially for testing the interaction), since our sample size was small. Biological measures (blood draws and 24-hour urine collections) were obtained before the first day of the control period and at the end of the month.

The 22 massage sessions were scheduled for four patients at a time with four licensed massage therapists (or therapists in advanced stages of training). Ses-

sions occurred at one of three times: (1) before work, (2) during lunch break, or (3) just after work (Monday through Friday). Patients had a different massage therapist each day. Most massage therapists volunteered 1 day a week for 4 weeks. The massage sessions followed a standardized protocol (see below), and instructions for the protocol were placed in clear view on the wall to serve as a reminder for the massage therapists. After each session, the patient rated the effectiveness of the relaxation produced by the massage.

The 45-minute massage protocol included the application of several types of strokes (e.g., stroking, stretching, rocking, squeezing, and holding) applied successively to several areas of the body: in the supine position—head and neck, arms, torso, and legs; and in the prone position—legs and back.

The immune measures selected represent measures important for cellular immunity, both functional, such as NKCC and enumerative (e.g., cells coexpressing the CD3 and CD4 marker and the CD3 and CD8 marker, NK cells with the CD56 marker, and cells expressing the CD56 marker but not the CD3 marker). Clinically, the measures chosen were relevant for fighting off viruses and tumors.[40] Measures also included those relevant in HIV disease progression—CD4 cells, CD8 cells, neopterin, and $\beta_2$microglobulin.[41] Soluble CD8 (sCD8) was also included, since this is a soluble form of T-cell receptors found on CD8 cells, which are shed when these cells are active. Since one subset of CD8 cells represents cytotoxic cells (those that coexpress the S6F1 receptors, also measured in this study), the information on sCD8 and numbers of $CD8^+S6F1^+$ cells could provide information relevant to the cytotoxic capacity of the immune system.

Researchers measured state anxiety with the State Trait Anxiety Inventory (STAI) and salivary cortisol before and after the first massage session to check whether the massage was both psychologically and physiologically relaxing. The 19 patients who filled out the STAI before and after the first massage experienced a significant decrease in anxiety. The patients (all HIV-positive) who provided salivary samples both before and after the first massage experienced significantly decreased cortisol values. Thus the massage appeared to have the expected effect—it decreased both anxiety and cortisol levels.

The effects of the month-long massage intervention are presented in Tables 12-4, 12-5, and 12-6 and in Figure 12-1.

TABLE 12-4

Anxiety and Relaxation Changes over the Course of the Month-Long Massage Period

Variables	Massage—subjects		n	t
	Pre Mean SD	Post Mean SD		
State anxiety	39.00 (10.5)	31.89 (8.6)	28	3.28*
POMS anxiety	11.20 (10.2)	6.50 (4.2)	20	2.10†
Relaxation	53.79 (22.4)	79.83 (19.0)	29	−5.14*

POMS, Profile of Mood States.
*$p < 0.01$.
†$p < 0.05$.

Table 12-4 shows a significant decrease in both state anxiety before and after massage for the entire sample of HIV-positive and HIV-negative participants and Profile of Mood States (POMS) anxiety for the subset of 20 HIV-positive participants. In addition, relaxation (measured on a graphic rating scale with a possible score between 1 and 100) significantly increased over the month-long period of massages. The greatest gain in relaxation occurred during the first week, which then was maintained at a high level.

Table 12-5 shows that massage had no effects on the immune measures related to disease progression in HIV. These included CD4 T-cell count, CD4/CD8 ratio, $\beta_2$microglobulin, and neopterin. However, NKCC significantly decreased during the control period and significantly increased during the massage period, showing a notable interaction.

The number of NK cells with the positive marker CD56 exhibited a significant interaction, and the lymphocyte subset of cells with the marker $CD56^+CD3^-$ exhibited a significant increase during the massage period. The activity of CD8 cells increased significantly, both for the HIV-positive group alone and the combined HIV-negative and HIV-positive groups. The subset of cytotoxic T cells (with the marker $S6F1^+CD8^+$) increased significantly during the massage period and decreased insignificantly during the control period, showing a significant interaction.

Urinary cortisol also showed a significant interaction, since it decreased significantly during the massage period and showed a marginally significant increase during the control period. Although there was a trend toward a decrease in catecholamines during the massage period, the change was not significant.

The massages were relaxing, both in terms of decreasing anxiety levels and decreasing stress hormone levels. Our sample as a whole had high stress levels initially (on the STAI) when compared with normal samples. In fact, they were about as stressed as the patients in another study, who had just been told 5 weeks before that they were HIV-positive.[38] After the massage, our sample was considerably less stressed, at about the level of HIV-negative persons. Our sample also had high cortisol levels initially, in comparison to Davidson and Baum's[42] sample and to the laboratory controls from the cortisol company.* Perhaps the massage intervention worked well because patients were at an initially high stress level.

The month of massage therapy was associated with improvement in several measures of immune function relevant to cytotoxic capacity. The importance of the maintenance of NK cell numbers and NKCC in HIV-positive persons is twofold. First, since the virus infects and destroys CD4 cells, the NK cells represent another type of immune cell that may still afford some protection. Klimas et al[43] found that NK cells are relatively unaffected during the early stages of HIV infection, although NKCC is lower in gay men in general. During later stages of HIV infection, researchers hypothesized that persons with low CD4 T-cell counts who remain asymptomatic may have greater NK cell function.[44]

---

*Diagnostic Products Corporation, "Count a Cortisol Manual," April 29, 1993.

TABLE 12-5

Immune Changes over the Course of the Month-Long Massage Period

Variables	Massage—all subjects Pre Mean (SD)	Post Mean (SD)	n	F	Massage positive f (mean Δ)‡	Massage negative f (mean Δ)‡	Control positive f (mean Δ)‡	Interaction§ f (mean Δ)‡
CD4/mm³	519.31 (267.1)	563.12 (391.6)	26	0.22	0.66	0.04	1.37	3.10
CD4/CD8	0.77 (0.5)	0.77 (0.5)	26	0.01	0.32	0.14	0.24	1.02
Neopterin (ng/ml)	4.31 (4.3)	3.54 (2.7)	29	1.82	1.54	0.32	0.08	3.65†† (−5.35)
(NK)CD56¶ /mm³‖	214.92 (161.1)	252.20 (142.8)	25	1.49	0.23	3.57	2.59	7.24** (89.45)
CD56⁺CD3⁻ #/mm³¶	101.71 (68.2)	157.00 (110.8)	24	7.90**	4.04** (47.44)	4.84** (78.83)	2.02	4.97†† (83.78)
NK cytotoxicity*	24.43 (16.4)	33.29 (19.5)	18	23.23#	23.23# (8.86)		7.95 (−8.05)	16.97** (18.36)
CD8#/mm³	751.77 (328.4)	821.46 (394.1)	26	1.14	1.69	0.37	20.88** (−176.18)	19.10** (369.78)
Soluble CD8 (U/ml)	606.46 (360.6)	812.16 (583.1)	29	7.40**	7.95** (293.03)	0.18	0.61	0.76
S6F1⁺CD8⁺/ Mm³†	686.55 (338.9)	881.18 (437.4)	11	5.02**	5.02** (194.63)		1.23	8.18** (274.38)

NK, Natural killer; SD, standard deviation.

*Because of the expensive nature of this assay, it was done for positives only.

†Because three-color flow was only available for the second cohort, n = 11.

‡There were 29 subjects: 20 massage-positive, 9 massage-negative, and 11 control-positive.

§The interaction was calculated for the second cohort and functionally compared the change during the massage period with the change during the control period. Nine subjects had data for all time points.

‖CD 56⁻ cells measured in the lymphocyte and monocyte gate.

¶CD 56⁺ CD3⁻ cells measured in the lymphocyte gate only.

#p <0.01.

**p <0.05.

††p <0.10.

TABLE 12-6

Neuroendocrine Changes over the Course of the Massage and Control Periods*

| Variables | Massage—positive | | f | Control | |
	Pre Mean SD	Post Mean SD		Positive f	Interaction f
Norepinephrine μg/24h	31.19 (13.2)	26.45 (16.9)	0.49	0.32	0.25
Epinephrine μg/24h	6.30 (4.9)	3.43 (3.0)	2.02	0.01	0.29
Cortisol μg/24h	44.09 (26.7)	23.51 (19.0)	5.52*	4.12*	11.22*

SD, Standard deviation.
*$p < 0.05$.

Second, NK cells are supposed to provide protection against both viruses and tumors.[40] Several malignant neoplastic diseases occur more frequently in AIDS patients.[45] The most common malignancy is Kaposi's sarcoma (KS), which occurs in 15% of AIDS patients; the next most common is non-Hodgkin's lymphoma, which is reported in 10% of AIDS patients. This population also experiences an increased incidence of melanoma, anal carcinoma, and adenocarcinoma of the liver.

Furthermore, NKCC may be important in other diseases, such as cancer. First, lowered NK activity is associated with the development of metastasis and shorter survival time in patients with cancer.[40,46,47] In animals, destruction of NK cells was associated with greater survival of intravenously injected tumor cells and a greater probability of the development of pulmonary metastasis. When NK activity was restored, resistance to metastasis occurred.[48,49] Second, NK activity is lower in individuals with tumor progression in breast cancer[50,51] and in those with a family history of breast cancer.[52] The lowered NK activity in persons with a family history of breast cancer may be due partly to distress-induced immunosuppression.[52] However, although distress contributed to the lower levels of NK activity found in women with a family history of breast cancer, differences still persisted, even when distress was taken into account.

The increase in soluble CD8 (which occurs when CD8 cells are active), together with a significant increase in the cytotoxic subset of CD8 cells (those with the S6F1 marker), suggests that an additional source of cytotoxic capability is enhanced by massage. Cytotoxic T cells tend to be virus-specific, as opposed to NK cells, which confer nonspecific immunity. Also, $CD8^+S6F1^+$ cells may fight against HIV-1. In a study in which activated autologous $CD8^+$ T cells (most of which were $S6F1^+$) and interleukin-2 (IL-2) were infused into AIDS patients, researchers observed clinical improvement in lymphoadenopathy, oral hairy leukoplakia, and KS.[53]

Several limitations of this study are apparent. First, the study is based on a small sample size and should thus be replicated. A randomized test of the efficacy of massage therapy is warranted, which would eliminate the potential problems of a within-subject design or of deciding how long an interval to leave to ensure that physiological measures return to baseline. The current design did not enable researchers to determine which ingredient of the massage intervention was potent. Other control groups that further studies might incorporate to answer this question include (1) a resting condition, (2) a muscle relaxation condition, or (3) an attention/social contact condition. Finally, a trial in a population of cancer patients, for whom cytotoxic capacity may be especially important, could be useful.

In conclusion, 1 month of massage was associated with improvement in several measures of immune function relevant to cytotoxic capacity. This potentially important preliminary finding may be the first step toward validating the health benefits of a procedure that has existed for a long time without clinical verification.

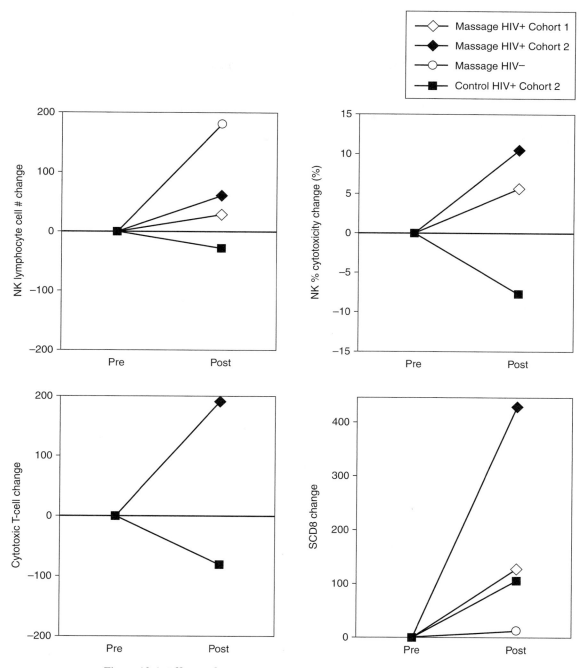

Figure 12-1 Effects of massage or control period on immune measures.

Thus, as these studies show, the clinical course of HIV can be improved. In young infants whose HIV status is unknown but who are reported to have growth and developmental delays through HIV-exposure, massage therapy can improve growth and development. Although the older men were severely immunocompromised, they too benefited clinically from the massage therapy, which led to an increase in NK cells and NKCC. NK cells ward off virus-bearing cells, suggesting that this form of treatment has good ripple effects, from simply making people "feel better" to significantly increasing the number of NK cells that destroy cancer cells. Further studies on the long-term effects of massage therapy on HIV-exposed infants are needed, including (1) whether immune function can be enhanced, (2) whether NK cell number and activity can increase, and (3) whether HIV infection can be prevented in HIV-exposed newborns. Massage therapy may also be effective in preventing developmental delays in infants who were exposed to HIV but did not become HIV-positive. Adults who are less immunocompromised should be studied to determine whether massage therapy can affect the disease markers (e.g., CD4/CD8 ratio), whether NK cells can somehow substitute for HIV-destroyed cells, and whether a continuing dose of massage therapy can prolong the lives of individuals infected with HIV.

References

1. Andiman WA: Medical management of the pregnant woman infected with human immunodeficiency virus type 1 and her child, *Semin Perinatol* 22:72-86, 1998.
2. Campbell T: A review of the psychological effects of vertically acquired HIV infection in infants and children, *Br J Health Psych* 2:1-13, 1997.
3. Gulgolgarn V, Ketsararat V, Niyomthai R, et al: Somatic growth and clinical manifestations in formula fed infants born to HIV-infected mothers during the first year of life, *J Med Assoc Thai* 82:1094-1099, 1999.
4. Berhane R, Bagenda D, Marum L, et al: Growth failure as a prognostic indicator of mortality in pediatric HIV infection, *Pediatrics* 100:E7, 1997.
5. Culnane M, Fowler M, Oleske J: Infant growth after in utero exposure: reply, *JAMA* 282:528-529, 1999.
6. Santacroce SJ: Uncertainty and mothering the HIV seropositive infant, *Dissertation Abstracts International: Section B-The Sciences and Engineering* 58:1806, 1997.
7. Byrne MW: Feeding interactions in a cross-section of HIV-exposed infants, *West J Nurs Res* 20:409-430, 1998.
8. Lester BM, Als H, Brazelton TB: Regional obstetric anesthesia and newborn behavior: a reanalysis toward synergistic effects, *Child Dev* 53:687-692, 1982.
9. Peckham CS, Tedder RS, Briggs M, et al: Prevalence of maternal HIV infection based on unlinked anonymous testing of newborn babies, *Lancet* 21:519-561, 1990.
10. Belman AL, Diamond G, Dickson D, et al: Pediatric acquired immunodeficiency syndrome, *Am J Dis Children* 142:29-35, 1988.
11. Diamond GW, Kaufman J, Belman AL, et al: Characterization of cognitive functioning in a subgroup of children with congenital HIV infection, *Arch Clin Neuropsychol* 2:245-256, 1987.
12. Epstein LG, Sharer LR, Oleske JM, et al: Neurological manifestations of human immunodeficiency virus infection in children, *Pediatrics* 78:678-687, 1986.
13. Nozyce M, Hittelman J, Muenz L, et al: Effect of perinatally acquired human immunodeficiency virus infection on neurodevelopment in children during the first two years of life, *Pediatrics* 94:883-891, 1994.
14. Mellins CA, Levenson RL, Zawadzki R, et al: Effects of pediatric HIV infection and prenatal drug exposure on mental and psychomotor development, *J Pediatr Psychol* 19:617-627, 1994.
15. Scafidi F, Field T: Massage therapy improves behavior in neonates born to HIV-positive mothers, *J Pediatr Psychol* 21:889-897, 1996.
16. Kletter R, Jeremy RJ, Rumsey C, et al: A prospective study of mental and motor development of infants born to HIV-infected intravenous drug abusing mothers, *Fifth Int Conf AIDS: Abstracts* 5:225, 1989 (abstract).
17. Cornell EH, Gottfried AW: Intervention with premature human infants, *Child Dev* 47:32-39, 1976.
18. Field T: Supplemental stimulation of preterm neonates, *Early Hum Dev* 4:301-314, 1980.
19. Gaiter J: Nursery environments: the behavior and caregiving experiences of full-term and preterm newborns. In Gottfried AW, Gaiter J, editors: *Infant stress under intensive care,* Baltimore, 1985, University Park Press.
20. Gottfried AW: Environment of newborn infants in special care units. In Gottfried AW, Gaiter J, editors: *Infant stress under intensive care,* Baltimore, 1985, University Park Press.
21. Masi W: Supplemental stimulation of the premature infant. In Field T, Sostek A, Goldberg S, Shuman HH, editors: *Infants born at risk,* New York, 1979, Spectrum.

22. Ottenbacher KJ, Muller L, Brandt D, et al: The effectiveness of tactile stimulation as a form of early intervention: a quantitative evaluation, *J Dev Behav Pediatr* 8:68-76, 1987.

23. Field T, Schanberg SM, Scafidi F, et al: Tactile/kinesthetic stimulation effects on preterm neonates, *Pediatrics* 77:654-658, 1986.

24. Kuhn C, Schanberg S, Field T, et al: Tactile/kinesthetic stimulation effects on sympathetic and adrenocortical function in preterm infants, *J Pediatr* 119:434-440, 1991.

25. Scafidi F, Field T, Wheeden A, et al: Behavioral and hormonal differences in preterm neonates exposed to cocaine in vitro, *Pediatrics* 98:851-855, 1996.

26. Blanche S, Rouzioux C, Moscato ML, et al: A prospective study of infants born to women seropositive for human immunodeficiency virus type 1, *New Engl J Med* 320:1643-1648, 1989.

27. Johnson JP, Nair P, Hines SE, et al: Natural history and serological diagnosis of infants born to human immunodeficiency virus-infected women, *Am J Dis Children,* 143:1147-1153, 1989.

28. Wheeden A, Scafidi FA, Field T, et al: Massage effects on cocaine-exposed preterm neonates, *J Dev Behav Pediatr* 14:318-322, 1993.

29. Porges SW: Method and apparatus for evaluating rhythmic oscillations in aperiodic response systems, United States Patent No. 4510944, 1985.

30. Ironson G, Field TM, Scafidi F, et al: Massage therapy is associated with enhancement of the immune system's cytotoxic capacity, *Int J Neurosci* 84:205-217, 1996.

31. Field T, Morrow C, Valdeon C, et al: Massage reduces anxiety in child and adolescent psychiatric patients, *J Am Acad Child Adolesc Psychiatry* 31:125-131, 1992.

32. Field T, Grizzle N, Scafidi F, et al: Massage and relaxation therapies' effects on depressed adolescent mothers, *Adolescence* 31:903-911, 1996.

33. Kiecolt-Glaser JK, Stephens RE, Lipetz PD, et al: Distress and DNA repair in human lymphocytes, *J Behav Med* 8:311-320, 1985.

34. Kiecolt-Glaser JK, Glaser R, Strain EC, et al: Modulation of cellular immunity in medical students, *J Behav Med* 9:5-21, 1986.

35. Fawzy FI, Kemeny ME, Fawzy NW, et al: A structured psychiatric intervention for cancer patients, *Arch Gen Psychiatry* 47:729-735, 1990.

36. Antoni MH, Goodkind K, Goldstein V, et al: Coping responses to HIV-1 serostatus notification predict short-term affective distress and one-year immunological status in HIV-1 seronegative and seropositive gay men, *Psychosom Med* 53:227, 1991 (abstract).

37. Ironson G, Schneiderman N, Kumar M, et al: Psychosocial stress, endocrine, and immune response in HIV-1 disease, *Homeostasis* 35:137-148, 1994.

38. Ironson G, LaPerriere A, Antoni M, et al: Changes in immune and psychological measures as a function of anticipation and reaction to news of HIV-1 antibody status, *Psychosom Med* 52:247-270, 1990.

39. Antoni MH, Schneiderman N, Fletcher MA, et al: Psychoneuroimmunology and HIV-1, *J Consult Clin Psychol* 58(1):38-49, 1990.

40. Whiteside TL, Herberman RB: The role of natural killer cells in human disease, *Clin Immunol Immunopathol* 53:1-23, 1989.

41. Lifson AR, Hessol NA, Buchbinder SP, et al: Serum β_2 microglobulin and prediction of progression to AIDS in HIV infection, *Lancet* 339:1436-1440, 1992.

42. Davidson LM, Baum A: Chronic stress and posttraumatic stress disorders, *J Counsel Clin Psychol* 54:303-308, 1986.

43. Klimas NG, Caralis P, LaPerriere A, et al: Immunological function in a cohort of human immunodeficiency virus type 1-seropositive and -negative healthy homosexual men, *J Clin Microbiol* 29:1413-1421, 1991.

44. Solomon GF, Benton D, Harker J, et al: Prolonged asymptomatic states in HIV-seropositive persons with 50 CD4$^+$ T cells/mm^3: preliminary psychoimmunologic findings, *J Acquir Immune Defic Syndr Hum Retrovirol* 6(10):1173, 1993.

45. Epstein JB, Scully C: Neoplastic disease in the head and neck of patients with AIDS, *Int J Maxillofac Surg* 21:219-226, 1992.

46. Pross HF, Baines MG: *Low natural killer cell activity in the peripheral blood of metastasis-free cancer patients is associated with reduced metastasis-free survival time.* In Nineteenth International Leukocyte conference, Alberta, Canada, 1988 (abstract).

47. Schantz SP, Goepfert H: Multimodal therapy and distant metastasis: the impact of natural killer cell activity, *Arch Otolaryngol Head Neck Surg* 113:1207-1213, 1987.

48. Gorelik E, Wiltrout RH, et al: Role of NK cells in the control of metastatic spread and growth of tumor cells in mice, *Int J Cancer* 30:107-112, 1982.

49. Hanna N: Inhibition of experimental tumor metastasis by selective activation of natural killer cells, *Cancer Res* 42:1337-1342, 1982.

50. Akimoto M, Ishii H, Nakajima Y, et al: Assessment of host immune response in breast cancer patients, *Cancer Detect Prev* 9(3-4):311-317, 1986.

51. Takasugi M, Ramseyer A, Takasugi J: Decline of natural nonselective cell mediated cytotoxicity in patients with tumor progression, *Cancer Res* 37:413-418, 1977.

52. Bovbjerg D, Valdimarsdottir H, Kash K, et al: Familial risk for breast cancer, psychological distress, and immune function, *Psychosom Med* 56:148, 1994 (abstract).

53. Klimas N, Patarca R, Walling J, et al: Clinical and immunological changes in AIDS patients following adoptive therapy with activated autologous CD8 T cells and interleukin-2 infusion, *AIDS* 8:1073-1081, 1994.

ACKNOWLEDGMENTS

These studies were funded by Johnson & Johnson and the Office of Alternative Medicine, NIH.

Special thanks are extended to the massage therapists from Educating Hands who contributed their time for the study.

Appreciation is expressed to J.B. Fernandez, K. Gamber, and R. Gamber for providing technical assistance.

Manual Therapy Interventions for People Living with HIV Disease

BRUNO CHIKLY

MARY LOU GALANTINO

JOHN E. UPLEDGER

ABSTRACT

Various pain syndromes and musculoskeletal alterations may occur throughout the spectrum of HIV disease. To minimize the use of pharmacological agents for pain management, manual therapies can be employed. These include (1) soft tissue mobilization, (2) muscle energy techniques, (3) strain/counterstrain, (4) myofascial release (MFR), (5) CranioSacral Therapy (CST), (6) visceral manipulation, and (7) lymph drainage techniques. Energy-based interventions include therapeutic touch (TT), Reiki, and healing touch. These complementary manual therapy techniques are multifaceted and originate from various philosophies. This chapter reviews aspects of HIV-related pain syndromes, a brief overview of various manual therapies, and existing research on their effects on pain modulation. Various practitioners are trained in one or more of these various techniques, and the reader is advised to inquire about the approach used in a manual therapy session.

Advances in the medical management of HIV disease have increased life expectancy. Quality of life (QOL) is becoming increasingly important to address in all dimensions of work and activities of daily living (ADLs). Therefore pain management must be integrated into the total care of patients with HIV disease.[1] The prevalence of pain in HIV-infected individuals varies according to the stage of disease and generally ranges from 25% to 80%, with the prevalence of pain increasing as the disease progresses.[2] Studies suggest that approximately 25% to 30% of ambulatory HIV-infected patients in early stages of the disease experience clinically significant pain.[3] People with AIDS who experience pain, like their counterparts with cancer pain, typically describe an average of two to three concurrent pains at a time.[4]

The opportunistic infections (OIs) and drug side effects that result from the treatment of HIV disease can have a direct effect on daily functional activities. Examples include peripheral neuropathy (PN) syndrome, rheumatological complications, Kaposi's sarcoma (KS), and various musculoskeletal alterations. The weakness, pain, and loss of range of motion (ROM) caused by these conditions can lead to changes in gait pattern, loss of function, and decreased QOL.[5] The role of pain management in treating these HIV complications requires various pharmacological and nonpharmacological approaches.

Federal guidelines developed by the Agency for Health Care Policy and Research (AHCPR) for the management of cancer pain also address pain management in the treatment of HIV/AIDS.[6] A multidimensional model acknowledges the interaction of emotional, cognitive, cultural, and environmental aspects of pain. An individual may experience various types of pain: (1) physical pain, (2) painful losses, (3) the pain of not knowing, and (4) social pain.[7] Optimal management of the person experiencing HIV-related pain may require a combination of pharmacological, cognitive-behavioral, psychological, psychotherapeutic, anesthetic, neurosurgical, and rehabilitative approaches. This chapter focuses on the manual therapy approaches of this multimodal intervention.

Various clinical problems that are often presented to the health care professional include the following:

1. Neurological deficits secondary to central nervous system (CNS) involvement with resultant neurocognitive and functional changes
2. PN secondary to drug toxicity and progression of HIV disease
3. Myopathies secondary to medication and direct HIV involvement
4. Arthrosis secondary to side effects of medication
5. Postural dynamics secondary to weight loss from protein-calorie malnutrition (PCM)
6. Past medical history of previous injuries that may be exacerbated during HIV disease

The typical description of a pain syndrome associated with HIV portrays a disorder producing a multitude of pathological changes and deficiencies of the immune system. The possible causes of most of the pain syndromes or sites are complex. Pain symptoms may be overshadowed by a constellation of other overwhelming problems, which may include OIs, diarrhea, dyspnea, anorexia, weight loss, and neuropsychological symptoms.

FEATURES OF HIV-RELATED PAIN SYNDROMES

Taking a careful patient history and giving the patient a physical and a differential diagnosis are important first steps. The pain etiology may stem from multiple sources, and the mechanism of pain must be determined before treatment is rendered. Medications, diagnostic procedures, and other interventions may cause pain. Patients may have a preexisting pain syndrome unrelated to the course of HIV disease.[8] Pain is also the most common reason for hospitalization of people with HIV/AIDS.[9]

Abdominal pain can have many causes: (1) lymphadenopathy from HIV infection or lymphoma, (2) KS, (3) infectious diarrhea, (4) organomegaly, and (5) nonspecific gastritis. Patients frequently experience pain of somatic and visceral origin.[10]

Neuropathic pain syndromes occur in up to 40% of HIV patients who report pain.[10,11] Neuropathic pain is often overlooked because the cause is often unknown in individuals with HIV/AIDS.[12] Various PNs are described with HIV disease.[13] These PNs include both acute and chronic inflammatory demyelinating neuropathies (IDPs). The most common PN is distal symmetrical PN (DSPN), which affects as many as 30% of HIV-infected persons (see Chapter 11). Lane et al suggest that AZT only causes a myopathy when underlying HIV-related IDP is present.[14] Wulff et al describe six patterns of HIV-associated PN: (1) DSPN, (2) IDP, (3) progressive polyradiculopathy, (4) mononeuropathy multiplex, (5) autonomic neuropathy (AN), and (6) diffuse infiltrative lymphocytosis syndrome (DILS). Unfortunately, patients with PN are often misdiagnosed or overlooked.[15]

Patients with HIV disease frequently report having headaches.[11] A differential diagnosis is necessary to rule out toxoplasmosis, CNS lymphoma, and cryptococcal meningitis. Nonspecific headaches may be caused by postural changes and muscular imbalances that can occur over the course of HIV disease.

Musculoskeletal changes and pain associated with HIV-related arthritis conditions may result in significant gait deviations.[16] Studies have demonstrated a predilection to primary involvement of the knees, ankles, and feet in HIV-positive individuals.[17] The proper implementation of orthotics and optimal footwear helps prevent further postural deficits. Modalities and manual therapy to modulate pain are incorporated into the rehabilitation approach.

HIV infection and fibromyalgia were studied by Simms.[18] The prevalence of fibromyalgia in this population is significant, since an estimated 5% of patients visit a general medical clinic, and 12% of patients visit a rheumatologist.[19,20] The treatment for fibromyalgia includes physical modalities, such as heat, ice, spray and stretch techniques, biofeedback, and manual therapy.[5]

Patients with HIV-related arthritis can be treated with a combination of appropriate medication and rehabilitation that focuses on enhancing functional outcomes.[21,22] If fatigue becomes an issue because of OIs, energy conservation techniques may be incorporated into the treatment plan. Since a rheumatological diagnosis represents one of many complications of HIV disease, practitioners should coordinate treatment with all the members of the health care team.

Using exercise intervention in combination with manual therapy techniques should be designed specifically to the patient's diagnosis, tolerance, and particular endurance needs (see Chapter 14). When prescribing an exercise program for patients with concomitant HIV disease, other neurological, cardiorespiratory (CR), gastrointestinal (GI), and musculoskeletal concerns should be considered. Self-mobilization techniques and gentle home exercises are also presented to the patient, and medication and patient counseling are recommended.[23] Treatment should be individualized and should address both pain and functional issues of the HIV-infected population.[24]

Musculoskeletal concerns for people living with HIV disease can be orthopedic. Patients with associated PN may often incur low back pain. Instead of being directly related to HIV disease, the pain may be the aftermath of an OI, which results in muscle spasms and postural changes. A constellation of problems may manifest in altered gait and difficulty with transitional positions. This leads to neuromusculoskeletal dysfunction, and traction produced by postural dysfunction on the sensory nerve elements within the connective tissue system may produce pain.

Soft tissue mobilization includes massage and MFR techniques. Fascial dysfunction caused by a number of external and internal insults to the body can contribute to changes in health.[25] MFR can be a direct or an indirect technique. The direct technique takes the tissue to the barrier on three planes, and the tissue or joints are loaded in the direction of least mobility, whereas the indirect technique moves in the direction of greatest mobility. A relaxation in tissue tension results from the treatment, and heat is released from the tissues.

Another technique for pain management, the strain/counterstrain technique, includes trigger point releases and can be included in the repertoire of manual therapy techniques. The strain/counterstrain technique was developed by Lawrence Jones, DO. It is a positional technique that results in the decrease or arrest of inappropriate proprioceptor activity of the muscle spindle.[26] This technique results in relaxation and elongation of the muscle fiber, which permits improved articular balance for increased joint mobility and ROM.

The muscle energy technique, which was developed by Fred Mitchell, DO, is a positional technique that facilitates the correction of biomechanical dysfunction by normalizing neuromusculoskeletal balance.[27] A three-planar model is used. Gentle, unidirectional, isometric resistance is conducted to restore normal articular balance and joint mobility. The joint is positioned on three planes in the direction of least mobility. The movement direction for the coronal plane is either right or left sidebending, whereas the movement for the saggital plane is either flexion or extension. The movement direction for the transverse plane is either right or left rotation. Therefore the movement is stacked on three planes. The movement is passively performed; there is no assistance for the movement and no resistance to the movement. The therapist's hands palpate for the first indication of tissue tension, which reflects resistance to a passive range of motion. The following brief series describes this technique:

1. The joint is positioned in an interbarrier zone on three planes.
2. The patient controls the position of the joint.
3. The patient makes an active contraction.
4. The contraction has a specific direction.
5. The therapist responds with a distinct counterforce.
6. The intensity of the contraction is controlled.

7. The resistance to the contraction is small.
8. The contraction is isometric.

Visceral manipulation is a manual therapy consisting of light, gentle, specifically placed manual forces that encourage normal mobility, tone, and inherent tissue motion of the viscera and their connective tissue.[28,29] People with HIV disease experience a host of GI problems from various OIs, and visceral manipulation may potentiate the normal physiological function of individual organs.

These techniques should not be used with patients who have an acute infection, however. Visceral motion can be divided into four categories, according to the system that influences or controls them: (1) somatic nervous system, (2) autonomic nervous system (ANS), (3) craniosacral rhythm, and (4) visceral motility.

CST is a gentle, noninvasive, yet powerful and effective treatment approach that relies primarily on hands-on evaluation and treatment. The hands-on contact is extremely tender and supportive. It is accompanied by a sincere intention to assist the patient in any way possible. In other words, the therapist facilitates the patient's own healing processes. The rapport that develops during the patient-therapist interaction lends itself to the positive therapeutic effect experienced by most patients. This gentle, caring approach is welcomed by the majority of people with HIV disease.[30-32]

The CST practitioner also does corrective work that is done on a basic physiological level by gentle hands-on manipulations applied both directly and indirectly to the craniosacral system. This system is essentially a semiclosed hydraulic system, the boundaries of which are formed by the dura mater throughout its extension within the cranial vault and the vertebral canal. It includes the dural sleeves, since they invest the spinal nerve roots outside of the vertebral canal as far as the intervertebral foramina, and the caudal end of the dural tube, which ultimately becomes the cauda equina and blends with the coccygeal periosteum. The fluid within the semiclosed hydraulic system is the cerebrospinal fluid (CSF). The choroid plexuses within the brain's ventricular system and the arachnoid granulation bodies regulate the inflow and outflow of the fluid, respectively. The latter structures are located largely within the venous sinuses that service the brain's circulatory system. To qualify as a semiclosed hydraulic system, the fluid inflow and outflow must be regulated. The model that has been presented, which attempts to explain the inflow control mechanisms, involves a feedback system from intrasutural stretch and compression receptors. These receptors communicate via the nervous system to the choroid plexuses and provide a rhythmically on-and-off activity for CSF production into the system. CSF outflow is not rhythmically interrupted, but its rate may be adjusted by intracranial membrane tension patterns, which are broadcast primarily via the falx cerebri and tentorium cerebelli to the anterior end of the straight venous sinus, where an aggregation of arachnoid granulation bodies is located. This concentration of arachnoid granulation bodies affects venous backpressure, which in turn affects the rate of reabsorption of CSF into the blood-vascular system. Also included in the structures of the craniosacral system are the bones of the cranium, as well as the second and third cervical vertebrae, the sacrum, and the coccyx.[30,31,33-37]

Both clinical research and observation demonstrate that dysfunctions of the craniosacral system manifest as a wide variety of syndromes, symptoms, and degenerative processes. The craniosacral system influences the physiological milieu in which the CNS lives. It also has a powerful influence over both the pituitary and pineal glands because of their anatomical intimacies. Therefore it has a powerful effect on both brain and spinal cord function, as well as on the endocrine system. CST has a positive effect on a diversity of brain dysfunctions, ranging from seizure problems to dyslexia and attention deficit disorder (ADD). It has a positive impact on the ANS, through both the central control nuclei in the brain stem and the spinal cord's segmental effects on the sympathetic nervous chains and ganglia. The latter effect is caused by the ability of CST to desensitize spinal cord segments that have become hypersensitized, or facilitated, secondary to chronic excessive input. These hypersensitive segments often result from chronic localized infections or painful musculoskeletal or myofascial dysfunctions. Hypersensitive or facilitated segments send an unwarranted and excessive outflow to their related end organs, which in turn send excessive sensory input back to these already hypersensitive segments. Thus the situation becomes self-propagating. In addition, the sympathetic system input from the related hyperactive segments is increased, thus raising total sympathetic tonus with all of its attendant problems. Thermography shows that hand warming occurs during CST, which indicates a reduction of sympathetic tonus. Concurrently, blood pressure and cardiac rate, when elevated (as is often the case in sympathetic hypertonus), move toward normal. Subjective pain improves almost invariably as CST treatment progresses.[30,33,35,38-48]

People with HIV disease, with their multitude of visceral dysfunctions and neuromusculoskeletal and myofascial problems (many of which are painful), clearly can be made more comfortable and functional through the regular application of CST.

In addition, clinical observation suggests that CST can enhance fluid motion on an interstitial level, as well as across cell membranes. CST also seems to enhance arteriovenous and lymphatic activity, as evidenced by the reduction of clinical edema during the treatment process. This reduction of edema is probably a result of its effect on the ANS. By whatever mechanism it occurs, this enhancement of the microcirculation of all fluids undoubtedly has a positive impact on the accumulated toxic waste products within static fluids. All patients, including patients with HIV disease, benefit when fluid stasis is transformed into fluid motion.

CST also appears to have a positive effect on immune response. A virally induced fever in typical childhood diseases frequently can be reduced by the use of CST. When this occurs, the child usually has no more febrile episodes after the fever reduction but instead begins the recovery phase. Experienced CST practitioners often witness this phenomenon. These observations justify a formal investigation into the effects of CST on the immune system.

Patients with HIV disease are best served by methods that allow them to rechannel energies that deal with pain and secondary dysfunction into more constructive directions that enhance body resistance. CST appears to be one of these methods.

LYMPH DRAINAGE THERAPY*

Nonspecific manual therapy practice is associated with stimulation of the immune system, enhancement of the lymphocyte cytotoxic response, an increase in the number of natural killer (NK) cells, a decrease in anxiety, and an increase in relaxation level.[49] In terminally ill AIDS patients, manual therapy modalities can also reduce pain level, swelling, joint stiffness, muscle spasms, skin pathologies, and sleeping disorders, as well as improve anxiety, self-esteem, and body image.[50]

Manual therapies include a large range of techniques that are beneficial in numerous therapeutic conditions. We focus on the principal applications of lymphatic drainage in the treatment of HIV/AIDS.

The main pathologies in HIV/AIDS infection are (1) immune system dysfunction, (2) defects in cell-mediated immunity, and (3) subsequent OIs by microorganisms, such as viruses, bacteria, parasites, and fungi, that can affect most of the systems of the body. We examine how these conditions are related to the lymphatic system and why HIV-infected patients can benefit from the many applications of lymphatic drainage techniques.

Basic History of the Discovery of the Lymphatic System and Lymphatic Drainage Techniques

Throughout the course of medical history, the lymphatic system mainly went unrecognized until the seventeenth century.[51,90] Gaspard Asselli (1581-1626) made the first historical discovery of the lymphatic vessels (the "white veins") in 1622. The use of gentle manual techniques to activate the lymphatic flow occurred toward the beginning of the twentieth century. Frederic P. Millard (1878-1951) began his lymphatic research around 1904. As founder and president of the International Lymphatic Society, he published *Applied Anatomy of the Lymphatics* in 1922.[52] He used the words *lymphatic drainage* in his research. Emil Vodder (1896-1986) was a Danish massage practitioner and a doctor of philosophy. Between 1932 and 1936, Vodder gained further insight into manual lymphatic drainage.[53,54,90] He developed a traditional manual technique for lymph drainage.

Lymph Drainage Therapy (LDT) is an original method of lymphatic drainage developed by French physician Bruno Chikly, MD.[55-57,90] LDT is original because it teaches the practitioner how to manually identify the specific rhythm, direction quality, and depth of the lymph flow consistent with scientific discoveries.[56-58,90] Advanced practitioners can assess and manually map the lymphatic circulation during sessions and find the most accurate pathway for drainage. Lymphatic drainage techniques can be a valuable addition to the treatment of HIV patients, but more scientific research regarding the applications of lymphatic drainage techniques on the different stages of HIV infection is required.

The Lymphatic System

Medical science is only beginning to fully understand the role that lymph plays in the body.[59-61]

Lymph is a fluid that originates in the connective tissue.[62-64] Interstitial liquid flows in connective tissue through unorganized pathways, sometimes called the "tissue canals" or **prelymphatic pathways.** Once it appears in the first lymphatic capillaries, this interstitial fluid or prelymphatic fluid is officially named **lymph.**

The lymphatic system transports water (96%), colloids, proteins, lipids (mainly free fatty acids [FAs] and lipoproteins), specific cells (about 85% of lymphocytes and 15% of macrophages), hormones, toxins, pieces of cell debris, waste, and dyes.

Lymph returns numerous substances that have escaped from the blood compartment to the circulatory system. The lymph nodes break down and destroy lymphatic foreign bodies and pathogenic agents so they can eventually be flushed out of the body through the organs of elimination (e.g., liver, kidneys, large intestine, skin, lungs).

The lymphatic system fine-tunes the drainage of the connective tissue and thus constitutes a sort of overflow, which evacuates water and excess substances (especially macromolecules and toxins) in the interstitial environment. Through this process, the lymphatic system maintains optimal functioning of the connective tissue and regulates the volume and pressure of tissue fluid.

Structure of the Lymphatic System

Lymphatic capillaries, which are made of a single layer of flat cells, have openings 4 to 7 times bigger than those of blood capillaries.[65,66,90] After prelymphatic fluid enters the lymph capillary, the flat cells of the lymph capillary wall close, working as inlet valves.[63,67]

Lymph precollectors and collectors are larger lymph vessels with valves. Located between two lymphatic valves, the lymphangions (intervalvular segments) of the lymph collectors are made of two or three layers of spiral smooth muscles that carry lymph to the neighboring lymph nodes. Like little pacemakers, these muscular units have an extensive innervation and produce peristaltic waves of contractions controlled by the ANS. The lymphatic system is precisely an active system. The rhythmical contractions of the lymphangions, which are located along the lymph collectors, are probably the most efficient factors that help lymph circulation.[68-72]

Lymph flow usually passes through one or more lymph nodes. Lymph nodes are part of the lymphatic system, and they are also part of the secondary lymphoid organs. This system comprises the various tissues and organs that are part of the immune system and amasses lymphocytes and related cells.

Lymph nodes have the following specific functions[73,90]:

1. They are filtration centers for the lymph circulation.
2. They regain and disable toxins of the body.
3. They produce mature lymphocytes. The production of lymphocytes is activated about threefold when the flow of lymph is increased through the nodes. This indicates the use of manual techniques, such as LDT, to increase the production of lymphocytes.
4. They concentrate lymph.

Lymphocytes (especially B lymphocytes) reproduce in the marginal center of the lymph node. The outer cortex of the nodes contains primary follicles with nonsensitive lymphoblasts, which are not exposed to antigen, and secondary follicles that contain sensitized T lymphocytes, some of which are already transformed in plasmocytes and memory T cells.

AIDS and the Lymphatic System: Histology

In HIV infection, the nucleus of the helper/inducer T4 lymphocytes is the primary target of HIV. The virus takes over the function of the infected cell and makes it work for its own benefit, producing an colossal amount of HIV. Studies suggest that as many as 2 billion lymphocytes (CD4) are produced every day to replace the losses induced by the virus.

Researchers know little about the way HIV disseminates through the lymphomyeloid complex. However, HIV infection involves the lymphatic system and represents an important reservoir for the virus.[74] The application of LDT or any other technique that stimulates fluid circulation, depending on the stage of the disease, must be chosen carefully.

Lymph Node Pathology in HIV Infections

In HIV infections, three morphological and immunopathological patterns can be observed in the lymph nodes.[75-78]

- Type I: extensive follicular hyperplasia associated with other simple tissue lesions. It is associated with the chronic polyadenopathies of HIV infection (persistent generalized lymphadenopathy).
- Type II: mixed hyperplasia, diffuse lymphoid hyperplasia, and loss of germinal centers.
- Type III: lymphocyte cell depletion. This may explain how, during the later stages of AIDS, adenopathy almost completely disappears in the absence of infectious complications. This variant is always associated with end-stage AIDS infection.

HIV initially stimulates and finally exhausts lymph nodes throughout the body. The number of T4 cells decreases and involves all sections of the nodes during the two latest stages of AIDS. T8-cell count, on the other hand, is only higher during the first two stages. The number of B cells is higher during the early stages of AIDS and is lower in lymphocyte depletion.

In clinical practice, the reaction of the patient during lymphatic drainage immune system stimulation may be different if the patient is in a hyperplasic or depleted stage. Thus it is always advised to shorten the first three or four sessions and observe the clinical reactions of the patient.

Lymphatic Drainage Techniques

Lymphatic drainage is a specialized manual therapy designed to activate lymph flow and cleanse the human fluid system. It has numerous applications and is probably one of the specific manual therapies that has received the most scientific documentation, at least in Europe. Studies can easily follow the pathway of lymph with markers and assess both immune system reactions and many specific clinical changes.[79-85] The first serious hospital research was performed by the German physician Johannes Asdonk in the late 1960s, who tested the technique on 20,000 patients. In Europe lymphatic drainage techniques are now commonly used in hospitals, prescribed by physicians, and reimbursed by medical insurance. In Florida, Medicare reimburses lymph drainage techniques primarily for the medical applications of the techniques, such as edemas and lymphedemas. Other applications of lymph drainage techniques are fairly new and require more scientific documentation.

Indications of Lymph Drainage Therapy

In clinical conditions, lymphatic drainage can alleviate various aspects of HIV infection when appropriate. It is impossible to make a list of all the possible applications of LDT for HIV infection in such a short article. The following general guidelines will help the reader understand the numerous applications of lymphatic drainage techniques.[79-82] Only trained therapists can work on a specific condition related to HIV infections. The guidance of a physician is strictly required for diagnosis and treatment of these conditions.

1. Stimulation of the immune system: In physiological conditions, lymphatic drainage techniques have an immune system stimulation effect and can be used both in active and preventive conditions: (1) chronic or subacute inflammatory processes (e.g., bacteria, virus, fungi, parasites, foreign substances)—when indicated, complications of *Candida albicans*, herpes simplex virus (HSV), Epstein Barr virus (EBV), varicella-zoster (VZ), cytomegalovirus (CMV), *Pneumocystis carinii*, *Cryptococcus*, toxoplasmosis, tuberculosis, other *Mycobacterium* species, histoplasmosis, listeriosis, *Salmonella*, fungi, autoimmune disease, and so forth, and (2) in different body systems—skin, lungs, eyes, CNS, and so forth. Always note the main contraindications of fever and acute infections.
2. Drainage of different substances:
   - Toxins: tissue cleansing
   - Macromolecules (proteins): trapped toxin-protein in the tissue, evacuation of fluid retention
   - Fat
3. Activation of fluid circulation (lymph and interstitial liquids, venous circulation, blood capillaries). Helps reroute stagnant fluid in:
   - Edema (chronic inflammation, trauma, postsurgery)
   - Secondary lymphedema
   - Circulation in the chambers of the eyes, joints, periosteum, muscles, viscera, and so forth
4. Stimulation of the parasympathetic system, which diminishes sympathetic tone. Natural steroid hormones are among the body's most active immunosuppressant substances. The deep parasympathetic relaxation of LDT can help. LDT has a direct impact on stress, anxiety, depression, and sleeping disorders.

5. Other aspects of parasympathetic stimulation include analgesic (antipain) and antispastic (antispasm) action. The constant stimulation of the skin C nociceptors, using lymphatic drainage techniques, has an inhibitory action on chronic pain.

Specific Applications of Lymph Drainage Therapy: Kaposi's Sarcoma

The origin of KS is unclear, and recent publications indicate that it may not be caused by the presence of HIV in the tissues.

KS was first described in 1872 by the dermatologist Moritz Kaposi. It is a pseudoneoplastic infection caused by a newly discovered herpes virus (e.g., herpes 8, human herpes virus 8 [HHV-8], KS-associated herpes virus [KSHV]). It may be an infectious disease rather than a malignancy. It can exist independently from AIDS, but it is the most frequent malignant lesion in HIV-positive patients.

KS is an aggressive pathology that develops widespread, multifocal lesions in the skin, oral mucosa, lymph nodes, lungs, large intestine, and other visceral organs. It may originate from the dedifferentiation and proliferation of the endothelium of a lymphatic or blood vessel. It is diagnosed by taking a biopsy of the lesion.

Lymphedema and KS

A common complication of KS is lymphostatic edema (LE). KS-associated LE usually affects the lower extremities but can occur in the upper extremities, face, neck, and thorax in exceptional cases. Lymphangioscintigraphy usually shows delayed lymph absorption, lymphatic vessels, and node abnormalities.

Combined decongestive physiotherapy (CDP; Box 13-1, Box 13-2) is a conservative approach and is usu-

---

BOX 13-2

CDP Hands-On Modalities

There are also different names to describe the hands-on modality of CDP.

Lymph Drainage Therapy (LDT)—Chikly
Manual Lymph Drainage (MLD)—originally Vodder
Manual Lymph Drainage Therapy (MLDT)
Manual Lymph(atic) Techniques (MLT)—treatment or therapy; a term used increasingly in scientific publications to avoid taking sides

---

BOX 13-3

CDP Treatment Problems

- There is a scarcity of available information and conflicting scientific information in the United States.
- The nature of lymphostatic edema (LE) is chronic: LE is a condition that generally grows worse over time if left untreated.
- Health care providers, patients, and insurance companies have limited knowledge about CDP.
- The patients' compliance and commitment is essential to success. Patients need to be well-educated about their illness and its treatment.
- Bandages and other medical external compression are sometimes difficult to accept as components of the treatment.
- LE usually requires lifelong care and psychological support.
- Insurance companies are reluctant to reimburse CDP in the United States.

BOX 13-1

Abbreviations

In the past, schools have used different names for CDP; however, all these terms are equivalent. This book uses the abbreviation CDP for simplicity.

Combined Decongestive Physiotherapy (CDP)—used by Medicare in Florida
Combined Decongestive Therapy (CDT)—Vodder
Complex Lymphatic Therapy (CLT)—Casley-Smith, Australia
Complex Physical Decongestive Therapy (CPDT)—Földi, Germany
Complex Physical Therapy (CPT)—Casley-Smith, Australia, 1980
Lymphedema Multimodal Therapy (LMT)
Lymphedema Therapy (LT)

ally the first treatment to consider in LE (Box 13-3). The LE in KS can be alleviated by CDP (Box 13-4). CDP, which is reimbursed by Medicare in Florida, includes skin care, external compression, exercises under compression, self-drainage, and other physiotherapy modalities and it is usually appropriate (see Box 13-4).

CDP is safe, noninvasive, effective, and cost-effective, but it must be applied by trained and skilled practitioners. It often does not cure LE but seeks to restore the normal size and function of the limb. The sooner the patient receives treatment (even preventively, before the onset of LE), the faster is the response to the treatment.

CDP Treatment of LE

Although all treatments for LE should be tailored to the patient, CDP treatment includes at least two

phases that are equivalent in all therapies. These two phases may need to be repeated after about 4 to 6 months.[90]

PHASE I: decongestive, acute phase. Phase I usually requires 2 to 4 weeks of treatment, until a plateau of decongestion has been reached. For cases of simple LE, it may take 5 to 25 sessions.

1. Patient education (e.g., contraindications, precautions, complications, self-bandaging, diet)
2. Skin care and skin precautions
3. Hands-on modality: manual lymph(atic) techniques (MLT) or LDT (once or twice a day, possibly as often as 5 to 7 days/week at some clinics)

The first objective of LDT, a manual component of CDP, is to do a superficial Manual Lymphatic Mapping (MLM), identify the direction of the

BOX 13-4

Kaposi's Sarcoma References

Papadopulos-Eleopulos E, Turner VF, et al: Kaposi's sarcoma and HIV, *Med Hypotheses* 39, 1992.

Witte MH, Witte CL: AIDS-Kaposi's sarcoma complex: evolution of a full-blown lymphological syndrome, *Lymphology* 21:4-10, 1988.

Witte MH, Witte CL, Way DL, et al: AIDS, Kaposi's sarcoma, and the lymphatic system: update and reflections, *Lymphology* 23:73-80, 1990.

Kurz I: *Textbook of Dr. Vodder's manual lymph drainage,* vol 1-3, ed 2, Heidelberg, 1990, Haug.

Leduc A: *Le drainage lymphatique: théorie et pratique,* Monographie de Bois-Larris, Masson, 1980.

Földi M, Casley-Smith JR: *Lymphangiology,* Stuttgart, Germany, 1983, Schattauer Verlag.

Wittlinger H et al: *Einführung in die Manuelle Lymphdrainage nach Dr Vodder,* Heidelberg, Germany, 1979, Grundkurs-Haug Verlag.

Collard M, Asdonk J, Bartetzko CH: Experimentalbeitrag zur Manuellen Lymph-drainage Lymphangiographischen Unter-suchungen, Vorträge auf der 4 und 6 wissen-schaftlichen Tagung der Gesellschaft für Manuelle Lymph-drainage in Saig 1972 und Hamburg, 1973.

Francois A: Use of isotopic lymphography in the evaluation of manual lymphatic drainage effects in chronic lower limb edema. In Partsch H, editor: *Progress in Lymphology,* vol 11, Excerpta Medica,

International Congress Series no. 779, Amsterdam, 1987, Elsevier Science Publishers.

Boris M, Weindorf S: Lymphedema reduction by noninvasive complex lymphedema therapy, *Oncology* 8(9):95-106, 1994.

Carriere B: Edema: its development and treatment using lymph drainage massage, *Clin Mgmt Phys Ther* 8(5):19-21, 1988.

Casley-Smith JR et al: *Modern treatment for lymphoedema,* Lymphedema Association of Australia, Adelaide, 1994, University of Adelaide.

Cluzan RV: Lymphatics and edema. In Cluzan RV et al, editors: *Progress in lymphology,* vol 13, Excerpta Medica, International Congress Series no. 994, Amsterdam, 1992, Elsevier Science Publishers.

Földi M: Treatment of lymphedema, *Progress in lymphology,* vol 12, Excerpta Medica, International Congress Series no. 887, Amsterdam, 1990, Elsevier Science Publishers.

Mortimer PS: Managing lymphoedema, *Clin Exp Dermatol* 20:98-106, 1995.

Kubik S, Manestar M: Anatomische Grundlagen der Therapie des Lymphödems, *Ödem* 19-31, 1986.

Chikly B: Silent waves: theory and practice of Lymph Drainage Therapy (LDT), Scottsdale, Ariz, 2001, IHH Publishing.

lymph circulation, and find the most efficient alternate pathways for activation of the lymphatic flow

4. Medical compression: bandaging
5. Psychological and stress management, if needed

Compliance. A home maintenance program involves:

1. Self-education of the patient
2. Hygiene and precautions
3. Self drainage, twice daily
4. Self-bandaging (facilitate with a companion)
5. Exercises under compression twice daily, breathing, and moderate exercise
6. Diet and weight loss if needed

Lymph drainage. Administer LDT once or twice a day. Rest, then walk or exercise for 15 to 45 minutes. During the first phase of acute decompression, the bandages are kept on the limb or limbs at all times, except during the MLT/LDT sessions.

Other modalities. Other possible modalities include medication, ultrasound, laser, hyperbaric chambers, and mercury bath.

PHASE II: rehabilitation, maintenance, and preservation phase. After the plateau of decompression, switch from bandages to compression garments during the day. The protocol is similar to that of Phase I, but the home program maintenance is much more extensive.

1. MLT/LDT is replaced by self-drainage twice daily. The therapist is seen much less often.
2. The bandages are replaced during the day by compression garments (sleeves or stockings) and other equipment (e.g., Reid sleeve, Legacy sleeve).

PHASE III: repetition of acute decongestion phase I. Phase I treatments may be repeated within 6 months.

Contraindications of Lymphatic Drainage Therapy

More information is needed about how HIV disseminates through the lymphatic system. Some contraindications and precautions, most of which involve common sense, should be strictly respected by trained therapists.[80,81,83,90] Some therapists may choose to avoid draining patients who were recently infected with HIV, and it is always advised to shorten the first few sessions.

Here are a few basic guidelines and contraindications associated with complications of HIV infection:

Contraindications:

1. Acute infectious or inflammatory processes

2. Serious circulatory problems (e.g., thrombosis, phlebitis)
3. Hemorrhage (bleeding): be absolutely sure that the bleeding has stopped
4. Malignant ailments (e.g., sarcoma, active cancer, leukemia)

A recent report from the International Society of Lymphology confirmed that scientific studies did not provide any evidence of aggravation or spreading of cancer with lymphatic drainage techniques. However, for their own protection, LDT therapists should not work on patients with either active cancer or cancer that is not medically under control, and they should always check with a physician.

Lymphatic Drainage Therapy: The Manual Technique

To practice an efficient LDT session, the following general points should be specifically observed[90]:

1. Rhythm and frequency of movements: LDT follows and enhances the patient's natural inner lymphatic rhythm. After advanced training, the subtle rhythm of the lymph flow can precisely move the practitioner's hands at the right time and in the right direction.
2. Hand pressure: Hand pressure should be very light. The ideal pressure is usually a maximum of 1 oz (0.5 to 2 oz)/cm^2, which is about 8 oz/in^2.
3. Direction of the flow of drainage: The lymph has to follow the specific direction of drainage, which is usually toward the node group responsible for its drainage. Precise anatomical and physiological knowledge is necessary to carry out this progression in an efficient manner.
4. Hand techniques: The wrists are very good indicators and activators of movement, and they are the best at moving the lymph
5. Duration of movements: The rhythm of the maneuver should match the natural rhythm of the flow of lymph. Hand movements have:
   - an active phase: a movement directed toward the nodes
   - passive phase: the tissue itself makes a passive return
6. Sequence of movements: The course of movements is usually carried out in a back to front fashion or in a retrograde (reverse) way. Drain from proximal to distal.

7. Contraindications of lymphatic drainage: respect the above list of precautions and contraindications.

Patients' Reactions

Patients may experience some detoxification reactions in the 2 to 6 days after LDT sessions. They may also experience a healing crisis, which should not last more than a few days. To prevent these crises, keep the length of the first sessions short, prepare the patient, and suggest that patients eat light, clean food and drink a lot of fluid before and after their sessions.

In summary, many manual therapy techniques exist that can be employed for specific painful conditions throughout the spectrum of HIV disease. The patient has many different options, and knowledge of these manual therapy techniques helps access these options from an informed perspective. We conclude with a brief review of energy-based interventions for pain management.

ENERGY-BASED SYSTEMS

The field of energy medicine is a diverse and ancient one, predating conventional modern Western medicine by thousands of years. Research results show that the practitioner does not need to physically touch the recipient to achieve the desired effects during and after a session.[86] Reiki, a Tibetan/Japanese technique, is an example of such an energetic intervention. Non-contact TT (NCTT) is another modality taught in nursing schools, and Dolores Krieger and Dora Kunz were the first persons to introduce health professionals to this ancient art. A critical factor in understanding the mechanisms that underlie the effects of NCTT stems from studies in quantum physics. Efforts to isolate possible mechanisms responsible for the relaxation outcomes experienced by NCTT recipients come from four main categories: (1) electromagnetic field studies, (2) pain studies, (3) stress and anxiety studies, and (4) wound healing.[87] Each of these areas has been studied, and outcomes have been measured. In a classic study, Krieger reported a significant increase in hemoglobin values in response to TT (treatment group) versus routine hospital care (control group).[88] These results have implications for the HIV-positive patient taking AZT, who may experience the side effects of anemia.

The procedure to conduct NCTT requires two conditions: (1) intentionality, a form of meditation and calming the mind so that the practitioner is non-judgmental and intends to help or heal and (2) assessment, which is performed by scanning over the person's body about 3 to 6 inches away from the skin to detect differences in temperature, electrical potential, or other perceivable sensations. The treatment involves transferring energy from the practitioner to the client.

Patients who experience hypersensitivity caused by DSPN can benefit by hand-mediated energetic healing techniques when they are unable to tolerate direct manual therapy techniques. People with HIV disease have explored these techniques. Because the recipient is not touched during a treatment, these techniques cannot be explained directly by physiological and psychological effects of physical touch, such as those described by psychoneuroimmunology (PNI). These techniques and responses suggest a twofold explanation based on both electromagnetic and quantum physics and transpersonal psychology.[89]

SUMMARY

This chapter focuses on manual and energy-based therapies for the management of various pain syndromes seen throughout the spectrum of HIV disease. Emphasis is placed on the use of CST and LDT, with a brief overview of energy-based interventions. However, a host of manual therapy techniques exist beyond the scope of this chapter that can provide beneficial effects for pain management and generalized relaxation. It is recommended that consumers of manual therapy interventions understand the specific techniques used in a therapeutic session. Asking questions and experiencing the physical, psychological, and spiritual effects throughout a session will foster both greater understanding and future manual therapy interventions.

References

1. Stine GJ: *Acquired immune deficiency syndrome: biological, medical, social, and legal issues,* Englewood Cliffs, N.J., 1993, Prentice-Hall.
2. Singer E, Zorilla C, Fahy-Crandon B, et al: Painful syndromes reported for ambulatory HIV-infected men in a longitudinal study, *Pain* 54:15-19, 1993.

3. Breitbart W, Passik S, Bronaugh T: Pain in the ambulatory AIDS patient: prevalence and psychosocial correlates, Proceedings of the thirty-eighth Annual Meeting of the Academy of Psychosomatic Medicine, Atlanta, 1991.

4. Breitbart W, Rosenfeld B, Passik S, et al: The undertreatment of pain in ambulatory AIDS patients, *Pain* 65:239-245, 1996.

5. Galantino ML, McCormack G: Pain management. In Galantino ML, editor: *Clinical assessment and treatment in HIV disease: rehabilitation of a chronic illness,* Thorofare, N.J., 1992, Slack, Inc.

6. Jacox A, Carr D, Payne R: Clinical practice guideline number nine: management of cancer pain, US Department of Health and Human Services, Public Health Service, Agency for Health Care Policy and Research, AHCPR Publication 94-0592, pp 139-141, 1994.

7. Galantino ML, Findley T, Kraft L, et al: Blending traditional and alternative strategies for rehabilitation: measuring functional outcomes and quality of life issues in an AIDS population, Proceedings of the eighth World Congress of International Rehabilitation Medicine Association, *Moduzzi Editore* 1:713-716, 1997.

8. Muma RD, Boruki MJ, Ayachi S, et al: Diagnosis and treatment of HIV-related conditions. In Muma RD, Lyons BA, Borucki MJ, Pollard RB, editors: *HIV manual for health care professionals,* Stamford, Conn, 1997, Appleton Lange.

9. Lewis M, Warfield C: Management of pain in AIDS, *Hosp Pract* 30:51-54, 1990.

10. Hewitt D, Breitbart W, Rosenfeld B, et al: Pain syndromes in the ambulatory AIDS patient, Proceedings of the thirteenth Annual Meeting of the American Pain Society, Miami, 1994.

11. Reference deleted in proofs.

12. Belgrade MJ: Following the clues to neuropathic pain, *Postgrad Med* 106(6):127-140, 1999.

13. Lange DJ, Britton CB, Younger DS, et al: The neuromuscular manifestation of human immunodeficiency virus infections, *Arch Neurol* 1084-1088, 1988.

14. Lane RJ, McLean KA, Moss J, et al: Myopathy in HIV infection: the role of zidovudine and the significance of tubuloreticular inclusions, *Neuropathol Appl Neurobiol* 19(5):406-413, 1993.

15. Wulff EA, Wang K, Simpson DM: HIV-associated peripheral neuropathy: epidemiology, pathophysiology, and treatment, 59(6):125-160, 2000.

16. Munoz-Fernandez S, Cardenal A, Balsa A: Rheumatic manifestations in 556 patients with human immunodeficiency virus infection, *Semin Arthritis Rheum* 21:30-39, 1991.

17. McReynolds M: The rheumatological manifestations of HIV disease. In Galantino ML, editor: *Issues in HIV rehabilitation,* Alexandria, Va, 1996, APTA—Oncology manuscript.

18. Simms RB, Zerbini CAF, Ferrante N: Fibromyalgia syndrome in patients infected with human immunodeficiency virus, *Am J Med* 92:368-374, 1992.

19. Berman A, Espinoza LR, Diaz JD, et al: Rheumatic manifestation of human immunodeficiency virus infection, *Am J Med* 85:(1)59-64, 1988.

20. Bennett RM, Smythe HA, Wolfe F: Recognizing fibromyalgia, *Patient Care* 23:60-83, 1989.

21. Alpiner N, Oh T, Hinder S, et al: Rehabilitation in joint and connective tissue diseases and systemic diseases, *Arch Phys Med Rehabil* 76(5S):32-39, 1995.

22. Gutierrez VFJ, Martinez-Osuna P, Seleznick MJ, et al: Rheumatological rehabilitation for patients with HIV. In Mukand J, editor: *Rehabilitation in patients with HIV disease,* New York, 1991, McGraw-Hill.

23. Goldenberg DL: Fibromyalgia and other chronic fatigue syndromes: is there evidence for chronic viral disease? *Semin Arthritis Rheum* 18:111-120, 1988.

24. O'Dell MW, Dillon ME: Rehabilitation in adults with human immunodeficiency virus-related diseases, *Am J Phys Med Rehabil* 71:183-190, 1993.

25. Barnes J: Myofacial release: the missing link in traditional treatment. In Davis C, editor: *Complementary therapies in rehabilitation,* Thorofare, N.J., 1997, Slack, Inc.

26. Jones L: *Strain and counterstrain,* 1981, The American Academy of Osteopathy.

27. Weiselfish S, Kain J: Introduction to developmental manual therapy: an integrated systems approach for structural and functional rehabilitation, *Phys Ther Forum* (6): 1990.

28. Barral JP: *Visceral manipulation,* Seattle, 1987, Eastland Press.

29. Barral JP: *Visceral manipulation II,* Seattle, 1989, Eastland Press.

30. Upledger JE: Thermographic view of autism, *Osteopath Ann* 118:356-359, 1983.

31. Upledger JE: *Craniosacral therapy II,* Seattle, 1987, Eastland Press.

32. Upledger JE: *Somatoemotional release and beyond,* Palm Beach Gardens, Fla, 1990, Upledger Institute Publishing.

33. Upledger JE: Relationship of craniosacral examination findings in grade-school children with developmental problems, *J Am Osteopath Assoc* 77(10):760-776, 1978.

34. Wallace, Avant, McKinney, et al: Ultrasonic measurement of intracranial pulsations at 9 cycles per minute, *J Neurol* 1985.

35. Roppel RM, Upledger JE: Bioelectric phenomena in relation to neural function, *J Am Osteopath Assoc* 1976.

36. Retzlaff EW, Roppel RM, Becker, et al: Craniosacral mechanisms, *J Am Osteopath Assoc* 76:288-289, 1976.

37. Retzlaff EW, Mitchell FL, Upledger JE, et al: Nerve fibers and endings in cranial sutures: research report, *J Am Osteopath Assoc* 77:474-475, 1978.

38. Upledger JE: The reproducibility of craniosacral examination findings: a statistical analysis, *J Am Osteopath Assoc* 76(12):890-899, 1977.

39. Upledger JE: Mechano-electric patterns during craniosacral osteopathic diagnosis and treatment, *J Am Osteopath Assoc* 78(11):782-791, 1979.

40. Upledger JE: Cranial therapy proves successful with some ADD children, *Assoc for Retarded Citizens Advocates* 1980.

41. Upledger JE: The therapeutic value of the craniosacral system, *Massage Ther J* 27(1):32, 1988.

42. Upledger JE: Cancer: now you see it, now you don't. In *The cancer chronicles*, 5:5-6, 1994, Equinox Press.

43. Karni Z, Upledger JE: *Early steps of cranial therapy in Israel*, 1979, Publication of Technion Institute.

44. Karni Z, Upledger JE, Mizrahi J, et al: Examination of the cranial rhythm in long-standing coma and chronic neurological cases, *J Israel Institute Technol* 1980.

45. Retzlaff EW, Upledger JE: Cranial suture pain, *J Am Osteopath Assoc.*

46. Vredevoogd J, Upledger JE: Management of autogenic headache, *Osteopath Ann* 1979.

47. Retzlaff EW, Vredevoogd J, Upledger JE: A proposed mechanism for drugless pain control, *J Am Osteopath Assoc* 1997.

48. Reference deleted in proofs.

49. Ironson G, Field T, Scafidi F, et al: Massage therapy is associated with enhancement of the immune system's cytotoxic capacity, *Int J Neurosci* 84(1-4):205-217, 1996.

50. Ruebottom A et al: Casey House Hospice, Inc., Toronto, June 4-9, vol 5, 1989.

51. Chikly B: Who discovered the lymphatic system? *Lymphology* 30(4):186, 1997a.

52. Millard FP: Applied anatomy of the lymphatics. In Walmstey AG, editor: *International Lymphatic Research Society*, 1922.

53. Vodder E: *Le drainage lymphatique, une nouvelle methode therapeutique, sante pour tous*, Paris, 1936.

54. Vodder E: Die manuelle Lymphdrainage—massage as an auxiliary therapy, Manual Therapy Congress, London, Sep 25-28, 1965.

55. Chikly B: Applications of pre and postsurgical lymph drainage therapy, *Massage Bodywork* 12(3):64-67, 1997b.

56. Olszewski WL, Engeset A: Intrinsic contractility of leg lymphatics in man: preliminary communication, *Lymphology* 12:81-84, 1979.

57. Olszewski WL, Engeset A: Intrinsic contractility of prenodal lymph vessels and lymph flow in human leg, *Am J Physiol* 239:775-783, 1980.

58. Olszewski WL, Engeset A: Studies on the lymphatic circulation of humans, In Johnston MG, editor: *Experimental biology of the lymphatic circulation*, Amsterdam, 1982, Elsevier Science Publishers.

59. Adair TH, Guyton AC: Introduction to the lymphatic system. In Johnston MG, editor: *Experimental biology of the lymphatic circulation*, Amsterdam, 1982a, Elsevier Science Publishers.

60. Guyton AC: *Textbook of medical physiology*, Toronto, 1988, WB Saunders.

61. Kubik S: *The lymphatic system*, New York, 1985, Springer Publishing Co., Inc.

62. Adair TH, Guyton AC: Lymph formation and its modification in the lymphatic system. In Johnston MG, editor: *Experimental biology of the lymphatic circulation*, Amsterdam, 1982b, Elsevier Science Publishers.

63. Hauck G, Castenholz A: Contribution of prelymphatic structures to lymph drainage, *Lymphology* 16(1):6-9, 1992.

64. Leak LV: Lymphatic endothelial-interstitial interface, *Lymphology* 20(4):196-204, 1987.

65. Casley-Smith JR, Florey HHW: The structure of normal small lymphatics, *Q J Exp Physiol* 46:101, 1961.

66. Castenholz A: Functional morphological features and flow dynamics of initial lymphatic structures. In *Progress in lymphology*, vol 12, Exerpta Medica, International Congress Series no. 887, Amsterdam, 1990, Elsevier Science Publishers.

67. Kubik S: Initial lymphatics in different skin regions. In Partsch H, editor: *Progress in lymphology*, vol 11, Exerpta Medica, Amsterdam, 1987, Elsevier Science Publishers.

68. Armonio S et al: Spontaneous contractility in the human lymph vessels, *Lymphology* 14:173, 1981.

69. Johnston MG: Involvement of lymphatic collecting ducts in the physiology and pathophysiology of lymph flow. In Johnston MG, editor: *Experimental biology of the lymphatic circulation*, Amsterdam, 1982, Elsevier Science Publishers.

70. Kinmonth JB, Taylor GW: Spontaneous rhythmic contractility in human lymphatics, *J Physiol* 133:3, 1956.

71. Wang GY, Zhong SZ: Experimental study of lymphatic contractility and its clinical importance, *Ann Plast Surg* 15(4):278-284, 1985.

72. Zawieja DC, Davis KL, Schuster R, et al: Distribution, propagation, and coordination of contractile activity in lymphatics, *Am J Physiol* 264:1283-1291, 1993.

73. Yoffey JM, Courtice FC: *Lymphatics, lymph, and lymphoid tissue*, London, 1956, Edward Arnold.

74. Yoffey JM: Cellular migration strains: the integration of the lymphomyeloid complex, *Lymphology* 18:5-21, 1985.

75. Diebold J, Marche C, Audouin J, et al: Lymph node modification in patients with acquired immune deficiency syndrome (AIDS or with AIDS-related complex): a histological, immunohistological, and ultrastructural study of 45 cases, *Pathol Res Pract* 180:6, 1985.

76. Ewing EP Jr, Chandler FW, et al: Primary lymph node pathology in AIDS and AIDS-related lymphadenectomy, *Arch Pathol Lab Med* 109:11, 1985.

77. Ost A, Baroni CD, Biberfeld P, et al: Lymphadenectomy in HIV infection: histological classification and staging, *APMIS* 97:7, 1989.

78. Pileri S, Rivano MT, et al: The value of lymph node biopsy in patients with acquired immune deficiency syndrome (AIDS or with AIDS-related complex): a morphological and immunohistochemical study of 90 cases, *Histopathology* 10:11, 1986.

79. Chikly B: *Lymph drainage therapy: study guide level 1 and 2,* Palm Beach Gardens, Fla, 1997c, Upledger Institute Publishing.

80. Kurz I: *Textbook of Dr. Vodder's manual lymph drainage,* vol 1-3, ed 2, Heidelberg, Germany, 1990, Haug.

81. Leduc A: *Le drainage lymphatique: theorie et pratique,* Masson, France, 1980, Monographie de Bois-Larris.

82. Foldi M et al: *Lymphangiology,* Stuttgart, Germany, 1983, Schattauer Veriag.

83. Wittlinger H et al: *Einfohrung in die Manuelle Lymphdrainage nach Dr. Vodder,* Heidelberg, Germany, 1979, Grundkurs-Haug Veriag.

84. Collard M, Asdonk J, Bartetzko CH: Experimentalbitrag zur Manuellen Lymphdrainage bell lymphangiographischen Untersuchugen, Vortage auf der 4 and 6 wissenschaftlichen Tagung der Gesellschaft for Manuelle Lymphdrainage in Said 1972 und Hamburg, 1973.

85. Francois A: Use of isoptic lymphography in the evaluation of manual lymphatic drainage effects in chronic lower limb edema. In Partsch H, editor: *Progress in lymphology,* vol 11, Exerpta Medica, International Congress Series no. 779, Amsterdam, 1987, Elsevier Science Publishers.

86. Quinn JF: Therapeutic touch as energy exchange: testing the theory, *Adv Nurs Sci* 6:42-49, 1984.

87. Quinn JF: Building a body of knowledge: research on therapeutic touch 1974-1986, *J Holistic Nurs* 6:37-45, 1988.

88. Krieger D: Healing by the "laying on" of hands as a facilitator of bioenergetic change: the response on in vivo human hemoglobin, *Psychoenergetic Syst* 1:121-129, 1979.

89. Slater VE: Healing touch. In Micozzi MS, editor: *Fundamentals of complementary and alternative medicine,* New York, 1996, Churchill-Livingstone.

90. Chikly B: Silent waves: theory and practice of Lymph Drainage Therapy (LDT), Scottsdale, Ariz, 2001, IHH Publishing.

Suggested Readings

Allen PJ et al: Lower extremity lymphedema caused by acquired immune deficiency syndrome-related Kaposi's sarcoma: case report and review of the literature, *J Vasc Surg* 22(2):178-181, 1995.

Casley-Smith JR: Prelymphatics. In Malek P, Bartos V, Weissleder H, Witte MH, editors: *Lymphology,* Stuttgart, Germany, Georg Thleme.

Evashwick CJ, Weiss LJ: *Managing the continuum of care,* Rockville, Md., 1987, Aspen Publishers, Inc.

Frans E, Blockmans D, Peetermans W, et al: Kaposi's sarcoma presenting as general lymphedema, *Acta Clin Belg* 49(1):19-21, 1994.

Frymann VM: Relation of disturbances of craniosacral mechanisms to symptomatology of the newborn: a study of 1250 infants, *J Am Osteopath Assoc* 65:1059, 1966.

LaPerriere A, Fletcher M, Antoni M: Aerobic exercise training in an AIDS risk group, *Int J Sports Med* 12:53, 1991.

Lubeck DP, Nobunaga AI, Williams CA, et al: Rehabilitation of selected nonneurological HIV disability. In O'Dell MW, editor: *HIV-related disability: assessment and management,* vol 7, Philadelphia, 1993, Hanley & Belfus, Inc.

McReynolds M: Rehabilitation management of the lower extremity in HIV disease, *J Am Podiatr Med Assoc* July, 1995.

Roppel RM, St. Pierre N, Mitchell FL: Measurement of accuracy in bimanual perception of motion, *J Am Osteopath Assoc* 77:475, 1978.

Upledger JE, Karni Z: Bioelectric and strain measurements during cranial manipulation, *J Am Osteopath Assoc* 77:476, 1978.

Upledger JE, Vredvoogd J: *Craniosacral therapy,* Chicago, 1983, Eastland Press.

Applications of Movement Therapy in HIV Disease

MARY LOU GALANTINO

ABSTRACT

Researchers have long appreciated the importance of exercise in maintaining health. Scientific evidence indicates that exercise training is not only appropriate but warranted for many chronic diseases. Exercise training can reduce the effects of stress and increase immune function in HIV/AIDS. Specific exercise prescriptions can be used across disciplines to implement exercise intervention programs for individuals at various stages of chronic HIV disease.

Traditional exercise encompasses weight training and aerobic exercise. Studies of these exercise interventions in asymptomatic HIV-positive individuals suggest improvements in mood, increases in cardio-vascular (CV) fitness, and a trend toward increased $CD4^+$ cell counts. This chapter presents a brief review of traditional exercise interventions and introduces analogous benefits from various movement strategies.

Exercise is a good example of a proven behavioral medicine intervention that requires establishing new partnerships and acquiring knowledge and skills across several disciplines. This chapter presents an overview of various movement therapies that are potential sources of alternative exercise interventions, such as Tai Chi, yoga, and Qigong. Clinicians who design exercise programs for people living with HIV disease may find it particularly interesting.

INTRODUCTION

Reports on physical activity and health often confirm that a daily regimen of moderate exercise reduces the risks of developing coronary heart disease, hypertension, colon cancer, diabetes, and depression.[1,2] In fact, insufficient physical activity is linked to the increased risk of developing disease and to a poorer prognosis for the management of many chronic diseases, including HIV/AIDS.[3] However, because HIV/AIDS patients' health "waxes and wanes," which is inherent in chronic disease and necessitates ongoing adaptations to the exercise prescription, terms such as *exercise* and *physical activity* may not be appropriate to fully describe this treatment. Therefore the term *Movement Therapy* is used to capture and convey the full range of available physical modality therapies for the rehabilitation of chronic disease. This chapter provides a sound rationale for the appropriate uses of Movement Therapy throughout the entire course of HIV/AIDS.

To accomplish these goals, this chapter first presents general background information for both the various physiological underpinnings of exercise and immunology as they relate to the spectrum of HIV disease and the stress associated with managing a chronic illness. Next, a brief review of the psychoneuroimmunology (PNI) literature serves as a framework for the use of exercise and Movement Therapy. Finally, guidelines for the design and implementation of a personalized program are provided. This chapter attempts to empower the HIV/AIDS population to incorporate Movement Therapy into their medical treatment plan. At the same time, this chapter also provides the professional medical community with the tools needed to assist them in their quest for implementation and further research.

BACKGROUND

The use of alternative therapies has increased during the HIV epidemic, some of which are more traditional than others.[4] Eisenberg[5] reported that a combination of prayer and exercise accounted for over 60% of all alternative therapies. Other alternative therapies include relaxation techniques (13%), massage (7%), imagery (4%), and spiritual healing (4%). Traditional exercises, such as aerobics and weight training, are incorporated in the medical model through exercise physiology and rehabilitation. However, various movement therapies (such as martial arts) are often viewed as being less traditional and outside the established medical model.

Substantial evidence suggests that traditional exercise, particularly aerobic exercise, provides substantial physiological and psychological benefits for most individuals, especially those with chronic diseases. However, the mode, duration, and intensity of many traditional standardized exercise programs may not always be appropriate during a chronic illness. The stage of disease and the type of illness may preclude more strenuous exercise activities at various times. During these times, less traditional movement therapies may be more appropriate and efficacious. In fact, movement therapy includes a number of constructs that are similar to those used in physical therapy, and it can complement an individual program of more traditional exercise.

Depending on the originating discipline, various types of movement therapy exist. Eastern thought perspectives dominate this area, and some examples include Feldenkrais,[6] Qigong,[7] and Tai Chi.[8,9] In a recent study by Bastyr University,[10] people living with HIV disease used various movement therapies. This study evaluated the use of alternative therapies within the past 6 months. Of the study's participants, 15.5% used yoga, 4.8% used Tai Chi, and 3.6% used Qigong. This chapter reviews each of these movement therapies in more detail.

STRESS AND EARLY PROGRESSION OF HIV DISEASE

Researchers have known for many years that depression or stress may exacerbate certain diseases, and certain alterations in immunity are associated with psychological conditions. The relationship between stress and immune functioning in other populations suggests that acute and chronic stress can impair or alter the immune response.[11,12] Some reports show that stress can increase the progression rate of early stages of HIV disease. In one study, patients received comprehensive medical, neurological, neuropsychological, and psychiatric assessments every 6 months, which included an assessment of stressful life events. The study was conducted over a 42-month period. The results demonstrated that the more severe the stressful event, the greater was the risk of early HIV disease progression. For every severe stress episode reported during a 6-month period, the risk of early disease progression doubled. Among the 66 patients who were monitored for 2 years or more, a logistic regression analysis was used to show that higher levels of severe life stress increased the odds of developing HIV progression by nearly fourfold. Therefore the researchers concluded that severe life-event stress is associated with an increased rate of early HIV disease progression.[13]

The psychological and physical consequences of HIV infection are associated with significant emotional distress and clinical syndromes in some patients, such as adjustment disorders, depression, and anxiety.[14,15] Focus is placed increasingly on the potential effect of HIV-related stress on the course of infection because of the observed and postulated relationship between psychosocial stress, neuropsychological functioning, and immune status.[16] Minimizing stressful events throughout chronic HIV disease can be managed in various ways, including meditation, relaxation, and various forms of exercise.

Literature Review on Exercise Studies and HIV Disease

Increases in physical fitness are often associated with improvements in certain chronic diseases, such as coronary heart disease and hypertension.[17] Evidence shows that exercise also influences the neuroendocrine and immune systems, resulting in a potential benefit to individuals with chronic immunodeficiency diseases.[18] Aerobic exercise training programs may enhance certain critical components of cellular immunity and act as a buffer for the detrimental mood changes that typically accompany stress, thus providing a behavioral approach to helping HIV-positive individuals.[19] The Bastyr study[10] delineated the use of aerobic exercise as one of the main movement modalities in alternative medicine research. Sixty-three percent of the participants stated that they used aerobic exercise during the past 6 months. The popularity of this intervention warrants continued outcome data from a physiological and quality of life (QOL) perspective.

Exercise and Anxiety

Exercise programs consisting of 6 weeks to 20 months of aerobic training have produced increased perceptions of well-being[20,21] and reductions in anxiety.[20,22,23] In addition, Morgan and colleagues have shown, dur-

ing almost 20 years of research, that state anxiety is reduced after an acute episode of physical activity.[24-26] The most consistent changes in affect occur in individuals who have at least moderate affective disturbances, rather than in those who score within the normal range.[21,24,27] These observations may have particular relevance for early symptomatic HIV-infected individuals. Exercise training for HIV-positive individuals, which has already been demonstrated as effective in reducing anxiety after a potent stressor,[19] also may reduce anxiety after each exercise session (three times/week). Exercise may therefore help early symptomatic HIV-1-positive individuals overcome anxiety produced by numerous stressors.

Exercise and Depression

Aerobic exercise training of various durations decreases depression.[21,28] After 10 weeks of aerobic exercise training, moderately depressed patients showed a significant decrease in depression as measured by the Beck Depression Inventory (BDI) and the Profile of Mood States (POMS).[29] Another study found that BDI scores were reduced from the moderately disturbed range to the normal range (less than 10) after moderate exercise training (as an adjunct to counseling therapy). In contrast, patients receiving counseling-only therapy showed a significantly smaller decrease in BDI (23 versus 19) scores. Previous research also showed that exercise training attenuates the depressive affect that accompanies a positive HIV diagnosis.[19]

Cardiopulmonary and Strength Improvements

Aerobic activity enhances the immune status and cardiopulmonary function of HIV-positive individuals.[19,30-32] Progressive resistance exercise programs for AIDS patients show improvements in strength, power, and endurance.[33] A study completed by Olsen, Wallace, and Carl[34] found that, among HIV-infected patients who were motivated to and capable of regular strenuous exercise, weight training offers a salutary benefit that is superior to intense running. Outcome measures included a mean change in $CD4^+$ percentage over a 24-month period. Other studies support the use of resistive exercise for complications of HIV wasting syndrome, lipodystrophy, and generalized conditioning.[35,36]

In addition to the use of various exercises, recombinant human growth hormone (rhGH; Serostim, Serano Laboratories, Norwell, Mass.) has been approved by the Food and Drug Administration (FDA) for the treatment of AIDS wasting. Schambelan et al[37] found that patients who received Serostim for 12 weeks had increased body weight (BW) and lean body mass (LBM) compared with the placebo group. Furthermore, patients on Serostim demonstrated increased work output, as measured during treadmill ambulation, which correlated with changes in LBM. These researchers also used a self-administered questionnaire, the HIV-Patient Assessed Report of Status and Experience (HIV-PARSE), but did not find that this measure changed as a result of Serostim use.

Other researchers have used similar patient questionnaires to examine the effect of exercise and hormone replacement therapy on QOL, such as the Medical Outcomes Study-HIV Specific Questionnaire (MOS-HIV) and the Health-Related Quality of Life Survey (HRQOL). However, they did not find significant treatment effects for these measures.[38,39] Various QOL measures can measure the impact of a particular type of exercise over time.

Hydrotherapy, or aquatic therapy, provides an environment for the benefit of aerobic and resistance exercise. Zacka[40] studied the effects of hydrotherapy and found that this type of exercise was also beneficial for persons with HIV disease. Physiological, psychological, and immunological variables were measured both at enrollment and completion of the 8-week study. At the end of the treatment, CD4$^+$ cell counts increased and almost reached significance for the hydrotherapy treatment group (but not the control group). Some of the psychological measures showed a similar pattern. By contrast, the hydrotherapy treatment group showed significant gains in muscle endurance and power as compared with the control group.[40]

Exercise Challenges

The chronic nature of HIV disease is replete with various opportunistic infections (OIs). Individuals may not be physically able to maintain an aerobic fitness level to sustain a significant change in the immune system. Only one study[31] investigated the effects of aerobic activity on the moderately-to-severely immunocompromised AIDS population. Physical function in the advanced disease state varied, since only six of the 25 patients were able to complete the 24-week exercise program.

The majority of exercise studies have been conducted with early-diagnosis HIV-positive individuals, since this population encounters very few OIs.[19] Because the progression of HIV disease involves increasing disability, advanced disease has an adverse effect on QOL and functional outcomes. Further research is needed to evaluate the benefits of alternative exercise programs for individuals living with AIDS who are unable to participate in a rigorous aerobic or progressive resistance exercise program. Exercising in a group fosters various social interactions, and benefits are also observed through physical and movement therapy interventions. Finally, as the health care market continues to change, group-oriented interventions, which are more cost-effective, may better serve this population and our health system.

Previous exercise studies have focused on the role of aerobic activity to enhance various immune markers and stave off OIs.[3,19] Aerobic studies have focused primarily on early-diagnosis HIV individuals from a preventive perspective.[19] OIs cause a great deal of fatigue, undermine an individual's continued capacity in the workplace, and compromise basic daily activities.[41,42] Few studies have documented exercise intervention from a group perspective.[43,44] Most group studies are conducted in the fields of health education and occupational therapy. Given the nature of chronic disability in an AIDS diagnosis, it is important to develop alternative interventions to evaluate improvement in functional outcomes of this population, such as movement therapy.

Psychoneuroimmunology

PNI investigates the interrelationships between psychological constructs (e.g., stressors, mood states) and the neuroendocrine and immune systems. Although the precise mechanistic links between these varied components of PNI are not yet fully elucidated, PNI provides a useful framework of our understanding of the role of stressors in immunomodulation. These effects may have a profound influence on the occurrence and progression of ill health in diseases such as HIV/AIDS.

Findings in PNI show that it is useful to evaluate the influence of behavioral factors on immune functioning and disease progression in HIV-infected individuals.[1,19,30,45] Behavioral interventions with immunomodulatory capabilities may restore competence and thereby arrest HIV at the earliest stages of disease progression.

As mentioned previously, a growing body of literature indicates that many different stressors have deleterious effects on the immune system.[46,47] Stressors in people living with HIV may be attenuated by an exercise training program. Research indicates that continued aerobic exercise training results in increased CD4 cell counts, immune surveillance, and slowed disease progression.[30] Other researchers have demonstrated similar benefits of exercise for advanced-stage HIV-infected individuals. However, these studies are conducted on traditional exercise methods. Exercise within the context of PNI appears to be a promising approach to the treatment of illness and the promotion of health.

Major findings of practical importance in terms of public health and athletic endeavor include the following: (1) In response to acute exercise (the most frequently studied area of exercise immunology), a rapid interchange of immune cells between peripheral lymphoid tissues and circulation occurs. (2) In response to long-term exercise training, the only congruent finding to date is a significant elevation in natural killer (NK) cell activity. Researchers have inconsistently reported changes in the function of neutrophils, macrophages, and T and B cells in response to exercise training, but they indicate that neutrophil function is suppressed during periods of heavy training. (3) Limited data suggest that unusually heavy or chronic exercise increases the risk of upper respiratory tract infection (URTI), whereas regular moderate physical activity reduces URTI symptomatology. (4) Work performance tends to diminish with most systemic infections. Clinical case studies and animal data suggest that infection severity, relapse, and myocarditis result when patients exercise vigorously.[2]

Evidence suggests that neuroendocrine pathways that are capable of influencing lymphocyte distribution and recirculation are disturbed in HIV-infected individuals. A study by Phillips et al[48] determined the effect of acute exercise in mobilizing and redistributing lymphocyte populations. Blood samples were obtained for serum cortisol, norepinephrine, and lymphocyte subsets at rest, immediately after exercise, and 20 minutes after exercise. Examination within the groups revealed that the HIV-positive group had significant increases in both CD8 and NK cells in response to exercise. In addition, the control group had a significant cortisol response to exercise, whereas the HIV-positive group did not. The trend continued 20 minutes after exercise. These results suggest that exercise-induced changes in lymphocyte subsets in HIV-positive asymptomatic persons are independent of cortisol but are dependent on catecholamine.

In a German cohort, lymphocyte subsets were determined by flow cytometry before and immediately after exercise. Investigators found that HIV infection not only results in changes in the proportion of peripheral lymphocyte populations but also results in altered recirculation after physical activity.[49] In a study by MacArthur, Levine, and Birk,[50] researchers evaluated the cardiopulmonary, immunological, and psychological responses to exercise training in HIV-positive persons. They concluded that exercise training is feasible, safe, and physiologically beneficial for many HIV-infected individuals. Individuals with CD4 cell counts less than $100/\mu l$ may be unable to complete an intensive program because of fatigue, disease progression, or other factors. Study lengths differ extensively and range from 6 weeks to 24 months. The acute and chronic effects of exercise also vary in the measurement of physiological and psychological parameters.

Little research has been done on the effect of exercise on viral load. One case study[51] reported a very low viral burden, which was expressed by an undetectable HIV ribonucleic acid (RNA) quantitative polymerase chain reaction (PCR). This patient was also taking zidovudine (AZT), lamivudine (3TC), and ritonavir (ABT-538). Case reports cannot prove causality, but this patient reported subjective and objective improvement in athletic performance and clinical parameters, which he attributed largely to a carefully tailored exercise training program.

A report at the Experimental Biology 1998 Meeting indicated that a high-intensity strength training program does not increase viral load in infected patients. Dr. Ronnenn Roubenoff of Tufts University investigated the effect of 15-minute training periods on viral load on 25 HIV-positive patients and concluded that the exercise actually led to a slight decrease in viral load. Judicious physical training programs that regularly monitor viral load and surrogate markers may warrant a higher profile in the clinical management and secondary prevention of HIV disease. Exercise profiles of long-term HIV/AIDS survivor populations deserve further study.

In summary, a review of all available literature reveals (1) no decline was seen in CD^+ cell counts in any of the studies, regardless of the initial stage of disease, level of $CD4^+$ cells, or symptomatology; and (2) a trend toward an increase in the number of $CD4^+$ cells in all but one study. This study showed that the more significant increases were seen in early-stage patients, and that homogeneous study samples were important when investigating the effects of exercise in a dynamic disease such as HIV/AIDS.[52] From a PNI perspective, psychological stress is one of the cofactors contributing to the immunological decline in HIV disease. Clinical evidence supports the stress-management role of exercise training as a means to explain the buffering of these suppressive stressor effects, thereby facilitating a return of the $CD4^+$ cells. Exercise intervention provides an opportunity to stave off OIs throughout the spectrum of HIV disease.

PSYCHOLOGICAL FINDINGS IN MOVEMENT THERAPY

Movement Therapy and Effects on Mood Alterations

A working definition of Movement Therapy includes an array of modalities. It can take the form of a dance therapy program, a particular technique (e.g., Feldenkrais, Alexander), or a martial art (e.g., Tai Chi, Qigong). The use of movement therapy has been advocated since the early part of the twentieth century. Empirical evidence of its beneficial effects on mood has accumulated slowly. Most of the relevant data come from studies on the effect of exercise on depression.[53]

The research literature that links movement and mood focuses on vigorous movement, such as aerobic exercise.[18] Studies conducted with patients who are not institutionalized but who fit the Research Diagnostic Criteria for major or minor depression found a comparable reduction in depression for both aerobic and anaerobic movement, as compared with sedentary controls.[54] This finding is significant because individuals suffering from chronic diseases are not likely to engage in vigorous aerobic movement because of symptoms and loss of energy for everyday activities.[55]

Professionals in clinical psychology and occupational therapy have studied group intervention from a psychosocial perspective.[56,57] Although many studies have documented patterns of emotional distress in persons with HIV disease, few controlled evaluations of therapy outcomes exist. Most of the reported studies concerned depressed HIV-positive individuals and the evaluation of a specific drug intervention. Symptoms of depression decreased and skills in active behavioral coping were noted.[58] Cognitive-behavioral and social support-group therapies produced reductions in depression, hostility, and somatization. Tests for clinical significance of change underscored the benefits of social support group intervention and long-term follow-up.[59]

However, literature on long-term AIDS survivors is replete with anecdotal evidence linking survival to one or more of the following: (1) having a positive attitude toward the illness, (2) participating in health-promoting behaviors, (3) engaging in spiritual activities, and (4) taking part in AIDS-related activities.[60-62] Positive relationships have been demonstrated between hardiness and perception of physical, emotional, and spiritual health, participation in exercise, and the use of special diets.[63-65]

The Use of Tai Chi as a Movement Modality

Eastern cultures have practiced the art of Tai Chi for centuries. The five schools of Tai Chi share three essential features: (1) the body is naturally extended and relaxed, giving priority to lissomeness; (2) the mind is tranquil but alert; and (3) body movements are slow, smooth, and well-coordinated throughout the exercise period.[9]

A limited number of studies found in Western literature have investigated the use of Tai Chi. Mianyu Qu[66] reported that 32 Chinese individuals (ranging from 50 to 89 years of age) who practiced Tai Chi for 5 to 6 months demonstrated significantly greater improvements in CV, metabolic, respiratory, and osseous measures, compared with 56 age-matched Chinese citizens who did not practice Tai Chi. Van Deusen and Harlane[67] noted that rheumatoid arthritis patients who participated in an 8-week home-based program of integrated Tai Chi and therapeutic dance had significantly greater upper extremity joint movement and reported greater enjoyment 4 months after treatment than did the control group. These findings have implications for patients living with

HIV who encounter HIV-related rheumatological complications.

The effects of balance and posture have also been explored through Tai Chi. Tse and Bailey[68] compared the performance of Tai Chi practitioners with that of nonpractitioners on five balance tests. The Tai Chi group did significantly better on three of the tests. Wolf et al[69] studied the effects of Tai Chi on the prevention of falls in elderly patients. The results for reducing the risk of falls in this population were significant.[70] Balance problems noted in the HIV population as a result of central or peripheral nervous system dysfunction may be augmented through the use of Tai Chi.

Cardiorespiratory (CR) responses to Tai Chi training have also been studied. One study examined ventilatory and CV responses to Tai Chi and found significantly lower ventilatory frequency, suggesting a better use of ventilatory volume than was anticipated from comparable exertional levels on a cycle ergometer.[71] Tai Chi practice resulted in findings of decreased depression, fatigue, and state anxiety. This result was demonstrated in a study of 96 experienced Tai Chi practitioners, which compared Tai Chi with meditation, brisk walking, and neutral reading.[72] Compared with a sedentary control group matched for age and gender, Tai Chi participants had a significantly higher VO_2, O_2 pulse, and work rate during Tai Chi exercise.

A recent study conducted with a group of AIDS patients compared the use of traditional aerobic exercise ($n = 13$) with Tai Chi ($n = 13$). A control group ($n = 12$) was also included. Outcome measures included the MOS-HIV, whereas functional measures included the functional reach, sit-up, and sit-and-reach tests. The physical performance test was used for general function. The MOS-HIV showed a significantly greater perception of overall health after the intervention. Significant differences were demonstrated in all functional measures compared with the control group. Both aerobic and Tai Chi exercise interventions benefited this group of AIDS patients.[73]

The Use of Yoga and Qigong as Movement Modalities

It is important to recognize the physiological similarities between these various movement therapies and the previous PNI perspectives in the traditional use of aerobic exercise. Qigong is one of the four aspects of Chinese medicine and is a spontaneous balancing and enhancing of the natural healing resources in the human system. The physiological mechanisms of Qigong are listed in Table 14-1.[74] Three areas delineated and enhanced through the practice of yoga and Qigong are (1) oxygen metabolism, (2) the lymphatic system, and (3) the nervous system. These systems include the use of several activities: (1) breathing practice, (2) visualization, (3) various postures, (4) concentrated movement, (5) self-massage, (6) relaxation, and (7) meditation.

Progressive relaxation and meditation alter heart rate (HR), brain wave activity, neurotransmitter profile, skin temperature, and muscle control.[75-77] These features are an integral part of yoga and Qigong, and both are influenced by voluntary control of the body's self-regulating mechanisms. Moderate body movement that occurs within a context of deep relaxation is common to both yoga and Qigong. Research on exercise, relaxed states, and other triggers of specific physiological responses are clearly implicated as useful resources that may help build the scientific information on the self-applied health maintenance methods of the Asian systems of traditional medicine.[74] Furthermore, research from Asian cultures is just beginning to be translated. The First World Conference on Academic Exchange of Medical Qigong was held in 1988 in Beijing, and 128 scientific papers have been translated into English.[78]

The challenge researchers face is the scientific interpretation of the *Qi* of the Chinese and the *Prana* of the Indians. However, literature in bioenergetic research is prolific. Electrodynamic fields have been studied by several researchers.[79-81] Nordenstrom[82] described the vascular interstitial closed circuit as a system of preferential ion conductance pathways comprising a network of biological circuitry. Jahnke[74] further explicated these factors in Table 14-1. Qigong and yoga activate a number of mechanisms associated with the lymphatic system, including lymph generation, lymph propulsion, immune function, cerebrospinal fluid (CSF) circulation, and nutritive function.[74]

Studies conducted on yoga are just beginning to emerge. Rehse[83] presented an experiential workshop at the International Conference on AIDS and reported improvements in self-confidence and a return to athletic activities after the intervention. Applications of yoga in the rehabilitation setting are

TABLE 14-1

Physiological Mechanisms of Qigong

Physiological mechanisms	Structures and substrates	Qigong activity
I. Oxygen		
1. Energy generation	Oxygen uptake	Movement/breath
2. Aerobic water	Oxygen uptake	Movement/breath
3. Immune enhancement	Oxygen uptake	Movement/breath
4. Free radical neutralization	Oxygen uptake	Movement/breath
II. Lymph		
1. Aerobic generation	Oxygen	Movement/breath
2. Propulsion		
(a) Aerobic	Oxygen	Movement/breath
(b) Intrinsic contraction	Interstitial fluid volume	Breath/relaxation
(c) Muscle pump	Muscle contraction	Movement
(d) Gravitational	Body position	Postures/movement
(e) Breath apparatus	Lungs, diaphragm, cisterna chyli	Breath activity
3. Immune function	Propulsion	Breath, movement, and posture
4. Cerebral fluid flow	Propulsion	Breath, movement, and posture
5. Nutritive function	Propulsion	Breath, movement, and posture
III. Nervous System		
1. Autonomic	Brain, neurochemistry, nervous system	Relaxation and breath
2. Neurotransmitter profile	Hypothalamus	Relaxation and visualization
3. Microcirculation	Hypothalamus	Relaxation
4. Immunity	Macrophages, leukocytes	Relaxation, meditation
5. Brain hemisphere control	Brain, nervous system	Alternate nostril breath and right and left side movement
6. Brain wave frequency	Brain, nervous system	Meditation
7. Neuroreflex stimulation	Neuroreflex system	Rubbing points
8. Brain structures	Hypothalamus, pituitary, pineal gland, third ventricle	Intention, meditation, and visualization

From Roger Jahnke, OMD: Physiological mechanisms triggered by the practice of Qigong, Tai Chi, yoga, and Pranayama. In *Most profound medicine,* Santa Barbara, Calif, 1996, Health Action Publishers.

currently being explored for several populations, including people living with HIV disease.[84] Yoga and Qigong have exciting applications in the management of HIV disease, and further research is warranted to evaluate the physiological underpinnings in various immunological markers, physical improvements, and QOL outcomes.

Exercise Precautions and Concerns

Any orthopedic concerns should be addressed before beginning an exercise or movement therapy program. If musculoskeletal problems exist or if other pain symptoms are present, a concerted effort to modulate pain is necessary for the successful completion of an exercise regimen.[85] If HIV-related peripheral neuropathy (PN) exists, it is important to implement proper foot care and wear supportive shoes when performing weight-bearing activities.[86,87]

Some concern exists about the ability of aerobic exercise to increase the body's metabolic rate and thus increase additional muscle loss. However, with a balanced high-calorie diet and a sound nutritional program, this should not pose a problem for asymptomatic persons with HIV disease. If wasting is present, the etiology should be addressed, and treatment should be rendered. One study determined the contribution of total energy expenditure (TEE) to weight changes in individuals with HIV-related wasting. The researchers observed a significant positive relation between TEE and the rate of weight change. During rapid weight loss, TEE fell from an average 2750 to 2189 kcal/day. The key determinant of weight loss in HIV-related wasting, researchers concluded, was reduced energy intake, not increased energy expenditure.[88]

Before beginning any exercise regimen, a differential diagnosis for fatigue must be made, including anemia, low testosterone levels, and specific vitamin deficiencies. Proper caloric intake is necessary for each type of exercise to meet the energy expenditure required for the activity. Seeking the advice of a nutritionist is recommended for proper guidance.

Evidence of autonomic neuropathy (AN) on provocative testing is common in HIV infection, with estimates ranging from 30% to 60%.[89,90] Underlying cardiac parasympathetic dysfunction may need to be assessed throughout the course of HIV disease. One method described by Mallet et al[91] is the use of a 4-speed exercise test, which consists in pedaling an uploaded ergometer at maximal individual speed from the fourth to the eighth speed of a 12-speed maximal inspiratory apnea. From an electrocardiogram (ECG), vagal activity is estimated by a ratio. In this study, patients were submitted to the respiratory sinus arrhythmia, which is a valid method to detect vagal dysfunction. Researchers found that there was a tendency for lower values of vagal function test in HIV-positive patients. It is prudent to monitor vital signs throughout any exercise regimen.

A supervised training program should be consistent with recommendations by the American College of Sports Medicine (ACSM). Guidelines have been established for the three stages of HIV disease.[52] Exercise is safe and beneficial for most individuals with

HIV disease; however, caution is warranted during Stages 2 and 3. Stage 1 (asymptomatic disease) has no limitations on maximum graded exercise testing. During this stage, all metabolic parameters are within normal limits for most individuals. During Stage 2 (symptomatic disease), reduced exercise capacity, VO_{2max}, and O_2 pulse$_{max}$ may exist, as well as elevated heart rate reserve and breathing reserve. Stage 3 (AIDS) presents with dramatically reduced exercise capacity, reduced vital capacity, VO_{2max}, and O_2 pulse$_{max}$. Elevated heart rate and breathing reserve persist during this stage. Therefore careful monitoring of stage 3 and various other OIs is an important factor in comprehensive exercise management.

Social Interactions and the Association with Disease Management

The amount of research documenting an association between the extent and quality of an individual's social relationships and improved health and longevity is growing.[92,93] Although the evidence linking social isolation or lack of social support to increased morbidity and mortality (M&M) risk is extensive, important questions remain concerning the mechanisms or pathways by which these social circumstances influence health outcomes.[92] Various hypotheses have been offered, including the possible influence of social ties on attitudes and behaviors relevant to health and longevity, as well as the possibility of a more direct effect of social ties on human physiology.[94]

Data that support the idea that social and psychological factors play a role in human physiology is derived from research traditions, including psychophysiology and psychosomatic medicine,[95] and sociological and social-psychological research on social ties, stress, and coping.[96] However, the idea that social relationships influence physiology is also congruent with a broader, evolutionary perspective of human physiology and its susceptibility to modulation by external social factors. Physiological homeostasis in humans, and ultimately health status as well, are influenced not only by the physical environment but also by the social environment.[97,98]

Research provides support for the hypothesis that interpersonal relationships influence patterns of physiological functions. Data from experimental studies show that social contact can reduce physiological stress responses.[99,100] Community-based studies also show negative associations between reported levels of support and physiological parameters, such as serum cholesterol, uric acid, and urinary epinephrine.[99] Studies of immune function demonstrate that social relationships have both positive and negative impacts on immune function. Losing a partner to cancer or HIV, caring for family members with Alzheimer's disease, and going through a divorce are negatively associated with immune function, whereas more supportive relationships are associated with better immune function.[47]

Exercise and movement therapy in a group context may provide the socialization necessary to foster these physiological changes and adherence to an exercise regimen. One study noted poor initial performance with individualized exercise programs. Individuals underwent four fitness tests, anthropometric measurements, and HR and oxygen saturation rate monitoring. Mean resting HR was 90 over 14. The researchers concluded that individuals with HIV exhibited poor overall fitness by YMCA age-adjusted standards. Mean resting HR was elevated, which is indicative of poor baseline function. Although follow-up was limited, a modest yet significant improvement occurred within 1 month.[101] If this study was evaluated in a group context, greater socialization could foster higher levels of adherence and functional outcomes.

Another area of potential socialization is the workplace. QOL issues of people with HIV/AIDS are becoming more complicated as more people with the disease achieve higher CD4+ cell counts and lower viral load levels. Improvement in health status is directly related to the improved effectiveness of newer treatment regimens, and many individuals are improving enough to consider reentering the work force. Exercise and movement therapy may augment the stress and fatigue that are associated with adjustment to the workplace.

AREAS FOR FUTURE RESEARCH

This chapter presents an overview of studies in the areas of aerobic and weight training exercise through a PNI approach. Studies on movement therapies, including Tai Chi, Qigong, and yoga, have similar findings; however, studies on specific immunological aspects of the HIV population are needed in these areas. Nevertheless, the use of these movement therapies by long-term survivors of HIV disease is increasing. Future research on movement therapies includes a heuristic model for further PNI explanation, a focus on outcome measurements, and perceptions of QOL through these and various other movement therapies.

References

1. Antoni MH, Schneiderman N, Fletcher MA, et al: Psychoneuroimmunology and HIV-1, *J Consult Clin Psychol* 58(1):38-49, 1990.
2. Nieman DC: Exercise immunology: practical applications, *Int J Sports Med* 18(suppl 1):91-100, 1997.
3. LaPerriere A, Antoni M, Fletcher MA, et al: Exercise training programs for health maintenance in HIV-1. In Galantino ML, editor: *Clinical assessment and treatment in HIV: rehabilitation of a chronic disease,* Thorofare, N.J., 1992, Slack, Inc.
4. Sande MA, Volberding PA: Alternative therapies in HIV. In *Medical management of AIDS,* ed 4, Philadelphia, 1995, WB Saunders.
5. Eisenberg DM, Kessler RC, Foster C: Unconventional medicine in the United States: prevalence, costs, and patterns of use, *New Engl J Med* 328:246-252, 1993.
6. Jackson O, Gula D, Kire A, et al: Effects of Feldenkrais practitioner training on motor abilities: a video analysis, Platform Presentation, APTA Annual Conference, Denver, June 14-18, 1992.
7. Kastner M, Burroughs H: *Alternative healing: the complete A-Z guide to over 160 different alternative therapies,* La Mesa, Calif, 1993, Halcyon Publishing.
8. Belyea C: T'ai Chi Ch'uan. In Hill A, editor: *A visual encyclopedia of unconventional medicine,* New York, 1978, Crown Publishers, Inc.
9. Cheng M-C: *Tai Chi: the supreme ultimate exercise for health, sport, and self-defense,* Upper Saddle River, N.J., 1986, Prentice Hall.
10. Standish LJ, Greene KB, Bain S, et al: Alternative medicine use in HIV-positive men and women: demographics, utilization patterns, and health status, *AIDS Care* 13(2):197-208, 2001.
11. McKinnon W, Baum A, Morokoff P: Neuroendocrine measures in stress. In Wagner HL, editor: *Social psychophysiology and emotion: theory and clinical application,* Chichester, UK, 1988, John Wiley & Sons, Inc.
12. Dobbin JP, Harth M, McCain GA: Cytokine production and lymphocyte transformation during stress, *Brain Behav Immun* 5:339-348, 1991.
13. Evans DL, Leserman J, Perkins DO: Severe life stress as a predictor of early disease progression in HIV infection, *Am J Psychiatry* 154:630-634, 1997.
14. Fitzgibbon ML, Cella DF, Humfleet G: Motor slowing in asymptomatic HIV infection, *Percept Mot Skills* 68:1331-1338, 1989.

15. Hinkin CH, Van Gorp WG, Satz P: Depressed mood and its relationship to neurological test performance in HIV-1 seropositive individuals, *J Clin Exp Neuropsychol* 14:289-297, 1992.

16. Wolf TM, Dralle PW, Morse EV: A biopsychosocial examination of symptomatic and asymptomatic HIV-infected patients, *Int J Psychiatry Med* 21:263-279, 1991.

17. American College of Sports Medicine (ACSM): *Guidelines for exercise testing and prescription,* ed 5, Philadelphia, 1995, Lea & Febiger.

18. Mackinnon LT: Clinical implications of exercise. In Exercise and immunology, *Human kinetics,* Monograph No. 2, 77-84, 1992.

19. LaPerriere A, Fletcher MA, Antoni MH, et al: Aerobic exercise training in an AIDS risk group, *Int J Sports Med* 12(suppl 1):53-57, 1991.

20. Goldwater B, Collis M: Psychological effects of cardiovascular conditioning: a controlled experiment, *Psychosoc Med* 47:174-181, 1985.

21. Morgan WP: Affective benefits of vigorous physical activity, *Med Sci Sports Exerc* 17:94-100, 1985.

22. Morgan WP: Anxiety reduction following acute physical activity, *Psychiatr Ann* 9:141-147, 1979.

23. Raglin J, Morgan WP: Influence of vigorous exercise on mood state, *Behav Therapist* 8:179-183, 1985.

24. Morgan WP, Goldston S: *Exercise and mental health,* New York, 1987, Hemisphere Publishing.

25. Morgan WP: Psychological factors influencing perceived exertion, *Med Sci Sports* 5:60-65, 1973.

26. Morgan WP: *Psychology Today* pp 92-98, July, 1980a.

27. Reference deleted in proofs.

28. Griest JH, Klein MH, Eischens RR, et al: Running as treatment for depression, *Compr Psychiatry* 20(1):41-54, 1979.

29. McNair D, Lorr M, Droppleman L: *EITS manual for the profile of mood states,* San Diego, 1981, Educational and Industrial Testing Service.

30. LaPerriere A, Ironson G, Antoni MH, et al: Exercise and immunology, *Med Sci Sports Exerc* 26(2):182-190, 1994.

31. MacArthur RD, Levine SD, Birk TJ: Supervised exercise training improves cardiopulmonary fitness in HIV-infected persons, *Med Sci Sports Exerc* 25:684-688, 1993.

32. Birk T, MacArthur R: Chronic exercise training maintains previously obtained cardiopulmonary fitness in patients seropositive for human immunodeficiency virus type 1, *Sports Med Train Rehabil* 5(1):1-6, 1994.

33. Spence DW, Galantino ML, Mossberg KA, et al: Progressive resistance exercise: effect on muscle function and anthropometry of a select AIDS population, *Arch Phys Med Rehabil* 71:644-648, 1990.

34. Olson PE, Wallace MR, Carl M: CD4+ correlates of weight training in HIV-seropositive outpatients, Second National Conference on Human Retroviruses and Related Infections, Jan 29-Feb 2, 155, 1995.

35. Roubenoff R, McDermott A, Weiss L, et al: Short-term progressive resistance training increases strength and lean body mass in adults infected with human immunodeficiency virus, *AIDS* 13:231-239, 1999a.

36. Roubenoff R, Weiss L, McDermott A, et al: A pilot study of exercise training to reduce trunk fat in adults with HIV-associated fat redistribution, *AIDS* 13:1373-1375, 1999b.

37. Schambelan M, Mulligan K, Grunfeld C, et al: Recombinant human growth hormone in patients with HIV-associated wasting, *Ann Intern Med* 125:873-882, 1996.

38. Bhasin S, Storer T, Javanbakht M, et al: Testosterone replacement and resistance exercise in HIV-infected men with weight loss and low testosterone levels, *JAMA* 283:763-770, 2000.

39. Strawford A, Barbieri T, Van Loan M, et al: Resistance exercise and supraphysiological androgen therapy in eugonadal men with HIV-related weight loss, *JAMA* 281:1282-1290, 1999.

40. Zacka M, Perdices M, Boycott N, et al: Hydrotherapy and HIV, Annual Conference of Australian Society of HIV Medicine, Nov 16-19, 7:91, 1995 (abstract no. 111).

41. Ragsdale D, Morrow JR: Quality of life as a function of HIV classification, *Nurs Res* 39(6):355-359, 1990.

42. Darko DF, McCutchan JA, Kripke DF, et al: Fatigue, sleep disturbance, disability, and indices of progression of HIV infection, *Am J Psychiatry* 149(4):514-520, 1992.

43. Rigsby LW, Dishman RK, Jackson AW, et al: Effects of exercise training on men seropositive for the human immunodeficiency virus 1, *Med Sci Sports Exerc* 24(1):6-12, 1992.

44. Florijn YC: Physical activity as a therapeutic measure for HIV-infected persons, *Int Conf AIDS* 1992 (abstract).

45. Reference deleted in proofs.

46. Kiecolt-Glaser JK, Speicher CE, Holliday JE, et al: Stress and the transformation of lymphocytes by Epstein-Barr virus, *J Behav Med* 7(1):1-12, 1984.

47. Kiecolt-Glaser JK, Glaser R: Stress and immune function in humans. In Ader R, Felten DL, Cohen N, editors: *Psychoneuroimmunology,* ed 2, New York, 1991, Academic Press.

48. Phillips EJ, Ottaway CA, Freedman J, et al: The effect of exercise on circulating lymphocyte redistribution in symptomatic HIV-infected subjects, Second National Conference on Human Retroviruses and Related Infections, Jan 29-Feb 2, 32, 1995.

49. Bogner JR, Middeke M, Weiss M, et al: Physical exercise in HIV infection: lymphocyte subset alteration depends on the degree of immunodeficiency, *Int Conf AIDS* 9(1):201, 1993 (abstract no. PO-A19-0402).

50. MacArthur RD, Levine SD, Birk TJ: Cardiopulmonary, immunological, and psychological responses to exercise training in individuals seropositive for HIV, *Int Conf AIDS* 8(3):103, 1992 (abstract no. Pub 7327).

51. Olson PE, Elrick H, Cohan GR, et al: Nondetectable quantitative HIV PCR in a long-term survivor triathalete, *Int Conf AIDS* 11(2):140, 1996 (abstract no. We.C.3472).

52. LaPerriere A, Klimas N, Fletcher MA, et al: Change in CD4+ cell enumeration following aerobic exercise training in HIV -1 disease: possible mechanisms and practical applications, *Int J Sports Med* 18(suppl 1):S56-61, 1997.

53. Lyons S, Pope M: Constructs in motion. In Kirkcaldy B, editor: *Normalities and abnormalities in human movement,* vol 26, New York, 1989, Karger.

54. Doyne EJ, Ossip-Klein DJ, Bowman ED, et al: Running versus weight training in the treatment of depression, *J Consult Clin Psychol* 55:748-754, 1987.

55. American Psychiatric Association (APA): *Diagnostic and statistical manual of mental disorders,* ed 3, rev, Washington, DC, 1987.

56. Duncombe LW, Howe MC: Group treatment: goals, tasks, and economic implications, *Am J Occup Ther* 49(3):199-205, 1995.

57. Trahey PJ: A comparison of the cost-effectiveness of two types of occupational therapy services, *Am J Occup Ther* 45(5):397-400, 1991.

58. Targ EF, Karasic DH, Diefenbach PN, et al: Structured group therapy and fluoxetine to treat depression in HIV-positive persons, *Psychosomatics* 35(2):132-137, 1994.

59. Kelly JA, Murphy DA, Bahr GR, et al: Outcome of cognitive-behavioral and support group brief therapies for depressed, HIV-infected persons, *Am J Psychiatry* 150(11):1679-1686, 1993.

60. Kendall J: Promoting wellness in HIV-support groups, *J Assoc Nurses AIDS Care* 3(1):28-38, 1992.

61. Lutgendorf S, Antoni MH, Schneiderman N, et al: Psychosocial counseling to improve quality of life in HIV infection, *Patient Educ Counsel* 24:217-235, 1994.

62. Nunes JA, Raymond SJ, Nicholas PK, et al: Social support, quality of life, immune function, and health in persons living with HIV, *J Holistic Nurs* 12(2):174-198, 1995.

63. Belcher AE, Dettmore D, Holzemer SP: Spirituality and sense of well-being in persons with AIDS, *Holistic Nurse Pract* 3(4):16-25, 1989.

64. Kendall J: Wellness spirituality in homosexual men with HIV infection, *J Assoc Nurses AIDS Care* 5(4):28-34, 1994.

65. Carson VB: Prayer, meditation, exercise, and special diets: behaviors of the hardy person with HIV/AIDS, *J Assoc Nurses AIDS Care* 4(3):18-28, 1993.

66. Qu M: Taijiquan: a medical assessment. In Chinese Sports Editorial Board, editors: *Simplified Taijiquan,* Beijing, 1986, China International Book Trading Corporation.

67. Van Deusen J, Harlane M: The efficacy of the ROM dance program for adults with rheumatoid arthritis, *Am J Occup Ther* 41:90-95, 1987.

68. Tse S-K, Bailey DM: Tai Chi and postural control in the well elderly, *Am J Occup Ther* 46:295-300, 1992.

69. Wolf SL, Coogler CE, Green RC, et al: Novel interventions to prevent falls in the elderly. In Perry HM, Morley JE, Coe RM, editors: *Aging and musculoskeletal disorders: concepts, diagnosis, and treatment,* 1995.

70. Province MA, Hadley EC, Hornbrook MC, et al: The effects of exercise on falls in elderly patients, *JAMA* 273(17):1341-1347, 1995.

71. Lai JS, Wong MK, Lan C, et al: Cardiorespiratory responses of T'ai Chi Chuan practitioners and sedentary subjects during cycle ergometer, *J Formos Med Assoc* 92:894-899, 1993.

72. Jin P: Changes in heart rate, noradrenaline, cortisol, and mood during Tai Chi, *J Psychosom Res* 36:361-70, 1989.

73. Galantino ML, Findley T, Krafft L, et al: Blending traditional and alternative strategies for rehabilitation: measuring functional outcomes and quality of life issues in an AIDS population, The eighth World Congress of International Rehabilitation Medicine Association, *Monduzzi Editore* 1:713-716, 1997.

74. Jahnke R: Physiological mechanisms operating in the human system during the practice of Qigong and Pranayama. In Jahnke R, editor: *The most profound medicine,* Santa Barbara, Calif, 1996, Health Action Publishers.

75. Benson H: *The relaxation response,* New York, 1975, Morrow.

76. Krippner S, Villoldo A: *The realms of healing,* Santa Barbara, Calif, 1976, Celestial Arts.

77. Green E, Green A: *Beyond biofeedback,* New York, 1977, Delacorte Press.

78. Collected Proceedings: The First World Conference for the Academic Exchange of Medical Qigong, Beijing, 1988.

79. Burr HS, Northrop FSC: The electrodynamic theory of life, *Q Rev Biol* 8:322-333, 1935.

80. Burr HS: *Fields of life,* New York, 1973, Ballantine Books.

81. Becker RO: *The body electric: electromagnetism and the foundation of life,* New York, 1985, William Morrow & Co., Inc.

82. Nordenstrom BEW: Biologically closed electrical circuits: clinical, experimental, and theoretical evidence for an additional circulatory system, Stockholm, 1983, Nordic Medical Publications.

83. Rehse A: Body movement workshop for people with HIV/AIDS, *Int Conf AIDS* 8(3):126, 1992 (abstract no. PuB 7464).

84. Telles S, Naveen KV: Yoga for rehabilitation: an overview, *Indian J Med Sci* 51(4):123-127, 1997.

85. Galantino ML: *Clinical assessment and treatment in HIV disease: rehabilitation of a chronic illness,* Thorofare, N.J., 1992, Slack, Inc.

86. Galantino ML, Pizzi M, Lehmann M: Interdisciplinary management of disability in HIV infection. In O'Dell MW, editor: *HIV-related disability: assessment and management,* vol 7, Philadelphia, 1993, Hanley & Belfus, Inc.

87. Galantino ML, Jermyn RT, Tursi FJ, et al: Physical therapy management for the patient with HIV: lower extremity changes, *Clin Pediatr Med Surg* 15:329-346, 1998.

88. Macallan DC, Noble C, Baldwin C: Energy expenditure and wasting in human immunodeficiciency virus infection, *New Engl J Med 333(2):83, 1995.*

89. Ruttimann S, Hilti P, Spinas GA, et al: High frequency of human immunodeficiency virus-associated autonomic neuropathy and more severe involvement in advanced stages of human immunodeficiency virus disease, *Arch Intern Med* 152:485-501, 1991.

90. Villa A, Foresti V, Confalonieri F: Autonomic nervous system dysfunction associated with HIV infection in intravenous heroin users, *AIDS* 6:85-89, 1992.

91. Mallet AL, Soares PP, Nobrega AC, et al: Cardiac parasympathetic function in HIV-infected humans, *Int Conf AIDS* 8(3):104, 1992 (abstract no. 7333).

92. Cohen S, Syme SL: *Social support and health,* Orlando, Fla, 1984, Academic Press.

93. House JS, Landis KR, Umberson D: Social relationships and health, *Science* 241:540-545, 1988.

94. Seeman M, Seeman T, Sayles M: Social networks and health status: a longitudinal analysis, *Soc Psychol Q* 48:237-248, 1985.

95. Weiner H: *Psychobiology and human disease,* New York, 1977, Elsevier North-Holland, Inc.

96. Thoits PA: Conceptual, methodological, and theoretical problems in studying social support as a buffer against life stress, *J Health Soc Behav* 23:145-159, 1982.

97. Bovard EW: A balance between negative and positive brain system activity, *Perspect Biol Med* 116-127, 1962.

98. Bovard EW: Brain mechanisms in effects of social support on viability. In Williams Jr RB, editor: Perspectives on behavioral medicine, vol 2, *Neuroendocrine control and behavior,* Orlando, Fla, 1985, Academic Press.

99. Thomas PD, Goodwin JM, Goodwin JS: Effect of social support on stress-related changes in cholesterol level, uric acid level, and immune function in an elderly sample, *Am J Psychiatry* 142:735-737, 1985.

100. Kamarck TW, Manuck SB, Jennings JR: Social support reduces cardiovascular reactivity to psychological challenge: a laboratory model, *Psychosom Med* 52:42-58, 1990.

101. Scott MK, Torbutn L, Neal BA, et al: Physical fitness testing in patients with HIV/AIDS: poor initial performance with improvement on follow-up, *Int Conf AIDS* 11(2):444, 1996 (abstract no. Pub.B.1040).

Suggested Readings

Agency for Health Care Policy and Research (AHCPR No. 94-0573): *Managing early HIV infection—clinical practice,* Guideline no. 7, Rockville, Md, 1996, 1994, US Department of Health and Human Services, Public Health Service.

Borg G: Perceived exertion as an indicator of somatic stress, *Scand J Rehabil Med* 2:92-98, 1970.

Borg G: Perceived exertion: a note on history and methods, *Med Sci Sports* 5:90-93, 1973.

Borg G: Psychophysical bases of perceived exertion, *Med Sci Sports Exerc* 14:377-381, 1982.

Bottomly JM: Tai Chi: choreography of body and mind. In Davis CM, editor: *Complementary therapies in rehabilitation,* Thorofare, N.J., 1997, Slack, Inc.

Carson VB, Green HG: Spiritual well-being: a predictor of hardiness in patients with AIDS, *J Prof Nurs* 8(4):209-220, 1992.

Ironson G, LaPerriere A, Antoni MH, et al: Changes in immune and psychological measures as a function of anticipation and reaction to news of HIV-1 antibody status, *Psychosom Med* 52:247-270, 1990.

Jin P: Efficacy of Tai Chi, brisk walking, meditation, and reading in reducing mental and emotional stress, *J Psychosom Res* 26(4):361-370, 1992.

Kirsteins AE, Deitz F, Hwang SM: Evaluating the safety and potential use of a weight-bearing exercise, Tai Chi Chuan, for rheumatoid arthritis patients, *Am J Phys Med Rehabil* 70:136-141, 1991.

Kobasa S: Stressful life events, personality, and health: an inquiry into hardiness, *J Pers Soc Psychol* 37(1):1-11, 1979.

Lai JS, Lan C, Wong MK, et al: Two-year tends in cardiorespiratory function among older T'ai Chi Chuan practitioners and sedentary subjects, *J Am Geriatr Soc* 43:1222-1227, 1995.

LaPerriere A, Antoni MH, Ironson G, et al: Exercise intervention attenuates emotional distress and natural killer cell decrements following notification of positive serologic status in HIV-1, *Biofeed Self-Regulat* 15(3):229-242, 1990.

Office of Alternative Medicine: *Functional description of the office,* Bethesda, Md, 1993, National Institutes of Health.

O'Sullivan S: Perceived exertion: a review, *Phys Ther* 64(3):343-346, 1984.

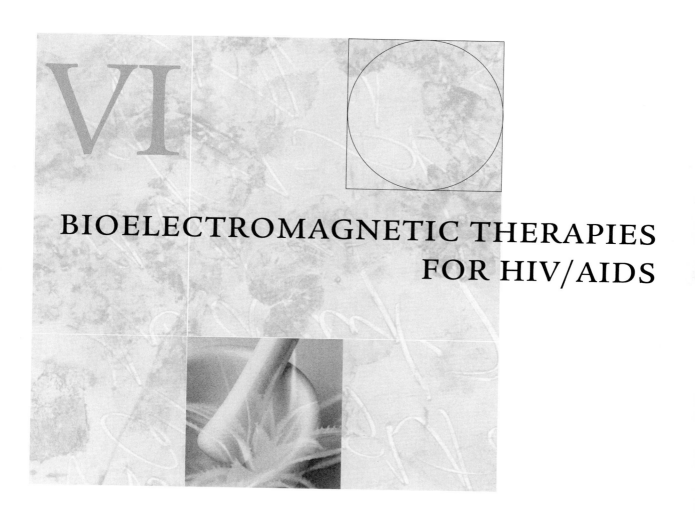

VI

BIOELECTROMAGNETIC THERAPIES FOR HIV/AIDS

15

Introduction to Electromagnetic Therapies in HIV/AIDS

LEANNA J. STANDISH

During the past 50 years, electromagnetic (EM) devices and technologies have been invented and implemented for both the diagnosis and treatment of disease, some of which have led to significant advances in conventional medicine. Examples include (1) magnetic resonance imaging (MRI), (2) transcutaneous electrical nerve stimulation (TENS), (3) electroencephalogram (EEG), (4) electromyography (EMG), and (5) direct current (DC) devices that facilitate bone union after complex fractures. The scientific literature on biomedical effects of nonthermal EM fields (EMFs) is growing. Preliminary evidence indicates that nonthermal EMFs exert biological effects, including effects on viral activity and immune cells in vitro. These EMFs include (1) DC, (2) extremely low frequency (ELF), (3) radio frequency (RF), (4) microwave (MW), (5) infrared (IFR), (6) ultra-violet (UV), and (7) visible light. Many EM medical technologies, however, remain within the domain of unproven unconventional methods. One of the best reviews of this field of alternative medicine was published as a 1992 *Report to the NIH on Alternative Medical Systems and Practices in the United States.*[1]

Various EM therapies have been prescribed for and used by HIV-infected persons during the past 15 years. Some of the better-known therapies include (1) Beck's device, (2) radionics, (3) the Rife machine, (4) cranio-electrical stimulation (CES), (5) electroacupuncture, (6) magnetically influenced homeopathic remedies (MIHR), and (7) electrodermal screening devices (EDSDs), including "Electroacupuncture According to Voll" (EAV). Although these modalities and devices have been used by HIV-positive patients, none of them, with the exception of electroacupuncture (see Chapter 11), have been subjected to controlled clinical trials. Nevertheless, of 1666 HIV-positive men and women participating in the Bastyr University Alternative Medicine Care Outcomes in AIDS study, 262 (16%) reported using some form of bioelectromagnetic therapy. The most commonly used therapies in this cohort included (1) EDSDs, (2) crystals, (3) CES, and (4) radionics.

Several new EM technologies combine EM diagnosis and treatment with homeopathy. For example, MIHR involves the injection of homeopathically prepared Chinese medicines into selected acupuncture points. These homeopathic medicines are subjected to a 5-gaussian magnetic charge as they are injected into each acupuncture point.

Several companies have developed the EAV into computerized technologies that are currently on the market. These entrepreneurial companies have produced computerized devices that measure the patient's DC charge and then select homeopathic remedies based on changes induced in the overall DC charge when the remedy is placed in the electrical circuit. Some of these technologies do not actually involve placing the remedy in an electrical circuit on the patient's body. Instead, a glass or plastic vial containing the medicine is placed either near the patient on a metal plate, through which DC flows, or in the patient's hand. Because the electrical resistance of glass is so high, it is unlikely that the current actually flows between either the equipment or the patient and the medicine. The validity of this technology is controversial.

Very little work has been published that investigates the internal and external validity and reliability of these devices. Calabrese et al[2] studied the reliability of one proprietary EAV device to measure EMFs in six human subjects. The source of greatest variability in this study did not come from the subjects, however, but from the operators. Like any diagnostic tool, this technology requires careful studies to determine both the sensitivity and specificity of each device. This research is necessary to determine whether these technologies also have therapeutic value.

Chapter 16 illustrates the methodological challenges of frontier CAM research. Although the implications of Dr. Brewitt's studies are scientifically significant, her research raises deep epistemological and methodological issues and rests on layers of interrelated assumptions. One must accept Dr. Brewitt's basic premise of acupuncture meridians, EAV and its relationship to specific organ systems, the algorithmic digital generation of RF signals that simulate homeopathic growth factors (hoGFs), the technology of the Life Information System

10 (LISTEN), and that hoGFs can exert immunological effects. These CAM diagnostic and treatment measures are used to study each other and correlate with immunological and clinical outcomes.

Dr. Brewitt has been a lone pioneer, making her own measurements of HIV-positive patients over the past decade. Like other CAM clinicians she has not had the luxury of double-blind, or even single-blind, testing. Many CAM researchers acknowledge the possibility that conscious intention on the part of researchers can influence biological systems, even remotely. What role did Dr. Brewitt's intention and her knowledge of and relationship with each patient play in the electrical conductance readings she derived for each patient at each Voll acupuncture point?

CAM research in its early stages is often based on consecutive case studies. In this chapter, Dr. Brewitt presents immunological T-cell data in two HIV-positive patients who received daily treatment with RF signals derived algorithmically from hoGFs. A theoretical model based on these two patients is then constructed when a causal link between the treatment and the immunological changes cannot be established without a randomized controlled trial with sufficient statistical power.

In addition, when Dr. Brewitt measured electrical conductance at 12 acupuncture points, she concluded that electrical conductance in HIV-positive and AIDS patients is different, and both differ from measurements taken in healthy controls. Making multiple comparisons increases the risk of type I statistical errors, which reject the null hypothesis when it is true and claim differences where there are none. Her work generates hypotheses instead of testing them.

Although this research raises complex methodological issues, it generates the intriguing testable hypotheses that (1) electrical conductance at acupuncture points may have diagnostic significance, (2) subtle RF signals may have immunological and clinical effects, and (3) RF signals derived from hoGFs and cytokines may have positive immunological effects on HIV-positive patients.

References

1. Rubik B, Becker RO, Flower RG, et al: Bioelectromagnetics: applications in medicine. In *Alternative medicine: expanding horizons. A Report to the NIH on Alternative Medical Systems and Practices in the United States,* 1991, Washington, DC, US Government Printing Office.
2. Calabrese C, Bier ID, Polissar N, et al: A preliminary study of reliability in an electrodermal screening device, Manuscript in preparation.

Bioelectromagnetic Medicine and HIV/AIDS Treatment

Clinical Data and Hypothesis for Mechanism of Action

BARBARA BREWITT

Every living thing is electromagnetic (EM). All living organisms survive by accumulating energy (and negative entropy) from Earth's external EM forces. The body's appropriate regulation of these extracellular signals is essential for successful development and survival. Changes within cell membranes or in cell surface receptors measurably shift EM parameters within normal, healthy limits.[1] Health, whether at the molecular, cellular, glandular, or systemic level, depends on optimal activation of EM potential.[2-7]

Bioelectromagnetic medicine is a logical choice for treating HIV and AIDS because all life forms, from humans to viruses, respond to both nonthermal and thermal EM fields (EMFs).[3,6,8,9] EM forces mediate chemical reactions, thus preceding biochemical reactions.[3,10,11] Extremely low EM forces regulate gene pro-

moters in thymocytes and cancer cell constructs, thus preceding DNA transcription.[12-14] EM forces also specifically activate HIV-derived DNA sequences that are incorporated into the host's DNA.[15,16] Ultraviolet (UV) light, a specific EM waveform, stimulates the HIV promoter and long-terminal repeat (LTR), thus further replicating HIV.[17] Maintenance of healthy homeostasis and well-regulated EM forces within the body may prevent HIV disease progression.

Abnormal alterations in EM forces surrounding healthy cell membranes can be quantified. Links between abnormal exposures to EMFs and the onset of cancer and leukemia are well documented.[18-25] New HIV treatment strategies were developed based on well-characterized anatomical and physiological changes that occur during disease progression. For example, bioelectric impedance analysis (BIA) of the skin gave insights into loss of lean body mass (LBM) during early stages of HIV infection, thus revealing the significance of nutrient uptake to maintain LBM.[26,27] Characterization of tissue histology during late stages of HIV/AIDS showed considerable tissue disruption within lymph nodes, signaling the degree of HIV immune destruction and the need for tissue-specific highly active antiretroviral therapies (HAART).[28] Now researchers are trying to derive other information from EM measurements.

Microscopic EM forces within us regulate healthy homeostasis.[29-30] The brain, for example, contains significant anatomical structures that pick up and respond to EM forces. The human brain's major functional areas contain over 5 million (4 ng/g) homogeneously distributed, prism-shaped magnetite crystals and over 20 million (70 ng/g) prism-shaped magnetite crystals in the brain's surrounding meninges.[31] These magnetite crystals are thought to be part of a universal biological regulating system, which is remarkably similar to the biogenic magnetites of bacteria and fish. The brain is very sensitive to radio frequency (RF) signals and uses ionic calcium as an important second messenger for signal transduction of EM messages.[32]

EM forces link information from the outside world to the innermost control area of cells. Cell models show how EM forces stimulate protein synthesis via virally derived DNA that is integrated into the host cell genome.[15] If we can recognize general principles from these models, we can gain greater insight into the healing impact of energy medicine on gene expression. From this point we can develop new and effective, yet nontoxic and affordable, HIV therapies.

CELLULAR EFFECTS

At the microscopic level, EMFs activate electrical potential in the cell membrane.[33] The cell membrane interfaces between the extracellular milieu and the inner workings of the cell via asymmetrical electrical surface potentials that are measurable and reproducible.[34] Ion channels and cell surface receptors contained in the cell membrane are integral to cellular communication. Cellular communication occurs by dispatching physical signal messengers such as chemokines, cytokines, growth factors (GFs), hormones, and neurotransmitters. These signals also can be EM.[35-37]

Signaling messengers need not enter the cell to communicate and transfer information,[38,39] nor are they directly needed to induce cellular changes or evoke DNA synthesis or cell division.[40] All that is necessary is activation of a receptor site at the cell surface via a conformational change. The receptor's conformational change then triggers an entire cascade of intracellular messengers that are directed to carry the extracellular signal to the DNA (Figure 16-1). Receptor activation occurs with electrical forces, single molecules, antibodies, and ligands.[41-44] HIV chronically activates the guanyl nucleotide-binding protein (G protein) signaling pathway shown in Figure 16-1, thus disturbing the inositol polyphosphate (P_i) metabolism. Abnormal P_i metabolism contributes to aberrant cell communication.[45,46] G proteins play a crucial role in regulating information flowing from outside the cell to the DNA inside the cell.

Many molecules, receptors, enzymatic processes, gene expressions, and structural organizations respond to weak EMFs (Table 16-1). EM forces stimulate cell changes through signals that are carried from the cell membrane to messengers that affect synthesis of RNA, DNA, and proteins.[39,47,48] Adenosine triphosphate (ATP) utilization, which provides energy for life processes, is as much a charge transfer process as it is a biochemical reaction.[3] Changes in protein kinase C (PKC), which consequently activates normal DNA transcription factor genes (proto-oncogenes) c-fos, c-jun, and c-myc, could be induced in a T-cell lymphoblastoid cell line (CCRF-CEM) by magnetic fields.[49] Abnormal expression of proto-oncogenes increases oncogene expression, the potential onset of cancer, and stimulation of the LTR promoter of HIV.[50]

Whether EM forces are large or small, the immune, nervous, and endocrine systems (often called the *neuroendocrine immune system*) are particularly sensitive to these subtle energy effects at cellular and subcellular levels.[51] The sensitivity of these systems stems from their complexity and regulatory feedback loops.

Studies document that stress and psychological concepts of reality have feedback loops that are easily regulated by EM forces. Additionally, immune and hormonal feedback loops are highly complex and respond to subtle energy signals. A few simple changes in feedback to the neuroendocrine immune system include the following[52]:

1. The nervous system[53-56]
2. Measurable mood changes, paranormal experiences, and psychological states[18,54,57-59]
3. Hormonal secretions and endocrine organ functioning[55,60-64]

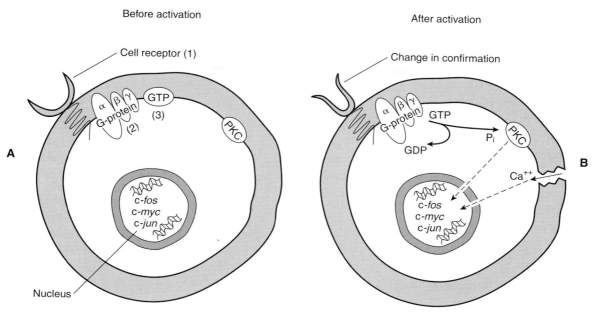

Figure 16-1 Cell receptor activation and simplified signal transduction via G proteins. Cell surface receptors contain both extracellular and cytoplasmic surfaces. EM signals, neurotransmitters, GFs, hormones, and HIV use a multistep process to carry signals from the extracellular surface to the cell and into the nucleus, where changes in DNA transcription occur. Classical "second" messengers that are activated through this G-protein cascade are cyclic AMP (cAMP), calcium (Ca^{++}), and polyphosphoinositide, an inorganic phosphate (P_i). Several plasma membrane-bound proteins are involved with receptor activation and consequential signal transduction: (1) a seven-transmembrane cell receptor; (2) G protein with the three subunits α, β, and γ; and (3) guanosine triphosphate (GTP). **A,** The inactivated receptor sits separated from the G protein that binds GTP in the inactivated state. **B,** The cell-receptor activated state occurs with either ligand binding or specific EM activity. Once the cell receptor is activated, its conformation changes, and a multistep process occurs in the lipid bilayer. This process initiates a cascade of second messengers for signal transduction. As the receptor is activated, the G protein binds to the cell receptor and simultaneously hydrolyzes GTP into guanosine diphosphate (GDP). This change releases P_i, which consequently activates protein kinase C (PKC). Simultaneously, both Ca^{++} influx and a change in the electrical potential of the cell membrane occur. Both Ca^{++} and PKC carry signals to the nucleus of the cell, where they activate proto-oncogenes such as *c-jun*, *c-fos*, and *c-myc*. These genes synthesize the transcription factor proteins C-Jun, C-Fos, and C-Myc, which bind to the DNA and regulate gene segment translation and transcription with consequential changes in cell behavior.

TABLE 16-1

Signaling Molecules and Enzymes Affected by Electromagnetic Forces

Molecules	Relevant examples	Authors
GFs, hormones, neurotransmitters	Cellular signals	Cossarizza A et al, 1989 Wilson BW et al, 1990
Receptors with 7 membrane domains	CC-CRK5 and fusin, HIV co-receptors, also used for GF signaling	Bistolfi F, 1987
Photoreceptors	Cones and rods for vision, phototransduction	Sopory SK, Chandok MR, 1996, Berridge MJ, Irvine RF, 1994, Alberts B et al, 1989
G Proteins	$CD4^+$ and $CD8^+$ T-cell receptor—$p56^{lck}$ HIV and GFs used for signal transduction	Berridge MJ, Irvine RF, 1994, Adey WR, 1988
Protein kinase C (PKC)	G protein's cascade for signal transduction	Adey WR, 1988 Phillips et al, 1992
cAMP-dependent protein kinase	G protein's cascade for signal transduction	Sopory SK, Chandok MR, 1996 Byus CV et al, 1984
Inositol phosphotide (P_i) turnover and diacylglycerol (DAG) messenger systems	G protein's cascade for signal transduction	Sopory SK Chandok MR, 1996, Berridge MJ, Irvine RF, 1994
Na^+, K^+, ATPase	Critical ion pumping enzyme at cell surface to activate energy	Liu DS et al, 1990
Lysosomes	Organelles used for intracellular digestion of macromolecules and bacteria	David SL et al, 1985
Chromosomes	Package DNA into units	
Chlorophyll	Photosynthesis	Alberts B et al, 1989
DNA transcription factors, c-myc, c-fos, c-jun—normal v-myc—viral derived	Regulate cell growth, death, or differentiation by determining which DNA sites are transcribed and amplified	Phillips JL et al, 1992 Lin H et al, 1994 Goodman R et al, 1994 Goodman R et al, 1989
DNA and α-RNA polymerase	Genetic material and regulatory sites for protein synthesis	Goodman R et al, 1994
Ca^{++} efflux	Second messenger for GF signaling	Sopory SK, Chandok MR, 1996; Walleczek J, 1992; Byus CV et al, 1984; Smith SD et al, 1987
Na^+, K^+, Li^+	Ions used for biological signaling	McLeod BR, Liboff AR, 1986

ATPase, Adenosine triphosphatase; cAMP, cyclic adenosine monophosphate; GF, growth factor.

4. White blood cell (WBC) and red blood cell (RBC) counts and lymphocyte activity[4,24,53,65-68]

Thus our ability to regulate subtle energy signals can either build or destroy communication processes within the immune, nervous, and endocrine systems.

CLINICAL AND IN VIVO EFFECTS

Clinical studies show that EM signals produced positive effects in a variety of illnesses. Nonthermal radio waves (10^4 to 10^9 Hz) effectively treated sinus infections, cellulitis, abscesses, bronchitis, tonsillitis, pain, staphylococci infections, and skin inflammations.[69] In the 1930s, AJ Ginsberg, MD proposed that the body acted like a partial condenser (capacitor) system that was surrounded by a field of EM waves with specific frequencies. The energy transmitted to cells was immediately dissipated to adjacent cells via adjacent cell membranes that became activated and carried signals from the outside of the cell to the inside. In contrast, pathogens, such as bacteria and parasites, formed very small, complete condenser (capacitor) systems that were unable to disperse transmitted energy, thus dying or self-destructing. In more biological terms, cell-to-cell communication and physical connections enable cells to resonate together, relieving any one cell of too much EM activity. A single HIV virion, however, is unable to dissipate or discharge excessive EM activity, and a frequency beyond the virion's capacity can cause it to self-destruct.

Using nonthermal RF waves can render HIV, other viruses, bacteria, and parasites less virulent or even destroy them. According to Dr. Ginsberg, "Every normal tissue or cell has a radio frequency of its own, and when these cells become changed, as a result of disease, the tissue frequency is also changed. . . . By application of ultrashort waves of the proper frequency to the abnormal tissue, it will be possible to restore diseased tissue to normal function." More recently, this idea was refined to include the concept that cells respond in specific ways to patterns of pulsed EM forces.[5,70]

Changing the cell's microenvironment with electrical forces demonstrates immune-related benefits. Immunological benefits, such as inhibition of bacterial growth and accelerated soft tissue healing, occur after exposure to a variety of electrical stimuli.[69,71-73] In England, EM therapy devices introduce negatively charged electrons into patients' skin and tissues to accelerate wound healing, treat inflammatory ailments, and relieve neuralgic pain.[74] In Bulgaria, the Odess Health Farm successfully treats chronic fatigue–like symptoms concomitant with viral hepatitis A infection by applying nonthermal EM radiation to the pyloro-duodenal area every other day for 10 treatments.[75] In the United States, tumor growth is more effectively inhibited by administration of direct current (DC) plus human interferon-alpha (INF-α) than by treatment with human INF-α alone.[76] Inhibition of tumor growth by the administration of DC has been reported since the 1950s.[77-80]

The nervous system also responds to EM forces. Pulsed magnetic forces applied to multiple sclerosis patients improved self-reported symptoms in eight different categories by 22% to 38% compared with none in the placebo group.[81] Rats with severed ulnar nerves that received pulsed EM energy experienced healing and improved physical functioning twice as fast as untreated rats.[82] Extensive research on RF signals and pulsed EMFs in vitro and in vivo consistently demonstrated accelerated nerve, bone, and wound healing.[4,53,83-84] The exposure of rats to static and oscillating EMFs simulated the same conditioned responses as those evoked by lithium ions. This effect occurred via increased sensitivity of G protein–coupled serotonin receptors and G protein–coupled alpha-adrenergic receptors within the brain.[54] Perceptual awareness and brain function are also extremely sensitive and responsive to EM forces.[53] Glial components within the central nervous system (CNS) are the target sites for these effects.

EM forces have clinical efficacy, ranging from surface wound healing to nervous and immune system healing, which can be traced to cellular and subcellular benefits. HIV disease is characterized by aberrant cell signaling and dysregulated cell functioning with consequential compromises in tissue integrity.[85] Reframing our knowledge of cell dynamics in the context of EM forces may lead to new subtle energy treatment strategies for HIV, as well as for other viral and bacterial infections.

THEORY

Bioelectromagnetic medicine is understandable from scientific and biophysiological perspectives. The theory of electrodermal screening (EDS) is based on findings that resistance at specific skin points (often acupuncture points) of approximately 450 μm to 1 cm^2 differs from the resistance adjacent to these skin points.[86-90] Reports of the magnitude of difference vary from twofold to sixfold on skin points[88,91] and greater than twentyfold on ear points.[92] Healthy skin resistance at specialized acupuncture/conductance points is reproducible at approximately 100,000 ohms versus 5,000,000 ohms at surrounding skin areas.[86,88,93-97]

Therefore specific acupuncture/conductance skin point resistance is fiftyfold lower than resistance at surrounding nonacupuncture points. Acupuncture/conductance points correlate to neurovascular bundles that contain high densities of cellular gap junctions.[98-100] The point names and organ and function associations for the skin points used in EDS were derived from Rheinhold Voll, MD. The validity of the associations between the organs and the point names discovered by Voll remains speculative; however, the diagnostic significance of specific hand and foot acupuncture/conductance points can be evaluated.

Many reports indicate that disease states can be characterized and even staged by measurements of electrical resistance.[6,101,102] Voll used EDS devices in the late 1940s and reported that pathophysiological states in humans could be characterized by measuring skin resistance at acupuncture points.[97,103] Using correlations between physical examinations and EDS measurements, Voll proposed that inflammatory states caused lower-than-normal skin resistance, whereas organ degeneration and tissue necrosis caused higher-than-normal skin resistance. The scientific weakness of Voll's English publications was his presentation of descriptive analyses of patients' conditions rather than factual data.

Dr. Helmut Schimmel, Voll's collaborator, proposed that diagnostic information was accessible through analyses of the temporal changes in amplitudes and fluctuations of electrical trace profiles.[93] Changes in EM frequencies in over 900 dogs and 135 humans discriminated accurately between health and disease states.[34] Dysregulated frequencies measured from the hollow organs of pathological small intestines and stomachs were restored to a healthy state by using low- and high-frequency EMF forces. Pathological conditions were also accurately detected from decreased resistance at auricular points.[104]

The healthy cell membrane contains a characteristic electrical potential at which it responds (i.e., at which the cell resonates).[34,102,105] All life forms therefore have a unifying principle of cell communication that responds to subtle energy field forces. For example, researchers in France show that biological information in a variety of cell systems can be transferred electromagnetically to induce specific cellular responses that mimic cholinergic signals of histamines, ovalbumin, and endotoxin.[36,37,106] Studies in the United States show that DC mimics nerve GF signals and significantly increases protein content in neuronal explants.[84]

EM frequencies also affect small polypeptides such as GFs and growth hormone (GH) (Table 16-1) because their tertiary structures contain electrically dynamic alpha-helical conformations that easily resonate at specific frequencies.[70,107,108] For example, GH contains many alpha-helix structures, thus it is activated by EM forces.[19] GH levels increased in healthy humans in response to electrical stimulation of auricular points.[109] Along with EM-responsive structures, GH and GFs have similar biological functions; they both optimize cell communication and maintain healthy homeostasis.[110] Brewitt and Standish[111] and Bellavite and Signorini[112] proposed that homeopathic GFs are ideal candidates to balance the immune system. In three different randomized, double-blind, placebo-controlled clinical studies, homeopathic recombinant human GH (HrGH) provided both physiological and psychological benefits to people between the ages of 18 and 72 years.[113]

Subtle energy forces, such as electrical signals and homeopathic GFs (hoGFs), were evaluated for their potential efficacy in treating HIV-positive individuals. Since viruses bind to the cell membrane, their viral coats may cause aberrant cell communication. Binding viral coats to cell membrane receptors changes the electrical charge that characterizes cell healthy resonance.[114,115] Several biological mechanisms transfer a broad array of information from the outside of the cell to the inside. One mechanism uses G proteins to guard the direct information that successfully transfers from the outside of the cell to the inside. HIV infection, EM signals, and GFs use G proteins to transmit their information through the cell membrane to impact DNA synthesis and cell behavior.

This chapter presents clinical data showing quantifiable differences in electrical conductance measurement at skin points between healthy controls and HIV-positive patients. Furthermore, data from two HIV-positive patients who received regular EM signals in the form of RF signals are presented. Peripheral blood lymphocyte counts, especially CD4$^+$ T-cell counts, improve when specific skin points that are characteristic of HIV infection are continually brought into a healthy, normal range. Finally, data are presented showing that HIV-positive patients treated with oral administration of hoGFs achieved normal EM profiles. After presentation of the data, a hypothesis was formed, stating that HIV infection can be effectively managed through regular use of subtle EM forces or other therapeutic interventions that effectively control G protein activities at the cell membrane.

Materials and Methods

Electromagnetic Measurements and Radio Frequency Signals

Electrical resistance was measured at specific skin conductance/acupuncture points using a computerized electrodermal screening (EDS) device called *LISTEN*.* This computerized ohmmeter device provides a maximal DC of 5 volts at 30 μA (maximum) to the skin, which is sufficient to overcome the 2.5 to 3.0 volts of background current (noise) produced by the skin. Electrical resistance was quantified by evoking a change in electrical potential at skin points through DC stimulation either during baseline evaluation or in response to treatment. Treatment was defined as RF signals emitted by a small radio emitter located in the central processing unit (CPU) of the computer hard drive.

The RF signals, which were contained in a database library, consisted of a unique pattern of eight or more binary numbers (0 or 1) contained in a discrete byte, each with a unique pattern of smaller bits. A serial shift register circuit received bytes of information and converted them to a transmitted pulsed square-wave signal with an amplitude of either 0 or 5 volts (similar to data transmitted repeatedly over a tele-

*BioMeridian, Inc, Orem, Utah.

phone modem). Each pulsed square wave was transmitted repeatedly and combined with other bytes to produce a broad range of EM frequencies, ranging from DC to 12 MHz. Each radio signal, which was associated with a name in ASCII characters, was transmitted repeatedly until the operator terminated the signal. When a signal was accepted for its ability to balance the patient's electrical conductance, its name appeared on the computer screen. When the name on the computer screen was selected, it transmitted a signal from the binary pattern to a shift register circuit.

Optimal resistance at an acupuncture skin point is 100,000 ohms,[116] scaled on the LISTEN device as 50 relative units of conductance. Electrical conductance is the inverse of resistance, and preliminary studies on healthy individuals, each of whom was measured at 28 different acupuncture points, determined that the mean maximum conductance was 50.3 ± 0.58 standard error of measurement (SEM) relative units.

General Protocol

Both RF signals of hoGFs and liquid preparations of hoGFs were evaluated for therapeutic efficacy in HIV-positive individuals. Four different studies were conducted, involving normal and HIV-positive persons. These four studies are summarized in Table 16-2. In Study A, 154 subjects, including healthy controls

TABLE 16-2

Study ID	Patient size	Patient status	Treatment type
Study A	$n = 117$	Healthy controls with some minor symptoms	Control
	$n = 37$	HIV⁺ asymptomatic	Baseline EDS measurement
Study B	$n = 2$	HIV⁺ with CD4⁺ T cells 130-180 cells/μl	Case studies RF signals of GFs to balance EDS readings 3-6 times/wk for 3 mos
	$n = 10$	HIV⁺ taking only natural therapies	Control for case studies
	$n = 11$	HIV⁺ taking only natural therapies	Control for case studies
Study C	$n = 11$	HIV⁺ CD4⁺ T cells 76-560 cells/μl	Control one-time RF signals to identify GF concentrations that balance EDS readings
Study D	$n = 10$	HIV⁺ CD4⁺ T cells 130-550 cells/μl	Original study—Double-blind, placebo-controlled study of 4 homeopathic GFs
	$n = 11$	HIV⁺ CD4⁺ T cells 130-550 cells/μl	Replication multisite studies— Double-blind, placebo-controlled study of 4 homeopathic GFs

($n = 117$) and HIV-positive patients ($n = 37$), were measured at several major acupuncture points to establish a baseline comparison. In Studies B and C, 23 and 11 HIV-positive patients, respectively, were evaluated for the effect of RF signals of GFs on disease state. Patients in Study B received treatment for 3 months, whereas those in Study C received only a single treatment. In Study D, 21 HIV-positive patients were orally administered liquid hoGFs (see Chapter 9). Disease state was monitored as in the three previous studies.

Hand and Foot Points with Their Organ Associations

Figure 16-2 shows the point locations and names of points that were identified by Voll.[117] Many conductance points coincided with classical Chinese acupuncture points and were mapped to specific organs and areas of the brain.[118-120] The points evaluated in these studies were selected by several criteria. First, these points had previously shown differences between healthy controls and persons with chronic inflammatory conditions, HIV infections, cancer, and AIDS.[2] Second, dielectric properties of lungs in vivo indicated that they responded to RF ranges from 10 kHz to 100 MHz,[121] which are sensitive to RFs. Third, both traditional acupuncture and the Voll points along the triple heater meridian (TH1), lung (LU10), and spleen (SP1L, SPCL, SP2L, SP3L, and SP4L)[122,123] are associated with significant acupuncture points related to HIV pathogenesis.[122] Finally, the neurovascular junctions and lymphatics of the spleen include vessels from the large toe of the left foot.[124] Thus an actual anatomical connection exists between the vessels of the left toe and the spleen.

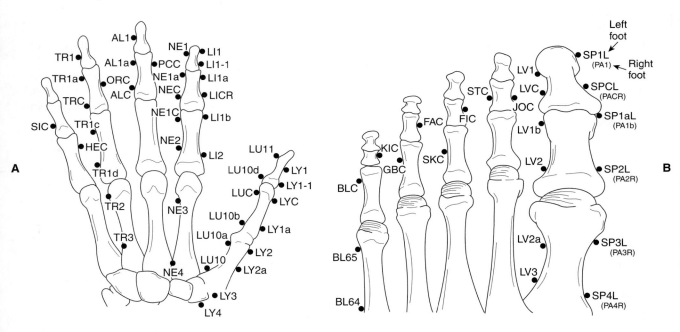

Figure 16-2 These point locations were assigned by Rheinhold Voll, MD, a German physician who trained and practiced in anatomy, acupuncture, electronics, and radio technology. Voll conducted major clinical research during World War II and mapped new anatomical locations of hand and foot points that differed from traditional Chinese acupuncture mappings. Each point is assigned two or three capital letters and a number. A small letter after the number denotes a significantly minor point. A capital L or R at the end of the notation denotes whether the point is exclusively related to the left or right side. **A,** Major hand conductance points measured in these studies were: (1) thumb points at its base LY4 and LU10; (2) index finger points NE3 and NE4; and (3) ring finger points TR1 and TR2. **B,** Major foot conductance points measured in these studies were: (1) large left toe SP1L, SPCL, SP2L, SP3L, and SP4L; (2) second toe JOC; and (3) middle toe FIC. See Table 16-3 for Voll's name and function associations (interpreted with modern context of histology).

Measuring Electrical Resistance and Providing Radio Frequency Signals

Each patient held either a source electrode or a brass bar covered with wet sterile gauze in one hand. The practitioner held either a second brass electrode or a pen-shaped probe and touched a specific acupuncture/conductance point on either the patient's hands or left foot (Figure 16-3). The acupuncture/conductance points were approximately 3 mm in diameter in healthy controls and were located in the epidermal layer of the skin. To obtain the most accurate and re-

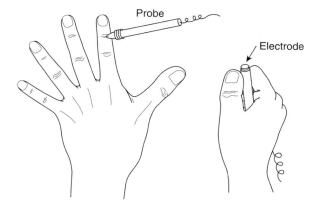

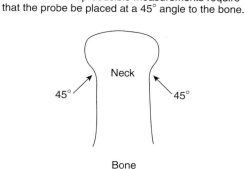

Accurate and reproducible measurements require that the probe be placed at a 45° angle to the bone.

Figure 16-3 Measuring electrical conductance correctly. In the upper figure, the patient holds a brass bar that is connected to a 5-volt DC at 30 µA source. This current creates an open circuit within the body. The practitioner holds a probe that completes the circuit when applied to the patient's skin. The patient's body elicits a measurable skin resistance to the voltage applied. The lower figure shows the correct positioning of the probe to acupuncture/conductance skin points and the angle at which it is applied (i.e., 45° at the neck of the bone).

producible measurements, the probe was placed at finger and toe points where the lowest resistance was found,[125] near the neck of the joints at a 45-degree angle to the bone.

The hand and foot skin points and their Voll-associated tissues and organs, some of which were measured in Studies A through D, are summarized in Table 16-3. Skin points whose values deviated from 45 to 55 relative units were measured again, coincidental with exposure to a broad band of RF signals associated with hoGFs (Studies B and C). The band of signals was given for a few seconds and was systematically reduced through repeated testing to one signal that produced a normal electrical conductance reading of 45 to 55 relative units (Study B). If chronically low or high conductance readings were not immediately brought into the normal range, additional RF signals were added until the abnormal skin points were brought back into the normal range. During Study C, subjects were exposed to a series of homeopathic potencies from all of the hoGFs that were used in Study B. The types of GFs and the concentrations that were most frequently reported to normalize electrical conductance were then prepared for physiological effects in terms of raising peripheral blood lymphocyte counts in Study D.

Baseline Evaluation: Study A

154 subjects (healthy, $n = 117$; HIV-positive, $n = 37$) were measured at skin conductance points located on the right side of the body plus the spleen acupuncture/conductance points located on the left toe (see Figure 16-2). All 117 of the healthy control subjects were evaluated for the major points: JOCR, FICR, SPCL, TH1R, and TH2R, and 60 of them (51%) were evaluated for all or most of the minor points of NE4R, LY4R, SP1L, SP2L, SP3L, SP4L, and LU10R. Healthy subjects were defined as persons visiting their health care practitioner for symptoms that did not include chronic DNA or RNA viral infections, cancer, or diabetes. HIV-positive patients had either CD4+ T-cell counts above 175 cells/µl without any major symptoms or were diagnosed with AIDS-defining illnesses ($n = 11$) with CD4+ T-cell counts below 150 cells/µl.

Treatment with Radio Frequency Signals: Studies B and C

Two different test groups were treated with RFs. The Study B group ($n = 23$) received signals regularly for 3 months, and the Study C group ($n = 11$) received

TABLE 16-3

Voll Tissue Names and Functions for Evaluated Hand and Foot Points

Voll point—location	Voll tissue name and function
JOCR—second right toe	Joints, master control point
LY4R—thumb—right side	Lymphatics related to lung
FICR—third right toe	Connective tissue
SPCL—large left toe	Spleen, master control point
SP1L—large left toe	Spleen lymphocytes homing to lymph nodes in upper body
SP2L—large left toe	Spleen lymphocytes homing to lymph nodes in lower body
SP3L—large left toe	Spleen—red blood cell formation
SP4L—large left toe	Spleen cells (macrophages and lymphocytes) related to phagocytosis and vascular functions
LU10R—base between right thumb and finger	Bronchi
TR1R—top of right ring finger (third finger)	Adrenals and gonadal function
TR2R—right ring finger	Thymus, thyroid, parathyroid
NE4R—second right finger, base of hand	Cranial nerves

signals for only 1 day. All RFs were pulsed signals with spatial modulation for maximal effectiveness and reproducibility.[87] In Study B, two HIV-positive patients who were not using antiviral (AV) therapy were evaluated for changes in T-cell counts (specifically $CD4^+$, $CD8^+$, and $CD3^+$ peripheral cell counts) after exposure to RF signals that simulated hoGFs. These two patients had been infected with HIV for more than 8 years and were given RF signals regularly to achieve optimal skin resistance at specific acupuncture/conductance points. Each radio signal simulated a different hoGF, and the unique radio signal that brought abnormal electrical conductance values back into the normal range was recorded in the software's memory system. Different RFs were administered to determine which GF signal or signals might best treat both persons. Lymphocyte counts were measured both before the treatment and after 3 months of treatment. $CD4^+$ T-cell counts collected from the two patients were compared to findings in two different double-blind, placebo-controlled clinical studies with HIV-positive patients who were on placebo ($n = 10$, $n = 11$) and received neither RF signals nor AV therapy.

In study B, electrical resistance was measured at points outside the normal range of 45 to 55 relative conductance units (inverse of resistance) on the LISTEN system. These points were associated with the spleen meridian (SP), environmentally related allergies (AL), lymph tissues in the lungs (LY4), the lymphatic system in general (LY), and the connective tissue (FIC) (see Figure 16-2 and Table 16-3). Each patient was treated for a 1-hour session for 3 months. Patient 1 was treated 3 to 5 days/week, and Patient 2 was treated 5 to 6 days/week.

In Study C, 11 HIV-infected individuals were delivered a wide spectrum of specific radio signals representing various potencies of hoGFs. Each response to a different potency (concentration) was quantified. This 1-day treatment identified the GF potency that normalized electrical resistance. HoGF potencies of 6 C (approximately 10^{-12} molar), 30 C (approximately 10^{-60} molar), 200 C (approximately 10^{-400} molar), and 1000 C, also known as 1 M (approximately 10^{-2000} molar, by the French method), were evaluated via RF signals.

Study D: Effects of Homeopathic Growth Factors on Electrical Conductance

The effectiveness of four hoGFs selected from Study C was tested in Study D ($n = 22$). HIV-positive individuals were examined for changes in electrical conductance over time during a 4-month, double-blind, placebo-controlled clinical study. Participants administered the treatment orally, swirling 10 drops around in the mouth from each of four bottles 3 times a day (40 drops tid). The bottles contained either one of the hoGFs at their concentrations (e.g., 1 M IGF-1, 30 C + 1 M PDGF-BB, 30 C + 1 M TGF-β1, and 200 C GM-CSF) or placebo. Measurements of electrical resistance at hand and foot points occurred every 3 weeks during the study. Changes in electrical resistance were compared with peripheral blood lymphocyte counts. HIV viral load testing was not available at this time.

Summary of Methods

The following step-by-step approach was used to research the effects of subtle energy medicine:

1. Identify key acupuncture/conductance skin points that are uniquely characteristic of HIV/AIDS patients versus those of healthy controls.
2. Identify specific RF signals that return abnormal skin conductance values to normal levels. Simultaneously measure changes occurring in peripheral blood lymphocyte counts of HIV-infected patients.
3. Identify specific homeopathic concentrations of GFs simulated by RF signals in a larger group of HIV/AIDS patients to bring abnormal skin conductance readings back into normal ranges.
4. Prepare some of the identified hoGFs into liquid preparations and evaluate their ability to restore EM skin conductance into the normal range and test the hypothesis in a double-blind, placebo-controlled clinical study (see Chapter 9).

Results

Study A: Electrical conductance readings of a minimum of 12 skin points in the 117 healthy controls were in the optimal range (48 to 52 relative units) 58% of the time and were in the normal range (45 to 55 relative units) 83% of the time (Figure 16-4, A). In the healthy controls, only two points, FICR and SP2L, were 17% and 12% higher than normal, respectively. None of the conductance readings were lower than normal levels. These measurements were compared with measurements of HIV-positive patients ($n = 37$, Figure 16-4, B) and patients diagnosed with AIDS-defining illnesses or with $CD4^+$ T-cell counts below 175 cells/μl ($n = 11$; Figure 16-4, C). Three of the 12 points measured, JOCR, SPCL, and SP3L, were not statistically different in any of the three groups. The other nine points were statistically higher or lower in HIV-infected patients. The findings were reproducible.

In asymptomatic HIV-positive patients, five points (42%) fell outside of the normal range, four of which were above the normal range: (1) LY4R ($+17\%$, $p = 0.01$), (2) LU10R ($+29\%$, $p = 0.002$), (3) TH2R ($+12\%$, $p = 0.0001$), and (4) NE4R ($+13\%$, $p = 0.0008$). One

point, SP1L (-12%), fell below the normal range, which Voll associated with splenic lymphocytes homing to the upper body (see Figure 16-4, B). Five points (42%) remained in the optimal range, and seven points (58%) fell into the normal range. Higher-than-normal electrical conductances suggest that the body is inflamed, which is a common general characteristic of HIV infection.

In general, the AIDS patients had statistically lower values of electrical conductance than both the control and asymptomatic HIV-positive groups (see Figure 16-4, C). Two points, LU10R ($+15\%$) and TH2R (12%, $p = 0.01$), were higher than those of controls. Five points (42%) were statistically lower than those of controls: (1) TH1R (-14%, $p = 0.058$), (2) SP4L (-18%, $p = 0.03$), (3) SP2L ($p = 0.004$), (4) SP1L (-23%, $p = 0.03$), and (5) FICR ($p = 0.008$). These AIDS patients had three points (FICR, NE4R, and SP3L; 25%) within the optimal range and seven points (58%) in the normal range. AIDS patients had three points with lower electrical conductances than HIV-positive patients (30%): (1) LY4R ($p = 0.04$), (2) SP4L ($p = 0.02$), and (3) TH1R ($p = 0.02$). The lower conductances in AIDS patients also characterized HIV disease progression.

Study B: T cells increased in those receiving simulated hoGFs. Both patients had $CD4^+$ T-cell counts below 200 cells/μl and were treated with RF signals for 30 to 60 minutes/day, 3 to 6 times/week, for 3 months. Patient 1 was treated with RF signals alone, and Patient 2 was treated with RF signals plus a combination of natural therapies. Table 16-4 shows the number of times that signals corresponding to specific GFs returned conductance readings to the normal range in acupuncture points associated with the lymphatics, spleen, TH1R, and lungs.

RF signals corresponding to NGF, IGF-1, αFGF, and TGF-α were the most effective and most frequently normalized the two patients' measurements. The patients' peripheral blood lymphocyte counts were measured for both many months before treatment and after 3 months of treatment (Figure 16-5). Before study entry, Patient 1's lymphocyte counts decreased until he was treated with a variety of different botanicals, especially bitter melon (*Momordica charantia*). Treatment with bitter melon in the previous 4 months was associated with $CD8^+$ and $CD3^+$ T-cell count increases of more than 30%. Total T-cell counts, however, did not have a significant effect on $CD4^+$ T-cell counts (Figure 16-5, A). Bitter melon treatment was discontinued for 1 month, and the administration

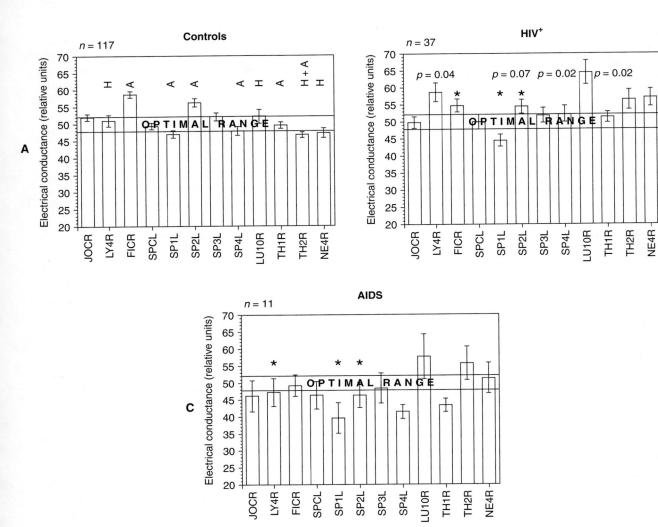

Figure 16-4 Electrical conductance measurements within the normal range were defined as 45 to 55 relative units, and optimal range was 48 to 52 relative units. The groups were: **A,** healthy control subjects; **B,** asymptomatic HIV-infected patients; and **C,** AIDS patients. Symbols above bars indicate statistical significance between control values and HIV (H) and AIDS (A). The * above the bars indicates reproducibility of measured values with findings previously reported by Brewitt.[2] Standard error bars are shown.

TABLE 16-4

Growth factor	Number of times GF balanced conductance	
	Patient 1	Patient 2
Nerve GF (NGF)	7	14
Insulin-like GF-1 (IGF-1)	8	4
Acidic fibroblast GF (α-FGF)	6	13
Basic fibroblast GF (β-FGF)	0	4
BB platelet-derived GF (PDGF-BB)	8	1
AA platelet-derived GF (PDGF-AA)	0	5
AB platelet-derived GF (PDGF-AB)	0	0
Transforming GF-alpha (TGF-α)	0	10
Epidermal GF (EGF)	0	3
Stem cell factor (SCF)	0	5
Transforming GF beta-1 (TGF-β1)	0	5
Transforming GF beta-2 (TGF-β2)	2	0
Granulocyte-macrophage colony-stimulating factor (GM-CSF)	2	0
Tumor necrosis factor-alpha (TNF-α)	0	0
Macrophage colony-stimulating factor (M-CSF)	0	0

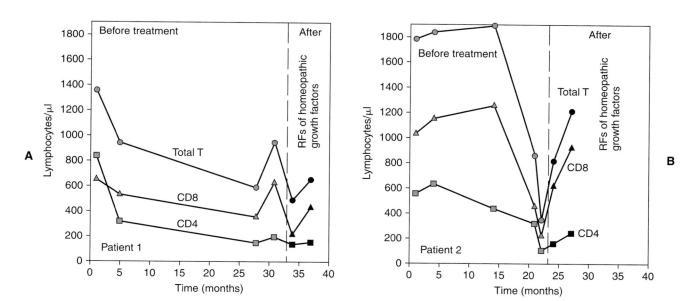

Figure 16-5 Peripheral blood T-cell counts in HIV-positive Patients 1 and 2 (**A** and **B,** respectively) in Study B, both before and after treatment. T-cell counts were recorded 4 to 5 times in the previous 24 months before treatment with RF signals and immediately after 3 months of treatment with regular RF signals of homeopathic GFs. The dashed line separates the monitoring period before RF treatment.

of RF signals of hoGFs began. This patient's immune parameters increased by 33% in CD8+ lymphocytes, by 102% in CD3+ lymphocytes, and by 16% in CD4+ lymphocytes during the next 3-month period without any treatment other than RFs.

Patient 2's immune parameters increased by 48% in CD8+ lymphocytes, by 50% in CD3+ lymphocytes, and by 50% in CD4+ T-cells (Figure 16-5, *B*). A long-term tracking of this patient's CD4+ T-cell counts over a 60-month period indicated that near-daily treatments with RF signals appeared to reverse his general downward trend in CD4+ T-cell counts and slowed disease progression (Figure 16-6). Monthly or bi-monthly treatments with RF signals of hoGFs were not sufficient to slow disease progression, and there was a downward trend in lymphocyte counts.

A general downward trend of -70 ± 50 CD4+ T-cells/μl in 4 months occurred when 21 HIV-positive

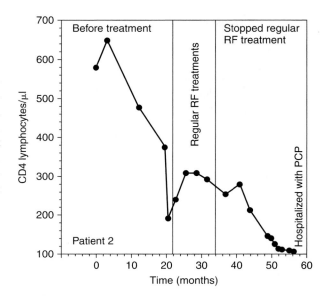

Figure 16-6 CD4+ T-cell counts in Patient 2 from Study B before RF treatment, during RF treatment, and after treatment. The patient's CD4+ T-cell count was followed for a 60-month period. The first 22 months had no RF signals, and the period of regular RF treatments 4 to 6 times/week are separated by lines. Irregular treatments of RF signals, which consisted of monthly or bimonthly visits, are identified. This patient was hospitalized with an opportunistic infection (OI) of *Pneumocystis carinii* pneumonia (PCP) and died shortly thereafter.

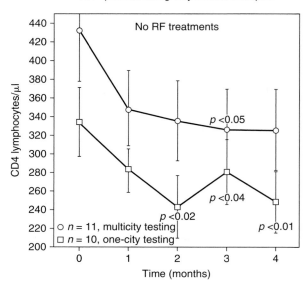

Figure 16-7 CD4+ T-cell counts in two placebo groups of double-blind, placebo-control design (squares represent single-site study, circles represent seven-city multisite study). The persons in these placebo groups were using only natural therapies. There was no uniform protocol of natural therapy, and no one was using HAART. Standard error bars are shown. Paired *t* test statistical differences from baseline measures are shown at specific time points.

patients used only natural therapies without other RF treatments (Figure 16-7). In general, HIV disease progression includes average losses of -85 to -100 CD4 cells/μl/year compared to -6 CD4 cells/μl/year losses in HIV-positive long-term nonprogressors or -7 CD4 cells/μl/year in healthy controls undergoing normal aging.[126] The increase in CD4$^+$ T-cell counts in both patients treated with RF signals was highly significant.

Study C: This study administered different RF signals of various homeopathic potencies of GF for a one-time event to 11 different HIV-positive patients with CD4$^+$ T-cell counts between 67 and 570 cells/μl. The findings from this study are shown in Table 16-5. A positive response was defined as the hoGF signal that brought the electrical conductance into the normal range of 45 to 55 relative units.

In 10 of the 11 patients (91%) treated, administration of the RF signal simulating IGF-1 brought the patient's electrical conductance back into the normal range. Most patients responded to more than one homeopathic potency for any single hoGF signal. RF signals representing PDGF in two of its isoforms, BB (82% of people responded positively) and AA (73% of

people responded positively), effectively normalized electrical conductance measurements. In general, 63% of HIV-positive patients responded to RF signals simulating the hoGFs of (1) IGF-1, (2) PDGF-BB, (3) PDGF-AB, (4) PDGF-AA, (5) NGF, (6) GM-CSF, (7) TNF-α, and (8) M-CSF. RF signals associated with higher potencies of GFs, such as 1000 C (1 M), normalized electrical conductance measurements of asymptomatic HIV-positive patients more effectively than RF signals associated with lower potencies of GFs. Homeopathic potencies of 6 C, representing picomolar (10^{-12} molar) concentrations of GFs, normalized electrical conductance readings in AIDS patients or symptomatic HIV-positive patients most frequently.

Study D: Electrical skin conductance measurements were taken of 22 patients who received four hoGFs. Baseline changes in electrical conductance measurements of 36 hand and foot acupuncture points were quantified every 3 to 4 weeks for 4 months (Figure 16-8). Points related to the hormonal, nervous, and immune systems along the SP, TR, and NE meridians of the second and fourth fingers and large left toe

TABLE 16-5

Growth factor	Number of people who responded/ total tested	Homeopathic potency			
		6 C	30 C	200 C	1000 C
Nerve GF (NGF)	7/11	3	2	1	4
Insulin-like GF-1 (IGF-1)	10/11	6	4	6	7
Acidic Fibroblast GF (αFGF)	6/11	2	3	1	5
Basic Fibroblast GF (βFGF)	6/11	2	2	5	4
Platelet-derived GF-BB (PDGF-BB)	9/11	3	5	1	5
Platelet-derived GF-AA (PDGF-AA)	8/11	3	4	3	2
Platelet-derived GF-AB (PDGF-AB)	7/11	3	5	3	4
Transforming GF-alpha (TFG-α)	5/11	2	2	4	3
Epidermal GF (EGF)	5/11	0	2	2	3
Stem cell factor (SCF)	5/11	3	1	3	2
Transforming GF beta-1 (TGF-β1)	6/11	3	3	1	6
Transforming GF beta-2 (TGF-β2)	4/11	1	2	2	1
Granulocyte-macrophage colony-stimulating factor (GM-CSF)	7/11	2	0	4	3
Tumor necrosis factor-alpha (TNF-α)	7/11	4	2	4	4
Macrophage colony-stimulating factor (M-CSF)	7/11	2	2	2	4

Column 1 = GF; Column 2 = number of individuals whose measurements normalized after exposure to a RF signal of a specific homeopathic GF. Columns thereafter show the number of people responding positively to each homeopathic potency.

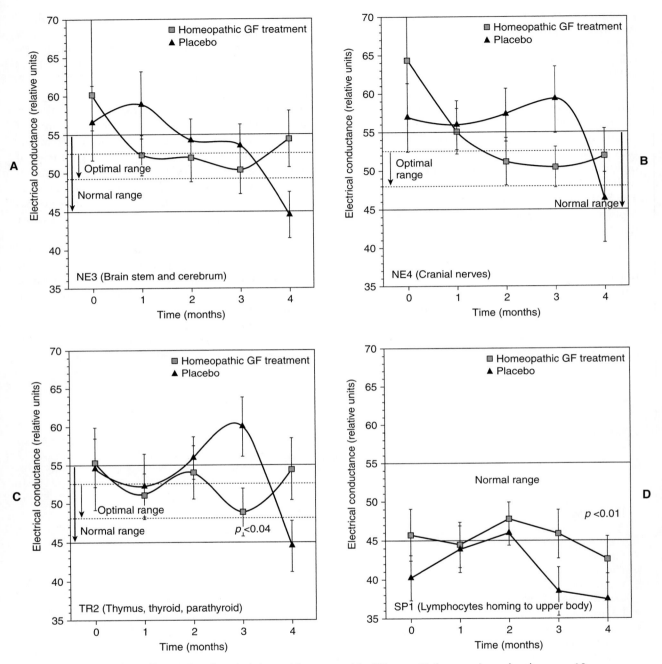

Figure 16-8 Effects of orally administered homeopathic GFs, *n* =11 (squares) or placebo, *n* = 10 (triangles) on electrical conductance in HIV-positive patients participating in a double-blind, placebo-controlled study. The points shown are: **A,** NE3; **B,** NE4; **C,** TR2; and **D,** SP1. Standard error bars are shown, as well as the time at which significance was determined.

were analyzed over time. There was no difference between normal treatment or placebo in 69% of these points.

The treatment caused points associated with (1) the brain stem and cerebrum (NE3), (2) cranial nerves (NE4), and (3) thymus, thyroid, and parathyroid glands (TR2 or triple heater two) to change from abnormal to repeatedly normal electrical conductance patterns. In contrast, the placebo had no effect on electrical conductance patterns, and the measurements remained out of balance throughout the study (see Figure 16-8). The NE3 point was higher than normal in both groups at study entry. Once treatment was initiated, the measurements for NE3 were normalized, and three of the measurements fell in the optimal range (Figure 16-8, A). In contrast, the measurements of subjects on placebo fell in the normal range twice, but none fell in the optimal range, and during the final month, the measurement fell below normal values. Similarly, NE4 point measurements that were very high at study entry fell into the normal range four out of five times with treatment of hoGFs (Figure 16-8, B). Initially high electrical conductance measurements in the placebo group continued to rise above normal levels until the end of the study, when they fell into the normal range one out of five times. The entry measurement of TR2 was near-normal in both the treatment and placebo groups (Figure 16-8, C). The treatment appeared to maintain the measurements within the normal range compared with placebo, in which measurements rose higher and fell lower than normal three out of five times. A statistical difference was measured between the two groups in month 3 ($p < 0.04$). The SP1 point measurements were lower than the other points before and after therapy. However, the measurements maintained greater stability in the treatment group than in the placebo group. ($p < 0.01$) (Figure 16-8, D).

Summary and Conclusions

The systematic methodology used to conduct these four small preliminary, Phase I and II clinical studies leads to new insights regarding the therapeutic efficacy of EM forces on HIV-positive patients. Preliminary data are adequate to form a hypothesis of the mechanism of action for nonthermal RF signals that effectively treat HIV-positive patients or other virally infected persons. Based on these findings, it is key to the hypothesis that homeostasis of energy fields be restored. Restoration of the body's healthy range of os-

cillating electrical resistance occurred through delivery of RF EM forces and through oral delivery of hoGFs.

The unique characterization of the body's energetic abnormalities enabled treatments to be more highly directed to specific corresponding tissues and organs. HIV/AIDS energetic abnormalities identified in these studies include meridians that Voll had assigned to the spleen, thymus/thyroid, lungs, and lymphatic system within the lungs and small intestines. These same organs and tissues are identified as early target sites for HIV infection and where pathological effects occur most often.[127-130]

Study A demonstrated the characteristic differences between specific acupuncture/conductance points in HIV-positive patients versus healthy controls. Other researchers have also measured differences in electrical parameters at skin points between healthy and disease states.[2,131-136] Disease states noted previously were (1) general inflammation, (2) HIV/AIDS, (3) Epstein-Barr virus (EBV), (4) cytomegalovirus (CMV), (5) cancer, (6) diabetes, (7) liver cirrhosis, (8) lung diseases, and (9) tumors. The current study, however, associates the organ/tissue names of the acupuncture/conductance skin points to Voll points. Voll points may follow along meridians that map particular organs or biological functions of the body, although these differ from traditional Chinese acupuncture maps.[117] Voll tissue names, however, correspond to organs and tissues that are affected during early stages of HIV infection, such as the lungs, nervous system, spleen, adrenals, thymus, and lymphatics.[127-130,137]

Measurements of specific points related to the spleen and connective tissue (i.e., FICR, SP2L, and SP1L) in Study A's larger study of HIV-positive and AIDS patients replicated earlier findings with a smaller sample size.[2] As previously asserted, asymptomatic HIV infection generally includes hyperconductance profiles.[2] Hyperconductance early in the HIV disease process is in keeping with findings by others using EDS and EM screening devices that note early stages of pathology.[2,6,96,138-142] Hyperconductance is associated with excessive fluid motion in malignant or inflamed tissue.[6,143]

AIDS patients generally had lower-than-optimal conductance readings. SP1L was the single point in both HIV-positive and AIDS patients that was lower than that in the control group. The spleen is one of the first targets for HIV infection, and this low measurement at the spleen skin points suggests that the spleen is one of the first organs to lose energetic vitality after infection. The spleen's loss of energetic vitality also supports the findings and conclusions reported earlier on EM readings in degenerative or progressed states of disease.[2,138] Chinese acupuncture points that are clinically significant to HIV infection include those related to the spleen, thymus, and lungs, which are similarly identified organs but not exactly the same points as those reported in this study.[122] Further characterization of the points identifying HIV infection and the specific treatment protocols that restore homeostasis to these specific organs is warranted.

CD4[+] T cells and other lymphocyte counts were raised by repeatedly stabilizing acupuncture/conductance skin points associated with the nervous and immune systems. The improvement in cellular immunity occurred by either delivery of RF signals simulating hoGFs or by delivery of oral administration of liquid hoGFs (Studies B and D). The specific skin points treated were associated with the spleen, thymus, and cranial nerves, all known as key reservoir organs for HIV residence.

Pulse waveforms, as occurs with radio waves, optimally transmit reliable and reproducible information from machines to humans.[87] Treatment with short-wave RFs and other EMF forces can improve conditions such as respiratory tract infections (RTIs), skin infections, general inflammatory conditions, sensory organ function, and psychophysical states of consciousness.[69,87,144-146] The studies presented in this chapter demonstrated how pulsed RF signals of hoGFs directed to specific target organ points strengthened both neurophysiological and immune responses of HIV-positive patients.

The study of two individual patients was preliminary by design; however, their gains in CD4[+] T-cell counts were significantly greater than the trends seen in two other studies of persons using placebos plus other natural therapies, without HAART or RF treatment. Losses in lymphocyte counts in persons taking a wide variety of natural supplements agree with previous reports by Standish et al[147] and Brewitt et al (see Chapter 9). HIV-positive patients using some natural therapies did not maintain stable CD4[+] T-cell counts over time. In contrast, the improvement in immune status in the two patients who were treated with RF signals occurred without HAART, without acupuncture, and with little supplementation of other botanicals, vitamins, or other hands-on therapies. Patient 2 improved more than Patient 1, suggesting that more frequent RF therapy plus supplementation with natural products is related to increased lymphocyte counts. Patient 2 was treated with the EM signals 35% more frequently than Patient 1. Further studies with this intervention in larger groups and with better controls are warranted to test reproducibility. The hoGFs that were the most effective at bringing the patients' electrical conductance into the normal range were (1) NGF, (2) IGF-1, (3) αFGF, and (4) TGF-α.

Specific RF signals simulating different hoGFs at separate concentrations were also identified in Study C for their ability to bring abnormally high or low points in HIV-infected patients back into the normal range. A majority of the people (63%) with HIV/AIDS responded to the RF signals associated with the hoGFs of (1) IGF-1, (2) PDGF-BB, (3) PDGF-AB, (4) PDGF-AA, (5) NGF, (6) GM-CSF, (7) TNF-α, and (8) M-CSF. Three of the GFs identified in Study B were also identified in Study C; namely, NGF, IGF-1, and TGF-α. Generally, the higher the potency (i.e., lower concentration), the more effective it balanced the EM field of the healthier HIV-positive individual. The lower potencies were more effective at treating HIV/AIDS patients with lower CD4[+] T-cell counts and greater disease progression.

Study D evaluated four of the hoGFs identified in Study C for their ability to improve electrical conductance profiles at specific Voll points associated with neuroimmune and endocrine functioning.[117] Oral administration of four hoGFs at potencies identified in Study C effectively balanced electrical skin conductance. This balance did not occur with persons using placebo and other natural supplements. Three skin points that significantly balanced over time in the treatment group compared with placebo were (1) TH2R, (2) NE3R, and (3) NE4R. These three points had statistically higher conductance values than those of healthy controls. Additionally, the variability around the mean value at the SP1L skin point was statistically more coherent on treatment than on placebo. This supports the premise that an autoregulatory process within the body's EM field occurred. The positive clinical results on immune parameters that also occurred with treatment of hoGFs are presented in Chapter 9.

The results from Studies B and D suggest that optimizing electrical conductance at hand and foot skin points via either pulsed RF signals or oral administration of hoGFs significantly improved the immune system of HIV/AIDS patients. The studies demonstrated that quantitative evaluation of acupuncture/conductance skin points can delineate subtle differences between HIV/AIDS patients versus healthy controls. Other studies have demonstrated distinct differences between states of health versus pathology and states of inflammation versus degeneration, including HIV/AIDS.[2,131,148] Cancer diagnosis has an electrical signature when six simultaneous abnormalities are found using an Nakatani neurometer at the traditional Chinese acupuncture meridians related to the pericardium, triple-heater, spleen-pancreas, kidney, and gall bladder.[139]

The patterns of electrical conductance of persons on placebo versus persons receiving oral administration of liquid hoGFs were significantly different. Autoregulatory functioning improved with oral administration of hoGFs. These hoGFs must have carried subtle energy signals, since the probability of them containing even one molecule of actual GF was less than one in 10^{400}. The measured positive effects originated from a solution with active ingredients that were no longer present, yet the solution carried clinically valuable potent biological information.

The model whereby information is transferred from the outside of the cell to the DNA inside the cell has been shown with EM stimuli via general mechanisms in the body that extend beyond the requirement for molecular binding to substrates. French immunologist Jacques Benveniste postulates that highly diluted compounds transfer information to cells via signal transduction pathways that are bioelectromagnetic.[37] Results from the studies presented in this chapter suggest the hypothesis that information is transferred from outside human cells to genetic DNA inside the cells via oral administration of hoGFs.

Biophysical mechanisms exerted positive immunomodulatory effects on HIV-positive patients who were not using HAART, most notably raising blood CD4$^+$ T-cell counts. These clinical findings open a new door for HIV infection treatment possibilities. Specifically, by balancing EM field rhythms at acupuncture/conductance skin points, measurable physiological and immunological benefits resulted. As skin point measurements associated with the thymus and cranial nerves were brought into homeostasis, immune cell counts simultaneously improved. These findings provide the perspective that treatment strategies for HIV infection happen at the cell receptor level. The subtle energetic approach evokes a cellular response from both the nervous and immune systems.

The reproducibility of the data from these clinical studies and from those presented in Chapter 9 demonstrate beneficial clinical effects from subtle energy forces.

A NEW HYPOTHESIS FOR EFFICACIOUS, NONTOXIC TREATMENT USING SUBTLE ENERGY MEDICINE

HIV competes for the same G-protein signaling processes that many GFs use. G proteins are requisite coreceptors for HIV that can infect human cells.[149-151] G proteins are the first site of information transfer from the cell membrane surface to its DNA.[152] The transfer of information from the outside of cells to their inner nucleus uses common pathways, such as G proteins. HIV, EM forces, and hoGFs use G proteins to transfer information to the DNA. Cells process a broad array of diverse extracellular signals into an appropriate small array of intracellular responses through only three types of signaling pathways: (1) receptors, (2) G proteins, and (3) effectors that direct the information from the receptor to the inside of the cell.[38,42,153] G proteins are part of a superfamily of proteins that are named by their binding and regulation by guanine nucleotides (which consists of a guanine, a sugar, and one or more phosphates). Three different subunits of G proteins[154] form a variety of combinations to direct various signals down specific pathways (see Figure 16-1). Over 320 heterotrimeric G proteins exist.[152,153] The signal transduction pathway of G proteins is already associated with numerous diseases.[155,156] HIV may activate G proteins in the same way as RF signals and hoGFs do. In fact, this signal transduction pathway may be used universally.

G proteins play an essential role during HIV infection. Researchers have known since 1986 that the CD4$^+$ T-cell receptor was not sufficient for the entry of HIV into human immune system cells.[151] This finding launched a decade-long search for the necessary "second receptor" for effective HIV infection of immune and nervous system CD4$^+$ T cells. In 1996 researchers identified at least two second receptors that enable HIV infection in human cells; both of them are transmembrane G proteins that couple with the CD4$^+$ receptor and are called *CC-CKR5* and *fusin*.[149,150] CC-CKR5 and fusin are now accepted as the second and final gate that HIV must pass through to enter macrophage and CD4+ T cells and to infect them by inserting viral genetic material into the cell's DNA.

G proteins take part in an enormous variety of biological sensing and communication systems. They help control everything from the successful entry of HIV into human immune cells, to mating in yeast, to egg-laying in the nematode *Caenorhabditis elegans,* to immune function, vision, and olfaction in humans.[157] G proteins are located within the cell lipid bilayer and are part of a superfamily of proteins.[158] G proteins couple with cell receptors to direct the flow of information from outside the receptor to inside the cell by converting the external signal into second messengers that regulate gene expression.[38,156] G-protein activation triggers signal transduction cascades, which regulate gene transcription, gene expression, protein synthesis, cell division, and cell death.[3,40,67,159] G proteins play significant roles during infection by viruses, such such as HIV and EBV, and by bacterial diseases, such as some lymphomas, whooping cough, and cholera. Other G protein–coupled-receptor disorders are well-known, such as retinitis pigmentosa (RP), stationary night blindness, color blindness, isolated glucocorticoid deficiencies, hyperfunctioning thyroidadenomas, and neonatal hyperparathyroidism. G proteins contribute significantly to receptor systems such as GFs, GH, chemokines, neurotransmitters, hormones, gonadotropin-releasing hormone (GnRH), pheromones, opsins, rhodopsins, melatonin, and serotonin.

Since EM forces are necessary cofactors for successful HIV infection, a new treatment strategy may include competitive G-protein signaling to inhibit HIV replication and activation. Further studies of approaches using homeopathic cell signaling proteins, such as hoGFs and homeopathic interleukins (ILs), both with and without EM signaling, are warranted given these positive preliminary findings.

References

1. Mathews AP: Electric polarity in hydroids, *Am J Physiol* 8:294-299, 1903.
2. Brewitt B: Quantitative analysis of electrical skin conductance in diagnosis: historical and current views of bioelectric medicine, *J Naturopath Med* 6(1):66-75, 1996.
3. Rubik B, Becker RO, Flower RG, et al: Bioelectromagnetics applications in medicine. In *Alternative medicine: expanding medical horizons, Report to NIH on Alternative Medical Systems and Practices in the United States,* Washington, DC, 1994, US Government Printing Office.
4. Becker RO: *Cross currents: the perils of electropollution, the promise of electromedicine,* Los Angeles, 1990, Jeremy P Tarcher.
5. Bassett CAL: Fundamental and practical aspects of therapeutic uses of pulsed electromagnetic fields (PEMFs), *Crit Rev Biomed Eng* 17:451-529, 1989.
6. Pethig R: Electrical properties of biological tissues. In Marino AA, editor: *Modern bioelectricity,* New York, 1988, Marcel Dekker, Inc.
7. Pilla AA: Mechanisms of electrochemical phenomena in tissue repair and growth, *Bioelectrochem Bioenerg* 1:227-243, 1974.
8. Tenforde TS, Kaune WT: Interaction of extremely low frequency electric and magnetic fields with humans, *Health Phys* 53:585-606, 1987.
9. Rosendal T: Studies on the conducting properties of the human skin to direct current, *Acta Physiol Scand* 5:130-151, 1942.
10. Liu K, Cruzan JD, Saykally RJ: Water clusters, *Science* 271:929-933, 1996.
11. Byus CV, Lundak RL, Fletcher RM, et al: Alterations in protein kinase activity after exposure of cultured lymphocytes to modulated microwave fields, *Bioelectromagnetics* 5:34-37, 1984.
12. Goodman R, Henderson AS: Transcription in cells exposed to extremely low frequency EM fields: a review, *Bioelectrochem Bioenerg* 25:335-355, 1991.
13. Lin H, Goodman R, Shirley-Henderson A: Specific region of the *c-myc* promoter is responsive to electric and magnetic fields, *J Cell Biochem* 54:281-288, 1994.
14. Liburdy R, Callahan DE, Harland J, et al: Signal transduction in the lymphocyte is influenced by 60 Hz magnetic fields, mitogen binding, calcium and mRNA induction, The Annual Review of Research on Biological Effects of Electric and Magnetic Fields from the Generation, Delivery, and Use of Electricity, Poster 12, San Diego, 1992.
15. Gold S, Goodman R, Henderson AS: Exposure of simian virus 40 transformed human cells to magnetic fields results in increased levels of T-antigen mRNA and protein, *Bioelectromagnetics* 15:329-336, 1994.
16. Goodman R, Wei L-X, Xu J-C, et al: Exposure of human cells to low frequency electromagnetic fields results in quantitative changes in transcripts, *Biochim Biophys Acta* 1009:216-220, 1989.

17. Libertin CR, Panozzo J, Groh KR, et al: Effects of gamma rays, ultraviolet radiation, sunlight, microwaves, and electromagnetic fields on gene expression mediated by human immunodeficiency virus promoter, *Radiat Res* 140:91-96, 1994.

18. Becker R: Electromagnetism and psi phenomena, *J Am Soc Psychical Res* 86:1-17, 1992b.

19. McLeod BR, Liboff AR: Dynamic characteristics of membrane ions in multifield configurations of low frequency electromagnetic radiation, *Bioelectromagnetics* 7:177-189, 1986.

20. Milham Jr S: Mortality from leukemia in workers exposed to electrical and magnetic fields, *N Engl J Med* 307(4):249, 1982 (letter).

21. Wright WE, Peters JM, Mack TM: Leukaemia in workers exposed to biolectrical and magnetic fields, *Lancet* 2(8303):1160-1161, 1982.

22. McDowell ME: Leukaemia mortality in electrical workers in England and Wales, *Lancet* 1(8318):246, 1983.

23. Coleman M, Bell J, Skeet R: Leukaemia incidence in electrical workers, *Lancet* 1(8331):982-983, 1983.

24. Wertheimer N, Leeper E: Electrical wiring configurations and childhood cancer, *Am J Epidemiol* 109:273-284, 1979.

25. Wertheimer N, Leeper E: Adult cancer related to electrical wires near the home, *Int J Epidemiol* 11(4):345-355, 1982.

26. Griffin GE, Paton NI, Cofrancesco Jr J, et al: Nutrition and quality of life in HIV infection: the roles of growth hormone in HIV-associated wasting, Update on AIDS wasting and lipodystrophy: one-day seminar, Twelfth World AIDS Conference, Geneva, June 28, 1998.

27. Ott M, Lembcke B, Fischer H, et al: Early changes of body composition in human immunodeficiency virus-infected patients: tetrapolar body impedance analysis indicates significant malnutrition, *Am J Clin Nutr* 57:15-19, 1993.

28. Pantaleo G, Craziosi C, Demarest JF, et al: HIV infection is active and progressive in lymphoid tissue during the clinically latent stage of disease, *Nature* 362:355-358, 1993.

29. Liburdy RP: Biological interactions of cellular systems with time-varying magnetic fields, *Ann N Y Acad Sci* 649:74-95, 1992.

30. Liboff AR, Williams Jr T, Strong DM, et al: Time-varying magnetic fields: effect on DNA synthesis, *Science* 223:818-820, 1984.

31. Kirschvink JL, Kobayashi-Kirschvink A, Woodford BJ: Magnetite biomineralization in the human brain, *Proc Natl Acad Sci U S A* 89:7683-7687, 1992.

32. Blackman CF, Benane SG, Rabinowitz JR, et al: A role for the magnetic field in the radiation-induced efflux of calcium ion from the brain tissue in vitro, *Bioelectromagnetics* 6:327-337, 1985a.

33. Adey WR: Collective properties of cell membranes. In Ramel C, Norden B, editors: *Resonance and other interactions of electromagnetic fields,* Oxford, UK, 1991, Oxford University Press.

34. Zukauskas G, Dapsys K, Ilgesviciute J: Quantitative analysis of bioelectrical potentials for the diagnosis of internal organ pathology and theoretical speculations concerning electrical circulation in the organism, *Acupunct Electrother Res* 13:119-130, 1988.

35. Adey WR: The cellular microenvironment and signaling through cell membranes, *Prog Clin Biol Res* 257:81-106, 1988.

36. Benveniste J, Aïssa J, Litime MH, et al: Transfer of the molecular signal by electronic amplification, *FASEB J* 8:A398, 1994 (abstract).

37. Aïssa J, Litime MH, Attias E, et al: Transfer of molecular signals via electronic circuitry, *FASEB J* 7:A602, 1993 (abstract).

38. Linder ME, Gilman AG: G proteins, *Sci Am* 267(1):56-64, 1992.

39. Blackman CF, Benane SG, House DE, et al: Effects of ELF (1 to 120Hz) and modulated (50Hz) radio frequency fields on the efflux of calcium ions from brain tissue in vitro, *Bioelectromagnetics* 6:1-11, 1985b.

40. Cone CD: Variation of the transmembrane potential level as a basic mechanism of mitosis control, *Oncology* 24:438-470, 1970.

41. Bourguignon GJ, Jy W, Bourguignon LYW: Electric stimulation of human fibroblasts causes an increase in Ca^{+2} influx and the exposure of additional insulin receptors, *J Cell Physiol* 140:379-385, 1989.

42. Restrepo D, Miyamoto T, Bryant B, et al: Odor stimuli trigger influx of calcium into olfactory neurons of the channel catfish, *Science* 249:1166-1168, 1990.

43. Dower SK, Kronheim SR, March CJ, et al: Detection and characterization of high affinity plasma membrane receptors for human interleukin 1, *J Exp Med* 162:501-515, 1985.

44. Belsham GJ, Brownsey RW, Hughes WA, et al: Anti-insulin receptor antibodies mimic the effects of insulin on the activities of pyruvate dehydrogenase and acetyl CoA carboxylase and on specific protein phosphorylation in rat epididymal fat cells, *Diabetologia* 18(4):307-312, 1980.

45. Nye KE, Knox KA, Pinching AJ: Lymphocytes from HIV-infected individuals show aberrant inositol polyphosphate metabolism which reverses after zidovudine therapy, *AIDS* 5:413-417, 1991.

46. Nye KE, Pinching AJ: HIV infection of H9 lymphoblastoid cells chronically activates the inositol polyphosphate pathway, *AIDS* 4:41-45, 1990.

47. Bourguignon GJ, Bourguignon LY: Electrical stimulation of protein and DNA synthesis in human fibroblasts in vitro, *FASEB J* 1:398-402, 1987.

48. Rodan GA, Bourret LA, Norton LA: DNA synthesis in cartilage cells is stimulated by oscillating electric fields, *Science* 199(4329):690-692, 1978.

49. Phillips JL, Haggren W, Thomas WJ, et al: Magnetic field-induced changes in specific gene transcription, *Biochim Biophys Acta* 1132:140-144, 1992.

50. Mercier G, Galien R, Emanoil-Ravier R: Differential effects of *ras* and *jun* family members on complex retrovirus promoter activities, *Res Virol* 145:361-367, 1994.

51. Michaelson SM, Houk WM, Lebola NJA, et al: Biochemical and neuroendocrine aspects of exposure to microwaves, *Ann N Y Acad Sci* 247:21-45, 1975.

52. Pert C: *The molecules of emotion,* New York, 1997, Scribner.

53. Becker RO: Modern bioelectromagnetics and functions of the central nervous system, *Subtle Energies* 3(1):53-72, 1992a.

54. Thomas JR, Schrot J, Liboff AR: Low intensity magnetic fields after operant behavior in rats, *Bioelectromagnetics* 7:349-357, 1986.

55. Becker RO, Selden G: *The body electric: electromagnetism and the foundation of life,* New York, 1985, William Morrow & Co, Inc.

56. Aleksandrovskaya M, Kolodov Y: The potential role of neuroglia in the onset of a bioelectrical reaction of the brain to a constant magnetic field, *Reports Acad Sci USSR* 170:482-485, 1966.

57. Wilson B: Chronic exposure to ELF fields may induce depression, *Bioelectromagnetics* 9:195-205, 1988.

58. Michaud L, Persinger M: Geophysical variables and behavior: alterations in memory for a narrative after application of theta frequency electromagnetic fields, *Percept Mot Skills* 60:416-418, 1985.

59. Reichmanis M, Perry F, Marino A, et al: Relationship between suicide and the electromagnetic field of overhead power lines, *Physiol Chem Phys* 11:395-403, 1979.

60. Goodman R, Weisbrot D, Uluc A, et al: Transcription in *Drosophilia melanogaster* salivary gland cells is altered after exposure to low-frequency electromagnetic fields: analysis of chromosome 3R, *Bioelectromagnetics* 13:111-118, 1992a.

61. Goodman R, Weisbrot A, Uluc A, et al: Transcription in *Drosophilia melanogaster* salivary gland cells is altered after exposure to low-frequency electromagnetic fields: analysis of chromosomes 3L and X, *Bioelectromagnetics* 28:311-318, 1992b.

62. Welker H, Semm P, Willig J, et al: Effects of an artificial magnetic field on serotonin, *N*-Acetyltransferase, and melatonin content of the rat pineal gland, *Exp Brain Res* 50:426-432, 1983.

63. Goodman R, Bassett CAL, Andrew L, et al: Pulsing electromagnetic fields induce cellular transcription, *Science* 220:1283-1285, 1983.

64. Semm P, Schneider T, Vollrath L: Effects of an earth-strength magnetic field on electrical activity of pineal cells, *Nature* 288(5791):607-608, 1980.

65. Cossarizza A, Monti D, Bersani F, et al: Extremely low-frequency pulsed electromagnetic fields increase cell proliferation in lymphocytes from young and aged subjects, *Biochem Biophys Res Commun* 160:692-698, 1989.

66. Cadossi R, Hentz VR, Kipp J, et al: Effect of low-frequency, low-energy pulsing electromagnetic fields (PEMF) on x-ray-irradiated mice, *Exp Hematol* 17(2):88-95, 1989.

67. Cadossi R, Emilia G, Ceccherelli G, et al: Lymphocytes and pulsing magnetic fields. In Marino AA, editor: *Modern bioelectricity,* New York, 1988, Marcel Dekker, Inc.

68. Liboff AR, Rozek RJ, Sherman ML, et al: $Ca^{2+}-45$ cyclotron resonance in human lymphocytes, *J Bioelectricity* 6(1):13-22, 1987.

69. Ginsberg AJ: Ultrashort radio waves as a therapeutic agent, *Med Record* 140:651-653, 1934.

70. Liboff AR: Geomagnetic cyclotron resonance in living cells, *J Biol Phys* 13:99-102, 1985.

71. Weiss DS, Kirsner R, Eaglstein WH: Electrical stimulation and wound healing, *Arch Dermatol* 126:222-225, 1990.

72. Rowley BA, McKenna JM, Chase GR, et al: The influence of electrical current on an infecting microorganism in wounds, *Ann N Y Acad Sci* 238:543-552, 1974.

73. Barranco SD, Spadaro JA, Berger TJ, et al: In vitro effect of weak direct current on *Staphyloccocus aureus, Clin Orthop* 100:250-255, 1974.

74. Head EL: An electrical therapy device, Patent #8326602, Croydon Printing Co, The United Kingdom Patent Office, London, 1984.

75. Odess Health Farm: Treatment in early convalesce after viral hepatitis—treating pyloroduodenal area with electromagnetic radiation in mm wave band, London, 1990, Derwent Publishing (abstract from patent #90-367065/49).

76. Sersa G, Miklavcic D: Inhibition of SA-1 tumor growth in mice by human leukocyte interferon alpha combined with low-level direct current, *Mol Biother* 2(3):165-168, 1990.

77. David SL, Absolom DR, Smith CR, et al: Effect of low-level direct current on in vivo tumor growth in hamsters, *Cancer Res* 45(11 pt 2):5625-5631, 1985.

78. Habal MB: Effect of applied DC currents on experimental tumor growth in rats, *J Biomed Mater Res* 14:789-801, 1980.

79. Schauble MK, Habal MB, Gullick HD: Inhibition of experimental tumor growth in hamsters by small direct currents, *Arch Pathol Lab Med* 101:294-297, 1977.

80. Humphrey CE, Seal EH: Biophysical approach toward tumor regression in mice, *Science* 130:388-389, 1959.

81. Richards TL, Lappin MS, Acosta-Urquidi J, et al: Double-blind study of pulsing magnetic field effects on multiple sclerosis, *J Altern Complement Med* 3(1):21-29, 1997.

82. Wilson DH, Jagadeesh P, Newman PP, et al: The effects of pulsed electromagnetic energy on peripheral nerve regeneration, *Ann N Y Acad Sci* 238:575-585, 1974.

83. Bassett CAL, Mitchell SN, Gaston SR: Pulsing electromagnetic field treatment in nonunited fractures and failed arthrodoses, *JAMA* 247:623-628, 1982.

84. Sisken BF: Effects of EM fields on nerve regeneration. In Marino AA, editor: *Modern bioelectricity*, New York, 1988, Marcel Dekker, Inc.

85. Margolick JB, Donnenberg AD: T-cell homeostasis in HIV-1 infection, *Semin Immunol* 9(6):381-388, 1997.

86. Jakoubek B, Rohlicek V: Changes of electrodermal properties in the "acupuncture points" in men and rats, *Physiologia bohemoslovaca* 31:143-149, 1982.

87. Kume Y, Ohzu H: Electrocutaneous stimulation for information transmission, I: optimum waveform eliciting stable sensation without discomfort, *Acupunct Electrother Res* 5:57-81, 1980.

88. Reichmanis M, Marino AA, Becker RO: Electrical correlates of acupuncture points, *IEEE Trans Biomed Eng* 22:533-536, 1975.

89. Saita HG: Modern scientific medical acupuncture, *J Am Osteopath Assoc* 72:685-696, 1973.

90. Borsavello LC: Acupuncture verifiee par l'electrique, *Science et Vie* 695:80-89, 1971.

91. Wulfsohn NL, Yoo JHK, Gelineau J: Twenty-seven acupuncture points and their electrical resistance. In Warren F, editor: *Handbook of medical acupuncture*, New York, 1976, Van Nostrand.

92. Hyvärinen J, Karlsson M: Low-resistance skin points that may coincide with acupuncture loci, *Medical Biology* 55:88-94, 1977.

93. Tiller WA: On the evolution of electrodermal diagnostic instruments, *J Advancement Med* 1(1):41-56, 1988.

94. Eory A: In vivo skin respiration CO_2 measurements in the acupuncture loci, *Acupunct Electrother Res* 9:217-223, 1984.

95. Becker RO, Marino AA: *Electromagnetism and life*, Albany, 1982, State University of New York Press.

96. Tiller WA: On the explanation of electrodermal diagnostic and treatment instruments, part I: the electrical behavior of human skin, *J Holistic Med* 4(2):105-127, 1982.

97. Voll R: The phenomenon of medicine testing in electroacupuncture according to Voll, *Am J Acupunct* 8:97-104, 1980.

98. Darras JC, de Vernejoul P, Albarède P: Nuclear medicine and acupuncture: a study on the migration of radioactive tracers after injection at acupoints, *Am J Acupunct* 20(3):245-256, 1992.

99. Darras JC: Isotopic and cytological assays in acupuncture. In Morton MA, Dlouhy C, editors: *Energy fields in medicine: a study of device technology based on acupuncture meridians and Chi energy*, Kalamazoo, Mich, 1989, The John E Fetzer Foundation.

100. Shang C: Singular point, organizing center, and acupuncture point, *Am J Chin Med* 17:119-127, 1989.

101. Swarup A, Stuchly SS, Surowiec A: Dielectric properties of mouse MCA1 fibrosarcoma at different stages of development, *Bioelectromagnetics* 12:1-8, 1991.

102. Smith SR, Foster KR, Wolf GL: Dielectric properties of VX-2 carcinoma versus normal liver tissue, *IEEE Trans Biomed Eng* 33:522-524, 1986.

103. Voll R: Twenty years of electroacupuncture diagnosis in Germany: a progress report, *Am J Acupunct* Special EAV edition 17(3):5-14, 1989.

104. Oleson TD, Kroening RJ, Bresler DE: An experimental evaluation of auricular diagnosis: the somatotopic mapping on musculoskeletal pain at ear acupuncture points, *Pain* 8:217-229, 1980.

105. Popp FA, Gurwitsch AA, Inaba H, et al: Biophoton emission, *Experientia* 44(7):543-600, 1988.

106. Aïssa J, Jurgens P, Litime MH, et al: Electronic transmission of the cholinergic signal, *FASEB J* 9:A683, 1995 (abstract).

107. Clackson T, Wells JA: A hot spot of binding energy in a hormone receptor interface, *Science* 267:383-386, 1995.

108. McDonald NOQ, Hendrickson WA: A structural superfamily of growth factors containing a cystine knot motif, *Cell* 73:421-424, 1993.

109. Debreceni L: The effect of electrical stimulation of the ear points on the plasma ACTH and GH level in humans, *Acupunct Electrother Res* 16:45-51, 1991.

110. Sorrentino V: Growth factors, growth inhibitors, and cell cycle control, *Anticancer Res* 9:1925-1936, 1989.

111. Brewitt B, Standish LJ: High dilution growth factors/cytokines: positive immunological, hematological, and clinical effects in HIV/AIDS patients, *Eleventh Intl Conf AIDS*, Vancouver, BC, Canada, July 7-12, 1996, pp 270-271.

112. Bellavite P, Signorini A: *Homeopathy: a frontier in medical science*, Berkeley, Calif., 1995, North Atlantic Press.

113. Brewitt B, Hughes J, Welsh EA, et al: Homeopathic human growth hormone for physiologic and psychologic health: three double-blind, placebo-controlled studies, *Alternative Complementary Therapies* 5(6):373-385, 1999.

114. Tucker SP, Thornton CL, Wimmer E, et al: Bidirectional entry of poliovirus into polarized epithelial cells, *J Virol* 67(1):29-38, 1993.

115. Christensen HH: A retrovirus uses a cationic amino acid transporter as a cell surface receptor, *Nutr Rev* 50(2):47-48, 1992.

116. Zong-Xiang Z: Research advances in the electrical specificity of meridians and acupuncture points, *Am J Acupunct* 9:203-216, 1981.

117. Voll R: *Topographic positions of the measurement points in electroacupuncture*, English ed 1, vols 1-4, plus suppl, Medizinisch Literarische Verlagsgesellschaft MBH, Uelzen, Germany, 1977, C Beckers Buchdruckerei GmbH & Co, KGM Sc. (Translated by H Schuldt).

118. Omura Y: Connections found between each meridian (heart, stomach, triple burner, etc.) and organ representation area of corresponding internal organs in each side of the cerebral cortex: release of common neurotransmitters and hormones unique to each meridian and corresponding acupuncture point and internal organ after acupuncture, electrical stimulation, mechanical stimulation (including shiatsu), soft laser stimulation, or Qigong, *Acupunct Electrother Res* 14:155-186, 1989.

119. Kendall DE: Understanding traditional energetic concepts. In Morton MA, Dlouhy C, editors: *Energy fields in medicine: a study of device technology based on acupuncture meridians and Chi energy,* Kalamazoo, Mich, 1989, The John E Fetzer Foundation.

120. Lu HC: *A complete translation of the yellow emperor's classic of internal medicine and the difficult classic,* Vancouver, Canada, 1978, Academy of Oriental Heritage.

121. Surowiec AJ, Stuchly SS, Keaney M, et al: Dielectric polarization of animal lung at radio frequencies, *IEEE Trans Biomed Eng* 34:62-66, 1987.

122. Van Benschoten MM: Acupoint biophoton diagnostics and HIV pathogenesis: a five-year review, *Am J Acupunct* 24(2/3):177-194, 1996.

123. ChuangY-M: *Chinese acupuncture,* Hanover, N.H., 1972, Oriental Publications (Translated by DK Skiu).

124. Chassee EE, Lytle IM: *Basic physiology and anatomy,* ed 4, Philadelphia, 1980, Lippincott-Raven Publishers.

125. Woolley-Hart A: The role of the circulation in measurements of skin conductivity, *Br J Dermatol* 87:213-226, 1972.

126. Buchbinder SP, Katz MH, Hessol NA, et al: Long-term HIV-1 infection without immunological progression, *AIDS* 8:1123-1128, 1994.

127. Fauci AS, Pantaleo G, Stanley S, et al: Immunopathogenic mechanisms of HIV infection, *Ann Intern Med* 124:654-663, 1996.

128. McCune JM: HIV-1: the infective process in vivo, *Cell* 64:351-363, 1991.

129. Stanley SK, McCune JM, Kaneshima H, et al: Human immunodeficiency virus infection of the human thymus and disruption of the thymic microenvironment in the SCID-hu mouse, *J Exp Med* 178:1151-1161, 1993.

130. Emilie D, Fior R, Crevon MC, et al: Cytokines from lymphoid organs of HIV-infected patients: production and role in the immune disequilibrium of the disease, *Res Immunol* 145(8-9):595-600, 1994.

131. Tsuei JJ, Lam FMK, Mi M, et al: Part II: Studies in bioenergetic correlations: study on bioenergy in diabetes mellitus patients, *Am J Acupunct* 17:31-38, 1989.

132. Anderson SB: The diagnosis and treatment of chronic fatigue syndrome with bioelectronic regulatory (BER) techniques, *Am J Acupunct* 16(3):225-234, 1988.

133. Bergsmann O, Woolley-Hart A: Differences in electrical skin conductivity between acupuncture points and adjacent skin areas, *Am J Acupunct* 1:27-32, 1973.

134. Langman L, Burr HS: A technique to aid in the detection of malignancy of the female genital tract, *Am J Obstet Gynecol* 57:274-281, 1949.

135. Burr HS, Smith GM, Strong LC: Electrometric studies of tumors induced in mice by the external application of benzpyrene, *Yale J Biol Med* 12:711-717, 1940.

136. Burr HS, Smith GM, Strong LC: Bioelectric properties of cancer-resistant and cancer-susceptible mice, *Am J Cancer* 32:240-248, 1938.

137. Reference deleted in proofs.

138. Tiller WA: What do electrodermal diagnostic acupuncture instruments really measure, *Am J Acupunct* 15:15-23, 1987.

139. Kobayashi T: Early diagnosis of microcancer by cancer check of related acupuncture meridian, *Am J Acupunct* 13:63-68, 1985.

140. Schepps JL, Foster KR: The UHF and microwave dielectric properties of normal and tumour tissues: variations in dielectric properties with tissue water content, *Phys Med Biol* 25:1149-1159, 1980.

141. Bottomly PA, Andrew ER: RF magnetic field penetration, phase shift, and power dissipation in biological tissue: implications for NMR imaging, *Phys Med Biol* 23:630-643, 1978.

142. Damadian R, Cope FW: NMR in cancer V: electronic diagnosis of cancer by potassium (^{39}K) nuclear magnetic resonance: spin signatures and T_1 beat patterns, *Physiol Chem Phys* 6:309-322, 1974.

143. Hazlewood CF, Change DC, Medina D, et al: Distinction between the preneoplastic and neoplastic state of murine mammary glands, *Proc Natl Acad Sci U S A* 69(6):1478-1480, 1972.

144. Mladejovsky MG: A computer-based brain stimulation system to investigate sensory prostheses for the blind and deaf, *IEEE Trans Biomed Eng* 23(4):286-296, 1976.

145. Dobelle WH, Mladejovsky MG: Phosphenes produced by electrical stimulation of human occipital cortex and their application to the development of a prosthesis for the blind, *J Physiol* 243(2):553-576, 1974.

146. Bach-y-Rita P, Collins CC, Saunders FA, et al: Vision substitution by tactile image projection, *Nature* 221(5184):963-965, 1969.

147. Standish L, Guiltinan J, McMahon E, et al: One-year open trial of naturopathic treatment of HIV infection Class IV-A in men, *J Naturopath Med* 3(1):42-64, 1992.

148. Sullivan SG, Eggleston DW, Martinoff JT, et al: Evoked electrical conductivity on the lung acupuncture points in healthy individuals and confirmed lung cancer patients, *Am J Acupunct* 13:261-266, 1985.

149. Feng Y, Broder CC, Kennedy PE, et al: HIV-1 entry cofactor: functional DNA cloning of a seven-transmembrane, G protein-coupled receptor, *Science* 272:872-877, 1996.

150. Alkhatib G, Combadiere C, Broder CC, et al: CC-CKR5: A RANTES, MIP-1α, MIP-1β receptor as a fusion cofactor for macrophage-trophic HIV-1, *Science* 272:1955-1958, 1996.

151. Balter M: A second co-receptor for HIV in early stages of infection, *Science* 272:1740, 1996.

152. Conklin BR, Bourne HR: Structural elements of Gα subunits that interact with Gβγ receptors and effectors, *Cell* 73(4):631-641, 1993.

153. Birnbaumer L: Receptor-to-effector signaling through G proteins: roles for βγ dimers as well as α subunits, *Cell* 71(7):1069-1072, 1992.

154. Rahmatullah M, Ginnan R, Robishaw J: Specificity of G protein α-γ subunit interactions, *J Biol Chem* 270:2946-2951, 1995.

155. Milligan G, Wakelam M, editors: *G proteins: signal transduction and disease,* New York, 1992, Academic Press.

156. Karin M: Signal transduction from cell surface to nucleus in development and disease, *FASEB J* 6:2581-2590, 1992.

157. Roush W: Regulating G-protein signaling, *Science* 27(5252):1056-1058, 1996.

158. Gilman AG: G Proteins: transducers of receptor-generated signals, *Ann Rev Biochem* 56:615-649, 1987.

159. Goodman EM, Greenebaum B, Marron MT: Magnetic fields after translation in *Escherichia coli, Bioelectromagnetics* 15:77-83, 1994.

References for Table 16-1

Adey WR: The cellular microenvironment and signaling through cell membranes, *Prog Clin Biol Res* 257:81-106, 1988.

Alberts B, Bray D, Lewis J, et al: *Molecular biology of the cell,* ed 2, New York, 1989, Garland Publishing, Inc.

Berridge MJ, Irvine RF: Inositol trisphosphate: a novel second messenger in cellular signal transduction, *Nature* 312:315-321, 1984.

Bistolfi F: Classification of possible targets of interaction of magnetic fields with living matter, *Panminerva Med* 29(1):71-73, 1987.

Byus CV, Lundak RL, Fletcher RM, et al: Alterations in protein kinase activity after exposure of cultured lymphocytes to modulated microwave fields, *Bioelectromagnetics* 5:34-37, 1984.

Cossarizza A, Monti D, Bersani F, et al: Extremely low-frequency pulsed electromagnetic fields increase cell proliferation in lymphocytes from young and aged subjects, *Biochem Biophys Res Commun* 160:692-698, 1989.

David SL, Absolom DR, Smith CR, et al: Effect of low-level direct current on in vivo tumor growth in hamsters, *Cancer Res* 45(11 pt 2):5625-5631, 1985.

Goodman EM, Greenebaum B, Marron MT: Magnetic fields after translation in *Escherichia coli, Bioelectromagnetics* 15:77-83, 1994.

Goodman R, Wei L-X, Xu J-C, et al: Exposure of human cells to low-frequency electromagnetic fields results in quantitative changes in transcripts, *Biochim Biophys Acta* 1009:216-220, 1989.

Lin H, Goodman R, Shirley-Henderson A: Specific region of the *c-myc* promoter is responsive to electric and magnetic fields, *J Cell Biochem* 54:281-288, 1994.

McLeod BR, Liboff AR: Dynamic characteristics of membrane ions in multifield configurations of low frequency EM radiation, *Bioelectromagnetics* 7:177-189, 1986.

Phillips JL, Haggren W, Thomas WJ, et al: Magnetic field-induced changes in specific gene transcription, *Biochim Biophys Acta* 1132:140-144, 1992.

Smith SD, McLeod BR, Liboff AR, et al: Calcium cyclotron resonance and diatom mobility, *Bioelectromagnetics* 8:215-227, 1987.

Sopory SK, Chandok MR: Light-induced signal transduction pathway involving inositol phosphates, *Blood Cell Biochem* 26:345-370, 1996.

Walleczek J: EM field effects on cells of the immune system: the role of calcium signaling, *FASEB J* 6:3177-3185, 1992.

Wilson BW, Stevens RG, Anderson LE, editors: *Extremely low frequency electromagnetic fields: the question of cancer,* Columbus, Ohio, 1990, Battelle Press.

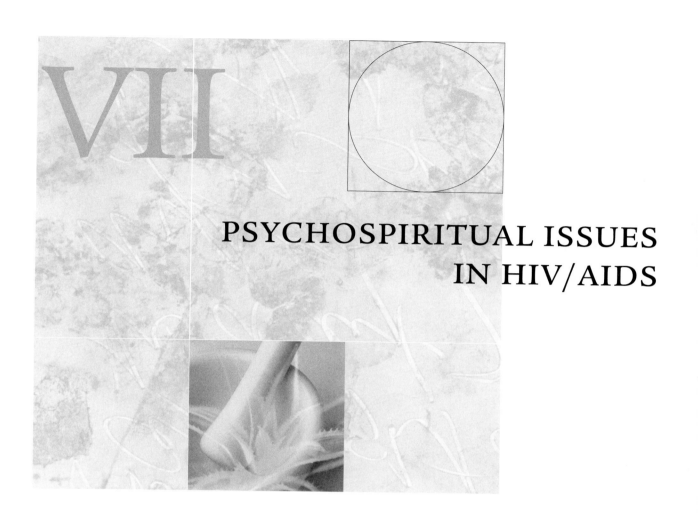

VII

PSYCHOSPIRITUAL ISSUES IN HIV/AIDS

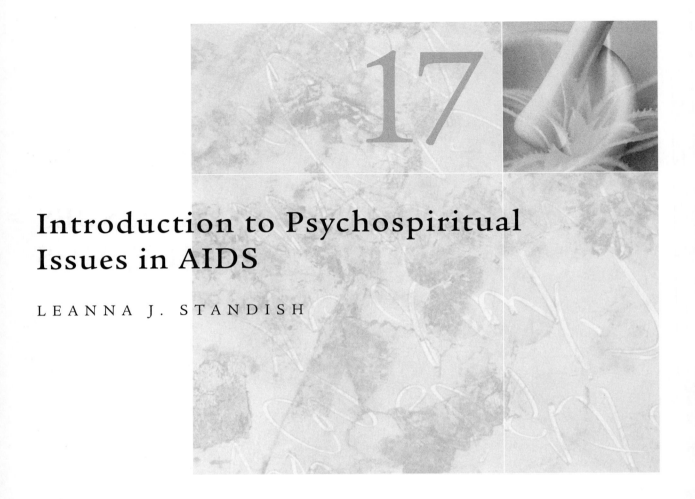

Introduction to Psychospiritual Issues in AIDS

LEANNA J. STANDISH

Receiving a diagnosis of a potentially life-threatening disease, such as AIDS or cancer, brings confrontation with one's mortality. In the face of death, most people experience fear, grief, loss, and anger. Some experience sublime transcendence. The very meaning and purpose of one's life is brought into question and review. Life-threatening disease, contemplating annihilation, and chronic suffering typically have a profound impact on one's spiritual orientation. The AIDS epidemic has been an impetus to a larger social movement in the United States that is reexamining the role of spirituality in health and illness. The health and psychological benefits of religiosity, spirituality, and a sense of meaning and purpose in life have been discussed widely in the United States since the 1960s. The AIDS epidemic accelerated this movement. Some proponents of the death and dying movement, which gained momentum during and partially as a result of the AIDS epidemic in the West, and the "near death experience" literature argue that there is some kind of life after death. When facing death, the question of whether some aspect of the self continues after biological death takes on an ontological urgency. Are the self and body one and the same? Can consciousness survive the death of the body? Data collected in preliminary well-designed, double-blinded, and statistically sound studies that are being performed in the Human Energy Systems Laboratory at the University of Arizona under the leadership of Gary Schwartz, PhD, and Linda Russek, PhD, suggest that some aspect of consciousness of deceased people may continue after biological death.

Early in the AIDS epidemic, Louise Hay and Elisabeth Kübler-Ross were two strong voices urging the

HIV-positive community to seek out a relationship with something beyond the self and to connect to experiences of the sacred. Kübler-Ross is well known for saying that death simply does not exist. We seem to be an entire culture now moving toward transcendence. AIDS helped get us there.

During the last decade, the scientific community began to examine and experiment with some of the fundamental concepts associated with spirituality. A number of theoretical physicists argue that data from quantum mechanical experiments validate some of the core precepts of Eastern mysticism.[1] Several popular and influential science writers, such as Fritzof Capra and Gary Zukav, point out the similarity between the conclusions about the nature of reality derived from two disparate fields—Eastern mysticism and quantum physics.[2,3] Scientific materialism is being questioned at a deep level. Many scientists who ask about the fundamental nature of reality are reexamining the basic tenet of materialistic biomedical science: that matter is primary and consciousness is an emergent epiphenomenon of matter in certain biological systems. Many philosophers and scientists, looking at the new data, conclude that consciousness, rather than matter, is primary in the universe. At the same time an increasing number of medical schools and hospitals are initiating spirituality and healing seminars and programs. The fundamental philosophy of monistic materialism that has dominated the biological sciences over the last 200 years is giving way to a modern form of monistic idealism. The fact of AIDS and the fact of many young people dying difficult deaths has changed the culture of biomedicine and made it more whole.

Prayer has become a topic of both casual and scientific conversation. Larry Dossey, MD, perhaps more than any other writer, brought the potential "power of" prayer and conscious intention to the attention of the scientific and medical community, as well as to the public.[4] The slowly growing literature on the remote effects of prayer begs a fascinating scientific question. Can internal biological and/or mental events, such as thoughts and emotions, influence external events and objects? Currently, the best overall review of the topic of "healing research" is by Daniel Benor.[5] His book describes the small but surprising number of controlled studies of the phenomenon in both in vitro and in vivo systems, including enzymes, one-celled yeast, bacteria, higher plants, and nonhuman and human animals. A systematic review of randomized clinical trials

(RCTs) in "distant healing" by Astin was published in 2000 by the *Annals of Internal Medicine.*[6] The study concludes that in a total of 23 published trials involving 2774 patients, 57% of the studies reported statistically significant findings with a mean effect size of 0.38. The authors conservatively suggest that the evidence warrants further investigation. A growing body of scientific data points to the notion that conscious intention can affect biological systems at a distance, and this may have far-reaching consequences for medicine.

One of the most interesting experiments in remote healing is the ongoing work of Elizabeth Targ, MD, in AIDS patients. Targ et al conducted a carefully designed study in which they ask if clinical outcomes can be altered by healers at a distance who have been assigned individual patients for whom they prayed on a daily basis.[7] The design of this experiment was meticulous. Subjects were 40 AIDS patients with CD4 T-cell counts below 200 and a history of at least one opportunistic infection (OI). These patients were stratified by severity of illness and randomized in a double-blind fashion to either the "healing group" or a control group. Forty experienced "healers" from many different traditions were given photographs and descriptions of subjects randomized to the healing group and asked to "direct intention for health and well-being" of the individual subjects to whom they have been assigned. The healers were assigned to the subjects on a rotating schedule, so that the subjects received healing intention for 1 hour per day, for 10 weeks, one at a time, from a total of 10 of the healers. All "healing" occurred at a distance, the subjects and healers never met, and subjects did not know to which group they had been assigned. Clinical, laboratory, and quality of life (QOL) outcome variables were measured at baseline and at the end of the 10-week experimental period.

Data from this small pilot study with a sample size of 20 in each group were sufficiently positive to warrant a larger study with major funding from the NIH. Dr. Targ and her group are now replicating their findings in a larger RCT with 150 HIV/AIDS patients currently receiving highly active antiretroviral therapy (HAART). The Bastyr University AIDS Research Center is collaborating with Targ's group to study the immunological correlates of measurable distant healing effects in this same group of study participants. Scientific evidence grows for the hypothesis that internal processes, such as thought or more specifically, silent prayer, can exert remote effects on biological systems, including humans.

Prayer and meditation are considered alternative therapies by many HIV-positive people. A full 58% of the Bastyr University cohort of HIV-positive men and women who use CAM report using prayer within the last 6 months as an alternative therapy for their illness, and 46% report using meditation as an alternative therapy. One of the goals of CAM research in HIV/AIDS is to discover if the use of prayer and meditation is associated with reduced morbidity and mortality (M&M). Do people who pray and/or meditate have either a longer life or a higher QOL than those who do not? What is the immunological and clinical impact of believing that consciousness survives biological death? The Bastyr University AIDS Research Center recently reported that the Alternative Medicine Care Outcomes in AIDS (AMCOA) cohort of 1036 HIV-positive men and women showed an association between the use of prayer and spiritual activities and improved self-reported mental health scores.[9]

Chapter 18 describes the rather large body of literature concerned with the psychospiritual dimension of coping with HIV infection and AIDS. Most studies investigate the relationship between spirituality/religiosity and psychological measures such as depression and anxiety. Fewer of the studies conducted in this area address the question of the relationship between spirituality and biomedical variables. What is the relationship between surrogate markers and spiritual maturity? Do Maslovian peak experiences or other types of transcendent experiences make a measurable biological difference? Do people who feel connected with a higher creative power in the universe maintain immunological health?

References

1. Goswami A: *The self-aware universe: how consciousness creates the material world,* New York, 1995, Jeremy P Tarcher.
2. Capra F: *The tao of physics: an exploration of the parallels between modern physics and eastern mysticism,* ed 3, Boston, 1991, Shambhala Publications.
3. Zukav G: *The dancing Wu Li masters: an overview of the new physics,* New York, 1994, Bantam Books.
4. Dossey L: *Healing words: the power of prayer and the practice of medicine,* New York, 1997, HarperCollins.
5. Benor DJ: *Healing research: holistic energy medicine and spirituality,* vol 1, Munich, 1992, Helix.
6. Astin J, Harkness E, Ernst E: The efficacy of "distant healing": a systematic review of randomized trials, *Ann Intern Med* 132:903-910, 2000.
7. Sicher F, Targ E, Moore D, et al: A randomized double-blind study of the effect of distant healing in a population with advanced AIDS, *West J Med* 169:356-363, 1998.
8. Schwartz G, Russek L: *The living energy universe,* Charlottesville, Va, 1999, Hampton Roads Publishing.
9. Standish LJ, Fitzpatrick A, Berger J, et al: Associations of mind-body interventions with quality of life in HIV-1-positive individuals, *Alternative Therapies* May/June, 2001.

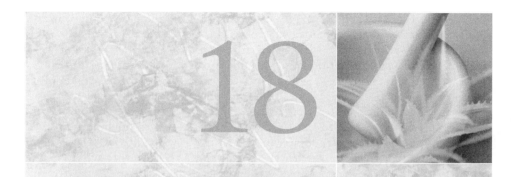

Psychospirituality and HIV/AIDS

A N N E E . B E L C H E R

As noted by Warner-Robbins and Christiana,[1] "Men, women, and children who have been diagnosed as having HIV/AIDS are confronted with many physical, psychological, sociological, and spiritual needs." Often, persons with HIV/AIDS first seek assistance for the spiritual aspect of their well-being. However, it is the spiritual aspect of a patient's care that is most often underemphasized or even overlooked.

Health care providers have not always been concerned with the care of the whole person—body, mind, and spirit. However, the devastation caused by HIV/AIDS has forced them to deal with those aspects of illness that are more elusive. Tibesar[2] notes that the distinctive nature of HIV/AIDS—transmissible, terminal, and stigmatizing—places an unusual burden on those who live with HIV disease and presents them with and health care providers with unique challenges. In addition, AIDS remains concentrated among the young, representing immeasurable cultural and economic losses. According to Carson et al,[3] this concentration challenges society "to examine persistent attitudes about sexuality, morality, the ministrations of compassion, acceptance of individual differences, and society's responsibility to deal with the suffering of its young." As Hinton observed,[4] younger persons are prone to be more anxious in terminal illness, since dying at an early stage of life disrupts many hopes, plans, and expectations. The person with HIV/AIDS is forced to confront existential issues such as a search for meaning, a purpose for the illness, and a clearer understanding of his or her place in the world.[5] Unresolved concerns and conflicts about life choices, as well as guilt regarding intravenous (IV) drug use or sexual activities that exposed them to HIV/AIDS, often compromise this task. Other complicating factors include low self-esteem, religious and social alienation and isolation, and public discrimination and condemnation.[6]

Travelbee[7] maintains that illness and suffering are spiritual encounters, as well as physical and emotional experiences. Travelbee[7] notes that the healthcare provider "must be prepared to assist individuals and families, not just to cope with illness and suffering, but to find meaning in these experiences." Care of the patient with HIV/AIDS poses a great challenge not only because of the severity of the disease and its treatment but also because of the patient's complex socioeconomic, educational, psychological, and spiritual needs.

Nursing has defined spiritual distress as "disruption in the life principle which pervades a person's entire being and which integrates and transcends one's biological and psychosocial nature."[8] The critical defining characteristic for this diagnosis is that it "expresses concern with meaning of life and death and/or belief systems." Health care providers working with persons with HIV/AIDS have often commented on the patients' discussion among themselves and with caregivers about their religious or spiritual experiences, involvement in faith healing, and other such activities in an effort to find meaning in and to maintain hope about their illness. In addition, a wide variety of publications for persons with HIV/AIDS include personal testimonials about spiritual issues and experiences, lists of spiritual healing groups and activities, and related articles.

Within a framework of holistic care, spirituality affects and is affected by psychosocial and physical domains. Thus one must help the patient explore his or her personal definition of spirituality, unique experiences as a person with HIV/AIDS, adequacy of support systems, and expectations of health care providers.

DEFINITIONS OF SPIRITUALITY

The 1971 White House Conference on Aging report included a definition of spirituality: "Man's inner resources, especially his ultimate concern, the basic value around which all other values are focused the central philosophy of life, which guides a person's conduct, the supernatural and nonmaterial dimension of human nature, including a person's need to find answers to questions about the meaning of life, illness, and death."[9] In contrast, religions are created to serve as a framework for a system of values, beliefs, rituals, and codes of conduct.

Reed[10] focuses on spirituality as an empirical indicator of the capacity for transcendence among terminally ill persons. Transcendence is defined as "a level of awareness that exceeds ordinary, physical boundaries and limitations," a crossing over or climbing beyond.[10] She believes that transcendent perspectives accrued throughout one's life, and especially during its last phases, may help one to maintain a sense of well-being when faced with the losses imposed by terminal illness. Reed perceives spirituality as personal views and behaviors that express a sense of relatedness to something greater than the self, which may include prayer, reading and contemplation, a sense of closeness to a higher being, and interactions with others. The relatedness "may be experienced intrapersonally (as a connectedness within oneself), interpersonally (in the context of others and the natural environment), and transpersonally (referring to a sense of relatedness to the unseen, God, or power greater than the self and ordinary resources.)"[11]

Colliton[12] defines spirituality as "the life principle that pervades a person's entire being, including volitional, emotional, moral-ethical, intellectual, and physical dimensions, and generates a capacity for transcendent values."[12] She believes that a person's spiritual dimension integrates and transcends his or her biological and psychosocial natures, which then gives the person access to such nonphysical realms as prophecy, love, artistic inspiration, and healing actions.

O'Brien[13] notes that a person is more direct in facing his or her spiritual side in times of crisis such as serious illness or possible death. "It is during such times that a person attempts to weigh and evaluate the essential and ultimate significance and intrinsic value of his life. . . ."[13] She defines spirituality as "that which inspires in one the desire to transcend the realm of the material."[13]

Hiatt[14] defines the spiritual dimension of an individual as that part "concerned with meaning" and thus a principal determinant of health-related attitudes and the worldview of both health care providers and patients. He further describes the spiritual dimension as focused on the search for "the absolute reality that underlies the world of the senses and the mind," which is reflected in the values one holds, one's sense of greater purpose, and the faith on which one's worldview and actions are based.[14] According to Hiatt,[14] faith is "a mental mechanism whereby the truth or no truth of events and their ascribed ultimate significance is ascertained by the mind." Thus faith plays an important role in the assignment of meaning. Spiritual development is a lifelong process that follows a cyclic and uneven course, with spiritual crises and encounters serving as nodal points. Assessment of a person's spiritual development includes the changes he or she has undergone, the issues being dealt with at the time, and the degree of unity in the personality.

According to Hiatt,[14] the relevant question regarding illness at a spiritual level is its purpose, not its mechanism. Illness is believed to occur because the self or spirit is seeking unity in one's being and needs to attract attention to factors that are preventing realization of that unity. By impairing the capacity to function, illness provides an opportunity for self-examination and initiation of changes that improve adaptation and promote unity.[14] Hiatt goes on to say that "suffering can be a powerful stimulus for perceiving the impermanence and relativity of certain percepts or life goals."[14] When people transcend suffering, they face it in clear perspective and then go beyond it to see the part of themselves that is not suffering and can still function and enjoy life.

Transcendence, as defined by Klass and Gordon,[15] is a "generalization of the many ways human beings have found to move beyond the banal, the profane, or the transitory into the meaningful, the sacred, or the eternal."[15] Transcendence during one's encounter with one's own death involves a transformation of perception, in that the problems of meaninglessness fear of nonbeing, and separation anxiety are overcome. Conrad[16] believes that transcendence is inherent in most forms of spirituality and becomes particularly important as one approaches the end of life. Peri[17] indicates "it is transcendence that restores wholeness to an individual after personal suffering." Smith[18] describes the relationship between transcendence and transformation as follows:

- One's field of perception is altered.
- The reality, significance, or importance of the facts is altered without changing the facts of present reality themselves.
- Present reality is changed intellectually.

Millison[19] notes that the terminally ill person experiences a crisis that "forces a redirection of emphasis away from career, success, and future." The person reviews life and begins to search for meaning and a sense of purpose. Millison defines spirituality as pertaining to the spirit or soul, as opposed to the physical nature. The spiritual dimension includes but is not confined to the religious because individuals can relate to some force beyond the self.

Vastyn[20] notes that life-threatening illness offers one of the few ways in which society sanctions a turning inward. Serious illness is considered justification for surrender of one's active side of life. Many persons do not seem able to experience this mode of living until illness strikes, thus the often-observed focus of the person with HIV/AIDS on self, illness, and the meaning of life and death, which occurs after the diagnosis has been made. Stark[21] defines three sources of meaning: (1) creative meaning, which is defined by accomplishment; (2) experiential meaning, which is based on personal experiences such as the birth of a child or the completion of a degree; and (3) attitudinal meaning, which involves assuming a positive attitude and deciding that fate cannot be changed.

Just as cancer "carries the indelible mark of our mortality"[20]—a stark reminder that individuals are subject to pain, suffering, and death—so does HIV/AIDS bring to the fore many questions about the meaning of life, purpose, value, and significance. In addition to the anticipated reactions of shock, denial, fear, and anger that accompany the diagnosis of AIDS, there is likely to be the spiritual phenomenon of profound personal crisis. The Greek meaning of *crisis* denotes a time for evaluation, judgment, and choice. This meaning may have particular relevance for the person with HIV/AIDS, who faces a time in life that marks a turning point, "one that inevitably involves change, one in which judgment and choice can be crucial."[20]

Epperly[22] identifies the following spiritual needs of persons with cancer that are also relevant to persons with HIV/AIDS:

- Relatedness, which is the need to feel that one has significance to those around them, particularly in light of changing roles and relationships
- Hope, which helps one to maintain the body's recuperative abilities
- Love, which one needs to give and receive

Clinebell[23] also defines spiritual need as the need for meaning and purpose in life, the need to give and receive love, and the need for hope and creativity. Wendle[24] indicates that HIV/AIDS "precipitates an unavoidable confrontation with one's own mortality" because death is a probable outcome. Many persons, he observed,[24] find strength in religion because they are seeking guidance, as opposed to their rather individualistic spirituality of the past." Warner-Robbins and Christiana[1] indicate that it is not uncommon for persons with AIDS (PWAs) to address issues never before confronted. "The spirituality of an individual is a special and private thing. It is absolutely critical that the individual spiritual beliefs of a PWA be respected at all times." The health care provider must never criticize, judge, or interpret the spiritual nature of the patient. As noted by Fortunato,[25] the spiritual issues that face the person with HIV/AIDS may be influenced by the mode of transmission of the disease. The PWA who is homosexual or bisexual may be faced with a religious reaction that blocks his or her efforts to meet spiritual needs. Much of Western religion has been so frightened by sexuality in general that it is repulsed by those whose sexuality is different. Gay persons may seek spiritual answers from the roots of their faith tradition rather than from the church.

Long-term survivors of HIV/AIDS have linked their personal well-being to their ability to respond to the existential challenge presented by the disease. These responses may include active participation in health care, involvement in HIV/AIDS activist organizations, support of other sufferers of HIV/AIDS, participation in research, and spiritual activities such as meditation, imagery, and prayer.

RELATED RESEARCH

Reed[26] examined the religious perspectives and sense of well-being of terminally ill adults who were ambulatory and not hospitalized. Fifty-seven terminally ill adults were matched with 57 healthy adults with regard to age, gender, education, and religious affiliation. The terminally ill subjects indicated significantly higher "religiousness" than did the healthy subjects. There was no difference between the groups in reported sense of well-being; however, there was a significant positive relationship between religiousness and well-being in the healthy group. A significant relationship existed between age and well-being in the terminally ill subjects, in which older terminally ill persons indicated a significantly higher sense of well-being than did younger persons. Reed recommended further study of terminally ill adults' potential for a sense of well-being. In a later study, Reed[10] surveyed three groups of adults: (1) 103 terminally ill hospitalized cancer patients, (2) 100 hospitalized patients who were not terminally ill, and (3)

100 healthy nonhospitalized persons. The groups were matched with regard to age, gender, years of education, and religious background. Terminally ill hospitalized adults indicated a greater spiritual perspective than either hospitalized adults who were not terminally ill or healthy nonhospitalized adults. There was also a positive relationship between spiritual perspective and well-being in the terminally ill hospitalized group.

Belcher, Dettmore, and Holzemer[27] found the theme of "connectedness" to others, both past and present, among a sample of 56 men with AIDS who were queried about their personal definitions of spirituality. Transcendence was expressed as "an ability now to observe life as a process." Religion was described as a framework that provided structure for spiritual concerns via rules, rituals, and traditions. Spiritual coping activities, such as meditating, reading spiritual literature, praying, and using guided imagery, were mentioned frequently, as was the value of social support from friends and significant others.

Warner-Robbins and Christiana[1] developed a questionnaire for the assessment of spiritual beliefs, issues, and concerns of PWA. Twenty-four forms (46% return rate) were analyzed. Findings were as follows: (1) respondents believed that a higher power cares for them as human beings; (2) respondents noted that although life has a worthwhile purpose, it was less important than just being alive; (3) respondents generally believed that gaining favor with a supreme being does not depend on attending religious services; (4) respondents believed that bad things have a purpose in their lives; (5) respondents felt that suffering for the purpose of gaining strength and belief in oneself had minimal value; (6) respondents felt that in no way were they being punished for a particular wrongdoing; (7) respondents felt that religious leaders provided less support to them than did the laity of their religious affiliation; (8) respondents felt strong support from their close friends; (9) respondents felt that involvement in a religious group was of lesser importance; (10) respondents felt it was very important to live according to their ethical beliefs; (11) respondents were unanimous in their answer to the question of the value of a clear conscience; (12) respondents indicated that they knew they were facing death; and (13) despite their present illness, respondents noted the presence of inner peace and their ability to identify a meaning and purpose for their lives. Although the sample size was small, these findings give health care providers many areas for further assessment and study.

Carson et al[3] studied a group of adult men with HIV/AIDS. More than 50% identified themselves as homosexual; another 17.5% were bisexual; and only five of the 65 subjects were IV drug users. This group of individuals was found to be both hopeful and spiritually well. The researchers believe that the patients' treatment in a large, well-known, and quite prestigious research center may have provided much of the hope they reported.

Perreault and Perreault[28] administered the Spiritual Orientation Inventory[29] to a convenience sample of 48 gay men living with HIV/AIDS and 47 men who indicated that they were HIV-negative and had never experienced a life-threatening illness. The groups differed significantly on transcendence, mission in life, sacredness of life, meaning in life, awareness, and idealism; these dimensions of spirituality were more important to gay men living with HIV/AIDS. Hall[30] interpreted the spiritual experiences of 10 men and women in advanced-stage HIV disease. Three themes were extracted: (1) purpose in life emerges from stigmatization; (2) opportunities for meaning arise from a disease without a cure; and (3) after suffering, spirituality frames the life.

SPIRITUAL ASSESSMENT

Health care providers often hesitate to ask patients about their spiritual well-being because they do not know how to conduct a spiritual assessment. Warner-Robbins and Christiana[1] indicate that a specific formula or an easy step-by-step model is unnecessary; rather, "what is important is that the patient be allowed to express his or her feelings and be granted an opportunity to talk." Questions should provide the patient with the "opportunity to share thoughts and feelings in an open and trusting manner" (Box 18-1). Kornfield[31] indicates that the way to a spiritual life centers on the following three questions, which could also provide the basis for a spiritual assessment: (1) did I love well, (2) did I live fully, and (3) did I learn to let go?

Piles[32] indicates that assessment skills necessary for the recognition of patients' spiritual needs include a listening ear and sensitivity to clues, such as noticing whether any religious articles are in the room or home and asking the patient about their significance. Another clue is listening to the patient who expresses a fear of dying (see Table 18-1 for other clues indicative of a spiritual need or crisis).

Guide to Assessing Spiritual Needs

When were you diagnosed with HIV?

How has HIV affected you, your family/significant others, and your everyday living?

Past experiences can affect present feelings. Do you have any memories of HIV?

Are you a member of any particular church? Do you have a religious background?

Do you have any religious practices? Have you been able to practice them now?

Who are your support systems? Are they available to you now?

How, if at all, has HIV affected what you believe?

Illness often compels a search for the meaning behind events; has HIV changed the meaning of your life?

What can we do to help you and yours?

Adapted from Carson VB: *Spiritual dimension of nursing practice*, Philadelphia, 1989, WB Saunders.

TABLE 18-1

Signs of Crisis from Patients in Spiritual Need

Spiritual need	Signs of crisis
Love	Expresses feelings of loss of faith
	Worries about separation from family at death
	Expresses guilt, shame, and anger with self or others
	Expresses loss of self-value and loneliness
	Expresses fear of dependence
Meaning	Expresses no reason to live
	Questions the meaning of suffering
	Expresses despair and detachment
Hope	Expresses fear of loss of control
	Denies reality of condition
	Depression
	Expresses lack of motivation
Dignity	Expresses anxiety about family roles
	Concern about inability to fulfill duties
	Fears loss of respect from others

Adapted from Johnson P: Spiritual health needs of oncology patients, *Nurs Interventions Oncol* 10:10, 1998.

SPIRITUAL INTERVENTIONS

Persons with HIV disease often want someone to assure them that it is not a sin to have this diagnosis and that this disease is not God's punishment against a person or group. Touch may be used to provide this assurance, since it is an important instrument of compassion and love.

Prayer is well received by many patients who have identified their need to communicate with God. Reading scripture may also be helpful, and patients may request a particular passage that brings them comfort. The value of distant prayer has received recent attention as well. Targ and Sicher[33] used 20 experienced healers who offered prayer or psychic healing on behalf of male volunteers with advanced AIDS. Results from the double-blind, randomized study are "highly promising."[34] Taylor and Gerszt[35] indicate that rituals such as prayer services held by and for persons with HIV/AIDS can bring a sense of unity by providing a link with the past and hope for the future.

Other activities that may help HIV-positive individuals include guided imagery, meditation, relaxation, Tai Chi, yoga, and other "mind-altering" strategies. Some persons with HIV/AIDS prefer reading religious or spiritual literature, attending healing or support groups that either address spiritual issues or incorporate spiritual practices, and participating in programs that serve others, such as Meals on Wheels.

Music and art are often soothing and healing to patients. Conducting a "life review" can help terminally ill patients recognize the significance of their lives; this process can be facilitated by sharing memories, photographs, and family stories.[36,37]

Referring the patient to a member of the clergy may be an appropriate intervention. Questions and challenges raised by PWAs and their family and significant others may require the professional guidance of a chaplain or another member of the clergy. The patient must give permission before this referral can be made.

Raleigh[38] believes that the individual who is without hope is in critical condition, because hope is a necessary condition for sustaining life. Limandri and Boyle[39] indicate that helplessness is frequently a precursor to hopelessness. Persons with HIV/AIDS undergo extensive tests and procedures and are exposed to complex equipment that invades their privacy, leading to perceived helplessness and loss of control. Although Marcel[40] claims that hope can be enhanced during times of personal trial and suffering, PWAs may not feel that the time they have after their diagnosis gives them much hope. However, for many persons, a belief in God is strongly linked to hope.[3] Religion offers one explanation for events that transcend one's own understanding.

Hall[41] focused on the experiences of men and women with HIV/AIDS via interviews. The participants identified four ways of maintaining hope: (1) miracles, (2) religion, (3) involvement in work or vocation, and (4) support of family and friends.

SOCIAL SUPPORT

Another important aspect of spiritual well-being is social support, which is correlated with increased survival time in terminally ill persons.[42] Evidence also exists that a nurturing social support network may have a positive effect on the immune system.[43,44] After a review of the literature on psychosocial variables and immunity, Jemmott and Locke[45] concluded that psychosocial factors, such as social support, interact with the human immune system in a positive way. Solomon[46] hypothesized that stress and psychosocial factors can influence the replication of HIV, the progression of AIDS, and length of survival. Solomon et al[47] reported that long-term AIDS survivors had more social support than did those who had a short survival time after their AIDS diagnosis.

As stated by McGough,[48] PWAs "often experience social stigma from family and friends, loss of lovers and significant others, loss of occupational and financial resources, denial of shelter and health care, and profound prejudice from society." Social abandonment may occur as a result of sexual abstinence, loss of significant others and friends who have died of AIDS, and alienation from natural parents and siblings.

Longo, Spross, and Locke[49] found "uncertainty of the future" among a sample comprised mostly of homosexual men, which was expressed in problems such as fear of dying, alienation from the church, and fear of being alone. Adaptive responses identified by these PWAs included reconciliation with church/religion, arrangements with friends and family for companionship, and use of coping strategies to increase hope and control. The researchers recommend that the health care provider elicit and document sources of support, among other interventions.

Assessment of social support is an essential first step in addressing the adequacy of and need for enhancement of the PWA's social network. The patient should list persons perceived to be in their network, which might include family members, friends, lovers, health care providers, employers, work associates, schoolmates, and neighbors. The next step in the process is evaluating the patient's perceptions of the network's availability and degree of supportiveness. These perceptions may be influenced by fear of stigma and prejudice, previous experiences (both positive and negative), fear of breach of confidentiality, cultural beliefs, costs, and expectations regarding the outcome of the illness.[48] Once the assessment is completed, the health care provider can assist the patient in identifying strengths and deficits in their social support system, with the emphasis on quality rather than quantity of perceived resources.

Goals that may be valuable to PWAs who have identified deficits in their social support network include (1) maintaining positive relationships, (2) nurturing the existing network, and (3) extending the network. Interventions by the health care provider that may be helpful to the patient in attaining these goals are (1) encouraging communication between the patient and members of the network; (2) helping the patient use appropriate resources for specific needs; (3) educating other health care providers to the social support needs of PWAs; (4) assisting the patient in contacting appropriate community resources; and (5) teaching the patient the anticipated course of illness and treatment. The size and quality of the social support network may change dramatically when the patient experiences a change in health status; the patient should be prepared to accept these changes and plan accordingly. For example, Di-Pasquale[50] notes the increasing number of support groups that have been established by agencies in an attempt to meet the psychospiritual needs of PWAs. Newmark[51] describes the effectiveness of such a group in providing strength and support for PWAs. Spector and Conklin[52] found that PWAs became strongly engaged with each other in group psychotherapy and experienced an easing of their distress. Ribble[53] suggests that some of the negative outcomes of stress and the anxiety of AIDS are reduced through support groups.

Individuals who are close to persons with HIV/AIDS may have their own spiritual questions and needs. Family members and significant others are often overlooked but also need the attention of spiritual leaders and health care providers. These individuals may ask, "Why is this happening to my loved one? Why is God doing this to us? What will others say? What am I going to do?" Often these persons do not want to hear specific words but instead want to vent their thoughts and feelings and to have someone listen to them and be available to them.[1]

OTHER ASPECTS OF SPIRITUAL CARE GIVING

Taylor[54] raises the ethical concern related to spiritual care giving: "How does (one) discuss spiritual or religious beliefs while being beneficent and respecting the autonomy of the patient?" She indicates that several factors contribute to this concern. Patients and their significant others or families are in a vulnerable position because of the nature of the illness; that is, persons with HIV/AIDS are physically, emotionally, and spiritually vulnerable. In addition, health care providers are socialized to behave as interventionists; that is, they may perceive themselves to be more knowledgeable than their patients regarding the "right thing to do." Health care providers often share their personal spiritual beliefs because of a sense of obligation to inform patients, a sense of duty to evangelize or "save" them, and a desire to comfort them. Health care providers may also share their beliefs in an effort to role-model the expression of honest feelings. In turn, patients may ask health care providers about their beliefs as a way of coping by seeking information. They may need to conduct what Taylor[54] calls a *safety check* to see if they will be secure in discussing such issues with the caregiver. She provides the following suggestions for dealing with this issue in an ethical manner:

- Balance the patient's autonomy with one's expertise and involvement or provide existential advocacy.
- Strive to maintain symmetry in one's relationships with patients.
- Question one's motivation when tempted to share personal spiritual beliefs.
- Follow the "Golden Rule" or proverbs that instruct one to consider how it would be to "walk in someone else's shoes."
- Consider developing answers to questions about personal spiritual beliefs that are broad enough to reflect agreement about some essential belief.

AREAS FOR FURTHER RESEARCH

The increasing interest in psychoneuroimmunology (PNI) has raised questions about its role in the resistance to HIV/AIDS and its value in long-term survival. O'Leary[55] suggests that different PNI processes may prevail at different stages of disease, thus researchers should explore factors that influence the impact of different interventions on patient outcome. These intervention studies may include the consequences of spiritual coping strategies for persons with HIV/AIDS. Kiecold-Glaser and Glaser[56] believe that a variety of health behaviors affect the role that PNI plays in resistance and response to illness—sleep, smoking, recent weight change, current health status, prescription medications, alcohol or drug use, caffeine intake—to which one could add psychological and spiritual status. Pelletier[57] also suggested that psychosocial interventions should be evaluated as tools for preventing or slowing the progression of HIV/AIDS.

Related areas for study that reflect anecdotal evidence or research cited here include but are not limited to the following:

- The value of suffering as perceived by the patient
- The relative importance of the support of religious leaders and the laity
- The types, quality, and quantity of social support perceived as useful to the patient
- Sources of hope

SUMMARY

There is no doubt that persons with HIV/AIDS face tremendous psychospiritual challenges during their experiences with the disease. The use of spiritual assessment and interventions, maintaining hope, and strengthening social support can make the journey less difficult and more rewarding. Ongoing research linking enhancement of PNI with spiritual coping strategies is essential.

References

1. Warner-Robbins CG, Christiana NM: The spiritual needs of persons with AIDS, *Fam Commun Health* 2:43-51, 1989.
2. Tibesar L: Pastoral care: helping patients on an inward journey, *Health Progress* 67:41-47, 1986.
3. Carson V, Soeken KL, Shanty J, et al: Hope and spiritual well-being: essentials for living with AIDS, *Perspect Psychiatr Care* 26:28-34, 1990.
4. Hinton J: *Dying*, Baltimore, 1972, Penguin Books.
5. Moynihan R, Christ G, Gallo-Silver L: Psychosocial, spiritual, and bereavement issues in the treatment of terminally ill people with AIDS, *Conference Proceedings from a North American Conference on Care of Terminally Ill Persons with AIDS*, Ottawa, 1987.
6. Kayal P: "Morals," medicine, and the AIDS epidemic, *J Religion Health* 24:218-235, 1985.
7. Travelbee J: *Interpersonal aspects of nursing*, Philadelphia, 1987, FA Davis.
8. Kim M, McFarland G, McLane A: *Pocket guide to nursing diagnoses*, St Louis, 1995, Mosby.
9. Moberg D: *Spiritual well-being: background and issues of the technical committee on spiritual well-being*, White House Conference on Aging, Washington, DC, 1971, US Government Printing Office.
10. Reed I: Spirituality and well-being in terminally ill hospitalized adults, *Res Nurs Health* 10:335-344, 1987.
11. Reed I: An emerging paradigm for the investigation of spirituality in nursing, *Res Nurs Health* 15:349-357, 1992.
12. Colliton M: The spiritual dimension of nursing. In Beland I, Possos J, editors: *Clinical nursing: pathophysiological and psychosocial approaches*, New York, 1981, Macmillan.
13. O'Brien M: The need for spiritual integrity. In Yura H, Walsh M, editors: *Human needs 2 and the nursing process*, Norwalk, Conn., 1982, Appleton-Century-Crofts.
14. Hiatt J: Spirituality, medicine, and healing, *South Med J* 79:736-742, 1986.
15. Klass D, Gordon A: Varieties of transcending experience at death: a videotape-based study, *Omega* 9:19, 1978.
16. Conrad NL: Spiritual support for the dying, *Nurs Clin North Am* 20:415-426, 1985.
17. Peri T-AC: Promoting spirituality in persons with acquired immunodeficiency syndrome: a nursing intervention, *Holistic Nurs Pract* 10:68-76, 1995.
18. Smith H: The reach and the grasp: transcendence today. In Richardson H, Cutler D, editors: *Transcendence*, Boston, 1969, Beacon Press.
19. Millison M: Spirituality and the caregiver, *Am J Hospice Care* 2:37, 1988.
20. Vastyn E: Spiritual aspects of the care of cancer patients, *CA Cancer J Clin* 36:110-114, 1986.
21. Starck PL: The human spirit: the search for meaning and purpose through suffering, *Hum Med* 8:132-137, 1992.
22. Epperly J: The cell and the celestial: spiritual needs of cancer patients, *J Med Assoc Ga* 72:374-376, 1983.
23. Clinebell H: *Basic types of pastoral counseling: new resources for ministering to the troubled*, New York, 1966, Abington.
24. Wendler K: Ministry to patients with acquired immunodeficiency syndrome: a spiritual challenge, *J Pastoral Care* 41:7, 1987.

25. Fortunato J: AIDS: *the spiritual dilemma,* San Francisco, 1987, Harper & Row.

26. Reed P: Religiousness among terminally ill and healthy adults, *Res Nurs Health* 9:35-41, 1986.

27. Belcher AE, Dettmore D, Holzemer SP: Spirituality and sense of well-being in persons with AIDS, *Holistic Nurs Pract* 3:16-25, 1989.

28. Perreault LT, Perreault M: A comparative study on the spirituality of men living with and without HIV/AIDS, *Int Conf AIDS* 11:404, 1996 (online abstract no. Tu.D.2834).

29. Elkins D, Hedstrom L, Hughes L, et al: Toward a humanistic-phenomenological spirituality: definition, description, and measurement, *J Humanistic Psychol* 28(4):5-18, 1988.

30. Hall A: Patterns of spirituality in persons with advanced HIV disease, *Res Nurs Health* 21:143-153, 1983.

31. Kornfield J: *A path with heart,* New York, 1993, Bantam Doubleday Dell.

32. Piles CL: Providing spiritual care, *Nurse Educator* 5:36-41, 1990.

33. Targ E: Evaluating distant healing: a research review, *Altern Ther Health Med* 3(6):74-78, 1997.

34. Schlitz MJ, Lewis N: The healing powers of prayer, *Noetic Sci Rev* 29-32, 1996.

35. Taylor PB, Gerszt GG: Spiritual healing, *Holistic Nurs Pract* 4:32-38, 1990.

36. Doka IJ: The spiritual needs of the dying. In Doka KJ, Morgan JD, editors: *Death and spirituality,* Amityville, N.Y., 1993, Baywood.

37. Burns S: The spirituality of dying, *Health Progress* 72: 48-54, 1991.

38. Raleigh E: An investigation of hope as manifested in the physically ill adult, *Dissertation Abstracts International* 41:1313-B, 1980.

39. Limandri B, Boyle D: Instilling hope, *Am J Nurs* 78:79-80, 1978.

40. Marcel G: *Homo viator: introduction to a metaphysic of hope,* Gloucester, Mass, 1963, Peter Smith.

41. Hall A: Ways of maintaining hope in HIV disease, *Res Nurs Health* 17:283-293, 1994.

42. Weisman A, Worden J: Psychosocial analysis of cancer deaths, *Omega* 6:61-75, 1975.

43. Pilisuk M, Froland C: Kinship, social networks, social support, and health, *Soc Sci Med* 12B:273-280, 1978.

44. Pilisuk M: Delivery of social support: the social inoculation, *Am J Orthopsychiatry* 52:20-31, 1982.

45. Jemmot J, Locke S: Psychosocial factors, immunologic mediation, and human susceptibility to infectious diseases: how much do we know? *Psychol Bull* 1:78-108, 1984.

46. Solomon G: Psychoneuroimmunologic approaches to research on AIDS, *Ann N Y Acad Sci* 496:628-636, 1987.

47. Solomon G, Temoshok L, O'Leary A, et al: An intensive psychoimmunologic study of long-surviving persons with AIDS, *Ann N Y Acad Sci* 496:647-655, 1987.

48. McGough KN: Assessing social support of people with AIDS, *Oncol Nurs Forum* 17:31-35, 1990.

49. Longo MB, Spross JA, Locke, AM: Identifying major concerns of persons with acquired immunodeficiency syndrome: a replication, *Clin Nurs Specialist* 4:21-26, 1990.

50. DiPasquale JA: The psychological effects of support groups on individuals infected by the AIDS virus, *Cancer Nurs* 13(5):278-285, 1990.

51. Newmark DA: Review of a support group for patients with AIDS, *Top Clin Nurs* 6:38-44, 1984.

52. Spector LC, Conklin R: AIDS group therapy, *Int J Group Psychother* 37:433-439, 1987.

53. Ribble D: Psychosocial support groups for people with HIV infection and AIDS, *Holistic Nurs Pract* 3:52-62, 1989.

54. Taylor EJ: Is sharing personal spiritual beliefs proselytizing or ethical spiritual caregiving? *Spiritual Care Special Interest Group Newsletter* 9:3, 1988.

55. O'Leary A: Stress, emotion, and human immune function, *Psychol Bull* 108:363-382, 1990.

56. Kiecold-Glaser JK, Glaser R: PNI: Can psychological interventions modulate immunity? *J Consult Clin Psychol* 60:569-575, 1992.

57. Pelletier KR: Mind-body health: research, clinical, and policy applications, *Am J Health Promotion,* 6:345-358, 1992.

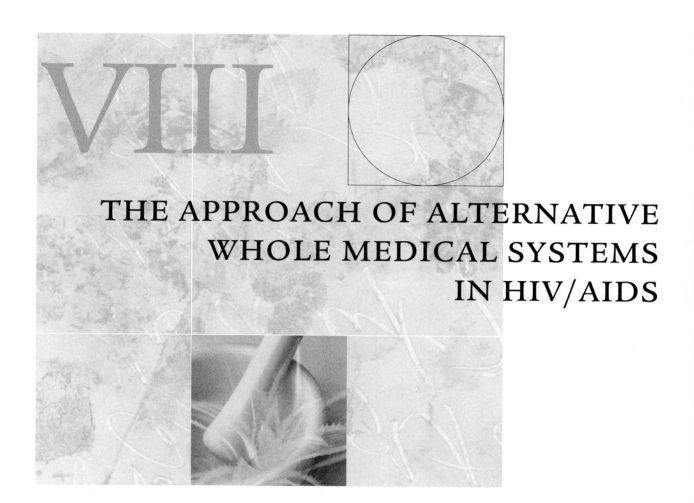

VIII

THE APPROACH OF ALTERNATIVE WHOLE MEDICAL SYSTEMS IN HIV/AIDS

19

Introduction to Alternative Medical Systems and AIDS

LEANNA J. STANDISH

An examination of alternative medicine must evaluate the impact that diverse alternative medical systems have had on the AIDS epidemic. A system of medicine may be defined as any set medical practice that has some defined theory of the causes and treatment of disease. Another important characteristic of medical systems is that in general they provide health care to a particular community. Globally, there are many medical systems in current practice. Which medical systems are considered "alternative" depends on the culture from which one views them. What is considered traditional medicine in many countries is what the industrialized world calls alternative medicine. Molecular medicine is an overarching term for the conventional Western medical system, although it is not the only the dominant molecular medical system of industrialized

nations that has provided health care for people with AIDS. Chinese medicine, Ayurvedic medicine, naturopathic medicine, and others are distinct medical systems with a distinct community of practitioners that have intervened in the AIDS epidemic. During the past 15 years, these systems of medicine have been practiced with greater prevalence and frequency, especially in the United States.

It would be fascinating to know if any of the traditional herbal medical systems that provide care to HIV-positive persons in Africa, Asia, and South America are capable of altering the markers that molecular medicine uses to track HIV progression: CD4+ T-cell count, viral load, and progression to AIDS rates. In the United States, two alternative medical systems, Chinese medicine and naturopathic medicine, "stepped up to the plate" early in the AIDS epidemic. Chapters 20 and 21 present the diagnostic and treatment methods used by two very different alternative medical systems. Chinese medicine originates from Asia and Asian philosophical views regarding the disease process and death. Chinese medicine and its underlying philosophy of medicine has a 2000-year history. Naturopathic medicine is far newer in the history of medicine, with at most a 200-year history. Historically, modern naturopathic medicine derives its core philosophy and methods from nineteenth century "nature cure" doctors in northern Europe. There has been a resurgence of interest in and practice of naturopathic medicine in the United States since the late 1970s.

The basic tenet of naturopathic medicine is a faith in the healing power of nature, *"vis medicatrix naturae,"* and the use of natural methods to treat disease, including plant medicines, hydrotherapy, homeopathy, nutritional medicine, and psychological counseling. Naturopathic doctors (NDs) are currently licensed in 13 US states. In several states, NDs are considered primary care physicians with third-party reimbursement. Modern naturopathic medicine has focused on using natural approaches to bring biochemical and physiological processes into homeostasis. Naturopathy, as taught in universities and colleges (four in the United States and one in Canada), is science-based natural medicine and thus has increasingly a molecular focus.

Chinese medicine does not refer to molecules at all. Naturopathic medicine does but uses natural, low-force methods for attaining biochemical changes that restore health. Many alternative medicine practitioners, including the authors of this book and the HIV-positive clinicians who treat patients who use these methods, would like to know if naturopathy or Chinese medicine offers useful medical care. More and more insurance companies and HMOs are asking if either of these systems of medicine have value in treating and managing HIV disease. Chapters 20 and 21 address that question.

Many living systems of medicine are currently in use in the world today. An incomplete list includes Chinese medicine, naturopathic medicine, homeopathy, herbal medicine, Shamanism, Tibetan medicine, Ayurvedic medicine, chiropractic medicine, and osteopathy. Naturopathic and Chinese medicine are covered here because many naturopathic physicians and Chinese medicine practitioners in the United States offered assistance to HIV-positive people in the gay, bisexual, African-American, Hispanic, and intravenous (IV) drug user communities. As early as 1984, small clinics were open to AIDS patients in most of the coastal US cities where AIDS cases were of frightening proportions. These clinics provided acupuncture, botanical medicine, nutritional supplements, body work, and group support.

Both the Chinese and naturopathic medical communities established centers for HIV alternative medicine care. Small research groups formed in Portland, Oregon; New York City; Chicago; San Francisco; and Seattle. Research was begun to examine efficacy. However, early on in the epidemic neither the naturopathic nor Chinese medical communities had the technical and financial resources to carry out controlled clinical trials. Nearly 15 years have passed, and much has been learned by acupuncturists, Chinese herbalists, and naturopathic physicians.

The following chapters review the diagnostic and treatment approach of two alternative systems of HIV/AIDS care and summarize the research that either underlies or validates the methods. As will be shown, there is a growing body of literature that suggests that these methods have value in the treatment and management of HIV disease. The preliminary evidence that Chinese medicine is helpful in treating several HIV-related conditions is stimulating for another reason: It suggests that the molecular model of conventional medicine is woefully incomplete.

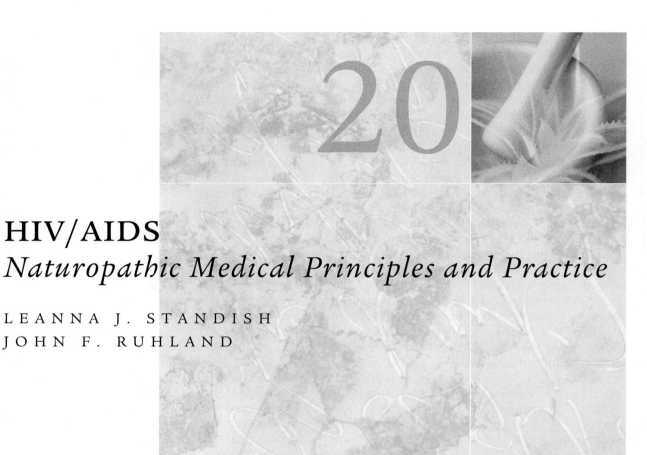

HIV/AIDS
Naturopathic Medical Principles and Practice

LEANNA J. STANDISH
JOHN F. RUHLAND

*A*IDS is a complex, multifactorial disease that has both immunodeficiency and autoimmune inflammatory aspects involving multiple systems of the body (e.g., immune, gastrointestinal (GI), genitourinary (GU), endocrine, dermatological, and nervous systems). Conventional medical management of HIV/AIDS revolves around two treatment principles: (1) inactivate or slow replication of HIV and (2) provide antibiotic prophylaxis for patients with abnormally low CD4+ T-cell counts. Naturopathic medical management revolves around several treatment principles that should guide the naturopathic physician in helping patients optimize their health, slow disease progression, improve quality of life (QOL), and possibly improve immune function.

FOCUS

This chapter is written for the naturopathic physician and other alternative medicine providers, although conventionally trained physicians may find the perspective, treatment principles, and some treatment suggestions useful. The field of HIV/AIDS medicine is rapidly changing. A dramatic change in the management of patients with HIV infection occurred in March 1996, when combination antiretroviral pharmaceutical therapy, which included protease inhibitors (PIs), was introduced. AIDS deaths have decreased dramatically in the last year with the introduction of highly active antiretroviral drug therapy (HAART). Conventional medical research has produced a breakthrough in drug therapy that lowers HIV replication as measured by reduction in HIV RNA viral load levels, and the lowering of viral replication appears to reduce morbidity and mortality (M&M) associated with HIV infection. HAART may also have benefit in immune restoration after long-term use in some patients. Nevertheless, complete immune restoration to pre-HIV levels has not yet been achievable. A central premise of naturopathic medicine and naturopathic medical research is that natural interventions may have an immunological impact and lead to slowed disease progression and improved QOL by optimizing immune and physiological function.

Although the International AIDS Conference was dominated in 1996 by the news that combination therapy with PIs was producing significant clinical benefits, interest in alternative medicine was high. Concerns continue to be expressed about the inaccessibility of expensive antiretroviral drug combinations to more than 90% of the world's HIV-positive people. Considerable interest and political action has focused on less expensive and more accessible alternative treatments, such as herbal medicines.

NATUROPATHIC TREATMENT PRINCIPLES

Conventional medical treatment for HIV infection and AIDS has two goals, or treatment principles: (1) inactivate the virus and (2) prevent opportunistic infections (OIs) through antibiotic prophylaxis. Naturopathic medicine takes a more comprehensive approach to the problem. The following nine treatment principles have been articulated and applied:
1. Reduce oxidant stress using antioxidants.
2. Optimize nutritional status by (a) improving GI nutrient absorption and mucosal integrity, (b) eliminating food allergens, (c) optimizing GI ecology, (d) eliminating GI pathogens, and (e) providing optimal therapeutic and dietary nutrition.
3. Eliminate cofactors (cofactor viruses, sexually transmitted diseases [STDs], and their residual, possibly miasmatic effects, as well as other pathogenic cofactors).
4. Provide botanical and hydrotherapeutic antiviral (AV) therapy.
5. Provide immunomodulation using botanical, nutritional, and hydrotherapeutic therapies.

6. Improve oxidation of tissues and manage stress through exercise.
7. Institute OI prophylaxis.
8. Provide a plan for psychoneuroimmunological (PNI) support.
9. Decrease toxicity and counter side effects for patients receiving pharmaceutical drugs (e.g., prophylactic antibiotics, antiretroviral drugs).

Diagnosis

A full naturopathic medical evaluation of HIV-infected patients requires additional history taking and testing beyond what is typically done in the conventional setting.

Health History

In addition to the standard medical history, it is important to obtain information about the factors listed in Box 20-1.

BOX 20-1

History of Sexually Transmitted Diseases in Chronological Order

- History of mononucleosis
- History of antibiotic courses for childhood and adult infections, including STDs
- Vaccination history and adverse reactions to vaccines
- History of cofactor viruses in chronological order (EBV; herpes I, II, 6, and 8; hepatitis A, B, and C; HPV; CMV)
- History of vaginal and GI yeast infections
- History of genital or anal warts and abnormal Pap smears
- Detailed 24-hour diet history ("Choose a typical day and tell me exactly what you ate and drank.")
- Exercise pattern
- History of psychoemotional trauma and issues (abuse history, anxiety, depression)
- Nature of the patient's spiritual life, if any, and felt purpose of the patient's life

CMV, Cytomegalovirus; *EBV*, Epstein-Barr virus; *GI*, gastrointestinal; *HPV*, human papilloma virus; *Pap*, Papanicolaou test, *STDs*, sexually transmitted diseases.

Laboratory Assessment

Box 20-2 lists the blood work essential for a full naturopathic evaluation of each HIV-positive patient.

Are There Risks of HIV Infection to Health Care Workers?

Some health care providers who are new to the field of HIV/AIDS health care have concerns about their safety. For those naturopathic physicians and CAM practitioners who have yet to treat HIV-positive patients, it is important to know that the risk of HIV infection from accidental needle sticks in the routine care of HIV-positive patients is relatively small. Nevertheless, it is important to follow standard safety procedures. Prospective studies indicate that the estimated risk for HIV infection after a percutaneous exposure to HIV-infected blood is approximately 0.3%.[1] Compare this

---

BOX 20-2

Essential Laboratory Assessments

Conduct These Assessments
- CBC with platelet count and ESR
- Full fasting chemistry and lipid panel (triglycerides, HDL, LDL)
- T and B lymphocyte/NK cell subsets (immune panel that includes $CD3^+$, $CD4^+$, $CD8^+$, $CD19^+$, and $CD56^+$ subsets)
- NK cell functional activity assay
- HIV RNA viral load
- DHEA (serum)
- Urinalysis with microscopic analysis (especially important in patients who are taking certain protease inhibitors)
- Serum *Candida* antibodies (IgA, IgG, IgM) and *Candida* antigen when available
- MAI blood culture if CD4 count is lower than 100 cells/ml
- Serum vitamin B_{12} (or methyl malonic acid) and folate
- For women, a recent Pap read by a thorough cytopathologist (i.e., in addition to the standard classification of cervical cells, the pathologist should look for and report koilocytotic changes, as well as make an assessment of bacterial dysbiosis)

CBC, Complete blood count; *DHEA,* dehydroepiandrosterone; *ESR,* erythrocyte sedimentation rate; *HDL,* high-density lipoprotein; *IG,* immunoglobulin; *LDL,* low-density lipoprotein; *MAI, Mycobacterium avium-intracellulare; NK,* natural killer; *Pap,* Papanicolaou test.

---

with the incidence of hepatitis C virus (HCV) seroconversion in health care workers reporting an occupational exposure in the 2 years between January 1992 and December 1993: There were 331 (51%) hollow-bore needle sticks, 105 (16.5%) suture needle or sharp object injuries, 85 (13%) mucous membrane contaminations, and 125 (19.5%) skin contaminations reported. Four HCV seroconversions were observed after hollow-bore needle sticks (1.2%; 95% CI 0.3% to 3.0%); no seroconversions occurred after other routes of exposure.[2] Although the exact numbers are unknown, many HIV-positive people are also coinfected with HCV.

Therapeutic Considerations

For each of the naturopathic treatment principles, the following therapeutic suggestions to attain each goal are described, including the scientific rationale for each treatment recommendation. This is not a protocol list, but suggestions only. Clinical management of HIV/AIDS is a rapidly changing field, and new ideas emerge and old ideas disappear rather quickly. One must individualize treatment. Although we have attempted to avoid naming specific products or companies, occasionally this is unavoidable, since the products are unique and available only by trade name through particular manufacturers. The Bastyr University Center for Natural Health in Seattle is a valuable resource for information on quality natural medicines.

A caveat: This chapter describes not only the published science for naturopathic medicines currently used by HIV-positive patients but also natural therapies that have been found to be useful in helping our patients. Not all of the treatments described in this chapter have been evaluated in clinical trials. Some researchers may argue that it is inappropriate to include such therapies in either a treatment or a book on AIDS treatment that is science-based. However, we decided to include some therapies that have no published data to support their use in medical management but nevertheless have proven to be safe and useful over the years.

Core Protocol

Although individualized treatment is essential to naturopathic management, patients are typically started on a core protocol that includes the following:
- Beta-carotene: 150,000 IU/day
- Vitamin C: 2000 mg tid

- Vitamin E: 400 IU bid
- Vitamin B complex: 1 capsule with breakfast
- Cod liver oil: 1 tablespoon/day
- Multiple vitamin and mineral supplement: 2 capsules bid with breakfast and lunch. If HIV viral load is high, vitamin supplementation without iron is wise.
- Balanced whole foods diet, modified as necessary (high fiber and complex carbohydrates, moderate fat and protein, low refined carbohydrates and sugar)
- Aerobic exercise: minimum 20 minutes 3 times/week
- Sleep/rest: minimum 8 to 10 hours daily
- Co-enzyme Q_{10}: 30 mg tid between meals
- SPV-30: 1 capsule tid if HIV viral load is detectable and/or if the patient has refused antiretroviral therapy (ART)
- Maitake mushroom extract: 10 drops bid
- *Glycyrrhiza glabra* (licorice) solid extract: ¼ to ½ tsp bid between meals

The scientific rationale for each item in the core protocol is provided in the following sections.

Treatment Principle 1: Antioxidant Therapy to Reduce Oxidative Stress

Oxidative stress may contribute to several aspects of HIV disease pathogenesis and progression, such as viral replication, inflammation, decreased immune cell proliferation, loss of immune function, apoptosis, weight loss, and increased drug toxicities. Since HIV-infected people are immunosuppressed, they are susceptible to inflammatory responses induced by oxidative stress resulting from exposure to viral and opportunistic pathogens and drugs. Inflammation is associated with the formation of reactive oxygen intermediates (ROIs), the secretion of cytokines such as IL-1, IL-2, and IL-6, granulocyte-macrophage colony-stimulating factor (GM-CSF), and tumor necrosis factor (TNF-α, TNF-β). HIV-positive patients have increased levels of TNF-α and IL-6 in their serum.[3] Even asymptomatic HIV-positive patients show elevated sedimentation rates.[4]

Evidence for oxidative damage in HIV-infected patients is provided by the finding that malondialdehyde (MDA), a by-product of lipid peroxidation (LP), is increased in HIV infection[5] and may play a role in stimulation of HIV replication. Allard et al measured antioxidant vitamin serum levels (e.g., vitamin C, vitamin E, and selenium) and found significantly lower concentrations compared with HIV-negative controls.[6] Lipid peroxides and breath pentane and ethane output were higher in HIV-positive patients. The authors concluded that HIV-positive patients have increased oxidative stress and a weakened antioxidant defense system. Breath alkanes, plasma lipid peroxides, and MDA are markers of oxidative stress in HIV disease, and Aghdassi and Allard reported that supplementation with vitamins C and E reduced these LP markers in HIV-positive patients.[7] Ample evidence now exists that oxidative stress is increased in HIV disease, and a smaller but growing body of data suggest that oral administration of antioxidant micronutrients have a beneficial role in medical management of HIV disease. The goal of antioxidant therapy is to quench free radicals (FRs) or ROIs produced by inflammation.

Beta-Carotene

HIV-infected people, including children and women, have been shown to have lower blood levels of beta-carotene (50,000 to 150,000 IU/day).[8,9] Some preliminary evidence shows that supplementation above the RDA level has immunological and clinical benefits.

Significantly lower plasma levels of carotenoids, including lutein, cryptoxanthin, lycopene, alpha-carotene, and beta-carotene, as well as vitamin C and cholesterol, have been found in HIV-positive patients.[8] Serum beta-carotene deficiency has also been reported in HIV-infected children, and it is even more pronounced in children with AIDS.[10] Serum vitamin A and beta-carotene are decreased in HIV-1-infected pregnant women in the first trimester who have CD4+ T-cell counts lower than 200.[11] Low blood levels of vitamins A (18%), E (27%), riboflavin (26%), B6 (53%), and B12 (23%), together with copper (74%) and zinc (50%) have been documented in HIV-1-positive patients.[12] Even asymptomatic patients may have a severe beta-carotene deficiency. Carotene deficit and an associated increase in FRs are potentially harmful, suppressing HIV latency in infected macrophages, stimulating viral replication, and decreasing cellular immunity.[13] Mean serum levels were significantly lower for vitamin A, folate, and carotene in patients with HIV wasting syndrome than in nonwasting patients with comparable CD4+ cell counts.[14] Selenium (Se) and beta-carotene improve the function of the enzymatic antioxidant system in blood and glutathione status in HIV-positive patients.[15] An intake of greater than two times the RDA of beta-carotene, as well as other micronutrients, is associated with increased survival in HIV-1-positive patients.[16]

In a small, randomized, controlled trial of HIV-positive patients, oral doses of beta-carotene at 180 mg/day increased CD4+ T-cell counts by 17% in 4 weeks.[17] However, Nimmagadda et al were unable to replicate these findings in a pilot open-label study in 21 HIV-positive patients.[18] In their study, beta-carotene supplementation of 180 mg/day for 4 weeks did not alter CD4 lymphocyte count or plasma HIV RNA copy number. Nor was a correlation found between presupplementation and postsupplementation beta-carotene or vitamin A plasma concentrations and presupplementation and postsupplementation CD4+ or HIV RNA measures. Coodley et al, in a prospective double-blind, placebo-controlled study ($n = 72$), compared patients who received 60 mg beta-carotene administered orally three times a day (tid) plus a multivitamin for 3 months with randomly assigned subjects who received only a multivitamin. The beta-carotene-plus-multivitamin group's results, with the exception of increased serum beta-carotene levels, did not differ from the multiple-vitamin-alone group in terms of T-cell quantitative subsets, natural killer (NK) cell numbers, and HIV RNA plasma levels. The authors hypothesized that adding the multivitamin to both arms of the study masked the effects of beta-carotene.[17] Another study reported that beta-carotene supplementation decreased fever, nocturnal sweating, diarrhea, and weight loss and that it improved mean CD4+ T-cell counts.[19]

Beta-carotene may also help prevent atherosclerosis. HIV-positive patients have an increased risk of atherosclerosis and have evidence of endothelium dysfunction that may be related to loss of antioxidants. Constans et al showed in a small study with 10 HIV-positive patients that supplementation of the antioxidants beta-carotene (30 mg bid) and Se (100 μg/day) reduced inflammatory markers associated with atherosclerotic process. For this reason, it may be prudent to advise supplementation of these antioxidants in HIV-positive patients who are receiving HAART therapy that elevates serum lipids and who may therefore be at additional risk for atherosclerosis and cardiovascular (CV) disease.[20]

Some published data indicate that synthetic beta-carotenoids may increase the risk of lung cancer in smokers.[21] Based on these findings from oncology research, controversy about the safety of beta-carotene now exists. Given these uncertainties, we use only natural carotenoids and inform our patients, particularly those who smoke, of the possible risks of taking beta-carotene. For patients who have doubts about the safety of taking supplemental beta-carotene, we recommend two glasses of fresh carrot juice/day instead.

Coenzyme Q10

Coenzyme Q10 (CoQ10; dosage: 30 to 100 mg tid) is a ubiquitously found cellular antioxidant that regulates adenosine triphosphate (ATP) synthesis within mitochondria. This nutrient is prescribed by naturopathic physicians for several disorders, including cancer and CV disease. It is often recommended to HIV/AIDS patients because data on HIV/AIDS patients suggest a blood deficiency of CoQ10 compared with HIV-negative controls.[22] CoQ10 (100 mg/day) was reported in one study to increase CD4+/CD8+ ratios in HIV-negative subjects.[23]

Vitamin C

Vitamin C (dosage: 2000 mg tid between meals) is commonly taken in high doses by HIV-positive individuals. The Bastyr University Alternative Medicine Care Outcomes in AIDS (AMCOA) study reported that, of 1016 HIV-positive participants in an observational study of CAM, vitamin C was the most frequently reported CAM substance, used by 65% of this nationwide cohort.[24] Despite its widespread use by HIV-infected persons, only one controlled trial of vitamin C in HIV disease has been reported. Allard et al presented a poster at the 1998 International AIDS Conference in Geneva.[25] Forty-nine HIV-positive patients were randomized to receive either 800 IU vitamin E and 1000 mg of vitamin C daily oral supplementation or placebo for 3 months. Vitamin C and E supplementation significantly reduced oxidative stress. There was also a trend toward lowered viral load in the treatment group.

Some in vitro work suggests that ascorbate can suppress HIV replication in both chronically and acutely infected T cells.[26] In addition, ascorbate saturation by lymphocytes is linked to enhanced immunocompetence.[27] More information about vitamin C in its role as an AV may be found in the later section on naturopathic AV therapy.

Health care providers offer differing recommendations regarding vitamin C dosing for HIV-positive patients. Some recommend a slow increase in oral dosing until bowel tolerance (6 to 20 g/day) is attained. We have noticed that patients with GI dysbiosis experience diarrhea from even the lowest recommended dose of vitamin C. This may indicate a need to perform a complete digestive stool test to assess GI candidiasis and inflammation.

Some of the AV PIs, such as indinavir, can induce nephrolithiasis. Although there have been no specific studies addressing the question of whether vitamin C adds to the risk of kidney stones in patients taking indinavir, there is some concern about adding excessive levels of ascorbic acid to the regimen of a patient taking this particular PI.

Bioflavonoids that are present in a number of plant species, including rosehips, may also be beneficial in HIV-positive patients. Flavonoid compounds inhibit HIV activation in latently infected cells.[28]

Vitamin E

Vitamin E (dosage: 400 IU/day) has been shown to have both immune-enhancing and antioxidant properties.[29] Reduced blood levels of vitamin E and polyunsaturated fatty acids (PUFAs) of phospholipids have been reported to favor the onset and the development of AIDS.[30] Data from another study suggested that vitamin A, E, and B_{12} deficiencies accelerated the development of AIDS.[31] In a sample of 296 HIV-positive men, the hazard of AIDS decreased as consumption of 11 micronutrients increased. This relationship was statistically significant for vitamin E, iron, and riboflavin.[32] Although there have been no published randomized controlled trials of vitamin E in HIV disease, some longitudinal studies have detected abnormalities in vitamin E levels in HIV-positive individuals. A study of 121 asymptomatic HIV-positive patients found that 22.3% had a deficient serum vitamin E level early in the course of the disease.[33] In 42 of the patients who were followed longitudinally, a significant decrease in vitamin E occurred over a 12-month period. In another study, serum levels of vitamin E were prospectively measured in 311 HIV-positive men over 9 years.[34] Results showed a 34% decreased risk of progression to AIDS and 34% decreased mortality in men in the highest quartile of serum vitamin E levels versus men in the lowest quartile.

Vitamin E has known immunomodulatory activity. Supplementation at high levels can modulate cytokine production by thymocytes.[35] In vitro, vitamin E restores retrovirus-suppressed splenocyte proliferation and NK cell cytotoxicity.[36] Vitamin E supplementation has been shown to partially reverse the myelosuppressive action of zidovudine (AZT) in HIV-positive patients.[37]

Selenium

Se deficiency and decreased glutathione peroxidase (GPX) activity is common in HIV infection and AIDS.[38-40] Both Se (dosage: 200 to 600 μg/day) and beta-carotene have been shown to improve the function of the enzymatic antioxidant system in blood and glutathione status in HIV-infected patients.[15] Measurements of plasma antioxidants and fatty acid (FA) composition of erythrocyte membranes and plasma antioxidants in HIV-positive patients show that Se is lower in patients with less than 400 CD4+ cells/mm³.[41] Some researchers have hypothesized that the latency period in HIV infection may be attributed to the period of time it takes to deplete the body of Se storage.[42] Stimulation of GPX activity with Se decreases HIV-1 activation after oxidative stress.[43] Moreover, in vitro experiments have demonstrated a dose-dependent inhibition by Se of nuclear factor kappa B (NF-κB)-controlled gene expression in HIV-1 replication.[44] An adequate supply of Se and antioxidant vitamins has been proposed to reduce the probability of the placental transmission of HIV in pregnancy.[45] For these reasons, Se intake is encouraged in HIV-positive patients either as a supplement or in food. Brazil nuts are high in Se.

N-Acetylcysteine

N-Acetylcysteine (NAC; dosage: 1000 to 4000 mg bid) is a sulfur-containing amino acid and glutathione precursor. Oral administration has been shown to elevate serum glutathione levels.[46] Orally administered glutathione is hydrolyzed in the stomach and is thus not absorbable. NAC, which is bioavailable after oral administration, is a therapeutic strategy to increase serum glutathione levels. In vitro studies show that NAC fully replenishes depleted reduced gluthathione (GSH).[47] Treatment with NAC improved cysteine and glutathione deficiency in AIDS patients.[48] A series of clinical studies and laboratory investigations suggests that AIDS may be, at least in part, the consequence of a virus-induced cysteine deficiency.[48] Oral administration of NAC in healthy persons increased the capacity of their peripheral blood mononuclear cells (PBMCs) to release anti-HIV chemokines.[49] By potentiating chemokine production, NAC may decrease susceptibility to infection. Two randomized clinical trials (RCTs) of NAC supplementation showed increased immunological functions as measured by NK cell and T-cell functions in HIV-positive patients.[50] Anti-HIV effects as measured by viral load were more variable in these studies but had a trend toward a decrease.

In vitro research shows some AV activity. For example, NAC (10 mM/L) caused a twofold inhibition of HIV and conferred a synergistic effect (approximately eightfold inhibition) when tested simultaneously with vitamin C (0.426 mM/L).[51] NAC reduces human immunodeficiency virus type 1 (HIV-1) replication in stimulated T cells. However, NAC and glutathione enhanced acute HIV-1 replication in monocyte-derived macrophages in vitro.[52] NAC appears to modulate HIV-1 replication in both chronically and acutely infected lymphocytes that produce high virus levels independently from cytokine activation. In both cases, NAC doses of 0.12 and 0.25 mM decreased, whereas doses from 0.5 to 2 mM increased the infectious HIV-1 yield.[53]

The relationship between HIV-induced cysteine deficiency and T-cell dysfunction also provides a rationale for treatment with NAC.[54] In one report, oral administration of NAC reversed loss in CD4+ T-cell count associated with change from optimal intracellular levels of glutathione and cysteine in HIV-positive individuals.[55]

Alpha-Lipoic Acid

Alpha-lipoic acid (lipoate, lipoic acid, dihydrolipoic acid, thioctic acid; dosage: 200 mg tid) was originally classified as a vitamin but later was found to be synthesized by animals and humans. It is unique in its ability to act as an antioxidant in fat- and water-soluble tissues in both its reduced and oxidized forms.[56] As an antioxidant, it is prescribed as a hepatoprotectant. Because of its in vitro anti-HIV activity, it is also prescribed to HIV-positive patients as one of many natural AV treatments. It is reported to prevent HIV activation in vitro and to react with reactive oxygen species.[57] Alpha-lipoic acid increases antioxidant recycling and reduces activation of HIV by reducing the NF-κB transcription factor.[58] To date, no published reports of clinical activity of alpha-lipoic acid in HIV have appeared in either a MEDLINE or an AIDSLINE database search. Given the effects that alpha-lipoic acid has on insulin sensitivity and glucose metabolism in diabetics, a clinical evaluation of clinical benefit in HIV-related diabetes and dysglycemias is in order.[59] There is justification for the hypothesis that alpha-lipoic acid may be useful in peripheral neuropathy (PN) in HIV based on the positive findings for alpha-lipoic acid on diabetic neuropathy at a dose of 600 mg tid for 3 weeks.[60]

Alpha-lipoic acid has been proposed as a potential treatment for depression, although no clinical studies have been published.[61] However, one study evaluated alpha-lipoic acid for its effects in HIV-related cognitive disorders based on the hypothesis, that antioxidant activity might be beneficial in the underlying pathophysiology of HIV-related dementia. In this study, alpha-lipoic acid (600 mg bid) was compared with L-deprenyl.[62] Alpha-lipoic acid had no detectable effect.

Alpha-lipoic acid also appears to inhibit HIV replication.[63] Preliminary evidence shows that alpha-lipoic acid prevents gene expression of HIV.[64] Of all the allyl compounds tested, thiamine disulfide, alpha-lipoic acid, and NAC significantly depressed HIV-1 *tat* activity.[65] The inhibitory action of alpha-lipoic acid was found to be very potent, since only 4 mM was needed for a complete inhibition, whereas 20 mM was required for NAC.[66] Alpha-lipoic acid has been shown to increase intracellular glutathione in human T cells.[67] In a small, open-label trial, lipoate increased plasma ascorbate (9 of 10 patients), total glutathione (7 of 7 patients), total plasma thiol groups (8 of 9 patients), T helper lymphocytes, and T helper/suppressor cell ratio (6 of 10 patients).[68]

Treatment Principle 2: Improve Nutritional Status

Optimizing nutritional status involves four components: (1) improving GI nutrient absorption and mucosal integrity, (2) eliminating food allergens and optimizing GI ecology health, (3) eliminating GI pathogens, and (4) providing optimal therapeutic and dietary nutrition. Therapeutic means for attaining each of these goals are described below.

Improving Gastrointestinal Nutrient Absorption and Mucosal Immunity

Lactobacillus acidophilus is frequently prescribed to HIV-positive patients for optimization of GI floral ecology. Many practitioners will prescribe one or two 500-mg capsules 1 to 3 times/day. It is often the first therapy offered for diarrhea associated with antiretroviral therapy (ART), antibiotic therapy, or the GI complication of HIV infection itself. *L. acidophilus* has been shown to persist in the stomach longer than other bacteria and may be useful in managing conditions associated with altered GI flora.[69]

Some NDs prescribe *L. acidophilus* when their HIV-positive patients begin Bactrim prophylaxis for *Pneumocystis carinii* pneumonia (PCP). Some evidence exists that oral administration of *L. acidophilus* may be clinically beneficial.[70] For example, *L. acidophilus* may influence survival of HIV in the female genitals.[71] Reports at the Twelfth International AIDS Conference indicate that bacterial vaginosis may be a significant cofactor in HIV infection risk among Ugandan women and that a deficiency in vaginal *L. acidophilus* is associated with a risk for bacterial vaginosis.

Butyric acid. Butyric acid is a source of energy for colonic epithelial cells, which are critical in mucosal immunity.[72] It is also a luminal trophic factor for the colonic and cecal mucosa.[73] Orally administered butyric acid has been used therapeutically in the treatment of colitis[74,75] and in other non-HIV conditions. Its use has been generalized to HIV-related GI mucosal disorders.

Glutamine. (500 to 1000 mg bid; tid in HIV wasting syndrome) Amino acid levels are implicated in HIV-related enteropathies, and amino acid supplementation has been proposed and used as prophylaxis and treatment for HIV-related colitis and diarrhea. A deficiency of the amino acid L-glutamine is associated with atrophy and degeneration of the small intestine.[76] Glutamine deficiency is hypothesized to be a causal factor in HIV-associated wasting.[77] Glutamine has been shown to be useful in treating malabsorption.[78] A study published in 2000 presented results of a placebo-controlled RCT ($n = 68$) of orally administered nutritional supplementation of the metabolites of three amino acids (methylbutyrate, L-glutamine, and L-arginine) for 8 weeks.[79] Patients who received amino acid nutritional supplementation had increased lean body mass (LBM) and a trend toward decreased viral load and increased immune status. Dietary sources of glutamine are available from oat bran and green cabbage.

Digestive enzymes. NDs often prescribe digestive enzymes (e.g., amylase, lipase, pancreatin) to HIV-positive patients who show signs or symptoms of maldigestion. Complete digestive stool analyses often detect poor pancreatic output in many patients with digestive complaints, including HIV-positive patients. Digestive enzymes taken with meals can assist enzymatic degradation of foods necessary for absorption. To date, no clinical trials have been published that describe evaluation of the efficacy of digestive enzyme supplementation in HIV-positive patients.

Treating Gastrointestinal Candidal Overgrowth

The presence of oral thrush indicates candidal overgrowth throughout the GI tract. Most NDs consider candidal infections important to treat regardless of the presence of symptoms. *Candida* organisms may be both the result and the cause of HIV-related health problems. Serum testing for *Candida* antibody titers and antigen levels can diagnose asymptomatic candidal infection. Nystatin, an FDA-approved antifungal medication, is often prescribed for thrush in a "swish and swallow" form. It also is prescribed orally if the *Candida* antigen is positive and/or if there are abnormally high levels of *Candida* antibodies, even in asymptomatic patients. Nystatin appears safe, since it is not absorbed into the circulation from the gut. Typical dosage is 500,000 U tid for a 30-day course. It has been shown to be efficacious in oral and gut antifungal prophylaxis[80] and effective in reducing yeast contamination in neonates,[81] as well as effective in eradicating systemic candidiasis.[82]

A number of botanicals are used by NDs to either prevent or treat candidal overgrowth, including oil of oregano, capryllic acid, pau d'arco (Teheebo), and te tree oil. However, no clinical trials have been published demonstrating efficacy of botanical treatments for *Candida* organisms. One part 5% hydrogen peroxide diluted with 2 parts water can effectively treat oral thrush. Te tree oil (an essential oil from *Melaleuca alternifolia*) has demonstrated in vitro activity against *Candida* organisms and fungal species,[83,84] and these data support the topical use of te tree oil on candidal superficial fungal infections.

L-carnitine. AIDS patients deficient in L-carnitine are at risk for alterations in fatty-acid oxidation and energy supply.[85] Also, L-carnitine deficiency can lead to critical metabolic dysfunctions.[86] De Simone et al compared L-carnitine supplementation (6 g/day) to placebo for 2 weeks, measuring the effects on serum and PBMC concentrations.[87] They reported that L-carnitine levels were lower in HIV-positive patients than in healthy controls and that there was a trend toward restoration of normal intracellular PBMC levels with supplementation. They also noted a strong reduction in serum triglycerides in the L-carnitine group. Some NDs prescribe oral doses of L-carnitine to HIV-positive patients who show signs of disordered fat metabolism, such as high serum triglycerides. It is frequently prescribed to patients who are diagnosed with HIV wasting syndrome. A small pilot study with five asymptomatic HIV-positive patients suggested that oral administration of 3 g/day of acetyl-L-carnitine prevented apoptotic loss of CD4 cells and increased serum insulin-like growth factor (GF).[88] Moretti et al studied the 4-month impact of L-carnitine infusions

(6 g/day) in 11 HIV-positive patients and reported an increase in absolute CD4 counts and reduced apoptosis.[89] A single case report suggests that L-carnitine may be a treatment for lactic acidosis induced by nucleoside analogues.[90]

Saccharomyces boulardii. *S. boulardii* is a nonpathogenic yeast that has been used in Europe as an antidiarrheal agent, and studies show that it significantly reduces antibiotic-associated diarrhea.[91,92] Oral administration of *S. boulardii* stimulates secretory IgA in the small intestine.[93] In a placebo-controlled RCT ($n = 128$), *S. boulardii* was found to prevent diarrhea in critically ill tube-fed patients.[94] *S. boulardii* has protective effects in *Clostridium difficile*-induced inflammatory diarrhea.[95]

Therapeutic and Dietary Nutrition

Most NDs assume that food sensitivities are more prevalent in HIV-positive patients, although there have been no systematic studies on this topic. A typical approach is to eliminate all gluten/gliadin grains, all milk and dairy products, and foods to which the patient has allergies or sensitivities for at least 2 weeks to observe change in symptoms. Chronic sinusitis in HIV-positive patients often responds to the elimination of common food allergens.

Whole foods. Dietary recommendations for HIV-positive patients are typically to reduce simple sugars, ensure essential fatty acids (EFAs), emphasize protein, eat clean fresh fruits and vegetables, increase variety of foods, and eliminate caffeine and alcohol.

Protein powder. Many HIV-positive patients have protein malnutrition secondary to malabsorption. NDs typically recommend protein powder supplementation for this reason. Patients are often recommended to prepare protein powder fruit smoothies consisting of 4 ounces of tofu or 2 scoops of protein powder with 1 cup nuts or nut butter (not peanuts), 1 cup yogurt, 1 cup fresh fruit or berries, 1 tbsp honey, and 1 tbsp flax oil; thin with rice milk or juice to make 24 fluid ounces; drink 8 oz tid.

Cod liver oil. Gamma linolenate selectively kills HIV-infected cells.[96] Oils rich in EFAs increase superoxide production of stimulated macrophages in mice.[97] These oils increase plasma EFAs and decrease urinary excretion of prostaglandin E_2.[98] A clinical study demonstrated that formula fortified with alpha-linolenic acid (1.8 g/day), arginine (7.8 g/day), and RNA (0.75 g/day) resulted in a statistically significant weight gain (+2.9 kg/4 months versus −0.5 kg/4

months with the control formula) in HIV-positive patients.[99] Reduced blood levels of PUFAs of phospholipids have been shown to be a risk factor for the onset and development of AIDS,[100] and a deficiency in two dietary EFAs, gamma-linolenic acid (GLA) and eicosapentaenoic acid (EPA), may determine individual susceptibility to AIDS.[101] FA composition of erythrocyte membranes in HIV-positive patients showed that saturated FAs are higher and PUFAs are lower than they are in controls.[41]

HIV-positive patients receiving total parenteral nutrition (TPN) may be at risk for omega-3 EFA deficits because TPN often contains high omega-6 and low omega-3 FAs.[102] Significant deficits of omega-3 EFAs have been measured in persons with neuropathy or impaired immune systems.

For the past decade, we have recommended that HIV-positive patients take 1 tbsp/day of high-quality cod liver oil, which is rich in omega-3 FAs, as well as vitamin A.

Oat bran. As a dietary supplement, oat bran (1 to 2 tbsp/day) can provide additional glutamine. Oat bran is rich in glutamine (as is green cabbage), contains water-soluble, fermentable-fiber beta-glucans, and may offer GI surface protection and mucosal reconditioning.[103]

Multiple vitamins and minerals. Many studies document nutrient deficiencies in people with AIDS. One study of dietary vitamin and mineral intake revealed that 88% of AIDS patients, 88% of HIV-positive patients, and 89% of ARC patients were ingesting less than 50% of the RDA for at least one nutrient. The mean number of deficiencies per patient was 1.8.[104] Another study found low blood levels of vitamins A (18%), E (27%), riboflavin (26%), B_6 (53%), and B_{12} (23%) together with copper (74%) and zinc (50%) deficiencies in HIV-1-positive patients. With the exception of riboflavin, zinc, and copper, a similar prevalence of abnormalities among HIV-1-negative controls was not observed.[14] Of a sample of 30 HIV-positive patients, percentages of patients with below-normal plasma concentrations of nutrients included zinc (30% of patients), calcium (27% of patients), magnesium (30% of patients), carotenes (31% of patients), total choline (50% of patients), and ascorbate (27% of patients). Percentages of patients with above-normal values included folate (37%) and carnitine (37%). Some patients with above-normal values for plasma vitamins reported self-supplementation, usually with large doses.[105]

In one epidemiological study, an intake greater than five times the RDA of vitamins B_1, B_2, and B_3 and an intake greater than two times the RDA of vitamin B_6 and beta-carotene were all associated with increased survival in HIV-1-positive persons. This study was unusual because it found that high doses of zinc were associated with poorer survival.[16] Deficiencies of vitamin B_{12}, folate, and thiamin may contribute to neurological impairment in HIV.[106] These studies clearly show that multivitamin supplementation can offset nutritional deficiencies. One study showed that daily multivitamin use was associated with a reduced hazard of AIDS.[107] For these reasons, a high-quality multivitamin is prescribed to all HIV-positive patients. For patients with wasting disease and malabsorption, liquid pediatric vitamins, which are more easily absorbed and tolerated, may be prescribed.

Folate. Absorption of folate (dosage: 400 μg/day) is significantly impaired in HIV.[108] Because folate deficiencies can cause anemias in HIV-positive patients already at risk for anemia by other causes, clinicians should assess serum levels of folate in HIV-positive patients. Increased incidence of bone marrow toxicity has been found in patients taking AZT when folic acid levels are low.[109] Folate supplementation is recommended if macrocytic anemia is present or after folate antagonist chemotherapy drugs have been used.

Vitamin B_1 (thiamin). Greater than five times the RDA of B_1 (dosage: up to 50 mg bid) has been associated with increased survival in HIV-1-positive persons.[16] The highest levels of total intake (from food and supplements) of vitamins C and B_1 and niacin were associated with a significantly decreased progression rate to AIDS.[110] In vitro, thiamin disulfide has been shown to be a potent inhibitor of HIV-1 production.[111]

Vitamin B_{12} (hydroxycobalamin). Decreased cobalamin levels are found frequently in HIV disease and occur at an early stage. Dosage of vitamin B_{12} is 1000 μg intramuscular (IM) 1 to 2 times/week in macrocytic anemia, PN, and depression. Low serum vitamin B_{12} concentrations are associated with faster HIV-1 disease progression.[31,34,108,112] Development of a deficiency of vitamin A or vitamin B_{12} was associated with a decline in CD4 cell count, whereas normalization of vitamin A, vitamin B_{12}, and zinc was associated with higher CD4 cell counts in 108 HIV-1-positive men.[113] Cobalamins also inhibit HIV-1 infection of normal blood monocytes and lymphocytes.[114] Vitamin B_{12} levels fall in most patients over time and may help predict which patients will experience disease progression most rapidly.[115] Vitamin B_{12} levels were low in 39% of 36 HIV-positive patients with chronic diarrhea.[116] A statistically significant relationship has been found between vitamin B_{12} deficiency, weight loss, and diarrhea in HIV-positive patients.[117] NDs often prescribe both oral doses and IM injections of 1000 μg of vitamin B_{12} on a weekly basis, especially for patients with anemia, PN, and depression.

Testosterone. Androgen deficiency combined with growth hormone (GH) resistance may contribute to the critical loss of lean body and muscle mass in hypogonadal men with AIDS wasting syndrome.[17] Most physicians routinely test serum testosterone levels and administer testosterone IM (usually weekly) if levels are low.

Intravenous nutrition. If wasting occurs, IV nutrition (e.g., vitamin C IV, cachexia formula, Myers cocktail, TPN) may be appropriate. The use of vitamin C infusion treatment has been shown to be beneficial in the clinical management of AIDS.[118] Eighty-two percent of patients with human T-cell leukemia virus-I (HTLV-I)-associated myelopathy had improved motor function with high doses of vitamin C.[119]

Treatment Principle 3: Clear Drug, Sexually Transmitted Disease, Yeast, and Viral Cofactors

Substantial evidence exists that other viral infections transactivate HIV infection (see Chapter 2). Many HIV-positive patients have a history of multiple viral infections, including (1) herpes simplex virus (HSV); (2) Epstein-Barr virus (EBV); (3) hepatitis A, B, or C; and (4) human papilloma virus (HPV; associated with condylomatous anal and genital warts). Optimization of health may require the control of these residual chronic viral infections. Thus elimination of cofactors, such as STDs and their residual, possibly miasmatic effects, is a treatment goal for NDs. Several methods are used to attain this goal, including homeopathic nosodes and botanical AV medicines. However, none have been subjected to clinical trials.

Many recreational drugs, including cocaine, amphetamines, and marijuana, have immunosuppressant effects.[120] Patients should be strongly advised to avoid recreational drugs, and if currently using, to enter detoxification and 12-step programs. Many people who use drugs, especially sympathomimetic substances such as cocaine and amphetamines, may be attempting to self-treat an underlying depression or anxiety. Helping patients get off drugs requires careful attention to the emotional etiology of the addiction. Be sure to treat the depression in such cases. Drug addictions can be related to deficiencies in amino acids essential for optimal neurochemical function. The clinician should also consider combination amino acid supplementation when a history of drug use is present. Auricular acupuncture also can be useful in treating drug dependency. A clinical program of repeated ear acupuncture has been demonstrated to be effective in treating cocaine addiction.[121-123] Many Seattle-area HIV-positive patients are referred for acupuncture therapy for not only drug detoxification but also for PN, depression, fatigue, and HIV-related diarrhea. Pilot data also suggest immune benefits of acupuncture. Traditional acupuncture increases both the concentrations of B-endorphins in mononuclear cells and T-lymphocyte proliferation in HIV-positive patients.[124]

Silymarin (in milk thistle and artichoke) has been used as a hepatoprotectant antioxidant botanical in HIV-positive patients with a history of drug abuse and hepatitis and in those who are currently receiving pharmaceutical drug treatment with associated risk for hepatotoxicity. Although there have been no clinical trials of silymarin in HIV-positive populations, silymarin-phosphatidylcholine complex is reported to improve liver function indices in patients with chronic active hepatitis.[125] Silymarin also has been shown to increase the superoxide dismutase (SOD) and antioxidant activity of blood cells of patients with liver disease.[126] Dosages of standardized silymarin of 160 mg tid are typically recommended.

Homeopathic Treatment for Drug and Viral Cofactors

Homeopathic nosodes have been used to reduce the complications of concurrent viral cofactors (e.g., HSV, human herpes virus 6 [HHV-6], herpes zoster [HZ], EBV, cytomegalovirus [CMV], and HPV), although no clinical trial results of this approach have yet been published. NDs use homeopathic nosodes based on homeopathic theory. We have been using increasing potencies of homeopathic preparations of inactivated viral antigens from 5X up to 200X with one dose/week for 10 weeks in ascending order of potency. Response can be objectively obtained by determining pretreatment and posttreatment serum antibody titers or antigen levels for those viruses to which each patient

has been exposed. Following the 10-week nosode treatment, retesting antibody titers and/or antigen levels should show lower levels of both. Anecdotally, this procedure has substantially decreased the frequency of herpetic outbreaks.

Some practitioners are using homeopathically prepared ultrahigh dilutions (UHDs) of *Cannabis sativa*, cocaine, amphetamines, LSD, heroin, amyl nitrate, and other drugs to help their patients detoxify from their specific addiction history. Similarly, some NDs use homeopathic preparations of prescription drugs to treat toxicities associated with their pharmacological use. For example, homeopathic trimethoprim/sulfamethoxazole (Bactrim, Septra, Cotrim) has been used successfully to desensitize HIV-positive patients to pharmacological doses required for PCP prophylaxis.[127] This approach may be used for controlling side effects or lowering toxicities associated with pharmaceutical drugs that a patient may have taken. In addition, unpublished in vitro data suggest that homeopathic doses of the immunosuppressant drug cyclosporin A, in keeping with the homeopathic law of similars, exert immune enhancement.[128]

Using Botanicals to Clear Cofactor Viral Infections (Herpes, HPV)

Glycyrrhiza glabra (licorice root) is used as a broad-spectrum AV botanical (see AV section). The solid extract, dosed at ¼ to ½ tsp bid, has been prescribed for controlling herpes and other DNA viral infections. Herpes outbreaks can be treated with combination botanical medicines. One formula developed by Eileen Stretch, ND, and used by clinicians in the Bastyr University HIV/AIDS clinic combines *Hydrastis canadensis*, *Lomatium dissectum*, *Passiflora incarnata*, *Taraxacum officinale*, *Astragalus membranous*, and *Gelsemium sempervirens*. During a prodrome, prodoses of 30 to 60 drops every 2 hours may prevent a full outbreak. The tincture is given qid during outbreaks. *P. incarnata* has antibacterial activity.[129] *A. membranous* injections have been shown to enhance antibody response to a T-dependent antigen (see *A. membranous* and *L. dissectum* in Treatment Principle 4).

NDs treat HPV infection with a combination of *L. dissectum* and *Thuja occidentalis*, although no clinical trials substantiate their use. *L. dissectum*, a botanical from Native American herbal traditions, is used for a variety of herbal infections, and recently it has been shown to inhibit HIV replication and suppress acute HIV-1 infections.[130] *T. occidentalis* also has a long history of traditional herbal use and has been shown to induce CD4$^+$ fraction of human peripheral blood T-cell subset and increase production of IL-1β, IL-2, IL-3, IL-6, interferon-gamma (IFN-γ), granulocyte colony-stimulating factor (G-CSF), GM-CSF, and tumor necrosis factor-beta (TNF-β).[131]

Treatment Principle 4: Provide Antiviral Therapy

With the advent of HAART, it is important to inform one's patients that pharmaceutical ART is effective in lowering HIV viral load, and, in many patients, modestly increasing CD4$^+$ cells. With each passing year, developments in ART are generating better drug combinations with fewer side effects. It is now common practice to use the term *HAART* when referring to antiretroviral therapy (highly active ART). Many HIV/AIDS conventional clinicians urge HIV-positive patients to initiate ART early in the course of their disease. Others recommend waiting until HIV viral load rises to moderate levels (depending on the clinician, 5000 to 30,000 copies/ml). It is important for the ND to know and communicate that no highly effective natural AV therapy for HIV/AIDS exists at this time. The following is a summary of botanical and nutritional therapies that may help slow viral replication. However, none of these natural therapies have been thoroughly evaluated in clinical trials and should not be used as substitutes for HAART.

Our approach has been to explain to patients the benefits and risks of HAART and refer the patient for comanagement with an MD experienced in HIV care who can provide individual consultation regarding initiation of ART. For patients who wish to try natural AV approaches, we recommend getting a baseline HIV RNA viral load, then prescribing adequate doses of concurrent multiple naturopathic AV medicines. A follow-up HIV RNA viral load should be repeated at 1 to 3 months after initiation of natural AV therapy. If viral load has not dropped one half (or by 0.3 log unit), one may conclude that the natural AV combination has not produced the intended benefit. The clinician should then reintroduce the decision to initiate ART or try another botanical combination. For example, we often start botanical AV therapy with SPV-30 (*Buxus sempervirens;* boxwood evergreen). If this proves ineffective in lowering viral load by 0.3 log unit, we then try a combination of licorice and *Hypericum perforatum,*

also known as St. John's wort (or start with *H. perforatum* with patients who have fatigue and/or depression, as well as detectable viral loads). Another combination to consider is garlic, *Curcuma longa* (curcumin or tumeric), and piperine (black pepper). Both animal and human pharmacokinetic data suggest that the bioavailability of curcumin may be enhanced with the addition of piperine.[132]

Bastyr University researchers are investigating the in vitro anti-HIV activity of combined botanicals with purported antiretroviral activity. More than 15% of higher plants have anti-HIV activity in vitro, although this is mostly small-to-moderate activity. Studies show that plants can interfere with HIV infection and replication at nine points in the virus's life cycle. If plants are screened and chosen wisely and adequate blood levels are attained from oral dosing, experimental combination botanical AV therapy may hold promise (see Chapter 6).

Glycyrrhiza Glabra (Licorice Root)

Licorice root is frequently used in both the naturopathic and Chinese botanical *materia medica* for a variety of conditions. Although there is evidence of anti-HIV activity for licorice in vitro, no definitive clinical trials have been conducted to assess the clinical value of this herb in HIV-positive patients. Lu Wei Bo in China reported positive clinical results on the treatment of 60 HIV-positive cases with Glyke, an orally administered combination traditional Chinese herbal therapy that contains *G. glabra.*[133] Licorice root is also prescribed by NDs because of *G. glabra's* adrenal effects. It is prescribed for "adrenal fatigue" as indicated by low serum DHEA (<200 ng/dl). Typical dosage is 500 to 1000 mg tid of crude root or ¼ to ½ tsp solid extract as tea bid. Because licorice root has been reported to have aldosterone-like effects and may produce or exacerbate hypertension, it is important to monitor the patient's blood pressure when prescribing this treatment.

One of the active constituents of licorice, glycyrrhizin (GL) has an inhibitory effect on several viruses, including HIV-1 and varicella-zoster virus (VZV). GL inhibits giant cell formation of HIV-infected cells.[134] In vivo inhibition of HIV-1 replication in AIDS has been demonstrated in patients by a Japanese research team.[135] GL showed significant effect in slowing progression to AIDS compared with placebo in a small, double-blind study.[136] In addition, GL has claimed some therapeutic and prophylactic effects on chronic active viral hepatitis. In one study, 0.2% GL dissolved in saline (2 mg/ml), supplemented with 2% glycine and 0.1% cysteine (Stronger Neo-Minophagen C, [SNMC]), was administered intravenously in a dose of 50 ml/day for a more than 1 week to three infants with CMV infection who exhibited abnormal liver function or hepatomegaly. Liver function became normal at the end of the course of SNMC. These findings suggest that GL has therapeutic effects on liver dysfunction associated with CMV infections.[137] GL has also been used in Japan and China to treat other viral infections, including hepatitis A, B, and C.

GL may also have immunomodulatory activity. Researchers from the University of Texas–Galveston presented some interesting animal data regarding glycyrrhizin at the Twelfth International AIDS Conference in Geneva in June 1998. They reported that glycyrrhizin restored resistance to *Candida albicans* in immune-deficient mice.[138]

Hypericum Perforatum (St. John's Wort)

The justification for using *H. perforatum* for HIV disease derives from preliminary in vitro data. Incubation of hypericin, one of the active constituents of *H. perforatum,* with HIV rendered the virus noninfectious.[139] Hypericin has been shown to inhibit binding and entry of HIV into host cells,[140] and also has been shown to cross the blood-brain barrier. This characteristic is important, since HIV virus often infects CNS macrophages. While hypericin may be anti-HIV in vitro, it is difficult to achieve sufficiently high blood levels via oral administration to produce AV activity. Thus clinicians use higher doses to treat HIV (1500 mg tid to qid of crude lyophilized extract) compared with doses used to treat depression (500 mg of crude extract tid). In the past hypericin was highly recommended as an antidepressant for HIV-positive patients. Be aware that *H. perforatum* can produce photosensitivity. Patients will tan and burn more rapidly and should be cautioned to use sunblock. Patients on HAART should be cautioned that coadministration of St. John's wort with the PI indinavir may accelerate liver metabolism of indinavir and thus possibly reduce the effectiveness of HAART.[142]

Buxus Sempervirens (Boxwood Evergreen; SPV-30)

SPV-30 is a popular botanical AV therapy and is available through several HIV buyers' clubs. SPV-30 is an extract of boxwood evergreen that has been evaluated in an open-label trial conducted by Mestman and Stokes.[143] By October 1995, 500 HIV-positive people

had enrolled. Results indicated stability of CD4+ T-cell counts, a slight rise in CD8+, and a drop in HIV RNA (69% decrease) after 2 months. A 1-year open-label evaluation of SPV-30 in 173 HIV-positive patients found that 63% of participants experienced a 0.3 log unit decrease in viral load after 6 months. Average CD4 counts appeared to stabilize, and CD8+ counts rose slightly over the 6-month period.[144] The dosage recommendation by the manufacturers of SPV-30 is 90 mg tid. To our knowledge, no further studies have been published on SPV-30, and its use has declined with the advent of HAART.

Curcuma Longa (Curcumin)

Curcumin has a long history of use as an antiinflammatory herb and is frequently prescribed to arthritis patients. It also shows anti-HIV activity in vitro by several mechanisms, including inhibition of HIV-1 by integrase inhibition,[145,146] inhibition of directed transcription,[147] and inhibition of HIV-2 protease.[148] If curcumin is used orally, it is advisable to coadminister black pepper to improve bioavailability. Both animal and human pharmacokinetic data[132] suggest that the bioavailability of curcumin may be enhanced with the addition of piperine.

Allium Sativum (Garlic)

Garlic has been reported to have immunomodulatory, AV, tumoricidal, and antimicrobial activity. Allicin and thiosulfinates present in *A. sativum* show AV activity in vitro against several viruses, including HSV- I, HSV-II,[149] and CMV.[150] A 1993 in vitro study showed that diallyl disulfide, another thiosulfinate constituent of garlic, can selectively kill HIV-1-infected cells.[65]

Quercetin

Quercetin is a bioflavonoid extracted from yellow onion and is commonly used in naturopathic medicine as an antiinflammatory with applications in allergy, asthma, arthritis, and autoimmune disorders. A proposed mechanism of action for its antiinflammatory action is the stabilization of membranes of histamine-secreting mast cells. In vitro data suggest that quercetin has AV activity against herpes simplex I and II.[151] It is also a strong inhibitor of HIV-reverse transcriptase (RT)[152] and a potent inhibitor of HIV-integrase,[153] DNA polymerase B, and RNA polymerase.[154] Many clinicians prescribe quercetin to their HIV-positive patients, but no clinical trials have been conducted to evaluate its effects on viral load or T lymphocytes.

Momordica Charantia (Bitter Melon)

Bitter melon was a popular AV herb used by many HIV-positive persons during the late 1980s and early 1990s, which was usually self-administered by rectal infusion. Some in vitro evidence of AV activity exists, but no formal clinical trials have been published. Protein constituents of *M. charantia* are shown to have abortifacient, antitumor, ribosome-inactivating, and immunomodulatory activities.[155] *M. charantia* was reported to contain a protein that inactivates viral DNA,[156] and a recombinant protein of *M. charantia* was found to have anti-HIV activity.[157]

Aloe Vera

Early in the epidemic, an aloe extract given the proprietary name Acemannan (ACE-M) was commercially developed by Carrington Laboratories and marketed as an effective treatment for HIV disease. Some HIV-positive persons began taking aloe extract as a drink, typically at a dose of 1 oz bid. Some preliminary evidence from in vitro studies shows that aloe has AV activity. For example, extracts of aloe were shown to inactivate HSV-I.[158] An in vitro study of ACE-M showed concentration-dependent inhibition of HIV replication,[159,160] and two controlled trials of ACE-M therapy in HIV-positive patients appeared in the peer-reviewed literature (see Introduction Chapter, Table I-1). Neither study showed significant effects on immune parameters or p24 antigen levels.

Whole-Body Hyperthermia

The Bastyr University HIV/AIDS clinic has been treating its HIV-positive patients with artificial fever therapy since the beginning of the epidemic. This form of hydrotherapy is one of the core modalities in naturopathic hydrotherapy and has a long history of use for treating both infectious diseases and malignancies. The rationale for using hyperthermia in HIV disease derives from the fact that HIV and other viruses are heat-labile and are inhibited by both natural and artificial fever.[161] Elevating the temperature to 42° C sensitized HIV-infected cells in vitro to subsequent oxidative stress by H_2O_2.

NDs induce artificial fever by immersing patients in heated whirlpool baths. The protocol is to elevate core temperature to 102° F for 20 minutes using bath water at 106° F. Hyperthermia treatments are typically given 2 times/week for 3 weeks. Unfortunately, there has never been a clinical study of hydrotherapeutic hyperthermia in HIV infection. With the introduction of HIV RNA viral load testing, it would be interesting to determine whether hyperthermia reduces viral load. There has been one report of whole-body hyperthermia in the treatment of Kaposi's sarcoma (KS). A 1991 single-patient study reported marked regression in KS and a 5% rise in $CD4^+$ count in an HIV-positive patient after hyperthermia treatments. Whole-body hyperthermia coinciding with beta-carotene supplementation in AIDS patients decreased HIV viral load and improved subjective life quality in a small study.[162]

There are studies of extracorporeal hyperthermia in HIV disease; however, this procedure is associated with greater risk than whole-body hyperthermia techniques. Systemic extracorporeal perfusion hyperthermia has been used with some apparent success in a small number of patients with KS.[163] Ash attempted to use this method to elevate temperatures to either 102° or 108° F.[164] The effects of one treatment that lasted 1 hour were tracked for 8 weeks. CD4, p24 antigen, and $\beta_2$microglobulin were tracked weekly. All markers improved in patients receiving the 108° F treatment, but the effect faded after 2 months. Although there were no detectable toxic effects at 102° F, no treatment effects were seen. At 108° F, however, clinically significant changes in blood chemistry were noted (e.g., a rise in creatine phosphokinase [CPK], serum glutamate pyruvate transaminase [SGPT], blood urea nitrogen [BUN]). A larger controlled trial of 30 patients with an average CD4 count of 120 yielded less positive findings: no change in CD4 counts and elevations in viral load at 3 months compared with an untreated control group. The results of elevating core temperature to 102° F casts doubt on the naturopathic strategy of elevating core temperature by whole-body immersion. Resolution requires a clinical trial of the naturopathic method in a controlled study with HIV-positive volunteers.

The enthusiasm for the use of whole-body hyperthermia in the treatment of HIV-positive patients has been dampened by the influence of Chinese medical practitioners who practice side by side with NDs in some alternative medicine clinics. Many HIV-positive patients are diagnosed as *Yin-Deficient* by their Chinese medical providers. Heat treatments such as hyperthermia are contraindicated in Yin-Deficient patients.

N-Acetylcysteine

NAC has been used by the HIV-infected community not only as an antioxidant but also for its potential as an anti-HIV agent. In vitro studies suggest that NAC has anti-HIV activity. For example, 10 mmol/L caused a nearly twofold inhibition of HIV and conferred a synergistic effect (approximately eightfold inhibition) when tested simultaneously with vitamin C (0.426 mmol/L).[51] NAC has also been shown to reduce HIV-1 replication in stimulated T cells[165] and to suppress HIV transcription in persistently infected cells.[166] Most NDs prescribe doses of NAC from 2000 to 8000 mg/day.

Vitamin A

Ample evidence exists that vitamin A deficiency is common among HIV-positive patients, even during the asymptomatic stage. Evidence also exists that vitamin A deficiency may be associated with immune dysfunction and higher rates of progression to AIDS among HIV-infected individuals. For example, vitamin A, E, and B_{12} deficiencies appear to be associated with accelerated development of AIDS.[31] Vitamin A deficiency is a predictor of mortality in HIV-infected IV drug users.[167] Development of deficiency of vitamin A or vitamin B_{12} was associated with a decline in $CD4^+$ cell count, whereas normalization of vitamin A, vitamin B_{12}, and zinc was associated with higher $CD4^+$ cell counts in 108 HIV-1-positive men.[40] Vitamin A deficiency is associated with decreased circulating CD4 T cells and increased mortality.[168] Vitamin A deficiency is also a risk factor for disease progression during HIV-1 infection,[168,169] and is lower in HIV-positive patients regardless of the $CD4^+$ cell count.[170] HIV-positive men require vitamin A intake far greater than the RDA to achieve normal plasma levels.[171] One study showed that, regardless of intake, AIDS patients may represent a population at considerable risk of vitamin A deficiency, since 27% of patients with "adequate intake" had serum retinol levels below the normal range.[172]

Evidence is strong that vitamin A deficiencies occur in HIV-infected individuals, even when their dietary intake seems adequate, and that these deficiencies are epidemiologically related to accelerated disease progression. However, there has been very little research that addresses the question of whether supplementation above RDA levels has clinical, immunological, or virological benefits. It is clear, however, that supplementation of vitamin A in HIV-positive pregnant women who have a deficiency of this antioxidant vitamin has a significant impact on the transmission of HIV to their neonates. Maternal vitamin A status inversely correlates with vertical transmission of HIV.[173] Some researchers have proposed that vitamin A may be more effective than AZT in preventing verti-

cal transmission of HIV, especially in malnourished women. Severe vitamin A deficiency (<20 μg/dl) was also associated with a twentyfold increased risk of having breast milk containing HIV-1 DNA among women with <400 $CD4^+$ cells/mm³.[174] A more recent study of 312 pregnant HIV-positive women in South Africa showed that vitamin A supplementation given in doses designed to decrease mother-to-infant transmission (5000 IU retinyl palmitate and 30 mg beta-carotene) did not result in either prenatal or postnatal HIV-symptoms in the mothers.[175]

Vitamin A may have a role in mucosal immune integrity. Detection of vaginal HIV-1 DNA in pregnant women is associated with severe vitamin A deficiency,[176] and reduced levels of vitamin A in women experiencing hypertension during pregnancy may place them at increased risk for mother-child transmission of HIV-1.[177] Serum vitamin A and beta-carotene are decreased in HIV-1-infected pregnant women in their first trimester with $CD4^+$ counts lower than 200.[178] Vitamin A supplementation for children of HIV-infected women appeared to be beneficial, reducing morbidity. This benefit was observed particularly in children with diarrhea.[179]

NDs typically prescribe vitamin A for a short course of 3 to 12 weeks and use oral doses of 25,000 to 100,000 IU/day. There has been some concern about potential toxicity with vitamin A, although it is rare. Symptoms of chronic overdose include headaches, body aches, and excessively dry skin.

Vitamin C

Vitamin C (dosage: 2000 mg bid/tid or to bowel tolerance) is used as an antioxidant by many HIV-positive patients. There is preliminary in vitro evidence of anti-HIV activity as well. Ascorbate exerts a posttranslational inhibitory effect on HIV by causing impairment of enzymatic activity.[180] Ascorbate diminishes HIV viral protein production in infected cells[26] and also suppresses extracellular levels of newly induced virus in unstimulated and latently infected cell lines.[180] In vitro studies suggest it works synergistically in controlling HIV infection in combination with NAC.[51] One recent controlled clinical study of combined vitamin C and E supplementation showed a trend toward lowered vital load compared with placebo.[25]

Vitamin E

Vitamin E acetate, or α-tocopheryl succinate, exerts a concentration-dependent inhibition of NF-κB activation.[181] Vitamin E supplementation (800 IU/day) when combined with vitamin C showed a trend toward lowered viral load in HIV-positive patients compared with placebo-treated subjects.[6,25] Typical doses prescribed to HIV-positive patients range from 400 to 800 IU/day.

Vitamin B$_3$ (Niacin)

Supplementation with several B vitamins may have clinical value in the management of HIV-positive patients. Intake of two to five times the RDA of B$_1$, B$_2$, B$_3$, and B$_6$ are all associated with increased survival in HIV-1-positive persons[16] and decreased progression rate to AIDS.[106] Some researchers have argued that HIV induces a state of intracellular pellagra that is reversed by the administration of nicotinamide. Nicotinamide, the amide form of niacin (dosage: up to 250 mg bid), inhibits HIV-1 infection in cell culture.[182] In vitro models of acute and chronic HIV infection are inhibited by nicotinamide, but not by nicotinic acid, in a dose-dependent manner.[183] In addition, HIV infection may cause chronic loss of tryptophan, thus causing decreases in niacin, which in turn may cause cachexia, dementia, diarrhea, and possibly immunosuppression of AIDS patients.[184] Because HIV disease has associated deficiencies in several of the B vitamins and because of the AV, neurological, and hematological effects of supplementation, an orally administered B complex vitamin taken with meals is recommended for all HIV-positive patients.

Antiviral Therapies to be Further Investigated

Ozone. Ozone became a popular alternative therapy for HIV disease, inspired partly by the growing European literature describing ozone treatment for cancer. Many HIV-positive patients have used rectal insufflation of ozone in an attempt to suppress HIV replication. Ozone, which is a strong oxidizer, can stimulate increased production of cellular antioxidant enzymes, eventually inhibiting the oxidative stress associated with infection and inflammation.[185] Inactivation of HIV-1 by ozone has been demonstrated in vitro[186] and at noncytotoxic concentrations.[187] Three of four patients with AIDS or ARC, with intractable diarrhea of unknown etiology and who were treated with daily colonic insufflation of medical ozone, experienced complete resolution, and one patient had marked improvement.[188] Many naturopathic physicians have been reluctant to administer ozone to their

HIV-positive patients because of the unknown effects of ozone on what is already excessive FR production and proinflammatory processes attendant with HIV disease.

Olea (olive leaf). Olive leaf has become a popular HIV treatment during the past several years. Although no controlled trials have been published, it has been reported to increase NK cell function, to be antiretroviral, and to be effective against HIV and herpes viruses.[189]

Treatment Principle 5: Immunomodulation

One of the most common reasons that HIV-positive persons use alternative therapies is the belief that certain nutrients, plants, and hormones can boost the immune system. It is not clear that general immune stimulation, were it achievable, would be beneficial to HIV-positive patients, who show not only immunodeficiency but clinical and immunological signs of inflammatory autoimmunity. Restoration of immune function in patients treated with ART is currently an area of intense research in the conventional AIDS biomedical community. There are a number of natural substances that have been used as alternative therapies for HIV/AIDS that have immunomodulatory activity when tested in vitro. Most of these approaches have not been subjected to clinical trial. Nevertheless, it is reasonable to hypothesize that the correct combination of natural immunoregulatory agents may be the basis for an immune therapy for HIV/AIDS. The following section discusses the scientific basis for the use of several nutrients, botanicals, hormones, and therapeutic modalities by naturopathic physicians in assisting their patients to maintain and improve immune function.

Coenzyme Q$_{10}$

CoQ$_{10}$ has been shown to protect against tumor growth and enhance viral immunity in animals.[190] When administered at 100 mg/day, CoQ$_{10}$ was shown to increase blood levels of CD4$^+$ lymphocytes in an uncontrolled study in HIV-positive patients.[191] It has also been shown to significantly increase levels of immunoglobulin G (IgG) in AIDS patients.[191]

N-Acetylcysteine
See previous section.

Vitamin B$_6$ (Pyridoxine)

In one epidemiological study, dietary intake and supplementation of vitamin B$_6$ (dosage: up to 100 mg bid) at twice the RDA was associated with increased survival in HIV-1-positive persons.[16] For HIV-positive men, immunodeficiency was associated with consumption of vitamin B$_6$ and zinc at only the RDA level.[192] Low blood levels of vitamin B$_6$ were observed in 53% of HIV-1-positive patients. A similar abnormality among HIV-1-negative controls was not observed.[12] Impaired immune responsiveness has been observed in HIV-1-positive patients with compromised vitamin B$_6$ status,[193] and vitamin B$_6$ status in HIV-1-positive patients was significantly associated with functional parameters of immunity.[194] Pyridoxine deficiency induces atrophy of lymphoid organs, markedly reduces lymphocyte numbers, and impairs antibody responses and IL-2 production.[195] Although it appears clear that HIV-positive individuals are at risk for vitamin B$_6$ deficiency, there have been no clinical trials to date evaluating the effects of supplementation. Nevertheless, since the vitamin B$_6$ levels in a high-quality B-complex multivitamin supplement are safe, it seems prudent to orally prophylax against possible deficiencies and their immunological and neurological sequelae.

Zinc

Zinc plays an important role in immune function. For example, the synthesis of thymic hormone requires zinc as an essential cofactor.[196] Low blood levels of zinc were documented in 50% of HIV-1-positive patients.[12] Of a sample of 30 HIV-1-positive patients, 30% were found to have below-normal plasma concentrations of several important vitamins and minerals, including zinc.[105] In another study, serum zinc levels were found to be lower in the HIV-positive progressors than in the HIV-positive nonprogressors and the HIV-negative subjects. Furthermore, higher serum copper and lower serum zinc predicted progression to AIDS independently of baseline CD4$^+$ lymphocyte level, age, and calorie-adjusted dietary intakes of both nutrients.[197]

A report by Mocchegiani and Muzzioli reemphasized the important role of zinc in immune deficiency and HIV disease.[198] They showed that HIV RNA plasma levels were inversely proportional to both CD4 count and zincemia values and that low zinc levels were associated with higher rates of OIs in HAART-treated patients.

Given the important value of zinc supplementation in other immune conditions and the risk of zinc deficiency in HIV-positive patients, many NDs prescribed megadoses of zinc (60 to 90 mg/day) early in the epidemic. However, few NDs prescribe zinc now because of one epidemiological study's surprising results, reporting that zinc intake above RDA levels was associated with higher disease progression rates and poorer survival rates.[16] In light of the inconclusiveness of the field and the uncertainty about the wisdom of supplementing zinc, most NDs choose not to prescribe megadoses of zinc. A safe compromise is to recommend to patients that, in addition to the zinc provided in multivitamin and mineral supplements, they should eat pumpkin seeds, which are a rich source of dietary zinc and EFAs.

Echinacea (for Acute Viral Symptoms; not for Chronic Use)

Echinacea is probably the best known and most commonly used botanical for "immune support." In vivo studies show that it increases the number of polymorphonucleocytes and monocytes, induces C-reactive proteins (CRPs), and elevates erythrocyte sedimentation rate (ESR).[199] In vitro, echinacea extracts stimulate phagocytic activity of macrophages.[200] It is remarkable that the use of echinacea is so widespread among Americans despite the lack of clinical evidence showing benefit.

Many HIV-positive people take echinacea for its immune stimulating effects, although there have been no clinical trials of echinacea in HIV/AIDS. Thirty-four percent of the Bastyr University nationwide AMCOA study cohort reported using echinacea for managing their HIV disease. Nevertheless, its use is controversial among CAM clinicians. Some have argued that the long-term use of this herb may be contraindicated in HIV/AIDS. The argument put forth by some clinicians is that, because this herb is purported to stimulate the production of T cells, its use may inadvertently increase the number of HIV-infected T cells. In addition, echinacea's reported effects on elevating CRPs and ESR indicate that its chronic use may exacerbate the inflammatory components of the HIV disease process. There have been to date no studies that address either issue.

At Bastyr University we have taken a conservative position on the use of echinacea for our HIV-positive patients. Our clinical experience tells us that short-term use of echinacea is effective for curtailing upper respiratory infections (URIs). We recommend only short-term use (3 to 7 days) of this botanical for our HIV-positive patients during the first sign of a respiratory infection, and we discourage chronic use of this plant for immune support.

Astragalus Membranous

A. membranous is also frequently used as an immune therapy by HIV-positive persons. Seventeen percent of the AMCOA cohort reported using it. This herb has a reputation among herbalists as an immune-stimulating botanical. It is purported to increase white blood cell (WBC) production. One animal study reported that injections in mice enhanced antibody response to a T-dependent antigen.[201] To our knowledge, no trials have been conducted in HIV-positive patients to assess the immunological effect of this herb.

Eleutherococcus Senticosus

E. senticosus, or Siberian ginseng, has immunomodulatory activity in vitro. For example, it has been shown to increase T helper cells, as well as cytotoxic and NK cells in vitro.[202] The clinical trial literature on ginseng is sparse, and no trials have been conducted with HIV-positive patients. Nevertheless, 12% of AMCOA participants report taking Siberian ginseng for their HIV/AIDS. Naturopathic physicians will frequently prescribe *E. senticosus* for the treatment of *adrenal fatigue,* a diagnosis frequently made by NDs for their HIV-positive patients.

Lentinus Edodes (Shiitake Mushroom)

Lentinan is believed to be the active immunomodulatory constituent of shiitake mushroom. There is some preliminary in vitro evidence for immunological and AV effects. For example, lentinan was found to increase host resistance to various bacterial, viral, and parasitic infections, including HIV.[203] In one murine study, it was reported to have marked antitumor and antimetastatic activity and prevented chemical and viral carcinogenesis.[204] With IL-2, lentinan was reported to stimulate CD8$^+$ cytotoxic T-cell antitumor activity in vitro.[205] Two phase I/II placebo-controlled trials of IV lentinan (1 or 5 mg) in a total of 98 HIV-positive patients have been conducted.[206] Although not statistically significant, a trends toward increased CD4 counts and neutrophils was observed in the patients receiving verum.

Grifola Frondosa (Maitake Mushroom)

This mushroom extract is being prescribed to HIV-positive patients with increasing frequency, although no clinical trials have been published. Its use is based on in vitro data that show that maitake extract can increase the activity of macrophages, NK cells, and cytotoxic T-cell populations. Significant immunostimulating activity has been confirmed in vivo as well, even with oral administration, including increased antitumor activity in vivo. In vitro, it has shown anti-HIV activity.[207] The most common commercially available form of maitake mushroom is a liquid extract D-fraction. Typical doses are 10 drops tid.

Adrenal Glandular

Oral administration of adrenal glandular material has been used for decades by NDs in an effort to improve adrenal gland function in patients diagnosed with adrenal fatigue. Adrenal dysfunction has been observed in HIV-positive patients (see the following section on DHEA). No clinical trials have been published to date that investigate the effects of oral administration of adrenal glandular material. There is some concern about viral and prion contamination in glandular products made from bovine sources. Such glandular medicines may be a dangerous source of cross-species viral contamination. Therefore it is important to use only products that have been adequately tested. Most NDs will use 1000 mg of crude lyophilized gland from New Zealand calves bid.

Dehydroepiandrosterone

The adrenal steroid hormone DHEA is an intermediate compound in the synthesis of testosterone and other steroid reproductive hormones. It should be used with caution in women who are at risk for hormone-sensitive cancers. Use of DHEA among HIV-positive men is now widespread (10% among AMCOA participants) and is based on published evidence of low levels of DHEA in the HIV-positive population and an association of low serum levels with progression to AIDS. A 1991 epidemiological study showed that decreased levels of serum DHEA was a predictor for progression to AIDS in asymptomatic HIV-positive men.[208] Other studies showed that both DHEA levels and CD4$^+$ counts were independent predictors of disease progression in HIV-positive men[209] and that low serum DHEA sulfate (DHEAS) is associated with markers of HIV disease, including low CD4 count and HIV symptom severity and is inversely correlated with HIV RNA.[210]

A correlational study of CD4$^+$ counts and serum cortisol and DHEAS showed a positive relationship between immune status as measured by CD4$^+$ count and DHEA, supporting the hypothesis that DHEA deficiency may worsen immune status in HIV-infected patients.[211] Abnormally low levels of DHEA were associated with low levels of serum IL-2,[212] and therefore low levels of DHEA may cause immunological deficits via deficient IL-2 production in lymphocytes. Direct murine lymphocyte exposure to DHEA at low concentrations (10^{-10} to 10^{-7} M) enhanced secretion of IL-2 after immunological challenge.[213] Christeff et al have reported that serum DHEAS levels are positively correlated with body cell mass (BCM) and negatively correlated with weight loss in HIV-positive men.[214] These authors also reported a decreased DHEA and increased cortisol (increased cortisol:DHEA ratio) in HIV-positive patients with advanced stages of disease and increased protein catabolism.

A phase I study evaluated the effects of oral administration of DHEA in 13 HIV-positive patients with baseline CD4$^+$ counts of 250 to 600 cells/mm^3. Five patients treated with the highest of three doses (750 mg/day) had CD4$^+$ cell increases at 8 weeks from a mean of 373/μl pretreatment to 463/μl after 8 weeks.[215] In another open-label, uncontrolled study in 12 HIV-positive patients, DHEA therapy (75 mg/day) increased CD4$^+$ and CD8$^+$ cell counts in the majority of patients.[216] A subsequent study evaluated escalating oral doses of DHEA (750 mg/day up to 2250 mg/day) for 16 weeks in 31 HIV-positive patients with baseline CD4$^+$ counts between 250 and 600 cells/μl. Dose proportionality was not evidenced by either serum DHEA or by DHEAS. No sustained increases in CD4$^+$ counts or decreases in serum p24 antigen or $\beta_2$microglobulin levels were observed. However, serum neopterin levels decreased transiently by 23% to 40% at 8 weeks.[215] In a small, open-label trial with 20 HIV-positive people, DHEA as monotherapy at a fairly high dose of 600 mg bid was shown to reduce viral load by 0.6 log unit in HIV patients with baseline CD4$^+$ counts of 50 to 300.[217] DHEA is a modest selective inhibitor of HIV-1 replication in human lymphocytes and macrophages. The AV mechanism does not appear to be mediated through reverse transcriptase inhibition (RTI), since DHEA did not inhibit HIV-1 RT enzymatic activity when tested up to 100 μm.

Acute infection of normal human lymphocytes was also inhibited by DHEA at 10 to 100 μm. In another in vitro experiment, DHEA at concentrations of 3 to 30 μg/ml produced 50% inhibition of macrophage HIV p24 expression.[218]

DHEA is frequently prescribed to, and self-prescribed by, many HIV-positive patients in the United States. Given the apparent safety of oral DHEA supplementation and preliminary data suggesting possible benefit, most NDs prescribe DHEA to their HIV-positive patients in doses ranging from 15 to 50 mg bid, especially when serum levels are low (less than 250 mg/dl). However, caution may be appropriate, since high serum DHEA levels have also been implicated in the pathogenesis of KS in HIV/AIDS. DHEA levels were significantly higher, as were testosterone and androstenedione, in 34 HIV-positive patients with KS versus 35 HIV-positive controls without KS.[219]

Thymic Fractions

The thymus gland has been implicated in HIV disease. The thymus regulates differentiation of T-cell precursors and can normalize the ratio between helper and suppressor subsets.[220] Thymic atrophy in postmortem autopsies was observed and reported early in the AIDS epidemic. Zinc is an essential cofactor in the synthesis of thymic peptide hormone. Both thymic and zinc deficiencies have been implicated in the pathogenesis of AIDS.[221] In 1987, one study reported that thymic hormone supplementation improved clinical symptoms and T-cell defects in early stages of HIV infection.[222] One thymic hormone, thymostimulin, was shown to increase CD4$^+$ lymphocytes in a small study of HIV-positive patients.[223] NDs use these preliminary data to support their use of glandular medicines. As with other glandular products, caution should be exercised when using thymic glandular products in the age of prions and cross-species viral contamination. Physicians should request viral contamination assays from manufacturers of glandular products. Typical dosages prescribed are 1000 mg of lyophilized glandular bid.

Constitutional Acupuncture

Chinese medicine is perhaps the most common form of alternative medicine used by HIV-positive Americans. Forty-five percent of the Bastyr AMCOA cohort reported seeing an acupuncturist. Treating AIDS by acupuncture has wide anecdotal support.[224] Chinese medicine, which includes acupuncture and herbal therapy, has been used in an attempt not only to manage symptoms of HIV disease and side effects of conventional therapy but also as a way of optimizing overall health and strengthening the immune system. One of the best treatises on the subject is the book *AIDS and Chinese Medicine* by Shattuck and Ryan, which offers a comprehensive discussion of traditional Chinese medicine (TCM) in the treatment of HIV/AIDS.[225]

There have been several clinical trials of Chinese medicine in HIV/AIDS (see Chapter 21 for an extensive review). For example, in a 12-week randomized, double-blind, placebo-controlled, clinical trial, 30 adults with symptomatic HIV infection with CD4+ counts between 200 and 499 received either a combination of 31 Chinese herbs or a placebo. Outcome measures included QOL, symptoms, weight, and CD4+ count. No differences between treatment groups attained statistical significance, but there were trends toward greater improvement among herb-treated subjects on all symptom subscales except dermatological.[226] An uncontrolled outcomes study reported that a 3-month treatment course of acupuncture and Chinese herbal therapy in HIV-positive patients statistically decreased symptom severity and improved QOL.[227] A study of 31 HIV-positive patients with PN showed that acupuncture alleviated pain or tingling in 38% of the patients.[228] One clinician, after treating 112 HIV/AIDS patients with a Chinese herbal formula called Glyke (60 mg bid) for 3 to 6 months, reported improvements in CD4+ counts and reduction in symptoms.[229]

Bastyr University clinicians have found Chinese medicine to be useful for treating depression, fatigue, diarrhea, sinusitis, and PN in HIV-positive patients.

Constitutional Homeopathy

Homeopathy, like Chinese medicine, has been used in an attempt to improve overall health and immune function of HIV-positive patients. To our knowledge, there have been only two papers published in a peer-reviewed journal that report the clinical effects of constitutional homeopathic treatment on HIV-positive patients. Both were conducted by Rastogi et al[230] in India, who reported on 129 asymptomatic HIV-positive patients treated with homeopathic medicines (potencies from 30 C to 1 M) on the basis of the individual's constitutional characteristics. They reported that 12 patients became enzyme-linked immunoabsorbent assay (ELISA)-negative after 3 to 16 months. In 1999, Rastogi et al[230a] published a controlled trial comparing the effect of individualized homeopathic medicines with placebo

in 100 HIV-positive patients from 17 to 50 years of age (71% men) randomized to receive either a single homeopathic remedy or placebo. The group receiving verum showed statistically significant increases in CD4+ T lymphocytes after 6 months. Another uncontrolled trial with 34 HIV-positive patients reported increased CD4+ counts in 23 patients and no change in 4 patients.[231]

Despite the few studies of classic homeopathy in AIDS, many NDs prescribe constitutional homeopathy for their HIV-positive patients. The Bastyr University Integrated Care HIV/AIDS Clinic learned some useful tips for classic homeopathic treatment from an Indian homeopathic physician, Dr. Pijush Kumar Mishra (Bastyr University AIDS Research Center Visiting Fellow 1996 to 1998):

- When skin symptoms predominate, consider sulfur, Psorinum, or HSV nosode (for herpes infection).
- When growths such as warts or condylomata predominate, consider *T. occidentalis,* nitric acid, or Medorrhinum.
- When GI symptoms predominate, consider Lycopodium, including Hepar sulph, or Mercurius (for liver symptoms).
- When neurological symptoms predominate, consider *Arsenicum alba, Aurum metallicum,* Bufo, Calcarea c, Cannabis i, Causticum, Kali phosphorus, Lachesis, Lycopodium, Mercurius sol, *Nux vomica,* Natrum muriaticum, opium, phosphorus, Phosphoricum ac, silica, Staphysagria, Stramonium, sulfur, Syphlinum, Tarentula c, *T. occidentalis,* or Thyroidinum.
- When respiratory and wasting symptoms predominate, consider Aurum m, *Arsenicum alba,* Tuburculinum, Iodum, Arsenicum iod, or Phosphoricum ac.
- With STD-related AIDS cases, consider using Medorrhinum and Mercurius sol intercurrently.
- For harmful effects of chemotherapy, steroids, AZT, and combination drugs, consider homeopathic x-ray.

Constitutional Hydrotherapy

The application of alternating cold and hot packs to the chest and back has been used in traditional naturopathic medicine for more than a century. In modern times, it is known that the skin plays a significant role in immune function.[232] This modality has been applied to the treatment of HIV-positive patients but has never been subjected to clinical trial. A few studies suggest that this treatment has general effects on immune function. For example, $\alpha_2$macroglobulins and complement factor C3 were increased after hydrotherapy treatments.[233] Hydrotherapy helps maximize circulation of well-oxygenated, nutrient-rich, and toxin-low blood.[234]

Promising Substances to be Further Investigated

Melatonin. Melatonin (3 to 5 mg before bedtime) is often prescribed for insomnia and may be useful for insomnia associated with HIV disease. There is growing literature showing immunomodulatory activity of melatonin. Melatonin has been reported to regulate not only neuroendocrine functions but also to exert immune-enhancing and antitumor effects.[235] Higher doses of melatonin (up to 25 mg before bed) have been studied in several human cancers. Preliminary data support the hypothesis that melatonin may have both immunomodulating and tumoricidal activity. The immunoregulatory potential of melatonin therapy in HIV has not yet been explored. It is safe to use melatonin at the lower doses for treating insomnia in HIV-positive patients. Some clinicians are conducting single-patient therapeutic trials of higher doses of melatonin and are monitoring changes in CD4+ T-cell counts and other pertinent immune parameters.

Treatment Principle 6: Increase Oxidation of Tissues and Manage Stress

Physical Fitness Program

Literature demonstrating the benefits of aerobic exercise in reducing stress, treating depression and anxiety, and improving immune function is growing. This area of HIV/AIDS research is reviewed thoroughly in Chapter 14. Researchers have observed that long-term AIDS survivors generally engage in 1.5 fitness or exercise programs.[236] Researchers have also found positive relationships between hardiness and perception of physical, emotional, and spiritual health; participation in prayer and meditation; and participation in exercise and the use of special diets.[237] Exercise may mitigate both the negative emotional response to and the immunological impact of being diagnosed as HIV-positive. Individuals undergoing aerobic training reported no increases in anxiety and depression in response to notification of HIV-1-positive status. In

another similar study, an exercise intervention attenuated emotional distress and NK cell decrements after notification of HIV-1-positive status.[238] An aerobic exercise training program may enhance certain critical components of cellular immunity and act as a buffer for the detrimental mood changes that typically accompany stress.[239] During the nonacute stage of AIDS, progressive resistance exercise induced physiological adaptation that improved muscle function and increased body dimensions and mass.[240] Although there are no convincing data that moderate exercise in patients with HIV is linked with improved T helper cell counts,[241] observational data in 156 HIV-positive homosexual men indicated that self-reported exercise 3 to 4 times/week was associated with slower progression to AIDS after 1 year.[242]

Treatment Principle 7: Opportunistic Infection Prophylaxis and Treatment

Viral, Bacterial, Protozoal, and Yeast Infections

Many AIDS-related OIs are successfully treated with conventional pharmaceutical drugs. In general, for those OIs that have effective conventional treatments, it may be inappropriate to delay therapy in order to try unproven naturopathic methods. Some naturopathic methods may help prevent the occurrence of OIs. Several OIs, such as cryptosporidioisis and *Mycobacterium avium-intercellulare* (MAI), are not successfully or completely treated by current conventional antimicrobials. There may be a place for naturopathic strategies to prevent and treat OI. A summary of such approaches follows.

General Opportunistic Infection Prevention Strategies

Zinc. Zinc supplementation (15 mg/day) may be useful as a general means of preventing some bacterial infections. Hypozincemia in 228 HIV-positive patients was associated with an increased incidence of concomitant systemic bacterial infections, but not PCP, viral, or fungal infections.[243]

Garlic. Garlic has broad-spectrum antimicrobial activity, and there is evidence, mostly from in vitro studies, of its antibacterial, AV, tumoricidal, and immunomodulatory activity. Fifty-one percent of the Bastyr University AMCOA cohort reported using it for treating their HIV disease.[244] Garlic extract has demonstrated AV activity against CMV[245] and has been shown to be cytotoxic against herpes virus, *Cryptococcus,* mycobacteria, and *Candida.*[246-251] It also has been shown to enhance NK cell activity in AIDS patients.[252] There is sufficient preliminary evidence for the effect of garlic in HIV disease to warrant a controlled clinical trial. Although it is impossible to know at this time what an adequate dosage might be for patients with HIV disease, it is reasonable to proceed with dosages used in treating other conditions. Typically, the equivalent of 8 garlic cloves/day is recommended for a medicinal dose. Garlic has also been shown to lower cholesterol and triglycerides in HIV-negative populations and has been proposed as a potential therapy for HAART-related hyperlipidemia. A controlled clinical trial is underway at Bastyr University.

Colloidal silver. Colloidal silver was commonly used by the HIV community in the 1990s to treat and prevent various bacterial infections. Among 1675 Bastyr University AMCOA participants, 8% reported using colloidal silver. Typical dosages are 1 tsp bid of 3 ppm solution. Electrochemical Ag^+ solutions exhibit antimicrobial effectiveness against *Escherichia coli, Pseudomonas aeruginosa, C. albicans,* and *Aspergillus niger.*[253]

Supersaturated potassium iodide. Supersaturated potassium iodide (SSKI) has a long history of use among naturopaths for preventing and treating bacterial infections. It is usually dosed at 8 drops/day. There have been no clinical trials in any human populations.

Vitamin D. Vitamin D has been shown to be useful in treating/preventing tuberculosis, although excessive dosages can compromise B and T lymphocyte efficiency.[254] In one study, AIDS patients with MAI infection had severely decreased serum vitamin D levels.[255] Supplementation in HIV/AIDS is usually not recommended for most patients, unless they have tuberculosis (TB), MAI, or psoriasis. Some in vitro reports claim that vitamin D can accelerate HIV replication, which has led clinicians to cease prescribing vitamin D supplementation in the general HIV-positive population. Moderate exposure of the skin to sunlight produces adequate vitamin D and is a healthy source. The hormonal form of vitamin D, $1,25(OH)_2D_3$, is involved in the regulation of the immune system.[256] A paper reporting that HIV-related psoriasis responded to a topical vitamin D analogue is of clinical interest.[257]

Fungal infections. Fungal infections can be an annoying problem for many HIV-positive patients. Toe-nail fungal infections are common and difficult to treat. *T. occidentalis* (cedar), *M. alternafolia* (te tree oil), and *Calendula officinalis* all have antifungal activity and are worth trying topically.

Parasitic infections. Parasitic infections of the GI system are also common among HIV-positive individuals. Pancreatic enzymes and *Artemesia absiunthium* (wormwood) have been anecdotally reported to be useful in treating GI parasites. CAM clinicians are advised to use appropriate stool tests to adequately diagnose GI problems. Although conventional antiparasitic drugs are not without their side effects and potential toxicities, it is inadvisable to delay effective conventional therapy for such infections, some of which have severe symptomatology.

***Pneumocystis carinii* pneumonia.** *P. carinii* pneumonia (PCP) has been successfully prevented in many HIV/AIDS patients by the prophylaxis with trimethoprim/sulfamethoxazole. Although it is not advisable to rely on natural medicines for this purpose, there is some preliminary evidence that gingko and zinc may be of additional value in preventing PCP. Gingko biloba shows in vitro activity against *P. carinii.*[258]

Cryptosporidiosis. Cryptosporidiosis in AIDS patients can lead to life-threatening diarrhea. Conventional medicine does not offer definitive therapy. An interesting innovative therapeutic strategy uses bovine colostrum, a natural medicine that has been in the naturopathic *materia medica* for 150 years. Colostrum from cows immunized against *Cryptosporidium* is lyophilized and has been given orally in 10 g doses reconstituted in water qid. Bastyr University and the University Health Clinic in Seattle were two national clinical sites evaluating the efficacy of hyperimmune bovine colostrum (Sporidin-G) in cryptosporidial diarrhea. In six patients treated in Seattle for 20 to 40 days, four had resolution of diarrhea and elimination of detectable *Cryptosporidium* oocysts in follow-up stool samples. It has also been shown that *Cryptosporidium* oocyst excretion in healthy human subjects exposed to a challenge with *Cryptosporidium parvum* showed was lower in those who received bovine hyperimmune anti-*Cryptosporidium colostrum* compared with placebo.[259]

Kaposi's sarcoma. KS is a neoplasm of endothelium that can appear in immunocompromised persons. KS prevalence among HIV-positive patients has been associated with certain sexual practices, and thus it has been hypothesized that an infectious agent is involved. KS has been difficult to treat by conventional methods. Some CAM therapies may be helpful in treating KS. EFAs formulated to increase the tissue levels of dihomogamma-linolenic acid (DGLA) relative to arachidonic acid were reported to cause a regression in early KS in a small, uncontrolled study.[260] *Chelidonium majus* has been tried in the treatment of KS. IV administration of 10 mg of *C. majus* every other day for 10 injections has been reported to diminish the size, thickness, and color of KS lesions in a small, controlled study of AIDS patients.[261] Retinoic acid may have an important place in KS therapy as well. Also, in a small uncontrolled pilot study conducted at Bastyr University, rectal insufflation of shark cartilage had no observable effect on shrinking lesions.

Treatment Principle 8: Psychoneuroimmunology

The past 20 years of research in neurochemistry and immunology have led to the conclusion that the central nervous system (CNS) and the immune system are interdependent systems. Immune cells have been found to have receptor sites for neurotransmitters, and cytokines secreted by the immune system affect brain physiology. The field of PNI is only about 30 years old. Candace Pert, PhD, codiscoverer of endogenous brain opiates, has written for both scientific and lay audiences about the complex interdependent network of the CNS and immune systems.[262] Currently Pert and her colleagues continue to work on the neurotransmitter peptide T as an AIDS therapy targeted at the CNS.

We now know that brain function affects the immune system and that the immune system affects brain function. A substantial base of research shows that stressors of various kinds can significantly alter immune function both in laboratory animals and humans. Animal experiments have demonstrated that stress can accelerate tumorogenesis, or tumor growth. The stress of hiding one's sexual orientation can have demonstrable consequences on health. For example, one study showed significantly elevated physical health risk among gay men who concealed their homosexual identity.[263]

Although physical and emotional stress appear to exert negative effects on immune function in several models, it is not clear that therapies, practices, and devices intended to reduce emotional stress will produce improved immune function or status. Preliminary research, however, looks promising,[264] and it is likely that future research will bear this out. While we wait for more definitive studies, it seems wise to assume that inner states have an impact on immune function and, hence, in HIV-positive people, on disease progression. Certain CNS states can alter immune function. It may not be such a long leap to suggest that engaging in practices or therapies that induce inner states of serenity may have a beneficial effect on HIV/AIDS. One of the most important research questions to be addressed is whether therapies and psychological programs that result in reduced experience of stress, depression, and hopelessness alter the clinical, virological, or immunological course of the disease.

There are many therapeutic approaches to stress, anxiety, and depression reduction by and for HIV-positive men and women, including (1) individual and group psychotherapy; (2) meditation; (3) yoga; (4) Tai Chi; (5) cranioelectrical stimulation (CES); (6) botanicals such as *Hypericum,* Valerian, and Kava Kava; and (7) amino acids and their precursors, such as 5-hydroxytryptophane; (8) vitamins, and (9) minerals.

Sleep

Many patients and their health care providers forget about the importance of regular sleep and rest in emotional health and immune system function. It is important to remind patients to get a minimum of nine hours of rest daily. If patients have difficulty sleeping, it is important that they rest. Sleep has been shown to increase circulating NK cells and lymphocytes.[265,266] Naturopathic physicians, being aware of the healing power of nature itself, emphasize sleep and rest, along with sunlight, fresh water, wholesome food, and exercise. It is also important to remind our patients of the wise words of psychotherapist Ann Wilson Schaef, PhD, that "it is fighting our feelings that causes our suffering, not our feelings."

Support Groups

Support groups for HIV-positive men and women sprang up in the United States from the very beginning of the epidemic. There are a number of studies of the psychological impact of such support groups. Support groups have been reported to measurably reduce depression, hostility, and somatization.[267] Another study showed that participation in an AIDS support group decreases levels of anxiety and hopelessness[268] and that long-term coping skills are fostered in HIV-positive support groups.[269]

Meditation and Spiritual Practice

When used as part of a stress-management program, meditation was reported to significantly reduce anxiety and to increase mood, self-esteem, and T-cell counts in HIV-positive patients.[264] Carson has explored the role of mediation and spiritual practice in HIV disease.[270] She demonstrated a positive correlation between hardiness and a patient's perception of spiritual health and participation in prayer and meditation.[270] Meditation in healthy volunteers has been shown in one study to increase corticotropin-releasing hormone immunoreactivity after meditation.[271] Standish et al have preliminary observational data to suggest that an association between improved mental health scores and meditation, prayer, and spiritual activities may exist.[272] Some evidence exists that the health of terminally ill patients is based more on spirituality and ability to relate to others than on pathology.[273]

Cranioelectrical Stimulation

CES has been used in the treatment of anxiety and depression. CES devices deliver microcurrent stimulation (0.1 mA, 100 Hz) to alligator clips attached to the ear lobes. Twenty minutes of treatment twice daily has been shown to be effective in treating anxiety and insomnia,[274] as well as depression.[275]

Hypericum Perforatum (St. John's Wort)

H. perforatum is commonly prescribed to HIV-positive patients for both its AV and its antidepressant action, although, to our knowledge, there have been no clinical trials in HIV disease. In 23 randomized trials with a total of 1757 patients on *H. perforatum,* the botanical was more effective than placebo and was similarly effective to standard antidepressants but with fewer adverse events.[276,277] Typical dosage for treating depression is 300 mg tid of extract standardized to contain 0.3% hypericin, one of the known active constituents. Given preliminary data that *H. perforatum* can affect plasma levels of the HAART drug indinavir, clinicians should exercise caution when prescribing this botanical.

Minerals and Vitamins

A variety of minerals and vitamins may affect CNS neurotransmission and therefore may be useful in managing stress, anxiety, and depression.

Magnesium. Magnesium (Mg) has been used and studied with HIV-positive patients. In one study, 59% of HIV-positive patients had low concentrations of Mg compared with 9% of controls. This deficiency, it has been hypothesized, may be relevant to HIV-related symptoms of fatigue, lethargy, and impaired mentation.[278] Absolute number of $CD4^+$ cells was directly correlated with the serum Mg concentration.[279] Most clinicians will prescribe magnesium doses of 1000 mg/day.

Vitamin B_6 and tryptophan. Vitamin B_6 (pyridoxine) and the amino acid tryptophan are also commonly prescribed to HIV-positive patients. One study of HIV-positive patients reported that psychological distress declined with normalization of vitamin B_6 status from inadequate to adequate status. A decrease in psychological distress was also observed with increased tryptophan intake in patients who were vitamin B_6 adequate.[280]

Vitamin B_1. Vitamin B_1 (thiamin) deficiency was found in nine out of 39 (23%) of patients with AIDS or ARC and with no history of alcohol abuse.[281] Wernicke's encephalopathy (WE) is a neuropsychiatric disorder caused by thiamin deficiency and may be found in undernourished AIDS patients. The triad of confusion, ataxia, and ophthalmoplegia may be present.[282] Thiamin deficiency was the identified cause of WE in two nonalcoholic patients with AIDS.[283]

Vitamin B_{12}. Vitamin B_{12} is frequently prescribed to HIV-positive patients. In patients with subtle signs of vitamin B_{12} deficiency, such as macrocytic anemia, or those with low serum levels of vitamin B_{12}, vitamin B_{12} supplementation found in a high-quality oral B-complex vitamin is usually adequate. Naturopaths will often initiate a therapeutic trial of vitamin B_{12} IM when patients show signs of fatigue and depression. Concurrent vitamin B_{12} deficiency may be a cofactor in subtle cognitive changes observed in the asymptomatic stages of HIV-1 infection.[284] IM vitamin B_{12} therapy may also be useful for PN. Numerous published studies lend support to this therapeutic strategy. For example, normalization of plasma cobalamin in vitamin B_{12}-deficient HIV-positive patients may provide a significant improvement in memory.[285] One case study reported reversal of apparent AIDS dementia complex in one patient following treatment with vitamin B_{12}.[286] Most vitamin B_{12}-deficient HIV-positive patients with neurological dysfunction had a therapeutic response with vitamin B_{12} supplementation.[287] In those patients with signs and symptoms of less-than-optimal levels of vitamin B_{12}, IM injection of 1000 μg/week for a course of 6 weeks is recommended.

S-adenosylmethionine. Deficiencies of folate and vitamin B_{12} have been found to reduce CNS *S*-adenosylmethionine (SAMe) concentrations. Deficiency of either folate or vitamin B_{12} may cause similar neurological and psychiatric disturbances including depression, dementia, myelopathy, and PN. Methyl donors, including SAMe, have a variety of pharmacological effects in the CNS, especially on monoamine neurotransmitter metabolism and receptor systems. SAMe has antidepressant properties, and preliminary studies indicate that it may improve cognitive function in patients with dementia.[288] Cerebrospinal fluid SAMe and glutathione concentrations decreased in HIV infection.[289] Plasma levels of methionine in HIV-infected patients were also found to be lower.[290]

Treatment Principle 9: Decrease Toxicity and Counter Side-Effects of Pharmaceutical Drugs

Occasionally naturopathic physicians receive feedback from their MD colleagues who are treating HIV-positive patients. A common statement is that naturopathic therapies seem to help with managing those symptoms of HIV disease, such as fatigue, diarrhea, and neuropathy, that are poorly treated by conventional methods. We also occasionally hear from both our patients and their MD practitioners that naturopathic treatment has been useful in managing some of the side effects of conventional therapies. The following therapies have been used over the past decade to lower the toxicities of ART. Unfortunately, controlled clinical trial data do not exist for these therapies. Their use is based only on clinical experience.

AZT Side Effects

AZT-induced myopathy, immunosuppression, and bone marrow suppression are common side effects of AZT monotherapy, and are also seen, although with less severity, when AZT is used in combination with triple therapy. AZT is documented to induce oxidative damage to muscle tissue.[291]

Coenzyme Q_{10} and L-carnitine. CoQ_{10} and L-carnitine have been prescribed to offset AZT-induced myopathy. There have been several reports that CoQ_{10} reduces Adriamycin-induced cardiomyopthy in cancer patients undergoing chemotherapy. This finding has been extended to HIV-positive patients taking AZT, some of whom may be at risk for cardiomyopathies related to HIV disease, and as an adverse effect of some AIDS drugs.[292] Tissue depletion of L-carnitine by AZT induces myopathies and impaired lymphocyte function.[293] A marked decrease in total and free L-carnitine was observed in 21 (72%) of AIDS patients taking AZT.[294]

Vitamin B_{12}. Vitamin B_{12} is prescribed because decreased cobalamin levels are found frequently in HIV disease, especially among those treated with AZT. Evidence of vitamin B_{12} malabsorption is found among patients with more advanced disease and GI symptoms. Serum homocysteine levels were significantly higher in patients with subnormal cobalamin levels.[295]

Vitamin E. Vitamin E tocopherol has been reported to partially reverse the myelosuppressive action of AZT in HIV-positive patients without interfering with its AV activity. Vitamin E was reported to increase AZT activity in a dose-dependent manner up to sixfold in a study of 296 patients.[296,297]

Zinc. AZT may also have an impact on zinc status. In one longitudinal study of asymptomatic HIV-positive patients, a large proportion of the AZT-treated participants exhibited decreased levels of zinc and copper. The level of plasma zinc appeared to be particularly important in maintaining immune function in the AZT-treated group.[298]

Crixivan/Indinavir Nephrotoxicity

Shortly after the PI indinavir (Crixivan) was approved by the FDA and was in widespread clinical use, an increased risk for nephrolithiasis was observed. Patients receiving indinavir therapy are advised by all health care professionals to drink at least 1 L of filtered water/day to reduce the risk. Naturopathic physicians at the Bastyr University Integrated Care Clinic formulated a "kidney tonic tea" for HIV-positive patients on indinavir therapy in an effort to prevent kidney stones. This formula is a decoction of *Arctostaphylus uva-ursi*, *Zea mays*, *Eupatorium perfoliatum*, *Equisetum arvense*, *Symphytum radix*, *Verbascum thapsus*, and *Barosma betulina* in equal proportions. Patients are advised to drink 1 cup tid. Since a clinical trial has not been performed, it is impossible to know whether this strategy helps. The botanical formula is based on sound botanical medical logic, and each herb has a long history of safe use. The risk of trying naturopathic therapies that have not been examined by clinical trials is sometimes smaller than the risk associated with trying synthetic pharmaceuticals used in conventional medicine, since most of the natural medicines used have a long history of safe traditional use. The application of traditional herbal medicine makes good sense in HIV/AIDS. Much of what is used in CAM treatment for HIV/AIDS is based on clinician experience, not on clinical trial results. The safety factor inherent in many, but certainly not all, natural medicines makes this possible.

Didanosine, Videx, Dideoxynosine

In the absence of any disease-induced pathology, didanosine (ddI; an antiretroviral RTI) and isoniazid (an antitubercular drug) can induce neuropathy. Myelin splitting and intramyelin edema were the most frequent abnormalities observed in the sciatic nerves of ddI-dosed rats, whereas whorls, extracellular debris, macrophages, and reduced myelinated axon numbers were seen after chronic isoniazid administration. Isoniazid also resulted in myelinopathy of the CNS.[299]

Omega-3 oils. The use of omega-3 oils may be helpful in mitigating the inflammation associated with neuropathy (GLA 500 mg bid). NDs will frequently prescribe 1 tbsp of cod liver oil/day to help prevent and treat drug-induced neuropathic inflammation.

Hepatoprotection

The hepatotoxic effects of ART may be exaggerated by the CAM community, although HIV-positive patients receiving combination ART frequently have high liver function tests. Elevated serum liver enzymes can result from a number of factors associated with HIV disease and its treatment. Many HIV-positive patients also have a history of or a current infection with hepatitis A, B, or C.

Silymarin. Naturopathic physicians typically prescribe the antioxidant and hepatoprotective plant flavonoid silymarin (milk thistle) to HIV-positive patients who are taking ART, antibiotics, or both. The hepatoprotectant properties of silymarin have been described in several studies, including case studies in the treatment of mushroom poisoning[300] and cirrhosis associated with hepatitis C.[301] Although its use in HIV has never been clinically evaluated, there is justification for its use from both data in other systems and hepatic insult. To date, there have been no clinical trials of silymarin's efficacy in improving liver function in the face of conventional AIDS drugs. Alpha-lipoic acid (see previous section) is also prescribed for this purpose.

Herb/Drug Interactions

Piscitelli et al showed that two botanicals commonly used HIV-positive patients, St. John's wort and garlic, may interact in complex ways with anti-HIV PIs. Oral administration of St. John's wort in HIV-negative volunteers reduced plasma levels of indinavir by 57%.[302] In 1998 Foster presented some preliminary evidence that garlic increases GI side effects of ritonavir, possibly because garlic inhibits cytochrome P-450 3A4, which is involved in hepatic metabolism.[303] Orally administered garlic has more recently been shown to influence the pharmacokinetics of saquinavir in HIV-negative, healthy volunteers.[304] The prudent approach when using any CAM substance that may affect drug absorption or liver metabolism is to measure HIV RNA viral loads frequently to ensure that viral resistance or breakthrough is not associated with use of botanicals or other CAM therapies.

Hypersensitivity Reaction to Sulfa Drugs (TMP, Bactrim, Septra)

Many HIV-positive patients who begin Bactrim prophylaxis against PCP experience hypersensitivity reactions. NDs often suggest ramping up slowly to the final dosage and to take high doses of vitamin C and quercitin, both of which are antiinflammatory in high doses (vitamin C 2000 mg every 2 hours and quercetin 1000 mg qid). Over-the-counter Alka Selzer Gold is also useful for reducing the hypersensitivity reaction. Homeopathically prepared Bactrim is useful for desensitizing HIV-positive patients who are taking pharmacological doses for PCP prophylaxis.[305]

Peripheral Neuropathy

PN usually presents as lower limb and feet tingling, burning, or numbness, which is usually bilateral. It can be a side effect of several of the pharmaceutical antiretroviral drugs and can also appear in the absence of causative drug treatment. Often the following orally administered treatment combination will help: (1) vitamin B_{12} (1000 μg IM bid for 6 weeks), (2) cod liver oil (1 tbsp bid), and (3) myelin basic protein (1000 mg bid) for oral administration. Acupuncture has been used to treat PN with some success. There is some preliminary indication that electroacupuncture is more effective.[306] A typical course of therapy would be 1 to 3 treatments/week for 6 weeks.

Colitis and Diarrhea Associated with HAART

A combination of the following can be helpful in treating diarrhea and colitis associated with ART:

1. Cod liver oil 2 tsp bid
2. Glutamine 2000 mg bid
3. Quercetin 1000 mg bid

We have noticed that calcium supplementation appears to mitigate diarrhea caused by the nonnucleoside reverse transcriptase inhibitor efavirenz (Sustiva).

Dental Amalgams. Some dental filling materials are considered toxic before they are placed in teeth and are considered hazardous waste once they are removed from teeth. Currently, the largest source of environmental mercury pollution is mercury fillings. It is illegal in several European countries to use mercury in fillings. The American Dental Association (ADA) was founded at the turn of the twentieth century as a lobbying group to promote inexpensive and easy-to-use mercury amalgam fillings. Before that time, it was illegal to use mercury fillings in the United States, and several dentists were arrested for using mercury fillings. Amalgam fillings have been shown to decrease CD lymphocytes in humans.[307,308] Alloyed metals have been associated with autoimmunity in laboratory animals and with immunosuppression in humans.[309] It is currently unclear whether removal of mercury fillings in HIV-positive patients produces a significant clinical difference that makes the expense and inconvenience of the procedure worthwhile. Therefore, although we do not recommend the removal of dental amalgams in our patients, if someone should ask whether it might be a good idea, the answer is probably yes. Such patients should be referred to a dentist who specializes in biological dentistry.

Vaccination

Conventional health policy recommends prophylactic vaccination of HIV-positive patients against hepatitis B, *Pneumococcus,* and *Haemophilus influenzae.* However, various reports show that immunization using vaccines may stimulate HIV replication.[310] Additionally, there have been some reports of serious complications following routine vaccinations.[311] In one double-blind, placebo-controlled trial involving 47 HIV-positive patients, immunization with the influenza vaccine resulted in increases in HIV RNA viral load from 23,892 to 135,873 copies/ml in the vaccinated group, whereas in the placebo group HIV RNA levels fell slightly from an average of 25,826 to 18,470.[312] Two more recent studies have not observed increased viremia after influenza vaccination in HIV-infected patients.[313,314] King et al randomized HIV-positive patients to receive trivalent attenuated influenza vaccine or placebo intranasally.[314] They found no increase in HIV RNA or lowered CD4 counts in those patients receiving verum.

Vitamin A supplementation may be advisable to those patients who opt for influenza vaccination. Hanekom et al have reported that vitamin A administered to HIV-positive children before influenza vaccination dampened the increase in the HIV viral load 14 days after immunization compared with placebo-treated children who showed an increase viral load of 0.14 log.[315]

Given the potential benefit of vaccination in immunocompromised patients and the potential risks of vaccination in HIV-positive patients, it is unclear how to advise patients as to whether they should be vaccinated against specific viruses. Naturopathic physicians have historically been concerned about the immunological impact of large-scale vaccination programs and have a philosophical distrust of vaccinations in general. The best strategy, given the lack of data and the uncertainly about what is best for the individual patient, is to provide information to the patient about the potential risks and benefits. It is also important to assess each individual's risk for particular infections. For example, if an HIV-positive patient does not use IV drugs and is either celibate or in a long-term monogamous relationship and/or has evidence of hepatitis B immunity via previous exposures, it seems unnecessary to receive the hepatitis B vaccine. Vaccination decisions should be made in close collaboration with HIV and infectious disease experts. For those patients who choose to be vaccinated, many naturopathic physicians will prescribe homeopathic *T. occidentalis* for vaccinosis (i.e., the ill effects of vaccination).

IS NATUROPATHIC MEDICAL TREATMENT EFFECTIVE?

The scientific basis for the treatments suggested in the preceding compendium of clinical recommendations is based almost exclusively on what some call "borrowed" science, or is some cases, on subjective clinical experience only. Scientific evidence for the naturopathic medical approach described in the preceding pages comes from in vitro studies, animal studies, epidemiologically reported associations, and uncontrolled clinical studies but rarely from RCTs. To date there has not been a single RCT that addresses the question of whether naturopathic medical care slows or halts disease progression or improves clinical, laboratory, or QOL outcomes for HIV-positive patients. Even uncontrolled clinical outcomes data are limited (see the following section), and it is unclear whether naturopathic or other kinds of holistic care produce similar, poorer, or superior health outcomes to standard conventional therapy, or are simply, as some conventional physicians have suggested, merely harmless placebo. There are three published uncontrolled studies that suggest that comprehensive natural medical care can benefit HIV-positive patients (see Chapter 24).[4,316,317]

HOLISTIC PROVIDERS AND COMPREHENSIVE HEALTH CARE PROGRAMS

Published Uncontrolled Studies

A comprehensive 1-year treatment program of naturopathic medicine was evaluated from 1989 to 1990 with an uncontrolled trial in 16 asymptomatic HIV-positive men.[4] Treatment modalities included botanical and nutritional medicine, whole-body hyperthermia, homeopathy, physical medicine, and psychological counseling. Symptomatic and neuropsychological improvement was observed, and morbidity and mortality rates compared favorably with 1-year results in similar patients treated with AZT, which was the only ART available at the time. Absolute $CD4^+$ cell counts rose transiently at 3 months, then subsequently declined to below baseline levels by month 12. The slope of $CD4^+$ decline was lower than in recently published AZT studies looking at survival rates in similar patients. In two published AZT studies, only 18% were still alive in the 26-month follow-up period, whereas 40% of the naturopathically treated cohort were still alive 54 months later.

In Los Angeles, Joan Priestley, MD, treated 225 HIV-positive patients at various stages of the disease from approximately 1988 to 1993 with a protocol that employed both conventional pharmaceutical ART and prophylaxis and nutritional supplementation (po and IV). She released some preliminary data, from which she concluded that maintenance of a stable body weight (BW) is influenced by the use of nutrient supplementation therapy. Even after $CD4^+$ cell counts dropped below 50, 58% of the patients on the protocol survived for at least another year. She also suggested that survival rates appeared to be higher among the group who had never taken AZT than among the group who had taken AZT.

Jon Kaiser, MD, described outcome data from his large HIV-positive practice in Los Angeles in his 1993 book *Immune Power: A Comprehensive Treatment Program for HIV*. Kaiser's treatment included ART; antibiotic prophylaxis combined with botanical and nutritional supplementation; moderate exercise; abstinence from cigarettes, drugs, and alcohol; stress reduction techniques; and participation in an emotional support group. He released data based on his private practice files during a surveillance period of 4.25 years (March 1987 to June 1991). He reports that, of 134 patients tracked (asymptomatic, symptomatic, and AIDS), 119 out of the 134 remained stable or improved their diagnosis during the 4.25 years with an overall survival rate of 98%. Kaiser compares the survival rates of his patients after AIDS diagnosis with data published in *JAMA* and by the Centers for Disease Control (CDC) data. Kaiser's patients showed an 80% survival at 27.3 months (1987 to 1992), whereas the *JAMA* data report 50% survival at 12.5 months (1981 to 1987), and CDC reports 50% survival at 22 months (1985 to 1990). Kaiser reports on 10 HIV-positive asymptomatic patients with mean $CD4^+$ cell counts at intake of 406 and a 96% preservation of mean CD4 count at the completion of a 30-month study period. He compares this to a CD4 cell count drop of 18% in a comparison group receiving only conventional therapy during the same period.

The nine naturopathic treatment principles proposed and described for the comprehensive treatment of HIV/AIDS seem sound. With rare exceptions, however, it has been difficult to achieve the implementation of all treatment principles. Often providing what an ND would consider adequate comprehensive treatment is simply not logistically achievable in most patients. In 10 years of working with HIV-positive patients, we have been able to implement what we consider to be truly comprehensive naturopathic care in only several cases. In some of those cases, stellar results have been obtained. However, for most HIV-positive patients, lack of financial resources is an obstacle to using the full potential of naturopathic medicine. Most insurance companies do not cover naturopathic medicines, and only a few in several states cover medical visits to licensed NDs. In addition, in many cases, the inability to establish true co-management among all of a patient's health care providers generates fragmentation of care. Implementation of many naturopathic therapies requires time, energy, and commitment on the part of the patient, each of which many be in short supply.

Now that nearly 15 years of the AIDS epidemic have passed, it seems appropriate for CAM clinicians and scientists to propose and obtain funding for a controlled clinical trial comparing comprehensive naturopathic care plus ART to conventional care. The design of such a trial is challenging but not impossible. By necessity, it will be an expensive and complex study, but, given the preliminary preclinical and clinical evidence, it is worth pursuing.

UNITED STATES NATIONAL INSTITUTES OF HEALTH OFFICE OF ALTERNATIVE MEDICINE/BASTYR UNIVERSITY HIV/AIDS RESEARCH CENTER

These three studies of clinical outcomes in HIV-positive patients treated with combination natural medicine protocols suggest that comprehensive care that is concordant with several naturopathic principles described in this chapter may be valuable in the clinical management of the HIV-positive patient. However, more research needs to be done to provide more certainty about which therapies in the field of alternative medicine are truly useful and which are not, or even worse, which are harmful. For this reason, the Bastyr University AIDS Research Center was established in 1994 through a cooperative agreement grant with the NIH's Office of Alternative Medicine (OAM) and administered through the National Institute of Allergy and Infectious Disease's Office of AIDS. Much of the work of the center has been focused on evaluating the clinical, laboratory, and QOL outcomes associated with use of complementary and alternative medicine in 1666 HIV-positive men and women enrolled in the Bastyr University Alternative Medicine Outcomes in AIDS.[244]

RESEARCH AGENDA FOR NATUROPATHIC MEDICINE

Now that we have the perspective of 15 years of watching the role of CAM in the treatment of HIV/AIDS, it is perhaps time to articulate a research agenda for naturopathic medicine in this area. Given what we know from the scientific literature, preliminary evidence, and clinical experience, the following research topics seem to be of the highest priority. The first area includes those CAM treatments that may be capable of reducing side effects of HAART, including garlic in the treatment of hyperlipidemia associated with PIs; alpha-lipoic acid in the treatment of HIV- and HAART-related dysglycemia, diabetes, and PN; and CoQ$_{10}$ in mitigating cardiomyopathy associated with both HIV disease itself and HAART. The second area is the study of the immunological activity of botanicals and biologicals toward the goal of protecting, improving, and restoring immune system function in HIV-infected populations (e.g., polysaccharides from medicinal mushrooms, ginseng, astragalus, melatonin, DHEA, and homeopathically prepared cytokines and GFs [see Chapter 9]). The third research area of promise is to determine if anti-HIV botanical medicines can be combined to produce a clinically significant AV effect.

More research needs to be done on CAM in the treatment of HIV/AIDS. Enthusiasm for CAM research may have been temporarily diminished in the CAM community by the success of combination HAART introduced in 1996. Nevertheless, the need for HIV/AIDS CAM research is now even greater in the following three areas: (1) mitigation of HAART-related side effects, (2) immune restoration, and (3) combination anti-HIV botanical therapy. CAM therapies may play a role in immune restoration and decrease the multiple side effects of HAART, including hyperlipidemia, diabetes, PN, anemia, and cardiomyopathy.

In the meantime, we urge physicians to apply the principles of naturopathic medicine in the care of their HIV-positive patients. These principles make theoretical sense, and many of the naturopathic therapies utilized rest on sound preliminary in vitro, animal, and, in some cases, preliminary human clinical data.

RESOURCES

It is usually considered bad form to provide information or recommendations about commercial sources of natural medicines. Since the natural health industry is not regulated, the quality of nutrients, botanicals, glandulars, and even homeopathics available over the counter is suspect. Aware of the potential problem, naturopathic physicians have established excellent collaborative relationships with a number of reputable and responsible companies. For CAM clinicians new to the field wishing to implement some of the principles and therapies described in this chapter, we recommend contacting the Bastyr University dispensary.

Dispensary

Products are available to patients with a physician prescription from Bastyr Center for Natural Health at (206) 834-4100, extension 4114.

Acknowledgment

The author wishes to thank Langley Douglass, Jung Kim, and Amanda Lien at the Bastyr University Research Institute for their assistance in the review of the scientific literature for this chapter. Special thanks to Tove Hansen and Heather Bradley for their bibliographic and technical assistance in the preparation of this manuscript.

References

1. Anonymous: Case-control study of HIV seroconversion in health care workers after percutaneous exposure to HIV-infected blood: France, United Kingdom, and United States, January 1988-August 1994, *MMWR Morb Mortal Wkly Rep* 44(50):929-933, 1995.

2. Puro V, Petrosillo N, Ippolito G: Risk of hepatitis C seroconversion after occupational exposures in health care workers: Italian study group on occupational risk of HIV and other bloodborne infections, *Am J Infect Control* 23:273-277, 1995.

3. Breen EC, Rezai AR, Nakajima K, et al: Infection with HIV is associated with elevated IL-6 levels and production, *J Immunol* 144:480, 1990.

4. Standish LJ, Guiltinan J, McMahon E, et al: One year open trial of naturopathic treatment of HIV infection class IV-A in men, *J Naturopath Med* 3:42-64, 1992.

5. Sonnerborg A, Carlin G, Akerlund B, et al: Increased production of malondialdehyde in patients with HIV infection, *Scand J Infect Dis* 20:287, 1988.

6. Allard JP, Aghdassi E, Chau J, et al: Effects of vitamin E and C supplementation on oxidative stress and viral load in HIV-infected subjects, *AIDS* 12(13):1653-1659, 1998.

7. Aghdassi E, Allard J: Breath alkanes as a marker of oxidative stress in different clinical conditions, *Free Radic Biol Med* 2(6):880-886, 2000.

8. Lacey CJ, Murphy ME, Sanderson MJ, et al: Antioxidant-micronutrients and HIV infection, *Int J STD AIDS* 7:485-489, 1996.

9. Mastroiacovo P, Ajassa C, Berardelli G, et al: Antioxidant vitamins and immunodeficiency, *Int J Vitam Nutr Res* 66(2):141-145, 1996.

10. Omene JA, Easington CR, Glew RH, et al: Serum beta-carotene deficiency in HIV-infected children, *J Natl Med Assoc* 88:789, 1996.

11. Phuapradit W et al: Serum vitamin A and beta-carotene levels in pregnant women infected with human immunodeficiency virus-1, *Obstet Gynecol* 87:564, 1996.

12. Beach RS, Mantero-Atienza E, Shor-Posner G, et al: Specific nutrient abnormalities in asymptomatic HIV-1 infection, *AIDS* 6:701-708, 1992.

13. Sappey C, LeClercq P, Coudray C, et al: Vitamin, trace element, and peroxide status in HIV seropositive patients: asymptomatic patients present a severe beta-carotene deficiency, *Clin Chim Acta* 230:35, 1994.

14. Coodley GO, Coodley MK, Nelson HD, et al: Micronutrient concentrations in the HIV wasting syndrome, *AIDS* 7:1595-1600, 1993.

15. Delmas-Beauvieux MC, Peuchant E, Couchouron A, et al: The enzymatic antioxidant system in blood and glutathione status in human immunodeficiency virus (HIV)-infected patients: effects of supplementation with selenium or beta-carotene, *Am J Clin Nutr* 64:101-107, 1996.

16. Tang AM, Graham NM, Saah AJ: Effects of micronutrient intake on survival in human immunodeficiency virus type 1 infection, *Am J Epidemiol* 143:1244-1256, 1996.

17. Coodley GO, Girard DE: Beta-carotene in HIV infection, *J Acquir Immune Defic Syndr Hum Retrovirol* 6:272-276, 1993.

18. Nimmagadda A, Burri B, Neidlinger T, et al: Effect of oral beta-carotene supplementation on plasma human immunodeficiency virus (HIV) RNA levels and $CD4^+$ cell counts in HIV-infected patients, *Clin Infect Dis* 27(5):1311-1313, 1998.

19. Bianchi-Santamaria A, Fedeli S, Santamaria L: Possible activity of beta-carotene in patients with the AIDS related complex, *Int Conf AIDS* 9:496, 1993.

20. Constans J, Seigneur M, Blann A, et al: Effect of the antioxidants selenium and beta-carotene on HIV-related endothelium dysfunction, *Thromb Haemost* 80(6):1015-1017, 1998.

21. DeLuca LM, Ross SA: Beta-carotene increases lung cancer incidence in cigarette smokers, *Nutr Rev* 54:178-180, 1996.

22. Folkers KF, Langsjoen P, Nara Y, et al: Biochemical deficiencies of coenzyme Q_{10} in HIV-infection and exploratory treatment, *Biochem Biophys Res Commun* 153:886-896, 1988.

23. Folkers KT, Hanioka T, Xia LJ, et al: Coenzyme Q_{10} increases T4/T8 ratios of lymphocytes in ordinary subjects and relevance to patients having the AIDS related complex, *Biochem Biophys Res Commun* 176:786-791, 1991.

24. Berger J, C Reeves, K Greene, et al: Literature review on the top 10 CAM substances used by HIV-positive participants in the AMCOA study, *J Naturopath Med* 9(1):20-31, 2000.

25. Allard JP, Aghdassi E, Narine N, et al: Effects of antioxidant vitamin supplementation in patients with HIV infection, *Int Conf AIDS* 1998 (abstract O-2).

26. Harakeh S, Jariwalla RJ, Pauling L: Suppression of human immunodeficiency virus replication by ascorbate in chronically and acutely infected cells, *Proc Natl Acad Sci U S A* 87:7245-7249, 1990.

27. Cameron E, Pauling L, Leibovitz B: Ascorbic acid and cancer: a review, *Cancer Res* 39(3):663-681, 1979.

28. Critchfield JW et al: Inhibition of HIV activation in latently infected cells by flavonoid compounds, *AIDS Res Hum Retroviruses* 12(1):39-46, 1996.

29. Wang Y, Watson RR: Is vitamin E supplementation a useful agent in AIDS therapy, *Prog Food Nutr Sci* 17:351, 1993.

30. Passi S, De Luca C, Picardo M, et al: Blood deficiency values of polyunsaturated fatty acids of phospholipids, vitamin E, and glutathione peroxidase as possible risk factors in the onset and development of acquired immunodeficiency syndrome, *G Ital Dermatol Venereol* 125:125-130, 1990.

31. Liang B, Chung S, Araghinikinam M, et al: Vitamins and immunomodulation in AIDS, *Nutrition* 12:1-7, 1996.

32. Abrams B, Duncan D, Hertz-Picciotto I: A prospective study of dietary intake and acquired immune deficiency syndrome in HIV-seropositive homosexual men, *J Acquir Immune Defic Syndr Hum Retrovirol* 6:949-958, 1993.

33. Pacht E, Diaz P, Clanton T, et al: Gadek J: Serum vitamin E decreased in HIV-seropositive subjects over time, *J Lab Clin* 130(3):293-296, 1997.

34. Tang AM et al: Low serum vitamin B_{12} concentrations are associated with faster human immunodeficiency virus type 1 (HIV-1) disease progression, *J Nutr* 127:345, 1997.

35. Yuejian W, Watson RR: Vitamin E supplementation at various levels alters cytokine production by thymocytes during retrovirus infection causing murine AIDS, *Thymus* 22:153, 1994.

36. Yuejian W, Huang DS, Wood S, et al: Modulation of immune function and cytokine production by various levels of vitamin E supplementation during murine AIDS, *Immunopharmacology* 29:225, 1995.

37. Geissler RG, Ganser A, Ottmann OG, et al: In vitro improvement of bone marrow-derived hematopoietic colony formation in HIV-positive patients by alpha-D-tocopherol and erythropoietin, *Eur J Haematol* 53:201-206, 1994.

38. Dworkin BM: Selenium deficiency in HIV infection and the acquired immunodeficiency syndrome (AIDS), *Chem Biol Interact* 91:181-186, 1994.

39. Dworkin BM, Rosenthal WS, Wormser GP, et al: Selenium deficiency in the acquired immunodeficiency syndrome, *JPEN J Parenter Enteral Nutr* 10(4):405-407, 1986.

40. Baum MK, Shor-Posner G, Lu Y: Micronutrients and HIV-1 disease progression, *Nutr Rev* 56:S135-S139, 1998.

41. Constans J, Pellegrin JL, Peuchant E: Membrane fatty acids and blood antioxidants in 77 patients with HIV infection, *Rev Med Interne* 14:1003, 1993.

42. Cheung N: Looking at dietary effects on weight loss and diarrhea in HIV seropositive patients: a pilot project, *Nutr Health* 10:201, 1995.

43. Sappey C, Legrand-Poels S, Best-Belpomme M, et al: Stimulation of glutathione peroxidase activity decreases HIV type 1 activation after oxidative stress, *AIDS Res Hum Retroviruses* 10:1451-1461, 1994.

44. Makropoulos V, Bruning T, Schulze-Osthoff K: Selenium-mediated inhibition of transcription factor NF-kappa B and HIV-1 LTR promoter activity, *Arch Toxicol* 70:277, 1996.

45. Schrauzer GN, Sacher J: Selenium in the maintenance and therapy of HIV-infected patients, *Chem Biol Interact* 91(2-3):199-205, 1994.

46. de-Quay B, Malinverni R, Lauterburg BH: Glutathione depletion in HIV-infected patients: role of cysteine deficiency and effect of oral N-Acetylcysteine, *AIDS* 6:815, 1992.

47. Raju PA, Herzenberg LA, Herzenberg LA, et al: Glutathione precursor and antioxidant activities of N-Acetylcysteine and oxothiazolidine carboxylate compared in in vitro studies of HIV replication, *AIDS Res Hum Retroviruses* 10:961-967, 1994.

48. Droge W: Cysteine and glutathione deficiency in AIDS patients: a rationale for the treatment with N-Acetylcysteine, *Pharmacology* 46:61-65, 1993.

49. Cavalline L, Alexandre A: Oral N-Acetyl-cysteome increases the production of anti-HIV chemokines in peripheral blood mononuclear cells, *Life Sci* 67(2):47-54, 2000.

50. Breitkreutz R: Improvement of immune functions in HIV infection by sulfur supplementation: two randomized trials, *J Mol Med* 78(1):55-62, 2000.

51. Harakeh S, Jariwalla RJ: Comparative study of the anti-HIV activities of ascorbate and thiol-containing reducing agents in chronically HIV-infected cells, *Am J Clin Nutr* 54:1231S-1235S, 1991.

52. Nottet HS, van Asbeck BS, de Graaf L, et al: Role for oxygen radicals in self-sustained HIV-1 replication in monocyte-derived macrophages: enhanced HIV-1 replication by N-Acetyl-L-cysteine, *J Leukoc Biol* 56:702-707, 1994.

53. Pani A, Marongiu ME, Lauterburg BH: Modulatory effect of N-Acetyl-L-cysteine on the HIV-1 multiplication in chronically and acutely infected cell lines, *Antiviral Res* 22:31, 1993.

54. Droge W, Eck HP, Mihm S: HIV-induced cysteine deficiency and T-cell dysfunction: a rationale for treatment with N-Acetylcysteine, *Immunol Today* 13:211-214, 1992.

55. Kinscherf R, Fischbach T, Mihm S, et al: Effect of glutathione depletion and oral N-Acetylcysteine treatment on CD4+ and CD8+ cells, *FASEB J* 8:448-451, 1994.

56. Nichols TW: Alpha-lipoic acid: biological effects and clinical implications, *Altern Med Rev* 2:177-183, 1977.
57. Packer L: Alpha-lipoic acid as a biological antioxidant, *Free Radic Biol Med* 19:227, 1995.
58. Packer L, Suzuki YJ: Vitamin E and alpha-lipoate: role in antioxidant recycling and activation of the NF-kappa B transcription factor, *Mol Aspects Med* 14:229, 1993.
59. Jacob S, Henrikesen EF, Schiemann AL: Enhancement of glucose disposal in patients with type 2 diabetes by alpha-lipoic acid, *Arzneimittelforschung* 45(8):872-874, 1995.
60. Ruhnau K, Meissner HP, Finn JR, et al: Effects of 3-week oral treatment with the antioxidant thioctic a (alpha-lipoic acid) in symptomatic diabetic polyneuropathy, *Diabet Med* 16(12):1040-1043, 1999.
61. Salazar MR: Alpha lipoic acid: a novel treatment for depression, *Med Hypotheses* 55(6):510-512, 2000.
62. Dana Consortium. *Neurology* 53:645, 1998.
63. Grieb G: Alpha-lipoic acid inhibits HIV replication, *Med Monatsschr Pharm* 5:243, 1992.
64. Merin JP, Matsuyama M, Kira T: Alpha-lipoic acid blocks HIV-1 LTR-dependent expression of hygromycin resistance in THP-1 stable transformants, *FEBS Lett* 394:9, 1996.
65. Shoji S, Furuishi K, Yanase R, et al: Allyl compounds selectively killed human immunodeficiency virus (type 1)-infected cells, *Biochem Biophys Res Commun* 194:610-621, 1993.
66. Suzuki YJ, Aggarwal BB, Packer L: Alpha-lipoic acid is a potent inhibitor of NF-kappa B activation in human T cells, *Biochem Biophys Res Commun* 189:1709, 1992.
67. Han D, Tritschler HJ, Packer-L: Alpha-lipoic acid increases intracellular glutathione in a human T-lymphocyte Jurkat cell line, *Biochem Biophys Res Commun* 207:258, 1995.
68. Fuchs J, Schofer H, Milbradt R: Studies on lipoate effects on blood redox state in human immunodeficiency virus infected patients, *Arzneimittelforschung* 43:1359, 1993.
69. Gismondo MR, Lo Bue AM, Chisari G, et al: Competitive activity of a bacterial preparation on colonization and pathogenicity of *C. pylori*: a clinical study, *Clin Ter* 134:41-46, 1990.
70. Olin BR et al: *Acidophilus,* St Louis, 1991, JB Lippincott Co.
71. Klebanoff SJ, Coombs RW: Viricidal effect of *Lactobacillus acidophilus* on human immunodeficiency virus type 1: possible role in heterosexual transmission, *J Exp Med* 174:289-292, 1991.
72. Kvale D, Brandtzaeg P: Constitutive and cytokine induced expression of HLA molecules, secretory component, and intercellular adhesion molecule-1 is modulated by butyrate in the colonic epithelial cell line HT-29, *Gut* 36:737-742, 1995.
73. Scheppach W, Bartram P, Richter A, et al: Effect of short-chain fatty acids on the human colonic mucosa in vitro, *JPEN J Parenter Enteral Nutr* 16:43-48, 1992.
74. Finnie IA, Dwarakanath AD, Taylor BA, et al: Colonic mucin synthesis is increased by sodium butyrate, *Gut* 36:93-99, 1995.
75. Assumpcao I, Rodrigues M, Barbieri D: Treatment of unspecific ulcerative rectocolitis in a child with enemas containing butyrate, *Arq Gastroenterol* 36(4):238-243, 1999.
76. Klimberg VS, Souba WW, Dolson DJ, et al: Prophylactic glutamine protects the intestinal mucosa from radiation injury, *Cancer* 66:62-68, 1990.
77. Shabert JK, Wilmore DW: Glutamine deficiency as a cause of human immunodeficiency virus wasting, *Med Hypotheses* 46:252-256, 1996.
78. Dwyer JT: Nutrition support of HIV-positive patients, *Henry Ford Hosp Med J* 39:60-65, 1991.
79. Clark R, Feleke G, Din M, et al: Nutritional treatment for acquired immunodeficiency virus-associated wasting using beta-hydroxy beta-methylbutyrate, glutamine, and arginine: a randomized, double-blind, placebo-controlled study, *JPEN J Parenter Enteral Nutr* 24(3):133-139, 2000.
80. Hoppe JE, Friess D, Niethammer D: Orointestinal yeast colonization of pediatric oncologic patients during antifungal prophylaxis: results of quantitative culture and *Candida* serology and comparison of three polyenes, *Mycoses* 38:41-49, 1995.
81. Damjanovic V, Connolly CM, van Saene HK, et al: Selective decontamination with nystatin for control of a *Candida* outbreak in a neonatal intensive care unit, *J Hosp Infect* 24:245-259, 1993.
82. Desai MH, Rutan RL, Heggers JP, et al: *Candida* infection with and without nystatin prophylaxis: an 11-year experience with patients with burn injury, *Arch Surg* 127:159-162, 1992.
83. Hammer KA, Carson C, Riley T: In vitro activity of essential oils, in particular *Melaleuca alternifolia* (tea tree) oil and te tree oil products, against *Candida* spp, *J Antimicrob Chemother* 42(5):591-595, 1998.
84. Concha J, Moore L, Holloway W: 1998 William J. Stickel Bronze Award. Antifungal activity of *Melaleuca alternifolia* (te tree) oil against various pathogenic organisms, *J Am Podiatr Med Assoc* 88(10):489-492, 1998.
85. DeSimone C, Tzantzoglou S, Jirillo E: L-carnitine deficiency in AIDS patients, *AIDS* 6:203, 1992.
86. DeSimone C, Tzantzoglou S, Famularo G: High dose L-carnitine improves immunologic parameters in AIDS patients, *Immunopharmacol Immunotoxicol* 15:1, 1993.
87. DeSimone C, Famularo G, Tzantzoglou S: Carnitine depletion in peripheral blood mononuclear cells from patients with AIDS: effect of oral L-carnitine, *AIDS* 8:655, 1994.

88. Di Marzio L, Moretti S, D'Alo S, et al: Acetyl-L-carnitine administration increases insulin-like growth factor 1 levels in asymptomatic HIV-1-infected subjects: correlation with its suppressive effect on lymphocyte apoptosis and ceramide generation, *Clin Immunol* 92(1):103-110, 1999.

89. Moretti S, Alesse E, Di Marzio L, et al: Effects of L-carnitine on human immunodeficiency virus-1 infection-associated apoptosis: a pilot study, *Blood* 91(10):3817-3824, 1998.

90. Claessens Y, Cariou A, Chiche J, et al: L-Carnitine as a treatment of life-threatening lactic acidosis induced by nucleoside analogues, *AIDS* 14(4):472-473, 2000.

91. McFarland LV, Surawicz CM, Greenberg RN, et al: Prevention of beta-lactam-associated diarrhea by *Saccharomyces boulardii* compared with placebo, *Am J Gastroenterol* 90:439-448, 1995.

92. Surawicz CM, Elmer GW, Speelman P, et al: Prevention of antibiotic-associated diarrhea by *Saccharomyces boulardii*: a prospective study, *Gastroenterology* 96:981-988, 1989.

93. Buts JP, Bernasconi P, Vaerman JP, et al: Stimulation of secretory IgA and secretory component of immunoglobulins in small intestine of rats treated with *Saccharomyces boulardii, Dig Dis Sci* 35:251-256, 1990.

94. Bleichner G, Blehaut H, Mentec H, et al: *Saccharomyces boulardii* prevents diarrhea in critically ill tube-fed patients: a multicenter, randomized, double-blind, placebo-controlled trial, *Intensive Care Med* 23(5):517-523, 1997.

95. Castagliuolo I, Riegler M, Valenick L, et al: *Saccharomyces boulardii* protease inhibits the effects of *Clostridium difficile* toxins A and B in human colonic mucosa, *Infect Immun* 67(1):302-307, 1999.

96. Kinchington D, Randall S, Winther M, et al: Lithium gamma-linolenate-induced cytotoxicity against cells chronically infected with HIV-1, *FEBS Lett* 330:219-221, 1993.

97. Berger A, German JB, Chiang BL, et al: Influence of feeding unsaturated fats on growth and immune status of mice, *J Nutr* 123:225-233, 1993.

98. Adam O, Wolfram G, Zollner N: Effect of alpha-linolenic acid in the human diet on linoleic acid metabolism and prostaglandin biosynthesis, *J Lipid Res* 27:421-426, 1986.

99. Suttmann U, Ockenga J, Schneider H, et al: Weight gain and increased concentrations of receptor proteins for tumor necrosis factor after patients with symptomatic HIV infection received fortified nutrition support, *J Am Diet Assoc* 96:565-569, 1996.

100. Passi S, De Luca C, Picardo M, et al: Blood deficiency values of polyunsaturated fatty acids of phospholipids, vitamin E, and glutathione peroxidase as possible risk factors in the onset and development of acquired immunodeficiency syndrome, *G Ital Dermatol Venereol* 125:125-130, 1990.

101. Begin ME, Das UN: A deficiency in dietary gamma-linolenic and/or eicosapentaenoic acids may determine individual susceptibility to AIDS, *Med Hypotheses* 20:1-8, 1986.

102. Holman R: The slow discovery of the importance of omega 3 essential fatty acids in human health, *J Nutr* 128(suppl 2):427S-433S, 1998.

103. Bengmark S, Jeppsson B: Gastrointestinal surface protection and mucosa reconditioning, *JPEN J Parenter Enteral Nutr* 19:410-415, 1995.

104. Dworkin BM, Wormser GP, Axelrod F, et al: Dietary intake in patients with acquired immunodeficiency syndrome (AIDS), patients with AIDS-related complex, and serologically positive human immunodeficiency virus patients: correlations with nutritional status, *JPEN J Parenter Enteral Nutr* 14:605-609, 1990.

105. Bogden JD, Baker H, Frank O, et al: Micronutrient status and human immunodeficiency virus (HIV) infection, *Ann N Y Acad Sci* 587:189-195, 1990.

106. Coodley G, Girard DE: Vitamins and minerals in HIV infection, *J Gen Intern Med* 6:472-479, 1991.

107. Beach RS, Morgan R, Wilkie F, et al: Plasma vitamin B_{12} level as a potential cofactor in studies of human immunodeficiency virus type 1-related cognitive changes, *Arch Neurol* 49:501-506, 1992.

108. Revell P, MJ OD, Tang A, Savidge GF: Folic acid absorption in patients infected with the human immunodeficiency virus, *J Intern Med* 230:227-231, 1991.

109. Israel DS, Plaisance KI: Neutropenia in patients infected with human immunodeficiency virus, *Clin Pharm* 10:268-279, 1991.

110. Tang AM, Graham NM, Kirby AJ, et al: Dietary micronutrient intake on survival in human immunodeficiency virus type 1 infection, *Am J Epidemiol* 143:1244-1256, 1996.

111. Shoji S, Furuishi K, Misumi S: Thiamine disulfide as a potent inhibitor of human immunodeficiency virus (type-1) production, *Biochem Biophys Res Commun* 205:967, 1994.

112. Paltiel O, Falutz J, Veilleux M, et al: Clinical correlates of subnormal vitamin B_{12} levels in patients infected with the human immunodeficiency virus, *Am J Hematol* 49:318-322, 1995.

113. Baum M, Cassetti L, Bonvehi P, et al: Inadequate dietary intake and altered nutrition status in early HIV-1 infection, *Nutrition* 10:16-20, 1994.

114. Weinberg JB, Sauls DL, Misukonis MA, et al: Inhibition of productive human immunodeficiency virus-1 infection by cobalamins, *Blood* 86:1281-1287, 1995.

115. Rule SA, Hooker M, Costello C: Serum vitamin B_{12} and transcobalamin levels in early HIV disease, *Am J Hematol* 47:167, 1994.

116. Ehrenpreis ED, Carlson SJ, Boorstein HL: Malabsorption and deficiency of vitamin B_{12} in HIV infected patients with chronic diarrhea, *Dig Dis Sci* 39:2159, 1994.

117. Balt, CA: An investigation of the relationship between vitamin B$_{12}$ deficiency and HIV infection, *J Assoc Nurses AIDS Care* 11(1):24-28, 31-35, 2000.

118. Kodama M, Kodama T: Vitamin C and the genesis of autoimmune disease and allergy, *In Vivo* 9(3):231-238, 1995.

119. Nakagawa M, Maruyama Y, Osame M: Therapy for HAM/TSP and AIDS, *Nippon Rinsho* 52:3019, 1994.

120. Root-Bernstein RS: *Rethinking AIDS,* New York, 1993, Free Press.

121. Washburn AM, Fullilove RE, Fullilove MT, et al: Acupuncture heroin detoxification: a single-blind clinical trial, *J Subst Abuse Treat* 10:345-351, 1993.

122. Avants SK, Margolin A, Holford TR, et al: A randomized controlled trial of auricular acupuncture for cocaine dependence, *Arch Intern Med* 160(15):2305-2312, 2000.

123. Russell LC, Sharp B, Gilbertson B: Acupuncture for addicted patients with chronic histories of arrests: a pilot study of the Consortium Treatment Center.

124. Bianchi M, Jotti E, Sacerdote P, et al: Traditional acupuncture increases the content of beta-endorphin in immune cells and influences mitogen induced proliferation, *Am J Chin Med* 19:101-104, 1991.

125. Moscarella S, Giusti A, Marra F, et al: *Curr Ther Res Clin Exp* 53:98, 1993.

126. Muzes G, Deak G, Lang I, et al: Effect of the bioflavonoid silymarin on the in vitro activity and expression of superoxide dismutase (SOD) enzyme, *Acta Physiol Hung* 78:3-9, 1991.

127. Bissuel F, Cotte L, Crapanne JB, et al: Trimethoprim/ sulfamethoxazole rechallenge in 20 previously allergic HIV-infected patients after homeopathic desensitization. *AIDS* 9(4) 407-408, 1995 (letter).

128. Mathur B: Personal correspondence, 1998.

129. Perry NB, Albertson GD, Blunt JW, et al: 4-Hydroxy-2-cyclopentenone: an anti-*Pseudomonas* and cytotoxic component from *Passiflora tetrandra, Planta Med* 57:129-131, 1991.

130. Lee TT, Kashiwada Y, Huang L, et al: Suksdorfin: an anti-HIV principle from *Lomatiumsuksdorfii,* its structure-activity correlation with related coumarins, and synergistic effects with anti-AIDS nucleosides, *Bioorg Med Chem* 2:1051-1056, 1994.

131. Offergeld R, Reinecker C, Gumz E, et al: Mitogenic activity of high molecular polysaccharide fractions isolated from the cuppressaceae *Thuja occidentalis L.* enhanced cytokine-production by thyapolysaccharide, g-fraction (TPSg), *Leukemia* 6(suppl 3):189S-191S, 1992.

132. Shoba G, Joy D, Thangam J, et al: Influence of piperine on the pharmacokinetics of curcumin in animals and human volunteers, *Planta Med* 64: 353-356, 1998.

133. Lu W: Treatment of 60 cases of HIV-infected patients with Glyke, *Chung Kuo Chung Hsi I Chieh Ho Tsa Chih* 13(6):324, 340-342, 1993.

134. Ito M, Nakashima H, Baba M, et al: Inhibitory effect of glycyrrhizin on the in vitro infectivity and cytopathic activity of the human immunodeficiency virus [HIV (HTLV-III/LAV)], *Antiviral Res* 7:127-137, 1987.

135. Hattori T, Ikematsu S, Koita A: Preliminary evidence for inhibitory effect of glycyrrhizin on HIV replication in patients with AIDS, *Antiviral Res* 11:255, 1989.

136. Ikegami N, Akatani K, Imai M, et al: Prophylactic effect of long-term oral administration of glycyrrhizin in AIDS development of asymptomatic patients, *Int Conf AIDS* 9:234, 1993.

137. Numazaki K, Umetsu M, Chiba S: Effect of glycyrrhizin in children with liver dysfunction associated with cytomegalovirus infection, *Tohoku J Exp Med* 172:147-153, 1994.

138. Utsunomiya T, Kobayashi M, Ito M, et al: Glycyrrhizin improves the resistance of MAIDS mice to opportunistic infection of *Candida albicans* through the modula of MAIDS-associated type 2 T cell responses, *Clin Immunol* 95(2):145-155, 2000.

139. Degar S, Prince AM, Pascual D, et al: Inactivation of the human immunodeficiency virus by hypericin: evidence for photochemical alterations of p24 and a block in uncoating, *AIDS Res Hum Retroviruses* 8:1929-1936, 1992.

140. Acosta EP, Fletcher CV: Agents for treating human immunodeficiency virus infection, *Am J Hosp Pharm* 51:2251-2267; quiz 2286-2287, 1994.

141. Reference deleted in proofs.

142. Miller J: Interaction between indinavir and St. John's wort reported, *Am J Health Syst Pharm* 57(7): 625-626, 2000.

143. Mestman B, Stokes D: Unpublished data, personal correspondence, 1995.

144. Pharo A, Salvato P, Thompson C, et al: Evaluation of the safety and efficacy of SPV-30 (boxwood extract) in patients with HIV disease, *XI Int Conf AIDS* 11:19, 1996 (abstract Mo.B. 180).

145. Mazumder AK, Raghavan K, Weinstein J: Inhibition of human immunodeficiency virus type-1 integrase by curcumin, *Biochem Pharmacol* 49:1165, 1995.

146. Li C: Three inhibitors of type 1 human immunodeficiency virus long-terminal repeat-directed gene expression and virus replication, *Proc Natl Acad Sci U S A* 90:1839, 1993.

147. Jordan WC: Curcumin: a natural herb with anti-HIV activity, *J Natl Med Assoc* 88:333, 1996.

148. Sui ZR: Inhibition of the HIV-1 and HIV-2 proteases by curcumin and curcumin boron complexes, *Bioorg Med Chem* 1:415, 1993.

149. Weber ND, Andersen DO, North JA, et al: In vitro virucidal effects of *Allium sativa* (garlic) extract and compounds, *Planta Med* 58(5):417-423, 1992.

150. Guo NL, Lu DP, Woods GL, et al: Demonstration of the antiviral activity of garlic extract against human cytomegalovirus in vitro, *Chin Med J (Engl)* 106:93-96, 1993.

151. Mucsi I, Gyulai Z, Beladi I: Combined effects of flavonoids and acyclovir against herpesviruses in cell cultures, *Acta Microbiol Hung* 39:137-147, 1992.

152. Ono K, Nakane H, Fukushima M, et al: Differential inhibitory effects of various flavonoids on the activities of reverse transcriptase and cellular DNA and RNA polymerases, *Eur J Biochem* 190:469-476, 1990.

153. Fesen MR, Kohn KW, Leteurtre F, et al: Inhibitors of human immunodeficiency virus integrase, *Proc Natl Acad Sci U S A* 90:2399-2403, 1993.

154. Ono K, Nakane H: Mechanisms of inhibition of various cellular DNA and RNA polymerases by several flavonoids, *J Biochem (Tokyo)* 108:609-613, 1990.

155. Ng TB, Chan WY, Yeung HW: Proteins with abortifacient, ribosome inactivating, immunomodulatory, antitumor, and anti-AIDS activities from *Cucurbitaceae* plants, *Gen Pharmacol* 23:579-590, 1992.

156. Bourinbaiar AS, Lee-Huang S: Potentiation of anti-HIV activity of antiinflammatory drugs, dexamethasone, and indomethacin, by MAP30, the antiviral agent from bitter melon, *Biochem Biophys Res Commun* 208:779-785, 1995.

157. Lee TT, Kashiwada Y, Huang L, et al: Suksdorfin: an anti-HIV principle from *Lomatium suksdorfii,* its structure-activity correlation with related coumarins, and synergistic effects with anti-AIDS nucleosides, *Bioorg Med Chem* 2:1051-1056, 1994.

158. Sydiskis RJ, Owen DG, Lohr JL, et al: Inactivation of enveloped viruses by anthraquinones extracted from plants, *Antimicrob Agents Chemother* 35:2463-2466, 1991.

159. Womble K, Helderman JH: The impact of Acemannan on the generation and function of cytotoxic T-lymphocytes, *Immunopharmacol Immunotoxicol* 14:63-77, 1992.

160. Kemp MC, Kahlon J, Carpenter R, et al: Concentration-dependent inhibition of AIDS virus replication and pathogenesis by Acemannan in vitro, *Int Conf AIDS* 6:315, 1990.

161. Owens SD, Gasper PW: Hyperthermic therapy for HIV infection, *Med Hypotheses* 44:235-242, 1995.

162. Pontiggia P, Bianchi Santamaria A, Alonso K, et al: Whole body hyperthermia associated with beta-carotene supplementation in patients with AIDS, *Biomed Pharmacother* 49:263-265, 1995.

163. Alonso K, Pontiggia P, Sabato A, et al: Systemic hyperthermia in the treatment of HIV-related disseminated Kaposi's sarcoma: long-term follow-up of patients treated with low-flow extracorporeal perfusion hyperthermia, *Am J Clin Oncol* 17:353-359, 1994.

164. Ash S, Steinhart C, Curfman M, et al: Extracorporeal whole body hyperthermia treatments for HIV infection and AIDS, *ASAIO J* 45(5):M830-M838, 1997.

165. Nottet HS, van Asbeck BS, de Graaf L, et al: Role for oxygen radicals in self-sustained HIV-1 replication in monocyte-derived macrophages: enhanced HIV-1 replication by N-Acetyl-L-cysteine, *J Leukoc Biol* 56:702-707, 1994.

166. Kinter AL, Poli G, Fauci AS: N-Acetyl-cysteine is a potent suppressor of human immunodeficiency virus transcription in persistently infected cells, *Trans Assoc Am Physicians* 105:36-43, 1992.

167. Semba RD, Caiaffa WT, Graham NM: Vitamin A deficiency and wasting as predictors of mortality in human immunodeficiency virus-infected injection drug users, *J Infect Dis* 171:1196, 1995.

168. Semba RD, Graham NM, Caiaffa WT: Increased mortality associated with vitamin A deficiency during human immunodeficiency virus type 1 infection, *Arch Intern Med* 153:2149, 1993.

169. Beach RS, Mantero-Atienza E, Shore-Posner G, et al: Specific nutrient abnormalities in asymptomatic HIV-1 infection, *AIDS* 6:701-708, 1992.

170. Constans J, Pellegrin JL, Pellegrin I, et al: Interferon and blood tumor necrosis factor in 95 patients with HIV infection, *Rev Med Interne* 14:1004, 1993.

171. Baum M, Cassetti L, Bonvehi P, et al: Inadequate dietary intake and altered nutrition status in early HIV-1 infection, *Nutrition* 10:16-20, 1994.

172. Karter DL, Karter AJ, Yarrish R: Vitamin A deficiency in non-vitamin-supplemented patients with AIDS: a cross-sectional study, *J Acquir Immune Defic Syndr Hum Retrovirol* 8:199, 1995.

173. Semba RD, Miotti PG, Chiphangwi JD: Maternal vitamin A deficiency and mother-to-child transmission of HIV-1, *Lancet* 343:1593, 1994.

174. Nduati RW, John GC, Richardson BA: Human immunodeficiency virus type 1-infected cells in breast milk: association with immunosuppression and vitamin A deficiency, *J Infect Dis* 172:1461, 1995.

175. Kennedy CM, Coutsoudis A, Kuhn L, et al: Randomized controlled trial asessing the effect of vitamin A supplementation on maternal morbidity during pregnancy and postpartum among HIV-infected women, *J Acquir Immune Defic Syndr* 24(1):37-44., 2000.

176. John GC, Nduati RW, Mbori-Ngacha D, et al: Genital shedding of human immunodeficiency virus type 1 DNA during pregnancy: association with immunosuppression, abnormal cervical or vaginal discharge, and severe vitamin A deficiency, *J Infect Dis* 175:57-62, 1997.

177. Ziari SA, Mireles VL, Cantu CG, et al: Serum vitamin A, vitamin E, and beta-carotene levels in preeclamptic women in northern Nigeria, *Am J Perinatol* 13:287-291, 1996.

178. Phuapradit W et al: Serum vitamin A and beta-carotene levels in pregnant women infected with human immunodeficiency virus-1, *Obstet Gynecol* 87:564, 1996.

179. Coutsoudis A, Bobat RA, Coovadia HM: The effects of vitamin A supplementation on the morbidity of children born to HIV-infected women, *Am J Public Health* 85(8pt1):1076-1081, 1995.

180. Harakeh S, Jariwalla RJ: Comparative analysis of ascorbate and AZT effects on HIV production in persistently infected cell lines, *J Nutr Med* 4:393, 1994.

181. Suzuki Y, Packer L: Inhibition of NF-kappa B activation by vitamin E derivatives, *Biochem Biophys Res Commun* 193:277-283, 1993.

182. Murray MF, Srinivasan A: Nicotinamide inhibits HIV-1 in both acute and chronic in vitro infection, *Biochem Biophys Res Commun* 210: 954-959, 1995.

183. Murray MF, Nghiem M, Srinivasan A: HIV infection decreases intracellular nicotinamide adenine dinucleotide (NAD), *Biochem Biophys Res Commun* 212:126-131, 1995.

184. Brown R, Ozaki Y, Datta S, et al: Implications of interferon-induced tryptophan catabolism in cancer, autoimmune diseases, and AIDS, *Adv Exp Med Biol* 294:425-435, 1991.

185. Bocci V: Does ozone therapy normalize the cellular redox balance? Implications for therapy of human immunodeficiency virus infection and several other diseases, *Med Hypotheses* 46:150-154, 1996.

186. Wells KH, Latino J, Gavalchin J, et al: Inactivation of human immunodeficiency virus type 1 by ozone in vitro, *Blood* 78:1882-1890, 1991.

187. Carpendale MT, Freeberg JK: Ozone inactivates HIV at noncytotoxic concentrations, *Antiviral Res* 16:281-292, 1991.

188. Carpendale MT, Freeberg J, Griffiss JM: Does ozone alleviate AIDS diarrhea? *J Clin Gastroenterol* 17:142-145, 1993.

189. Walker M: Antimicrobial attributes of olive leaf extract, *Townsend Lett* 7:80-85, 1996.

190. Tanner HA: Energy transformations in the biosynthesis of the immune system: their relevance to the progression and treatment of AIDS, *Med Hypotheses* 38:315-321, 1992.

191. Folkers K, Morita M, McRee J Jr: The activities of coenzyme Q_{10} and vitamin B_6 for immune responses, *Biochem Biophys Res Commun* 193:88-92, 1993.

192. Baum M, Cassetti L, Bonvehi P, et al: Inadequate dietary intake and altered nutrition status in early HIV-1 infection, *Nutrition* 10:16-20, 1994.

193. Vitamin B_6 and immune function in the elderly and HIV-seropositive subjects, *Nutr Rev* 50(5):145-147, 1992.

194. Baum MK, Mantero-Atienza E, Shor-Posner G, et al: Association of vitamin B_6 status with parameters of immune function in early HIV-1 infection, *J Acquir Immune Defic Syndr Hum Retrovirol* 4:1122-1132, 1991.

195. Harbige LS: Nutrition and immunity with emphasis on infection and autoimmune disease, *Nutr Health* 10:285-312, 1996.

196. Ripa S, Ripa R: Zinc and immune function, *Minerva Med* 86:315-318, 1995.

197. Graham NM, Sorensen D, Odaka N, et al: Relationship of serum copper and zinc levels to HIV-1 seropositivity and progression to AIDS, *J Acquir Immune Defic Syndr Hum Retrovirol* 4:976-980, 1991.

198. Mocchegiani E, Muzzoli M: Therapeutic application of xinc in human immunodeficiency virus against opportunistic infections, *J Nutr* 130(suppl 5S):1424S-1431S, 2000.

199. Roesler J, Emmendorffer A, Steinmuller C, et al: Application of purified polysaccharides from cell cultures of the plant *Echinacea purpurea* to test subjects mediates activation of the phagocyte system, *Int J Immunopharmacol* 13:931-941, 1991.

200. Luettig B, Steinmuller C, Gifford GE, et al: Macrophage activation by the polysaccharide arabinogalactan isolated from plant cell cultures of *Echinacea purpurea*, *J Natl Cancer Inst* 81:669-675, 1989.

201. Zhao KS, Mancini C, Doria G: Enhancement of the immune response in mice by *Astragalus membranaceus* extracts, *Immunopharmacology* 20:225-233, 1990.

202. Bohn B et al: Flow-cytometric studies with *Eleutherococcus senticosus* extract as an immunomodulatory agent, *Arzneimittelforschung* 37:1193, 1987.

203. Chihara G: Recent progress in immunopharmacology and therapeutic effects of polysaccharides, *Dev Biol Stand* 77:191-197, 1992.

204. Suzuki M, Takatsuki F, Maeda YY, et al: Antitumor and immunological activity of lentinan in comparison with LPS, *Int J Immunopharmacol* 16:463-468, 1994.

205. Suzuki M, Kikuchi T, Takatsuki F, et al: Curative effects of combination therapy with lentinan and interleukin-2 against established murine tumors, and the role of CD8-positive T cells, *Cancer Immunol Immunother* 38:1-8, 1994.

206. Gordon M, Bihari B, Goosby E, et al: A placebo-controlled trial of the immune modulator, lentinan, in HIV-positive patients: a phase I/II trial, *J Med* 29(5-6):305-330, 1998.

207. Nanba H, Yamasaki P, Shirota M, et al: Immunostimulant activity (in vivo) and anti-HIV activity (in vitro) of 3 branched B 1.6 glucan extracted from Maitake mushroom *(Grifola frondosa)*, *Int Conf AIDS* 8:30, 1992.

208. Jacobsen M, Fusaro R, Galmarini M, et al: Decreased serum dehydroepiandrosterone is associated with an increased progression of HIV virus infection in men with CD4 cell counts 200-499, *J Infect Dis* 164:864-868, 1991.

209. Mulder JW, Frissen PH, Krijen P, et al: Dehydroepiandrosterone as predictor for progression to AIDS in asymptomatic human immunodeficiency virus-infected men, *J Infect Dis* 165:413-418, 1992.

210. Ferrando S, Rabkin J, Poretsky L: Dehydroepiandrosterone sulfate (DHEAS) and testosterone: relation to HIV illness stage and progression over one year, *J Acquir Immune Defic Syndr* 22(2):146-154, 1999.

211. Wisniewski TL, Hilton CW, Morse EV, et al: The relationship of serum DHEA-S and cortisol levels to measures of immune function in human immunodeficiency virus-related illness, *Am J Med Sci* 305:79-83, 1993.

212. Suzuki N, Suzuki T, Engleman Eg, et al: Low serum levels of dehydroepiandrosterone may cause deficient IL-2 production by lymphocytes in patients with systemic lupus erythematosis, *Clin Exp Immunol* 99:251-255, 1995.

213. Daynes R, Dudley DJ, Araneo BA: Regulation of murine lymphokine production in vivo II: DHEA is a natural enhancer of interleukin 2 synthesis by helper T cells, *Eur J Immunol* 20:793-802, 1990.

214. Christeff N, Melchior J, Mammes O, et al: Correlation between increased cortisol: DHEA ratio and malnutrition in HIV-positive men, *Nutrition* 15(7-8):543-549, 1999.

215. Dyner TS, Lang W, Geaga J: An open-label dose-escalation trial of oral dehydroepiandosterone tolerance and pharmacokinetics in patients with HIV disease, *J Acquir Immune Defic Syndr HumRetrovirol* 6:459-465, 1993.

216. Hasheeve D, Salvato P, Thompson C: DHEA: a potential treatment for HIV disease, *Int Conf AIDS* 1994 (abstract PB0322).

217. Salvata P, Thompson C, Keister R: Viral load response to augmentation of natural dehydroepiandrosterone (DHEA), *XI Int Conf AIDS* 11:124, 1996 (abstract We.B.3385).

218. Schinazi RF, Eriksson B, Arnold B, et al: Effect of DHEA in lymphocytes and macrophages infected with HIV-1, *Int AIDS Conf* 1994 (abstract MCP 55).

219. Christieff N, Gharakhanian C, Thobie N, et al: Differences in androgens of HIV-positive patients with and without Kaposi's sarcoma, *J Clin Pathol* 48:513-518, 1995.

220. Trainin N: Prospects of AIDS therapy by thymic humoral factor: a thymic hormone, *Nat Immun Cell Growth Regul* 9:155-159, 1990.

221. Ripa S, Ripa R: Zinc and immune function, *Minerva Med* 86:315-318, 1995.

222. Valesini G, Barnaba V, Benvenuto R, et al: A calf thymus acid lysate improves clinical symptoms and T-cell defects in the early stages of HIV infection: second report, *Eur J Cancer Clin Oncol* 23:1915-1919, 1987.

223. Carco F, Guazzotti G: Therapeutic use of thymostimulin in HIV-seropositive subjects and with lymphadenopathy syndrome, *Recenti Prog Med* 84:756-764, 1993.

224. Dui J: Exploration of treating AIDS by acupuncture, *Chen Tzu Yen Chiu* 15:250-251, 1990.

225. Shattuck AD, Ryan MK: *Treating AIDS with Chinese medicine,* Berkeley, Calif., 1994, Pacific View Press.

226. Burack JH, Cohen MR, Hahn JA: Pilot randomized controlled clinical trial of Chinese herbal treatment for HIV-associated symptoms, *J Acquir Immune Defic Syndr Hum Retrovirol* 12:386-393, 1996.

227. Moffett H, Sanders P, Sinclair T, et al: Using acupuncture and herbs for the treatment of HIV infection, *AIDS Patient Care* 194, 1994.

228. Goh M: Acupuncture treatment for neuropathy—patients with HIV infection, International Symposium on Viral Hepatitis and AIDS, April 1991.

229. Lu Wei Bo: Personal communication, 1995.

230. Rastogi DP, Singh VP, Dey SK: Evaluation of homeo pathic therapy in 129 asymptomatic HIV carriers, *Br Homeopath J* 82:4, 1993.

230a. Rastogi DP, Singh VP, Singh V, et al: Homeopathy in HIV infection: a trial report of double-blind, placebo-controlled study, *Br Homeopath J* 88(2):49-57, 1999.

231. Wolffers I, de Moree S: Use of alternative treatments by HIV-positive and AIDS patients in the Netherlands, *Ned Tijdschr Geneeskd* 138(6):307-310, 1994.

232. Edelson RL, Fink JM: The immunologic function of skin, *Sci Am* 252:46-53, 1985.

233. Ring J, Teichmann W: Immunological changes during hydrotherapy, *Dtsch Med Wochenschr* 102:1625-1630, 1977.

234. Licht S, editor: *Therapeutic heat and cold,* New Haven, Conn., 1965, E Licht.

235. Kancheva RL, Zofkova I: Melatonin: the hormone of darkness, *Cas Lek Cesk* 135:231-235, 1996.

236. Solomon GF: Psychosocial factors, exercise, and immunity: athletes, elderly persons, and AIDS patients, *Int J Sports Med* 12(suppl 1):S50-S52, 1991.

237. Carson VB: Prayer, meditation, exercise, and special diets: behaviors of the hardy person with HIV/AIDS, *J Assoc Nurses AIDS Care* 4:18-28, 1993.

238. LaPerriere AR, Antoni MH, Schneiderman N, et al: Exercise intervention attenuates emotional distress and natural killer cell decrements following notification of positive serologic status for HIV-1, *Biofeedback Self Regul* 15(3):229-242, 1990.

239. LaPerriere A, Fletcher MA, Antoni MH, et al: Aerobic exercise training in an AIDS risk group, *Int J Sports Med* 12(suppl 1):S53-S57, 1991.

240. Spence DW, Galantino ML, Mossberg KA, et al: Progressive resistance exercise: effect on muscle function and anthropometry of a select AIDS population, *Arch Phys Med Rehabil* 71:644-648, 1990.

241. Nieman D, Pedersen B: Exercise and immune function. Recent developments, *Sports Med* 27(2):73-80, 1999.

242. Mustafa T, Sy F, Macera C, et al: Association between exercise and HIV diesease progression in a cohort of homosexual men, *Ann Epidemiol* 9(2):127-131, 1999.

243. Koch J, Neal EA, Schlott MJ, et al: Zinc levels and infections in hospitalized patients with AIDS, *Nutrition* 12:515-518, 1996.

244. Standish, LJ, Greene K, Bain S, et al: Alternative medicine use in HIV-positive men and women: demographics, utilization patterns, and health status, *AIDS Care* 13(2):197-208, 2001.

245. Guo NL, Lu D, Woods GL, et al: Demonstration of the antiviral activity of garlic extract against human cytomegalovirus in vitro, *Chin Med J (Engl)* 106:93-96, 1993.

246. Abdullah TH, Kandil O, Elkadi A, et al: Garlic revisited: therapeutic for the major diseases of our times? *J Natl Med Assoc* 80(4):439, 1988.

247. Frontling RA, Blumer GS: In vitro effect of aqeous extract of garlic on the growth and viability of cryptococcus neoforms, *Mycopathologia* 70:397-405, 1978.

248. China HMCo: Garlic in *Cryptococcal meningitis*: a preliminary report of 21 cases, *Chin Med J (Engl* 93:123, 1980.

249. Tsai Y et al: Antiviral properties of garlic: in vitro effects on influenza B, herpes simplex 1, and coxsackie viruses, *Planta Med* 27:460-461, 1985.

250. Delaha EC, Gargusi VL: Inhibition of mycobacteria by garlic extract *(Allium sativum), Antimicrob Agents Chemother* 27:485-486, 1985.

251. Rao RR et al: Inhibition of *Mycobacterium tuberculosis* by garlic extract, *Nature* 157, 1946.

252. Abdullah TH, Kirpatrick DV, Carter J: Enhancement of natural killer cell activity in AIDS with garlic, *Deutsche Zeit Onk* 21:52, 1989.

253. Simonetti N, Simonetti G, Bougnol F, et al: Electrochemical Ag$^+$ for preservative use, *Appl Environ Microbiol* 58:3834-3836, 1992.

254. Lochner JD, Schneider DJ: The relationship between tuberculosis, vitamin D, potassium, and AIDS: a message for South Africa? *S Afr Med J* 84:79-82, 1994.

255. Haug CJ, Aukrust P, Lien E, et al: Disseminated *Mycobacterium avium* complex infection in AIDS: immunopathogenic significance of an activated tumor necrosis factor system and depressed serum levels of 1,25 dihydroxyvitamin D, *J Infect Dis* 173:259-262, 1996.

256. Thomasset M: Vitamin D and the immune system, *Pathol Biol (Paris)* 42:163-172, 1994.

257. Gray JD, Bottomley W, Layton AM, et al: The use of calcipotriol in HIV-related psoriasis, *Clin Exp Dermatol* 17:342-343, 1992.

258. Atzori C, Bruno A, Chichino G, et al: Activity of bilobalide, a sesquiterpene from *Ginkgo biloba*, on *Pneumocystis carinii, Antimicrob Agents Chemother* 37:1492-1496, 1993.

259. Okhuysen P, Chappell C, Crabb J, et al: Prophylactic effect of bovine anti-*Cryptosporidium* hyperimmune colostrum immunoglobulin in healthy volunteers challenged with *Cryptosporidium parvum, Clin Infect Dis* 26(6):1324-1329, 1998.

260. *Int Conf AIDS* 5:479, 1989 (abstract Th.B.P.381).

261. Martinez G, Albarracin C, Liepins A: Effect of the alkaloid derivative Ukrain in AIDS patients with Kaposi's sarcoma, *Int Conf AIDS* 9:401, 1993.

262. Pert CB: *Molecules of emotion: why you feel the way you feel,* New York, 1997, Simon & Schuster.

263. Cole SW, Kemeny ME, Taylor SE, et al: Elevated physical health risk among gay men who conceal their homosexual identity, *Health Psychol* 15:243-251, 1996.

264. Taylor DN: Effects of a behavioral stress-management program on anxiety, mood, self-esteem, and T-cell count in HIV-positive men, *Psychol Rep* 76:451-457, 1995.

265. Born J, Lange T, Hansen K, et al: Effects of sleep and circadian rhythm on human circulating immune cells, *J Immunol* 158(9):4454-4464, 1997.

266. Moldofsky H: Sleep and the immune system, *Int J Immunopharmacol* 17(8):649-654, 1995.

267. Kelly JA, Murphy DA, Bahr GR, et al: Outcome of cognitive-behavioral and support group brief therapies for depressed, HIV-infected persons, *Am J Psychiatry* 150:1679-1686, 1993.

268. DiPasquale JA: The psychological effects of support groups on individuals infected by the AIDS virus, *Cancer Nurs* 13:278-285, 1990.

269. Hedge B, Glover LF: Group intervention with HIV seropositive patients and their partners, *AIDS Care* 2:147-154, 1990.

270. Carson VB: Prayer, meditation, exercise, and special diets: behaviors of the hardy person with HIV/AIDS, *J Assoc Nurses AIDS Care* 4:18-28, 1993.

271. Harte JL, Eifert GH, Smith R: The effects of running and mediation on beta-endorphin, corticotropin-releasing hormone, and cortisol in plasma, and on mood, *Biol Psychol* 40:251-265, 1995.

272. Standish LJ, Fitzpatrick A, Berger J, et al: Associations of mind-body interventions with quality of life in HIV-1 positive individuals, International Scientific Conference on Complementary, Alternative, and Integrative Medicine Research, San Francisco, 2001, (submitted for presentation).

273. Fryback PB: Health for people with a terminal diagnosis, *Nurs Sci Q* 6:147-149, 1993.

274. Philip P, Demotes-Mainard J, Bourgeois M, et al: Efficiency of transcranial electrostimulation on anxiety and insomnia symptoms during a washout period in depressed patients: a double-blind study, *Biol Psychiatry* 29:451-456, 1991.

275. Healy D: Rhythm and blues: neurochemical, neuropharmacological, and neuropsychological implications of a hypothesis of circadian rhythm dysfunction in the affective disorders, *Psychopharmacology (Berl)* 93:271-285, 1987.

276. Linde K, Ramirez G, Mulrow CD, et al: St. John's wort for depression: an overview and meta-analysis of randomized clinical trials, *Br Med J* 313:253-258, 1996.

277. Linde K, Mulrow C: St. John's wort for depression, *Cochrane Database Syst Rev* 2:CD00448, 2000.

278. Skurnick JH, Bogden JD, Baker H, et al: Micronutrient profiles in HIV-1-infected heterosexual adults, *J Acquir Immune Defic Syndr Hum Retrovirol* 12:75-83, 1996.

279. Beck KW, Schramel P, Hedl A, et al: Serum trace element levels in HIV-infected subjects, *Biol Trace Elem Res* 25:89-96, 1990.

280. Shor-Posner G, Feaster D, Blaney NT, et al: Impact of vitamin B_6 status on psychological distress in a longitudinal study of HIV-1 infection, *Int J Psychiatry Med* 24:209-222, 1994.

281. Butterworth RF, Gaudreau C, Vincelette J, et al: Thiamine deficiency and Wernicke's encephalopathy in AIDS, *Metab Brain Dis* 6:207-212, 1991.

282. Andersson JE: Wernicke's encephalopathy, *Ugeskr Laeger* 158:898-901, 1996.

283. Schwenk J, Gosztonyi G, Thierauf P, et al: Wernicke's encephalopathy in two patients with acquired immunodeficiency syndrome, *J Neurol* 237:445-447, 1990.

284. Beach RS, Morgan R, Wilkie F, et al: Plasma vitamin B_{12} level as a potential cofactor in studies of human immunodeficiency virus type 1-related cognitive changes, *Arch Neurol* 49:501-506, 1992.

285. Shor-Posner G, Morgan R, Wilkie F, et al: Plasma cobalamin levels affect information processing speed in a longitudinal study of HIV-1 disease, *Arch Neurol* 52:195-198, 1995.

286. Herzlich BC, Schiano TD: Reversal of apparent AIDS dementia complex following treatment with vitamin B_{12}, *J Intern Med* 233:495-497, 1993.

287. Kieburtz KD, Giang DW, Schiffer RB, et al: Abnormal vitamin B_{12} metabolism in human immunodeficiency virus infection: association with neurological dysfunction, *Arch Neurol* 48:312-314, 1991.

288. Bottiglieri T, Hyland K, Reynolds EH: The clinical potential of ademetionine (*S*-adenosylmethionine) in neurological disorders, *Drugs* 48:137-152, 1994.

289. Castagna A, Le Grazie C, Accordini A, et al: Cerebrospinal fluid *S*-adenosylmethionine (SAMe) and glutathione concetrations in HIV infection: effect of parenteral treatment with SAMe, *Neurology* 45:1678-1683, 1995.

290. Muller F, Svardal AM, Aukrust P, et al: Elevated plasma concentration of reduced homocysteine in patients with human immunodeficiency virus infection, *Am J Clin Nutr* 63:242-248, 1996.

291. de la Asuncion JG, del Olmo ML, Sastre J, et al: AZT treatment induces molecular and ultrastructural oxidative damage to muscle mitochondria: prevention by antioxidant vitamins, *J Clin Invest* 102(1):4-9, 1998.

292. Lewis W: Cardiomyopathy in AIDS: a pathophysiological perspective, *Prog Cardiovasc Dis* 43(2):151-170, 2000.

293. Mintz M: Carnitine in human immunodeficiency virus type 1 infection/acquired immune deficiency syndrome, *J Child Neurol* 10(suppl 2):S40-S44, 1995.

294. DeSimone C, Tzantzoglou S, Jirillo E: L-carnitine deficiency in AIDS patients, *AIDS* 6:203, 1992.

295. Paltiel O, Falutz J, Veilleux M, et al: Clinical correlates of subnormal vitamin B_{12} levels in patients infected with the human immunodeficiency virus, *Am J Hematol* 49:318-322, 1995.

296. *Med Trib* Sep 9, 34(17):18, 1993.

297. Gogu SR, Beckman BS, Rangan SR, et al: Increased therapeutic efficacy of zidovudine in combination with vitamin E, *Biochem Biophys Res Commun* 165(1):401-407, 1989.

298. Baum MK, Javier JJ, Mantero-Atienza E, et al: Zidovudine-associated adverse reactions in a longitudinal study of asymptomatic HIV-1-infected homosexual males, *J Acquir Immune Defic Syndr Hum Retrovirol* 4:1218-1226, 1991.

299. Schmued LC, Albertson CM, Andrews A et al: Evaluation of brain and nerve pathology in rats chronically dosed with ddI or isoniazid, *Neurotoxicol Teratol* 18:555-563, 1996.

300. Pizzorno JE, Murray MT: *A textbook of natural medicine*, Seattle, 1987, John Bastyr College Publications.

301. Berkson B: A conservative triple antioxidant approach to the treatment of hepatitis C: C alpha lipoic acid (thioctic acid), silymarin, and selenium: three case histories, *Med Klin* 94(suppl 3):84-89, 1999.

302. Piscitelli SC, Burstein AH, Chaitt D, et al: Indinavir concentrations and St. John's wort, *Lancet* 355(9203):547-548, 2000.

303. Foster et al: Seventh Annual Conference HIV/AIDS Research, 1998.

304. Piscitelli SC, Gallicano KD: Interactions among drugs for HIV and opportunistic infections, *N Engl J Med* 344(13):984-986, 2001.

305. Bissuel F, Cotte L, Crapanne JB, et al: Trimethoprim/sulphamethoxazole rechallange in 20 previously allergic HIV-infected patients after homeopathic desensitization, *AIDS* 9(4):407-408, 1995 (correspondence).

306. Galantino M, Eke-Okoro S, Findley T, et al: Use of noninvasive electroacupuncture for the treatment of HIV-related peripheral neuropathy: a pilot study, *J Altern Complement Med* 5(2):135-142, 1999.

307. Eggleston, David, DDS: Effect of dental amalgam and nickel alloys on T lymphocytes: preliminary report, *J Prosthet Dent* 51(5):617-623, 1984.

308. Lorscheider FL, Vimy MJ, Summers AO: Mercury exposure from "silver" tooth fillings: emerging evidence questions a traditional dental paradigm, *FASEB J* 9(7):504-508, 1995.

309. Enestrom S, Hultman P: Does amalgam affect the immune system? A controversial issue, *Int Arch Allergy Immunol* 106(3):180-203, 1995.

310. Sax P, Singer M: Routine immunization in HIV: helpful or harmful? *AIDS Clin Care* 8(2):11-15, 1996.

311. Talbot EA, Perkins MD, Fagundes S, et al: Disseminated bacille Calmette-Guerin disease after vaccination: case report and review, *Clin Infect Dis* (6):1139-1146, 1997.

312. Tasker S et al: Effects of influenza vaccination in HIV infected patients: a double-blind placebo controlled trial, Abstracts of the 35th ICAAC, 1995 (abstract LB-11).

313. Fuller J, Craven D, Steger K, et al: Influenza vaccination of human immunodeficiency virus (HIV)-infected adults: impact on plasma levels of HIV type 1 RNA and determinants of antibody response, *Clin Infect Dis* 28(3):541-547, 1999.

314. King J, Treanor J, Fast P, et al: Comparison of the safety, vaccine virus shedding, and immunogenicity of influenza virus vaccine, trivalent, types A and B, live cold-adapted, administered to human immunodeficiency virus (HIV)-infected adults, *J Infect Dis* 181(2):725-758, 2000.

315. Hanekom W, Yogev R, Heald L, et al: Effect of vitamin A therapy on serologic response and viral load changes after influenza vaccination in children infected with the human immunodeficiency virus, *J Pediatr* 136(4):550-552, 2000.

316. Kaiser J: *Immune power: a comprehensive treatment program for HIV,* New York, 1993, St Martin's Press.

317. Priestley J: Personal communication, 1992.

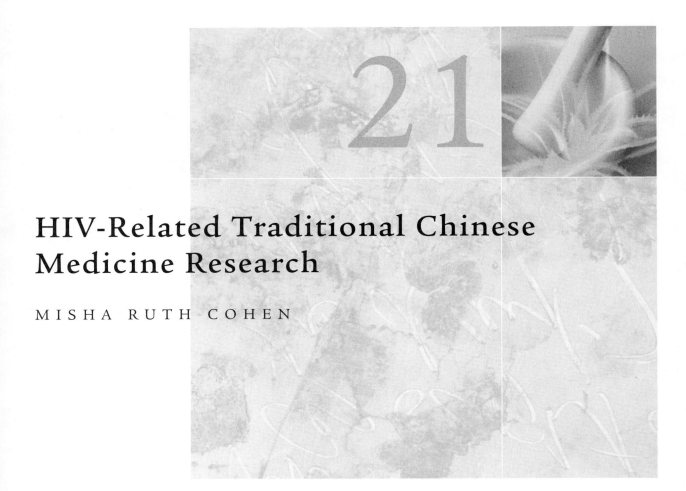

HIV-Related Traditional Chinese Medicine Research

MISHA RUTH COHEN

ABSTRACT

This chapter gives an overview of HIV/AIDS as it is perceived through the eyes of a traditional Chinese medicine (TCM) practitioner who also does Western-style medical research.

Clinical practice is outlined and includes a review of traditional Chinese diagnostics, according to the Chinese theories of Spleen/Stomach and Toxic Heat disorders, in an immune deficiency disease with a viral component.

Both completed and ongoing clinical research (controlled and uncontrolled studies) is extensively covered through the use of abstracts, with commentary on the abstracted material. Questions are raised concerning how Chinese medicine research can be performed in the future, including examples of study outcomes.

CLINICAL PRACTICE IN AN EPIDEMIC DISEASE

In ancient China the people by the riverside became very sick in epidemic proportions. Was this sickness caused by the external pernicious influence Summer Heat? Instead, it may have been the epidemic factor of Toxic Heat, its associated syndromes, and other patterns specific to the nature of the particular epidemic as it manifested on an individual basis. These syndromes were treated with herbal formulas that matched the pattern of the epidemic disease, as well as the variations associated with the individual's particular idiosyncratic manifestation of the epidemic illness.

Although HIV/AIDS was a new disease in the twentieth century, the application of diagnosis and treatment, according to epidemic disease patterns, in conjunction with individual patterns most closely explains the manifestation of both the vast similarities and the vast differences found in people living with HIV/AIDS today.

In China 2000 years ago, most people with an epidemic pattern of illness suffered from similar symptoms. Today we are struggling with a similar situation of epidemic disease—HIV/AIDS—in which many individuals have a similar disease pattern. Through the combination of classic Chinese herbal formulations, Western research, and vast clinical and observational experience, clinical protocols have been developed that are apparently effective and safe for treatment in the syndromes associated with the HIV/AIDS epidemic.

In ancient China—as in the modern world of AIDS—people were understood to have individual constitutional patterns and other patterns of disease in conjunction with the epidemic disease. Therefore Chinese medicine theory posits that the best form of treatment is to modify, alter, or give adjuncts to the base formulas for individuals with epidemic disease patterns. We are applying tried and true diagnostic patterns and treatments to a modern epidemic.

CLINICAL PRACTICE VERSUS RESEARCH

Although we can have much confidence in our clinical treatment of HIV/AIDS through our observation, diagnoses, and practice of Chinese medicine, research using Western scientific methods is quite another story. The main question is: How do we study people in the real world, whether they are using Chinese or Western medicine? There are many different treatment strategies with varied outcome results. Also, individuals have many different levels of adherence to a treatment plan.

A position paper recently published by the National Institutes of Health (NIH) Office of Alternative Medicine (OAM),[1] states that studies must be designed that approximate potential human functions and limitations in daily life. Research should be designed to either develop effective new treatments or test old ones. We are trying to eliminate treatments that are ineffective, dangerous, or too costly. Therefore research must be based on a clear understanding of the medicine being studied, as well as the proper methods for studying any given condition, or in more complex situations, the proper methods for studying a medical system's approach to disease.

THE GOAL OF TRADITIONAL CHINESE MEDICINE

The primary goal of TCM is to create wholeness and harmony within a person, allowing the person's body to heal itself. Traditional Chinese philosophy states that there are two polar principles of life, Yin and Yang, which are dialectically opposed to each other.

An imbalance of Yin and Yang within an individual is reflected as physical illness because the body is considered a microcosm of the world. TCM defines the physiological components of illness, using concepts such as Qi (Vital Energy), Xue (Blood), Jin-Ye (Body Fluids), Jing (Essence), and Shen (Spirit), as well as Organ Systems. Organ Systems are domains within the body that govern particular body tissues, emotional states, and activities.

For example, the Kidney Organ System manages fluid metabolism, which is associated with the interpretation of kidney activity by Western medicine. However, TCM also regards the Kidney Organ System as responsible for reproduction, growth, and regeneration. The bones, inner ear, marrow, teeth, and lumbar area are all associated with the Kidney System. Lack of maturation, frequent urination, lower back pain, and weakened vision, as well as fear and the will, are also part of this abbreviated version of the patterns of disharmony associated with the Kidney Organ System. All Organ Systems have functions that govern several areas.[2,3]

TCM theory postulates that the body's internal ability to remain strong is the key to health. According to this theory, people are born with a certain amount of Original Qi (Yuan Qi), which is easily depleted as energy is used by the body and not replaced. It is not easy to increase Original Qi, and a person must work hard during life just to retain it. Exercise, such as Tai Chi and Qigong, as well as proper eating and sleeping habits, are recommended for maintaining Original Qi. If a person consistently lacks sleep and proper nutrition, abuses drugs or alcohol, or has excessive or unsafe sex, he or she becomes deficient. When weakened and deficient, the person is more susceptible to infection by harmful external elements.[3]

TRADITIONAL CHINESE MEDICINE DIAGNOSIS IN HIV/AIDS

Toxic Heat

In Western medicine, extremely harmful elements would include severe bacterial or viral infections, like HIV, but the terms *virus* and *bacteria* are not part of the terminology and theory of TCM. Although a modern Chinese medicine practitioner understands that pathological organisms exist, when describing a viral disease like HIV, "Chinese medicine theory recognizes the existence of Pestilences—called *li qi* or *yi qi*. These are diseases that are not caused by the climatic factors of heat, cold, wind, dampness, or Summer Heat dryness, but by external infectious agents [...] that are severely toxic because they strike directly at the interior of the body."[4,5] In the case of HIV, the particular pestilence is identified as Toxic Heat, which is considered by TCM to be both an Epidemic Factor (i.e., something seen in a large number of patients) and its own individual, treatable syndrome.[6]

When Toxic Heat enters the body, it manifests with feelings of warmth, sweating, agitation, hot sensations, and pruritus. Examination may reveal a rapid pulse and a red tongue, and in all cases of chronic infection, TCM examination is likely to find little red spots on the tongue. (A review of over 5000 tongue slides from HIV-infected patients in a Chinese herbal treatment protocol conducted at Quan Yin from 1988 to 1990 revealed that little red spots—whether very visible or barely noticeable—were a nearly universal finding).[7]

After many years of clinical observation, treatment, and research, it is our view that HIV is a Toxic Heat epidemic factor that attacks initially the Spleen and Stomach Organ Systems described by TCM. This leads to a cascade of development of pathology of Organ System and Substance (e.g., Qi, Jing, Xue, Shen) imbalances. Our Chinese medicine treatment and herbal research is based on these premises.[8]

In a series of papers in 1988, Dr. Wei Bei Hai—a senior professor at the Beijing College of Traditional Chinese Medicine and a specialist in chronic viral disease—hypothesized from the point of view of Chinese medicine theory that HIV/AIDS was basically a disorder of the Spleen and Stomach. In 1989 Dr. Wei visited the United States and presented these papers translated from Chinese.[9] His theory was derived from the important work of Li Dong Yuen and others, who developed the Spleen and Stomach theory.

In the Yuen Dynasty, Dr. Li established the Spleen and Stomach theory. He wrote: "The Stomach Chi is the Root. When you eat, you digest and accumulate the food and become strong. Those who cannot eat or are unable to properly digest and assimilate their food will die. All five solid and six hollow organs receive their Chi from the Spleen and Stomach."[10]

During the Ching Dynasty, Dr. Yeh concluded that Dr. Li had emphasized the treatment of the Spleen but neglected the Stomach. Dr. Li promoted the treatment of *warming* and *tonification* but, according to Dr. Yeh, he did not use *moistening* and *tonifying* methods. According to TCM theory, the Spleen is a Yin Organ; it likes dryness and detests wetness. The Stomach is a Yang Organ; it likes wetness and moisture and detests dryness, so it is important to tonify the Stomach Yin.[10] Dr. Li's method of tonifying the Center and benefiting Yin is beneficial for Yang deficiency and Qi weakness of the Spleen. It is also effective for cold and wetness attacking the Middle Warmer.* When we speak of Spleen disorders today, we must also include the Stomach in our discussion.

Now let us look at the traditional characteristics of the Spleen and Stomach as Organ Systems and the pathologies that exist when the Spleen and Stomach systems are disturbed:

1. The chief functions of the Spleen and Stomach Organ Systems are associated with the digestive system. The Spleen and Stomach govern the transformation of food energy and Fluid. These organs are governed by the Earth phase of the Five Phases.
2. The generation and control of Blood is the second function of the Spleen and Stomach.
3. The Spleen and Stomach benefit the Qi.

In summary, together the Spleen and Stomach store or ingest the food and fluids, extract the essence of food and fluids, generate and control the Xue (Blood), and moisten and nurture the Organ Systems and the vessels.

According to the Ling Shu: "The Stomach is the Sea of the five solid and six hollow Organs. All food and grains enter into the Stomach."[11]

The Stomach governs the ingestion of food, whereas the Spleen governs its transportation and

---

*This includes the Spleen, Stomach, and Liver. The Middle Warmer is at the center of the body and is responsible for creating and maintaining enough digestive fire to absorb food and transform food energy (Qi) into Qi and other substances in the rest of the body.

transformation. There are two ways in which damage may occur to the Spleen and the Stomach:

1. From the Six External Evils
2. From the Internal Evils

Traditionally, if we remove the External Evil that causes abnormal ingestion and transportation of food energy, the functions will normalize. When we look at the pathogenic factor in HIV disease as the virus itself, a form of Pathogenic Heat called Toxic Heat, we can see how this rings true. If the ancient Chinese had known about viruses and bacteria, they would have classified them as External Evils. Internal damage may be caused by the Stomach or Spleen or by other Organs.

The symptoms associated with abnormal Stomach ingestion include:

1. Poor appetite, decreased intake of food, inability to eat, and gas after eating
2. Increased appetite, eating too much, and frequent hunger

The symptoms of abnormal Spleen transformation are:

1. Distention after a meal
2. Becoming sleepy or falling asleep after a meal
3. Emaciation despite eating enough food
4. Fatigue in the extremities

Turning to the function of the Ascending and Descending energy as it relates to the Earth Organ Systems, the Stomach is responsible for descending, whereas the Spleen is responsible for ascending. The Spleen is responsible for raising up the essence of Qi from the food, whereas the Stomach is responsible for moving food that lacks Qi downward. If the Spleen is not acted on properly by the Yang of the Stomach Qi, the Spleen Qi will collapse downward. The Stomach needs the Yin of the Spleen for movement. Therefore when the Spleen Yin is Deficient, the individual has constipation associated with the lack of Stomach Qi moving downward because of the Deficiency of Spleen Yin.

Now we turn to Qi problems of the Spleen and Stomach. The most common symptoms and signs associated with Spleen and Stomach Deficiency are (1) lack of Spirit, (2) lethargy, (3) weakness, (4) inability to eat, (5) decreased food intake, (6) distention of the epigastric area, (7) indigestion, and (8) loose stools or diarrhea. If severe sinking of Qi occurs, uterine or intestinal prolapse and urinary frequency or incontinence may result.

The Organ Systems affected by HIV, according to TCM, are initially the Spleen and Stomach, although all Organ Systems are eventually involved. The Spleen and Stomach Organ Systems influence the patient's digestion and appetite, lymph system, and muscle mass.

CHINESE DIAGNOSTIC PATTERNS FOUND IN HIV/AIDS

The two primary Chinese diagnostic patterns found in HIV disease are Toxic Heat and Spleen/Stomach Disharmony or Deficiency.

Toxic Heat

Symptoms: fevers, itching, sensations of heat, agitation
Tongue: red spots and red body
Pulse: rapid
Note: Toxic Heat is often associated with chronic viral or bacterial infection.

Spleen/Stomach Disharmony or Deficiency

Symptoms: lack of appetite, loose stools or diarrhea, nausea, flatulence, weight loss, decreased muscle mass, muscle weakness, dull pain, and bloating in the abdomen
Tongue: pale and swollen, lack of coating in center
Pulse: weak and deep

ADDITIONAL PATTERNS IN HIV/AIDS

Some examples of additional Organ and Qi, Xue, and Jing-Ye Patterns include (but are not limited to) Deficient Xue, Spleen Yang Deficiency, Liver Qi Stagnation, and Yin Deficiency.

Deficient Xue

Symptoms: fatigue, anemia, pale face and lips, lusterless complexion, pale nails
Tongue: pale
Pulse: thready and weak

Spleen Yang Deficiency

Symptoms: watery diarrhea with undigested food in stool, chronic cold feeling
Tongue: pale, swollen, scalloped
Pulse: slow or tight, deep

Liver Qi Stagnation

Symptoms: irritability, depression, premenstrual syndrome, dysmenorrhea, flatulence, costal tenderness or pain
Tongue: normal or purplish/dusky
Pulse: wiry
Sometimes, the following pattern is predominant (especially in intravenous [IV] drug users, warmer climates, and later-stage disease).

Yin Deficiency

Symptoms: night sweats, afternoon and evening fevers, chronic sore throat, restlessness and fatigue, wakes up during night
Tongue: red tip and pale body or light red or glossy
Pulse: thready and rapid

MODALITIES USED IN TRADITIONAL CHINESE MEDICINE

The various modalities of traditional Chinese medicine include dietary therapy, massage therapy, heat therapies, exercise, meditation, and acupuncture.

Heat therapies include the use of **moxibustion,** which is the burning of the common herb mugwort over certain areas of the body to stimulate or warm these areas.

Moxibustion has been found to raise the Qi and strengthen the Xue. In Chinese studies, it has been shown to stimulate white blood cells and help with T-cell transformation.

Exercise therapy ranges from martial arts to more subtle forms of movement, such as Tai Chi and Qigong.[12]

Acupuncture, which is perhaps the most well-known form of TCM in the United States, is the art of inserting fine sterile metal filiform needles into certain points to control the flow of energy in the meridians. Acupuncture, which also includes electrostimulation and hand stimulation, is most appreciated for its ability to relieve pain. According to TCM theory, it is also able to help the body change its energy patterns to heal itself of organic syndromes and symptoms. In these treatments, TCM does not often distinguish energetic effects from physiological effects.

These various modalities of TCM have different aims. Some focus on balancing the body's energy, whereas others focus on building the physical body and adding substances to both balance and change the body materially.

For example, in the Enhance herbal preparation (used widely in HIV),* herbs are used to tonify the Spleen Qi. When the Qi is tonified, the body is affected energetically by a rise in the amount of energy available for certain functions. Qi tonic herbs often have specific effects of increasing digestion and food absorption, thereby increasing the quality of the blood.

Acupuncture is associated with balancing the body's energy levels, whereas herbal substances are more like drugs or food in that they have specific organic effects.

In addition, breathing exercises are known to strengthen Qi (*Qi* is equivalent to the word for air in Chinese). By learning how to breathe correctly, the individual will have more available oxygen entering the bloodstream.

According to TCM, the various patterns (also described as syndromes) associated with HIV have been described in Chinese medical texts and by Chinese medicine practitioners for over 2000 years. TCM treatments that have been used over the past millennia are considered to be generally safe and effective for all patients suffering from HIV syndromes. However, in ancient China as well as in the modern world of AIDS, TCM recognizes that people have individual constitutions and patterns of disease that exist in conjunction with age-old syndromes. Therefore TCM posits that the best form of treatment is to modify, alter, or give adjuncts to the base TCM therapies.

Chinese medical theory states that HIV/AIDS is not a singular disease but combinations of syndromes. The diagnostic patterns in HIV are determined by using tongue observation and other observation techniques, by feeling the pulse and other palpation tech-

---

*Enhance is made by Health Concerns.

niques, and by questioning. These methods are the cornerstones of Chinese medicine diagnosis.

COMPLETED AND ONGOING TCM RESEARCH

The next section of this chapter covers studies that have Chinese medicine as a main component, which can mean very different things. Some studies study a modality for a specific symptom, with or without using a TCM diagnosis. Some studies cover more general aspects of Chinese medicine, and some exist within the Chinese *materia medica* but are far removed from current clinical Chinese medicine practices.

The abstracts included in this chapter are written in the words of the study investigators. Some antiquated terms, such as AIDS-related complex (ARC), are no longer used throughout the spectrum of HIV disease but were commonly used at the time of the studies. The studies may be difficult to follow in some places; however, many of them are repeated verbatim from their original sources. Passages that paraphrase the authors or summarize the original text to clarify the meaning and to remove extraneous material have been noted.

We have also included commentary to help the reader understand each study both individually and in the context of the chapter.

COMPLETED IN VITRO CHINESE HERBAL HIV STUDIES

Before discussing clinical trials, we mention an vitro study conducted with traditional Chinese herbs. There have been a few studies similar to this one; however, this study is the most prominently quoted and is characteristic of in vitro studies.

In a study conducted at the University of California–Davis and the Chinese University of Hong Kong, the following summary was given:

Twenty-seven medicinal herbs reputed in ancient Chinese folklore to have antiinfective properties were extracted by boiling under reflux. The extracts were tested for inhibitory activity against HIV in the H9 cell line at concentrations nontoxic to growth of H9 cells.

Using a significant reduction (>standard deviation [SD] below the mean) in the percentage of cells positive for specific viral antigens in three successive

assays indicative of activity against the virus, 11 of the 27 extracts were found to be active.

One of the extracts *(Viola yedoensis)* was studied in greater depth. At a subtoxic concentration, this extract completely stopped the growth of HIV in virtually all experiments. It did not inactivate HIV extracellularly, did not induce interferon (INF), and did not inhibit the growth of herpes simplex, polio, or vesicular stomatitis viruses in human fibroblast culture.

Chinese medicinal herbs appeared to be a rich source of potentially useful materials for the treatment of HIV infection.[13]

CHINESE MEDICINE CLINICAL TRIALS

Completed Controlled Clinical Trials

A few completed controlled Chinese medicine trials have been conducted in HIV disease. The following section includes presented abstracts and ongoing Chinese medicine research.

The first completed controlled herbal trial was a randomized, double-blind, placebo-controlled pilot study that took place at San Francisco General Hospital from 1992 to 1993. This study was led by Dr. Jeffrey Burack, along with Dr. Misha Cohen and Dr. Donald Abrams. The summary of that clinical trial is as follows.

Pilot Randomized, Controlled Trial of Chinese Herbal Treatment for HIV-Associated Symptoms

Objective. We wished to determine the short-term safety and efficacy of a Chinese medicinal herb preparation in treating symptoms of HIV infection in a 12-week randomized, double-blind, placebo-controlled clinical trial in a university-affiliated AIDS clinic at a public general hospital.

Methods. Thirty adults with symptomatic HIV infection, no previous AIDS-defining diagnosis, and $CD4^+$ counts from 0.200 to 0.499 $\times$ 10^9/L (200 to 499/mm^3) received 28 tablets/day of either a standardized oral preparation of 31 Chinese herbs or a cellulose placebo.

Results. The primary outcome measures were (1) changes in life satisfaction, (2) perceived health, and (3) number and severity of symptoms. Other outcome measures included adherence, changes in weight, $CD4^+$ count, depression, anxiety, physical and social function, and mental health. Two placebo-treated subjects and no herb-treated subjects had mild adverse events (AEs). Subjects on both arms of the study reported taking 94% of prescribed tablets. No differences between treatment groups reached the $p < 0.05$ level. Life satisfaction improved in herb-treated subjects (+0.86, 95% confidence interval [CI]: +0.29, +1.43) but not in placebo-treated subjects (+0.20, 95% CI −0.35, +0.75). Number of symptoms was reduced in subjects receiving herbs (−2.2, 95% CI −4.1, −0.3) but not in those receiving placebo (−0.3, 95% CI −3.2, +2.7). There were trends toward greater improvements among herb-treated subjects on all symptom subscales except dermatological. The belief that one was receiving herbs was strongly associated with reporting that the treatment had helped ($p < 0.005$), but not with changes in life satisfaction or symptoms.

Conclusions. Patients receiving the herbal therapy reported improvements in life satisfaction and disease symptoms. Whether Chinese herbs are effective in the management of symptomatic HIV infection can be adequately addressed only by larger trials of longer duration.[14]

This trial of Enhance and Clear Heat combination treatment was the first of its kind. It had less-than-positive results because it was a study of a natural therapy for HIV/AIDS, not a study of TCM. Although we need studies of nontoxic substances that many people use as part of their treatment, this study did not use TCM diagnosis as part of its premise nor did it evaluate variations in treatment based on diagnosis and prognosis from a TCM point of view.

However, because the study was evaluated rigorously by a research institution (University of California) and had some mildly positive effects, it was a good precedent for the ongoing study of Chinese herbal medicine for the treatment of HIV disease.

Another completed trial took place in Portland, Oregon. This study was a comparison of herbal medicine versus dinitrochlorobenzene (DNCB) plus herbal medicine and was conducted by Dr. Subhuti Dharmananda.[15]

Another completed Chinese herb trial was conducted the at Community Consortium in San Francisco, funded by the University of California–San Francisco (UCSF) AIDS Clinical Research Center. This study was led by Dr. Donald Abrams and Dr. Misha Cohen. The following section gives the initial summary of that trial (includes 13 patients, although 16 have currently completed the trial) before publication of results.

Use of a Chinese Herbal Medicine in the Treatment of HIV-Associated *Cryptosporidium*-Negative Diarrhea

Objectives. To assess the effectiveness and safety of a Chinese herbal formulation (Source Qi) in reducing the number of stools/day related to HIV-associated *Cryptosporidium*-negative diarrhea, as well as relief of other associated symptoms.

Methods. Sixteen male patients received treatment with Source Qi in an 8-week open-label study. Study participants could receive Western pharmaceutical treatment if they were on a stable antidiarrheal regimen, having failed first-line therapy. The primary outcome variable was the number of diarrhea stools/day (as noted in a daily diary). Other outcome variables included changes in stool formation (as measured by the Thygeson Stool Tool and noted in the daily diary) and relief of associated symptoms. Patients tested negative for *Cryptosporidium* and had chronic diarrhea, defined as having three or more loose stools/day for at least 14 days (and no other treatable causes for the diarrhea).

Results. Of the 13 patients who completed the study, there was a reduction in average numbers of stools/day (from −0.2 to −0.8). The apparent benefit appears unlikely to be due to a placebo effect, because it is not present in week 1 and is maintained until at least week 6 ($p = 0.0096$). Regression to the mean also seems unlikely because of the long lag time between recruiting subjects and beginning treatment, and that benefit is not seen in week 1.

Conclusions. These results suggest some benefit from Source Qi* in reducing the number of stools/day in patients with HIV-associated *Cryptosporidium*-negative diarrhea, as well as relief of associated symptoms. A larger study is required to confirm these results.[16]

The Source Qi trial was originally intended to be a double-blind, placebo-controlled study. However, both patients and doctors refused enrollment, since they wanted to have the possibility of the person receiving placebo for 8 weeks because diarrhea is such a severe,

---

*Source Qi is made by Health Concerns.

debilitating problem. Therefore the study was re-designed as an open-label trial and quickly enrolled HIV-positive patients.

Another randomized placebo-controlled study that has been completed in Chinese herbal medicine for HIV was led by Rainer Weber, MD, a Western medical doctor, with Chinese medicine doctors Silvio Schaller, MD, and Misha Cohen, OMD, at the University Hospital in Zürich, Switzerland. Their preliminary findings follow.

In this study, a component of Chinese medicine—tongue diagnosis—was evaluated at the beginning and end of the study. All participants' tongues were photographed and reviewed by the investigators, who were blinded to whether a participant was on herbal medication or placebo. However, there was no individual diagnosis made by a practitioner.

Protease inhibitors (PIs) were released in Switzerland for study at the same time as the beginning of this study. The release of PIs created a major problem, causing the study enrollment to be far below expected numbers. This problem greatly reduced the number of people interested in participating in the study, since people could not enter both types of studies at the same time. It also reduced the high hopes for efficacy of the new powerful drugs.

Treatment of HIV-Infected Persons with Chinese Herbs: A Randomized, Placebo-Controlled Trial*

Context. CAM remedies that have not been scientifically tested are nonetheless widely used to treat chronic illnesses, particularly if curative options are limited.

Objectives. To assess the effectiveness of Chinese herbs in reducing symptoms and improving the quality of life (QOL) of HIV-infected persons.

Design. Prospective, placebo-controlled, double-blind study.

Setting. University-based HIV outpatient clinic.

Patients. Sixty-eight HIV-infected adults with CD4 cell counts $<0.59 \times 10^9$/L.

Intervention. Participants received 7 pills qid containing either a standardized preparation of 35 Chinese herbs or placebo for 6 months.

---

*Weber R, Loy M, Christen L, Schaller S, Christen S, Joyce CRB, Cohen MR.

Main Outcome Measures. Symptoms, HIV disease progression, HIV-1 RNA plasma viral loads, CD4 and CD8 cell counts, and scores on standard questionnaires for QOL, depression, anxiety, and coping.

Results. Baseline data of the two groups were equal regarding previous antiretroviral therapy (ART) (74% versus 79%), median CD4 cell counts (0.20×10^9/L versus 0.25×10^9/L), and median HIV-1 plasma viral loads (35,612 copies/ml versus 52,027 copies/ml). At enrollment, none of the subjects was seriously ill or depressed, and average coping and QOL scores were normal. In all, 53 (78%) participants completed the study. Patients taking Chinese herbs reported significantly more gastrointestinal disturbances (79% versus 38%; $p = 0.003$) than those receiving placebo. No therapy-related toxicities were observed. At study end, no significant differences between the intervention and placebo groups were found regarding plasma viral loads, CD4 cell counts, symptoms, and psychometric parameters. HIV-1 RNA level was unchanged at study end. Among participants who were not on concomitant ART, median CD4 cell counts declined by 0.05×10^9/L in both study groups.

Conclusions. This standardized formulation of Chinese herbs for HIV-infected persons did not improve QOL, clinical manifestations, plasma viral loads, or CD4 cell counts. The data suggest that this formulation is not effective when administered in a Western medicine setting. The study has to be interpreted in consideration of historical perspectives because it was planned, approved, and initiated before antiretroviral triple-drug combination therapy was available.[17]

Another controlled clinical pilot study was completed in 1995. This trial consisted of studying acupuncture in HIV-positive persons who were also diagnosed with chronic viral hepatitis, and it was conducted at the Quan Yin Healing Arts Center by Misha Cohen, OMD. The following abstract was presented at a Satellite conference of the Geneva AIDS Conference in 1998.

In the following study, there has not yet been a statistical analysis of the groups. It is likely that they may only show trends as opposed to statistical significance, considering the small size of each study group. However, this type of anecdotal information is helpful in guiding us both in treatment and in developing more comprehensive studies that truly test Chinese medicine treatment for serious problems such as those associated with chronic viral hepatitis, with or without concomitant HIV infection. However, this type of analysis is generally not considered to be "gold-standard" by Western researchers.

Acupuncture Treatment in HIV-Positive Patients with Hepatitis C or Hepatitis B Virus Coinfection and Elevated Transaminases*

Objectives. To compare the results of acupuncture treatment versus no treatment in patients infected with both HIV and hepatitis C virus (HCV) or hepatitis B virus (HBV) and who have elevated hepatic transaminases.

Design. Prospective, randomized, controlled pilot study.

Methods. Fifteen patients with confirmed HIV and either HBV or HCV were enrolled into a 16-week pilot study to determine whether acupuncture treatment was useful in reducing elevated hepatic transaminases. Included were patients whose alanine aminotransferase (ALT) levels were more than 2.5 times normal levels. Patients were excluded who were already receiving acupuncture treatment, herbal treatment, or pharmaceutical treatment for chronic viral hepatitis. A substudy compared a group receiving Korean acupuncture treatment versus Chinese acupuncture treatment. Subjects were tested at week 0 and week 17 for ALT levels.

Results. Of the 15 patients enrolled, eight were randomly assigned to the acupuncture group and seven were assigned to the control group. In the acupuncture group, five out of eight patients (62.5%) had significant drops in ALT levels, with two patients (25%) whose levels dropped to within the normal range. All eight patients in the acupuncture group completed treatment. Also, two (25%) of the acupuncture group had ALT levels that dropped more than 200%. There was no difference between the Korean style and Chinese style treatments. In the control group, there was only one patient (14%) whose ALT level dropped, but not significantly. In the control group, four persons (57%) did not complete the study. There were 2 dropouts, 1 death, and 1 person too ill to complete laboratory testing at the end of the study. In natural history studies, only 10% of untreated infected patients have a significant drop in ALT levels over a 1-year study period.

*Cohen MR, Wilson CJ, Surasky A.

Conclusion. Treatment with acupuncture appears to have some success in reducing ALT levels in persons infected with both HIV and chronic viral HCV or HBV. A larger study is indicated in order to confirm these results.[18]

Some Uncontrolled Chinese Medicine Trials

One of the earliest reports on the use of TCM research in HIV/AIDS was in 1989 by Dr. Jin Lin Wang, in which he gave the following conclusions:

1. In persons using TCM alone, CD4 count increased: 66.02%, CD4 count decreased 9.71%, and CD4 count maintained 24.27%.
2. In persons using TCM with Western medicine (AZT), CD4 count increased: 29.6%, CD4 count decreased 25.51%, and CD4 count maintained 44.89%.
3. In certain cases, TCM can delay progression of disease.
4. TCM should be used on a continuous basis to maintain effect.
5. Treatment needs to be according to TCM diagnosis.

The preceding report may be useful to clinical practitioners in learning some ways to follow treatment interventions. However, there was no testable hypothesis but only a following of anecdotal case reports. It was also difficult to tell what the comparison groups truly were. Western researchers do not develop studies in this manner. These reports could be presented as anecdotal reports that may provide information for follow-up with a research protocol. This type of report is often discounted by Western scientific researchers.[19]

The following abstract was presented in China at the International Symposium on Viral Hepatitis and AIDS in 1991 after a 2-year observational treatment group by Quan Yin Healing Arts Center in cooperation with the Institute for Traditional Medicine.

Herbal Therapies For HIV Disease

Objectives. The main purpose of this research was to test Chinese herbal formulas for effectiveness in HIV treatment. The second purpose was to determine which formulas were most effective. Formulas were developed according to TCM theory and contained herbs that are known to be antiviral (AV) in vitro.

Methods. Four hundred ninety-six persons participated in an herbal treatment program over a 2-year period. Participants were followed for blood work parameters, as well as for symptom signs. All herbs were given in pill form at an average of 20 g/day. A general herbal protocol consisting of 21 700-mg tablets was given in conjunction with an adjunctive formula of 6 to 9 700-mg tablets.

Results. The vast majority (>80%) of participants reported feeling more healthy and having increased energy. Some preliminary evidence of slowed-down disease process and reduced symptoms exists. Stabilization of white blood cell (WBC), red blood cell (RBC), and hematocrit (Hct) counts was noted. Some anecdotal evidence of T-cell stabilization was noted, although there was difficulty in regularly attaining T-cell counts. Participants were able to take the pills on a long-term basis. The average treatment time was 6 months, although many participants were able to continue taking herbs during the 2-year period. Adjunctive formulas appear to reduce specific symptoms and signs.

Conclusion. Persons at all stages of HIV disease may benefit from the use of Chinese herbal formulas. Compliance and optimum dosage are best achieved in pill, powder, or concentrate form. Blood parameters tend to stabilize in persons taking herbs. Further research is needed to establish whether Chinese herbs are AV, particularly anti-HIV, in vivo.[20]

The preceding abstract reflects the type of observational group study that was popular at this time. This was before major treatment using any combination therapies. The purpose of the project was clear—to develop herbal formulas that may effectively treat HIV disease.

However, no control group was reported, although there was a comparison later made to a natural history study at UC–San Francisco. There was no clear hypothesis with which to adequately compare the groups, and no statistical analysis was performed.

Although these studies lacked much of what is needed for true scientific validity, when added together with the number of people involved, there was an impressive amount of data with which to inform clinical practice and to later develop scientifically sound studies.

From a similar perspective, the following abstract summarizes an uncontrolled study carried out in New Mexico by Makima Hawkins in the early 1990s.

The Use of a Chinese Herbal Composition for the Treatment of HIV: A Descriptive Study*

Methods. Fifty-nine persons at various stages of infection with HIV were recruited into a 6-month descriptive study in which they received a specified combination of Chinese herbs, Composition A, which was developed on the principles of TCM. Each participant received 26 g of the combination, in addition to adjunctive formulas that were selected according to traditional Chinese therapeutics. Laboratory analyses for CD4 lymphocytes, complete blood counts (CBCs), and chemistry profiles were performed both at baseline and at the conclusion of the study. Participants also rated the severity of a variety of symptoms related to HIV disease.

Fifty-two persons (88%) completed the study, and four (6.7% of the total) dropped out because they experienced side effects of the herbs.

Results. All symptoms improved while taking the herbal preparation. Half of the symptoms, including fatigue, night sweats, fever/chills, anxiety, depression, lymphadenopathy, and headache were statistically significant, with p-values ranging from 0.02 to 0.0000008. There was no evidence of measurable toxicity associated with the use of the study herbs.

This study clearly demonstrated that the use of Composition-A† provides beneficial improvements in symptoms associated with HIV infection.[21]

Conclusions. Without a control group or a comparison group, we cannot say that this study clearly demonstrated any conclusive results. However, the study was done was before combination therapies had been established, as well as before the advent of PIs. There also appeared to be no analysis of the laboratory values that were collected in the abstract or the presented paper. No separation was made between self-limiting symptoms and ongoing, chronic, illness-related symptoms. However, because so many symptoms were significantly reduced, the conclusion could indicate that further study is needed.

The following section is a summary of an uncontrolled American Foundation for AIDS Research (AMFAR)-funded acupuncture trial conducted in Boston from 1991 to 1992 for the treatment of peripheral neuropathy (PN).[22]

---

*Hawkins M, Hawkins T, Voorhees R, Smith J, Djordjevich P.
†Composition A is made by Seven Forests (Institute for Traditional Medicine).

A Pilot Study of Acupuncture for the Symptomatic Treatment of HIV-Associated Peripheral Neuropathy

Objective. To study the outcome of patients receiving acupuncture treatment for the symptomatic treatment of HIV-related PN not caused by drug toxicity. We evaluated objective and subjective nerve function and QOL measurements.

Methods. Thirty-nine patients received acupuncture twice weekly for 6 months in a nonrandomized observational study. No particular prescription was used, and the treatment choice was left to the practitioner's discretion. Neurological and QOL assessments were completed at entry and at months 2 and 6.

Summary. Twenty-six patients returned for the first follow-up at 2 months. The 13 patients lost to follow-up had more severe neuropathy and lower QOL scores than those who completed the treatment. Significant improvement was found for the quantitative sensory test (QST) of the toe ($p = 0.05$). No trends were found in the subjective symptom list. Five of seven QOL scales showed improvement (none significant).

Conclusions. This study suggests that there may be a role for acupuncture as a treatment for PN. Future controlled studies may help further define the efficacy of this method.

The preceding pilot study shows potential to study PN using TCM diagnosis and treatment. However, the pilot study was too short and uncontrolled to lead to any real conclusion. In neuropathy, 8 weeks may be too short a time to see statistically significant differences. However, the conclusion appears to be consistent with this observation.

The following abstract was presented as a poster at the International AIDS Symposium in Berlin, 1993. It reports on a retrospective questionnaire compiled in San Francisco.

The Effect of Chinese Herbs on the Symptom Levels of HIV-Positive Patients with CD4 Counts Greater Than 200*

Objective. To investigate the effect of Chinese herbs on the symptom level of HIV-positive patients with CD4 cell counts greater than 200.

Methods. A quota sample of 175 volunteer participants responded to a questionnaire by mail. Of the responses, 54 were not used because participants had either CD4 counts less than 200 or a social desirability response bias. Of the 121 remaining participants, 56 were taking the Chinese herbal formula and 65 were not. The Seven Forest herbal formula, Composition A, and Seven Forest adjunct formulas were used. Participants had been taking 26 g/day of Chinese herbs for at least 12 weeks: 7 tablets of Composition A tid and 7 tablets of an adjunct formula for their specific temperament once a day. The Composition A formula contains 28 herbs, including *Ganoderma, Astragalus, Isatis,* and *Milletia.* Questionnaires asked for the following variables: (1) age, (2) sex, (3) race/ethnicity, (4) risk group, (5) educational status, (6) current CD4 cell count, (7) health-promotion activity level, and (8) symptom level.

Results. The two groups were compared using analysis of variance (ANOVA) tests to identify significant variable differences between them. Patients taking Chinese herbs had fewer symptoms (Scheffe F test $= 7.73$, $p = 0.006$, $df = 1119$) and higher socioeconomic status (SES) (Scheffe F test $= 4.89$, $p = 0.029$, $df = 1119$) than those not taking Chinese herbs. No other significant differences were found between the two groups for any of the other variables ($p > 0.2$).

Conclusions. For this group of 121 HIV-positive patients with CD4 counts greater than 200, those taking Chinese herbs for at least 12 weeks had significantly fewer symptoms than those not taking Chinese herbs.

The preceding study is interesting for several reasons. First, it was one of the few TCM presentations at the 1993 International AIDS Symposium in Berlin. However, there are some obvious questions. One of the study's weaknesses is that it is not a prospective study but a by-mail retrospective questionnaire. This can lead to bias through self-selection and self-reporting. Also, it is unclear how the groups were chosen and whether or not there were people in the "nonherb" group who had previously taken herbs or were taking other herbal formulations. However, this study suggests that certain herbal formulations may decrease symptoms in HIV disease, which can lead to the development of more specific studies for definitive symptoms. It would be helpful to know which specific symptoms were reported to have significant decreases to follow-up on this study more effectively.

The following section is a summary of uncontrolled observations reported in 1994 from the former director, Michael Young, LAc, at the Immune Enhancement Project in San Francisco.

---

*Baker D, Copeland DR, Independent HIV Health Educators, San Francisco.

Chinese Herbal Therapies in HIV

Methods. One hundred ninety-three HIV-positive persons were recruited into 12-week research programs using traditional Chinese herbal therapies. The formulas used were developed at the Institute for Traditional Medicine in Portland, Oregon. The formulations were selected on the basis of the principles of TCM and supporting research from the scientific literature.

The formulas were prepared using a combination of extract and powdered herbal material. Patients were asked to consume 7 tablets qid allowing for a total intake of 26 g of herbal material/day.

Results. Of the 193 participants, 43 were unwilling or unable to complete the 12-week program by filling out the final questionnaire forms at the end of the program. Of the remaining 150 participants, many reported a reduction of chronic HIV-related complaints and improvement in QOL variables.

One variable relating to participation was then isolated—the concurrent use of nucleosides (AZT, didanosine [ddI], or zalcitabine [ddC]). The results of patients using nucleosides were compared with their counterparts who were not using nucleosides and were found to be similar, suggesting that the action of the herbal formulas occurs independently of nucleoside usage.

Conclusions. An analysis of the records of persons who did not complete the study and their reasons for discontinuing is given.

Laboratory parameters were monitored whenever possible; however, no conclusions could be obtained based on the data collected.[23]

One obvious observation is that the abstract has no hypothesis to be proved or disproved. Therefore this is not a study but a compilation of material from a treatment intervention. The bias of a retrospective analysis is present, and the original hypothesis is not known. After reading the data carefully, it is difficult to determine specific symptoms that may have improved that were not self-limiting, which is a flaw in the design of the analysis. Also, there is no reason given for not providing any conclusions about collected laboratory data. However, it is apparent that some positive anecdotal data on symptomatic response to treatment could be clarified with additional controlled or uncontrolled studies.

The following trial was an uncontrolled observational study that included review of clinical records and surveys were undertaken and analyzed at the American College of Traditional Chinese Medicine (ACTCM) Clinic in San Francisco. Howard Moffet, LAc, MS, MPH, was the principal investigator. The following section is extracted from that study published in *AIDS Patient Care*, August 1994.

Using Acupuncture and Herbs for the Treatment of HIV: The American College of Traditional Chinese Medicine Experience*

Methods. The ACTCM HIV Clinic program provided weekly acupuncture and herbal medicine services. Monitoring of 63 patients was done through weekly TCM evaluations, a complete physical examination by a nurse practitioner, CBC and T-cell counts, and monthly symptom and QOL surveys.

There were 19 HIV-positive, 6 ARC, and 38 AIDS Western-diagnosis patients. The most common Chinese diagnoses were Spleen Qi Deficiency, Liver Qi Congestion, and general Qi and Yin Deficiency.

Results. The benefits of treatment . . . include alleviation of symptoms. In this uncontrolled study, patient-reported symptoms were reduced both in severity and number of symptoms. There were statistically significant ($p < 0.05$) improvements in symptoms of fatigue, loss of appetite, lymphadenopathy, neuropathy, low-grade fever, skin irritation, and infection.

Benefits were also noted in QOL surveys . . . the trends were toward improvement in the measure of physical functioning ($p = 0.07$), social functioning ($p = 0.0003$), health perceptions ($p = 0.06$), and pain relief ($p = 0.06$).

Conclusions. It cannot be known exactly which factors may account for any improvement in patient conditions, since this study has no control group. However, the trends observed are very persuasive and clearly indicate the need for further, better-controlled studies.[24]

The preceding ACTCM observational study was a well-organized review of a relatively large number of patients undergoing treatment in a community clinic. This study helps us conclude which Chinese medicine diagnoses are most commonly seen in the clinic—a help to practitioners, researchers, and herbal developers alike.

Another uncontrolled trial was the study of Allicin, a component of garlic. Garlic is part of the Chinese pharmacopoeia, as well as part of Western herbalism. However, the substance was given in a pharmaceutical

---

*Moffet H, Sanders P, Sinclair T, Ergil K.

manner, not as a Chinese herbal formula or as part of a total Chinese medicine treatment plan. The trial was conducted by a community-based research organization called the AIDS ReSearch Alliance in California.

Garlic for Cryptosporidosis

Issue. Cryptosporidiosis is an infection of the gut caused by a parasite called *Cryptosporidium,* and the main symptom is prolonged diarrhea that leads to weight loss.

Methods. The trial used a garlic concentrate called Allicin, which is available in the United States in 30-mg glass vials imported from China. In this study, 30 mg of Allicin was mixed with 90 ml distilled water. This mixture was taken bid.

Results. Twenty persons enrolled in the study. The only major side effect, as expected, was a strong garlic smell and taste. This side effect was a problem for about a third of the participants and led at least one person to drop out of the study. After 6 weeks, there were 16 persons remaining in the study. Ten of these individuals had less diarrhea and fewer watery stools and had stable or increased body weight (BW).

Conclusions. The most significant finding of the study was that, in four out of eight subjects who chose to remain on the study for longer than 8 weeks, stool tests were repeatedly negative for the *Cryptosporidium* parasite. The average T4 cell count of subjects in this study was less than 30, and most had tried and failed the standard cryptosporidiosis treatment, Humatin. Clearance of *Cryptosporidium* organisms was not reported before in persons with such low T4 cell counts.[25]

From 1997 to 1998, Carla Wilson, executive director at Quan Yin Healing Arts Center, conducted a chart review and persons surveys to determine the use and possible efficacy of a combination of TCM techniques in the management of PN. The following is a summary abstract.

Chinese Medicine in the Treatment of Peripheral Neuropathy*

Issue. PN in the HIV/AIDS population is a serious and debilitating problem that requires an effective treatment protocol.

Project. At Quan Yin Healing Arts Center—a nonprofit, community-based, complementary medicine clinic that has delivered Chinese medicine for over 13 years in San Francisco—533 HIV/AIDS clients were treated in 1996, which was 66% of its client base. Over 75% of the people with HIV/AIDS had PN, from mild to severely debilitating. All women and men with PN received a combination of treatments, including one or more of the following interventions: (1) acupuncture, (2) electroacupuncture, (3) massage therapy, (4) moxibustion (an herbal heat therapy), and (5) herbal medicine. Clients received treatment in time intervals from twice a month to 3 times/week.

Results. Chart reviews and surveys conducted by the Executive Director revealed that over 75% of HIV-positive patients who were reviewed had reduced symptoms, including decreased pain, reduced numbness, and increased mobility (including walking and running when unable to do so previously). Variations in response were related to the total number of treatments, the number of weeks of treatment, compliance with self-care (such as self-moxibustion), and the combination of medications that caused PN. Some patients were able to discontinue PN treatments after several sessions, since they no longer had neuropathy-related complaints. Others needed ongoing care for PN, especially those who continued on drug combinations that were highly likely to cause neuropathy.

Conclusions. A combination of Chinese medicine therapies appears to have a high rate of efficacy in decreasing symptoms in HIV-positive patients with the serious and debilitating problem of PN. With the apparent rate of clinical success in a large number of clients, a controlled pilot study is recommended as a follow-up to this chart review and collection of surveys.[26]

Interestingly enough, the previous uncontrolled observational study points to a possible design for a clinical trial for PN that is quite different from the completed NIH funded study that failed. It is more similar to the brief study by Jonathan Ammen reported earlier in this chapter. This idea will be discussed in more depth later.

Ongoing Chinese Medicine Trials

Other studies are currently in progress:

An uncompleted controlled study (as of this writing) is a study of HIV-related sinusitis using acupuncture and Chinese herbs versus antibiotic therapy. This

---

*Wilson CJ, Quan Yin Healing Arts Center, San Francisco.

study is taking place at the Immune Enhancement Project (IEP) in San Francisco with Thomas Sinclair, LAc, MA, as principal investigator. It is funded by an NIH OAM grant.

Acupuncture and Herbal Treatment of Chronic HIV Sinusitis

Objective. To find out if traditional Chinese medicine or an antibiotic medicine (e.g., Augmentin) is better at reducing symptoms of sinusitis, and at preventing sinusitis from returning.

Methods. Patients will be randomly assigned to receive either acupuncture and Chinese herbs or Augmentin. The study lasts 12 weeks, with 8 weeks of treatment and 4 weeks of no treatment. Study visits will be weekly. Patients will be required to have an examination of their nasal cavity, as well as a CAT scan of their nasal passages. These examinations will be repeated 30 days after the study ends. Use of any antibiotics other than Septra/Bactrim or use of acupuncture/Chinese herbs not prescribed as part of the study is not allowed during the study.

Required:
- CD4 cell (T-cell) range: at least 50
- HIV-positive
- History of recurrent sinusitis

Not Allowed:
- Active infection with fever over 102°F
- Any active OI
- Pregnant or nursing women[27]

In the following personal communication, Mr. Sinclair of IEP has described the problems that were part of the process of that study. The problems he describes can be helpful for all of us in understanding the universal problems which face researchers when designing a Chinese medicine study—that the design must take into consideration the type of volunteers for such studies, the role of the Western and Eastern practitioners and researchers, and adequate funding, among others. Mr. Sinclair states:

"IEP is conducting a study comparing antibiotics to herbs and acupuncture in the treatment of HIV chronic sinusitis. Several problems have emerged.

1. At initial recruiting, many individuals were only interested in receiving acupuncture, not in being randomized. This occurred despite published information that explained study requirements. To correct this, we instituted much more careful prescreening of potential candidates.

2. Many candidates were on antibiotics at the time of screening, which were not allowed in the study. They were asked to return after completing the course of antibiotics and were often lost to follow-up.

3. Advent of PIs and new drug therapies played a role in decreasing the general level of interest in alternative therapies.

4. Screening requirements were difficult. We required a prescreen, an initial visit to a physician, and a CT scan of the sinus, followed by randomization. This could take up to 4 weeks before randomization and entry into the study. Many patients lost interest or had other health status changes.

5. Lack of adequate personnel. This study was woefully underfunded for the ambitious scale of the project. More staff time was required than was often available.

6. Coordination with the Western physician's office was often difficult, and many patients "no-showed" for their appointments with the MD.

7. Many patients were screened, had their CT scan, and were ready to be randomized when they were put on antibiotics by their primary care physician.

8. This study required a tremendous amount of staff time related to the approval process. We had to obtain an investigational new drug (IND) application with the FDA, as well as the standard IRB approval. In the future, I would run any studies conducted by IEP through an outside administrative agency.

That summarizes the major problems of the study."[28]

The following open-label anemia study is being conducted by the UCSF Community Consortium, funded by Bastyr University through its NIH OAM grant. This study is led by Dr. Donald Abrams and Dr. Misha Cohen.

This is the first Chinese herbal medicine study to incorporate some Chinese diagnosis as part of the study in order to begin to make guesses from a TCM diagnosis about whether or not there will be benefits from the study medication.

This study began as a double-blind, placebo-controlled study but (similar to the above IEP study) could not accrue participants; therefore it was necessary to alter the study midstream to complete the enrollment. The following is a summary of the current study.

A Pilot Study of Chinese Herbs in Mild-to-Moderate HIV-Associated Anemia

Purpose. The purpose of this prospective double-blind, placebo-controlled pilot study is to assess the activity of a standardized Chinese herbal formula in the treatment of mild-to-moderate anemia in persons with HIV disease.

Primary objective. To evaluate the effectiveness of a Chinese herbal formulation on changes in hemoglobin in patients with HIV-associated mild-to-moderate anemia.

Secondary objectives:

1. To evaluate the impact of a Chinese herbal formulation on WBC
2. To evaluate the effectiveness of a Chinese herbal formulation on relief of symptoms (i.e., fatigue) associated with mild-to-moderate HIV-associated anemia
3. To assess the safety of a Chinese herbal formulation in HIV-infected patients with mild-to-moderate anemia
4. To compare QOL between treated and placebo groups
5. To correlate TCM syndromes at baseline (through tongue and pulse diagnosis) with clinical observations and measurements over time

The following uncontrolled study may technically be called a Chinese herbal study, since it is using moxibustion, a Chinese herb used externally to produce warmth and tonification when used over certain areas or points. It is sponsored by the Center for Holistic Medicine on Long Island in New York.

Treatment: Acupuncture, moxibustion. This trial will study acupuncture and moxibustion for the treatment of diarrhea related to chronic malabsorption and HIV. All participants will be treated with acupuncture around the digestive area and moxibustion.

Moxibustion occurs when a mixture of a root and herb called *moxa* is lit, the flame is blown out, and the warm smoke is moved around the area being treated. The treatment is being done by the Dean of the Center for Holistic Medicine on Long Island. Treatments take place at Columbia Presbyterian Hospital. Participants will be paid $60.

Participants must be HIV-positive males of 18 years of age or older who have experienced 3 or more episodes of diarrhea over a 24-hour period for 3 weeks or more.

HOW DO WE DO RESEARCH IN CHINESE HERBAL MEDICINE AND TRADITIONAL CHINESE MEDICINE AS A WHOLE?

What is Meant by Traditional Chinese Medicine?

When we refer to TCM, are we referring primarily to the theory of TCM, or are we also referring to the practices of TCM? Or must we include both theory and practice when we refer to the study of TCM?

For example, if the theory of TCM is what we mean when we speak of TCM, then a study design must include a diagnosis using Chinese patterns in order to test the outcomes. If the practices or modalities of TCM are what we mean when we refer to TCM, then we could study, for example, acupuncture for neuropathy regardless of the TCM diagnostic pattern. We would expect one point prescription to be effective for all neuropathy, regardless of syndrome or channel theory, which may not work.

The failure of the PN acupuncture study funded by the NIH is case in point.[29]

For example, a study examining the treatment of neuropathy with ashi points along with appropriate channel points might be effective (which gives a channel diagnosis, but not necessarily a TCM pattern diagnosis). If we included TCM diagnostic patterns, we could determine particular types of treatment that might be effective. For example, in neuropathy, one Chinese pattern might include Cold stagnation, and it would make sense to use warming therapies as part of the treatment plan, according to the TCM diagnosis.

Designing research often can be contradictory because there are two aspects of TCM. First, we most often diagnose and treat according to TCM patterns. One example is the theory of stages of Cold disease developed in the Shang Han Lung for herbal treatment. There are also herbal theories based on stages of Warm disease, which are separate theories of herbal medicine.

Acupuncture texts contain several theories, including theories of the channels. If the practitioner treats a point on the channel, the point treats the channel. For example, an acupuncturist can treat a distal point on the channel. In acupuncture one can also treat ashi points, which are points of pain or sensitivity that may or may not be located on a channel. Other theories state that the practitioner can treat problems with points located on the opposite side of the body. In TCM acupuncture, we treat according to the Chinese pattern diagnosis.

When designing research of TCM for Western evaluation, we ask the following questions: (1) Will the TCM modality effect likely be equal or superior to the current Western treatment? (2) Is there a Western treatment available? For example, with HCV there is often no effective Western treatment, whereas TCM has a rich history of the treatment of syndromes and symptoms found in hepatitis. When Western treatment is effective, it often has intolerable side effects, whereas TCM theory posits that we can treat and allow for continuation of the Western therapy.

Can we study one part of TCM when we study a particular treatment? For example, in the Swiss Chinese herbal study described above, tongue diagnosis is made both before and after the study, and the researchers are blinded. This method helps us find out if there is a correlation with tongue diagnosis and whether or not the person is improving on TCM herbal treatment, as well as whether the tongue diagnosis reflects disease severity. Are the patterns we have determined as HIV-related patterns reflected by our tongue diagnosis?

In our study designs, we always try to include TCM diagnosis. However, TCM is limited by funding because it is labor-intensive, and it is often limited by investigator bias.

An Example Of Determining Outcome Measures

In one particular study design, the Western researchers delineated the following outcome parameters for evaluation:

- Primary: HCV RNA and elevated transaminases
- Secondary: QOL, symptom changes, CD4 count
  Taking our TCM experience into account, our ranking was a bit different:
- Primary: QOL, symptom changes, elevated transaminases
- Secondary: HCV RNA, CD4 count
  Chinese medicine informs us in a holistic world view, and, in research, in a controlled environment. Our TCM experience also told us that HCV RNA is

not likely to change, so our primary research outcome should not be something that may be set up for failure.

After discussion with the other researchers, we re-ranked the study. Now the outcomes are:

- Primary: QOL and elevated transaminases
- Secondary: Symptom changes, HCV RNA

This method would not ordinarily have been done in our Western-based research, and it represents true progress and change for both systems of medicine.

There is also room for studies of substances, such as herbal formulas, for specific Western diseases. For example, in the Source Qi study described earlier, we were studying one herbal formulation for chronic, nonpathogenic HIV-related diarrhea. We received positive results—interestingly enough, the results were even more specific—the Source Qi appeared to have a specific effect in reducing the side effect of diarrhea associated with the intake of the PIs. Because large numbers of people are using PIs as part of their AV HIV regimen, the Source Qi may be a very important tool, since it appears to be a nontoxic alternative to the toxic antidiarrhetic Western pharmaceuticals.

The Fantasy for the Future

If we had enough financial resources, we could begin to do studies that would provide the most useful information to both HIV providers and people with HIV/AIDS. We could do studies that included TCM diagnosis and the proper treatment for that diagnosis, and compare it to either a randomized control group or an existing comparison group. Ideally, we could study TCM as a system, not only its subset modalities in isolation. However, the study of modalities is also appropriate. There may be specific symptoms that could be studied easily and inexpensively and provide high-quality information that could be used clinically. For neuropathy symptoms, it would be valid to study acupuncture and moxibustion, either separately or in combination.

Although double-blind, controlled studies cannot be performed for acupuncture, they can be performed for herbal medicine. Double-blind studies also cannot be performed for either dietary therapy or Qigong.

The Questions Raised When Designing Research in TCM

What is the Methodology for Studying TCM?

Without attempting to fully answer the following questions, we are asking these questions as both TCM practitioners and Western scientific researchers so that we as a community can come together and begin to answer them.

Question 1: Can we study TCM with Western methodology? Does this mean using the scientific method, which could involve double-blind studies? Can we study TCM using randomized studies, studies with various control groups, or studies of individual substances for specific symptoms or Western disease diagnoses? Can we, in practice, truly study the diagnostic procedures and outcomes of TCM using the Western scientific method?

Question 2: Can we study TCM using Chinese methodology? Can we use diagnostic methods of TCM, such as tongue diagnosis, pulse diagnosis, facial colors, and abdominal palpation to determine outcomes that can be measured statistically?

Question 3: Can we study the various practices of TCM individually? Can we separate Chinese herbal medicine, acupuncture, or dietary therapy from the rest of TCM? Also, when we study Chinese herbal medicine, how do we study it?

To answer these questions, we must define the outcomes of research, which means we must define what we are studying. Many practitioners and researchers realize that when we study just one substance for a Western-defined disease process—whether it is one Chinese herbal formula, one herb, or one set of acupuncture points—this is not studying Chinese medicine in its entirety. When using no Chinese diagnosis to determine the study intervention, this should be seen as a study of a natural herbal substance or an HIV-related symptom therapy (i.e., using Source Qi for diarrhea), or in the case of one set of acupuncture points for several types of neuropathy (see the NIH-sponsored acupuncture/Elavil study), or a broader study of QOL and symptomatology using a natural herbal medicine (i.e., the SFGH study of Enhance/Clear Heat combination). Although some components of TCM are used, the use of Chinese diagnosis and the application of a diagnosis when designing an individual treatment plan is not employed in these studies.

Do We Always Need to Use a Full TCM Diagnosis in the Study Design?

Many of the controlled studies cited earlier in this chapter are studies of either a single substance/formula or a single set of acupuncture points given across the board to people with HIV without any individualized Chinese diagnosis. These studies do not have the fullness of TCM, in which we give a diagnosis and treat an individual according to that diagnosis. However, they are legitimate studies of the epidemic factor in disease, in which we may define the disease in terms of Chinese medicine patterns associated with the epidemic disease (in this case HIV), not the individual's constitution or patterns. Of course, in the clinical practice of TCM, however, we always diagnose an individual and look at his or her patterns, as well as the epidemic pattern of disease.[4]

So, What Are We Studying?

Are we studying Chinese medicine in its traditional form, using a Chinese herbal formula for a Western disease, or doing something else entirely?

The following are examples of each type of research study from the point of view of outcomes.

PRIMARY OUTCOME EXAMPLES

Chinese Treatment for a Western Diagnosis: Source Qi for HIV-Related Diarrhea

The first example is the Source Qi study for diarrhea mentioned earlier. The question is: Does Source Qi relieve HIV-related diarrhea? In this study, the researchers tried to determine efficacy in relief of a certain symptom and its associated symptoms with a specific Chinese herbal formula.

Source Qi was designed for Spleen Qi and Yang deficiency with severe diarrhea, with or without parasites. It was not designed for people with Heat-associated severe diarrhea. Therefore we had to be creative with the design of the study to exclude people who, from a Chinese viewpoint, could have Heat-related diarrhea. Because of several factors, we did not do individual diagnosis using questioning, tongue examination, and pulse diagnosis. However, we created an exclusion criteria—including using stool tests for pathogens—that in all likelihood would exclude people with heat diarrhea, although it could possibly still exclude some persons with underlying Spleen Qi deficiency. In this form, this study can be duplicated by Western scientists with absolutely no understanding of TCM. As a interesting subnote, those Heat-type diarrheas are more likely to be acute bacterial infections and would probably benefit from Western antibiotic therapy.

With enough money and people, we would design studies differently. Each person would be diagnosed individually to determine TCM patterns and would be treated with a formula that is specific for those patterns. The controls could be either a placebo or a comparison group. We could also create $n = 1$ studies and compare the subjects with themselves as their own placebos.

However, given the limitations of money and other factors, we were able to creatively use the resources we had to design some built-in Chinese diagnostic factors into this study. Again, doing research that studies a group of people is different than the clinical practice of treating an individual. This is true whether studying Chinese or Western medicine.

To carry out the study optimally as well as we could without using Chinese diagnostic techniques, we recognized that—as a whole—people who have severe diarrhea without bloody stools and fever usually have Spleen Qi and Yang Deficiency. We tried to design the study to rule out people with Heat conditions.

Therefore, although we took into account some TCM factors, this method used Chinese herbal medicine to treat a Western diagnosis.

If we established a Chinese diagnosis by using all the parameters of Chinese medicine and incorporating Chinese medicine as a whole, we would also offer dietary suggestions, as well as acupuncture and moxibustion treatment when appropriate. This could be the design of a broader study that may include other outcomes as well.

Chinese Treatment for a Chinese Diagnosis: Xiao Yao Wan for HIV-related PMS

Another approach would be to take a group of people, give a Chinese diagnosis, and then give the persons who fit specific Chinese diagnostic patterns an herbal formula appropriate for that diagnosis. For HIV-positive women with bloating and increased PMS symptoms, we might test Xiao Yao Wan to see if it alleviates Liver Qi Stagnation. This is an example of Chinese diagnosis/Chinese treatment approach.

SECONDARY OUTCOME EXAMPLE

A secondary outcome could be related to determining the correlation of a Chinese diagnosis (or a diagnostic technique) to a specific Western disease. For example, in the Source Qi study, a secondary outcome could be to ask if there is a correlation of a swollen, pale, wet tongue in chronic HIV-related diarrhea. This secondary outcome question would answer a strictly Chinese medicine question.

HOW DO WE DETERMINE THE RESEARCH METHOD?

There are several methodologies for doing research in TCM.

TCM Treatment Versus Western Treatment

We can compare a standard Western treatment with TCM. One example would be to compare Source Qi with standard antidiarrheal drugs, or to test acupuncture and herbs versus antibiotics for chronic sinusitis.

TCM Treatment Versus TCM Treatment

We could also compare two different herbal formulas that may have been chosen for efficacy in similar situations, such as studying Marrow Plus versus Ji Xue Teng Gao (*Milletia* gel) for AZT or chemotherapy-related anemia. Measurement outcomes can be evaluated for one set of acupuncture points against another for chronic hepatitis.

TCM Treatment Versus Placebo

We could also compare an herbal formula with a placebo, such as in the Swiss herb study and the SFGH herb study. There are many problems with this method, especially the challenge of recruiting people who do not want to join placebo studies. We had great difficulty in both the Marrow Plus anemia study and the Source Qi diarrhea study until we changed the studies to open-label studies; the herb studies then accrued individuals who were not previously interested. Open-label studies are more nebulous in some cases, so we as researchers need to creatively address the concerns of the researchers and persons with HIV/AIDS wanting definitive answers.

TCM Treatment Versus Control

We could also test a treatment that can be used by either a group being followed for natural history or a group receiving no treatment. David Baker's retrospective questionnaire study of Chinese herbs for symptoms and the Marrow Plus study for anemia are examples of this approach. If a group was being followed in a natural history study for recurrent herpes outbreaks, we could also test Chinese herbs against this group.

HOW DO WE CHOOSE WHICH TREATMENT TO STUDY?

Another question of concern for practitioners is: How do we choose a particular herb or herb formula, a set of acupuncture points, or moxibustion techniques for study?

The five ways we determine this are:
1. Based on clinical experience
2. Based on Western research
3. Based on Chinese or other reports
4. Based on classic use of points or herbs
5. Based on Chinese theoretical suppositions

All the above methods have advantages and disadvantages.

OTHER QUESTIONS

In conclusion, we address a few other issues that must be resolved as we conduct research. Other questions in understanding TCM research include those in Box 21-1.

BOX 21-1

Other Questions in Understanding Traditional Chinese Medicine Research

How Do We Determine the Target Population?
- Inclusion criteria
- Exclusion criteria

How Do We Determine Study Group Size?
- Need a biostatistician
- Need to estimate treatment effect
- Pilot study: Group size can be small or large—cannot necessarily determine trends; used to determine treatment effect for a larger study
- Treatment study: Group size must be large enough to determine treatment efficacy
- Be able to recruit study participants
- Be sure funding is available

Other Needs
- Find a source of funding
- Develop study questionnaire
  - Use previous study questionnaires
  - Use validated questionnaires
- Develop study protocol
- Advertise study and recruit participants
- Hire staff
- Implement study
- Complete study
- Evaluate data
- Publish results

SUMMARY

Let us come together—practitioners and researchers, East and West—for it will allow us to become more adept at answering the profound and difficult questions that we face in this devastating modern disease called AIDS.

References

1. Reference deleted in proofs.
2. Kaptchuk TJ: *The web that has no weaver,* New York, 1983, Congdon and Weed.
3. Cohen MR: *The Chinese way to healing: many paths to wholeness,* New York, 1996, Perigee Books.

4. Cohen MR: *The HIV wellness sourcebook: an East/West guide to living with HIV/AIDS and related conditions,* New York, 1998, Henry Holt.
5. Dicussion of *Warm epidemics* (Chinese medical text), 1642.
6. Macocia G: *The practice of Chinese medicine: the treatment of diseases with acupuncture and Chinese herbs,* New York, 1997, Churchill Livingstone.
7. Cohen MR: Review of tongue photos in HIV-positive persons participating in the Quan Yin Herbal Treatment Protocol for HIV-positive Persons, 1990 (unpublished).
8. Cohen MR: The spleen and stomach in HIV disease, *JNAAOM* 2(2):9-15, 1995.
9. Bei Hai W: Series of papers and lectures presented at The Immunity Symposium, Quan Yin Healing Arts Center, San Francisco, April 1989.
10. Feng ZH: Spleen and stomach in traditional Chinese medicine, *J Am Coll Trad Chin Med* 2:33, 1982 (translated by Cheung CS et al).
11. Reference deleted in proofs.
12. Cohen K: *The way of Qigong: the art of Chinese energy healing,* New York, 1999, Ballantine Books.
13. Chang RS, Yeung HW: Inhibition of growth of human immunodeficiency virus in vitro by crude extracts of Chinese medicinal herbs, *Antiviral Res* 9:163-176, 1988.
14. Burack J et al: Chinese herbal treatment for HIV-associated symptoms, *J Acquir Immune Defic Syndr Hum Retrovirol* 12(4):386-392, 1996.
15. Reference deleted in proofs.
16. Cohen MR, Mitchell TF, Bacchetti P, et al: Use of a Chinese herbal medicine for treatment of HIV-associated pathogen-negative diarrhea, *Integr Med* 21(2):79-84, 2000.
17. Weber R, Loy M, Christen L, et al: Randomized, placebo-controlled trial of Chinese herb therapy for HIV-1-infected individuals, *J Acquir Immune Defic Syndr* 22(1): 56-64, 1999.
18. Cohen MR, Wilson C, Surasky A: Acupuncture treatment in people with HCV and HIV coinfection and elevated transaminases, International AIDS Symposium, Geneva, 1998, abstract no. 60211.
19. Wang JL: Chinese herbs and acupuncture to treat ARC and AIDS, *J Acupunct Sci* Dec 12, 1989.
20. Cohen MR: Herbal therapies for HIV disease, International Symposium on Viral Hepatitis and AIDS, Beijing, April 15-18, 1991, (abstract).
21. Hawkins M, Hawkins T, Voorhees R, et al: The use of a Chinese herbal composition for the treatment of human immunodeficiency virus infection. In *HIV and Chinese medicine conference handout book,* San Francisco, 1993, ACMI.
22. Tosches WA, Cohen CJ, Day JM: A pilot study of acupuncture for the symptomatic treatment of HIV-associated peripheral neuropathy. In *HIV and Chinese medicine conference handout book,* San Francisco, 1993, ACMI.
23. Young MG: Chinese herbal therapies and HIV infection: a clinical report. In *HIV and Chinese medicine conference handout book,* San Francisco, 1993, ACMI.
24. Moffet H: Acupuncture and AIDS, *J Assoc Nurses AIDS Care* 7(3):54-56, 1996.
25. Reference deleted in proofs.
26. Wilson CJ: Chinese medicine in the treatment of peripheral neuropathy, International AIDS Symposium, Geneva, 1998 (abstract).
27. UCSF Community Consortium yearly trials search.
28. Sinclair T: Executive Director, Immune Enhancement Project (San Francisco), personal communication, January 1998.
29. Reference deleted in proofs.

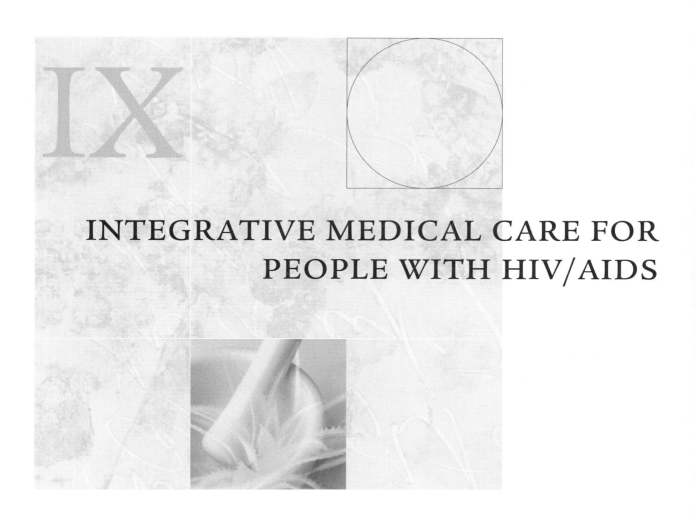

INTEGRATIVE MEDICAL CARE FOR PEOPLE WITH HIV/AIDS

22

Introduction to Integrative Approaches to the Treatment of HIV/AIDS

LEANNA J. STANDISH

The American medical movement to "integrate" CAM and conventional medicine is now in full swing. Many hospitals, clinicians, and medical schools are attempting to include CAM in their systems to provide integrated care. There seems to be a longing for truly integrated medical care in our communities. Although the integrative medicine movement continues, the recognition of definitional confusion is clear to nearly all persons involved. Does integrative medicine mean allowing patients access to multiple modalities? Or does it mean collaboration between both conventional and alternative health care providers, each respecting the other's specialty and the boundaries between them? Does it mean holistic, whole-person care in the con-

text of a strong patient-doctor therapeutic alliance? Does it mean the integration of philosophies and methods in the same physician's practice, or integration through teams of specialists?

The impetus for integrative medicine comes from health care consumers who pay health insurance premiums and health maintenance organization (HMO) fees. There is increasing national sentiment that many practices of alternative medicine are valuable and should be included in conventional health care settings and paid for by third-party payers. The impetus also comes from the growing alternative medical disciplines's demand for equity and full participation in the larger arena of the medical system in the United States. The CAM disciplines that seem to be making the greatest inroads toward the mainstream are (1) chiropractic, (2) acupuncture, (3) massage, (4) psychoneuroimmunology (PNI), (5) nutrition, and (6) naturopathic medicine.

It is not yet clear whether comprehensive, integrated care that combines both conventional medicine and alternative medicine improves what we care most about in medicine—longer and higher-quality lives. The answer to this question requires systematic research in the form of outcome studies and clinical trials. In the treatment of HIV/AIDS, we have learned over the past 15 years approximately how to measure and quantitate HIV/AIDS clinical progression in quality of life (QOL) instruments and laboratory and clinical endpoint measures of disease progression and survival. There is nearly global agreement on which treatment measures in HIV/AIDS seem to be best correlated with a longer and higher QOL. All AIDS clinicians and scientists can interpret studies performed in different countries because they have general agreement about the biological markers and categorization schemes for HIV disease. For example, most clinical studies of HIV treatments use CD4 as a measure of immune status, HIV RNA polymerase chain reaction (PCR) as a measure of virological activity, and body mass index (BMI) and progression rates using the American Centers for Disease Control (CDC) system as measures of clinical status.

Integration and evaluation must go together. We will always need to know which treatments help or do not help and which combinations of therapies seem to help the most. Integrative AIDS care is a useful model in which to study the impact of integration of CAM therapies with conventional care on morbidity, mortality, and QOL.

Chapters 23 and 24 are both excellent examples of the efforts that both small groups and individual practitioners have made toward providing integrated care to the HIV/AIDS community. The pioneering efforts by CAM providers and their patients in the HIV community to offer low-cost (often free) acupuncture therapy set the stage for the wider movement to integrate alternative medicine into major hospitals, HMOs, and medical insurance plans. Arthur Shattuck, LAc and Ryan Less are leaders in the development of free AIDS Chinese medicine clinics. For years they have been working to integrate acupuncture and other aspects of Chinese medicine into the community care system for people living with HIV. They feel confident that, although Chinese medicine may not be able to cure AIDS, it can help alleviate symptoms that are inadequately dealt with by conventional medicine (e.g., fatigue, nausea, neuropathy, depression, diarrhea, insomnia, night sweats) and mitigate side effects of conventional therapy.

In Chapter 23, Shattuck and Less discuss the problems that have confronted the integration of Chinese medicine into the mainstream system of care for HIV-positive people. The larger biomedical community is slowly beginning to accept the reality and efficacy of Chinese medicine in certain conditions, most notably in pain management. Although the process of bringing acupuncture and Chinese medicine care to the HIV community has been slow and often painful, many American acupuncturists have undergone substantial parts of their clinical training in AIDS clinics that specialize in Chinese medicine. These clinics are now more common in conventional AIDS clinics as well, and we are learning how to integrate care so that the benefits of both forms of medicine are enhanced and synergy occurs. Shattuck and Less give a historical account of the struggles to provide acupuncture and Chinese herbs for HIV-positive persons from the perspective of participant observers.

The 1997 National Institutes of Health (NIH) Consensus Report on Acupuncture concludes that sufficient evidence exists to suggest that acupuncture is both effective and less associated with adverse reactions than many accepted medical procedures. A review of the literature for the efficacy in specific HIV-related conditions suggests that sufficient preliminary evidence exists to justify the inclusion of acupuncture and Chinese herbs in the overall management of all symptomatic (and asymptomatic) HIV-positive patients. This review is presented in Chapter 21. Preliminary evidence from scientific studies argues for benefit in the treatment of certain HIV-related conditions, such as altered liver function, neuropathy, and cryptosporidial diarrhea. Nevertheless, acupuncture treatment for HIV/AIDS is still considered alternative by many groups of clinicians and patients. It is unavailable to many HIV-positive people living in some rural areas, and only a few insurance carriers provide coverage. However, as Chinese medicine continues to be used and practitioners of acupuncture and Oriental medicine continue to provide care, this system of medicine will be integrated more and more fully into the Western medical system.

Jon Kaiser's work is an excellent example of the integration of state-of-the-technology conventional medicine with nutritional and Chinese medicine. As

Dr. Kaiser describes in Chapter 24 on integrated HIV/AIDS care, it has been possible to combine aspects of both antiretroviral and antibiotic treatment and prophylaxis and CAM with HIV-positive patients. Not only is it possible, he argues, but the clinical results are superior to conventional care. Dr. Kaiser has conducted both a retrospective outcomes study and his own program of care with his HIV-positive patients, which combines antiretroviral therapy (ART) when appropriate and a natural therapy program consisting of nutrition, nutrient supplementation, acupuncture and herbs, exercise, hormone therapy, and stress reduction. His clinical outcomes in a sample of 74 patients treated and observed over a 2-year period are remarkably good and are superior to a case control group of matched HIV-positive patients receiving treatment in a clinic that specializes in conventional HIV care. Although these data may be viewed as preliminary, they are sufficiently intriguing to warrant further investigation through a controlled, prospective clinical trial.

Such a trial requires in vitro standardization of all herbs and nutrients, and establishing an adequate control will be difficult. The successful execution of a clinical trial of any integrated combination therapy for HIV requires combined research-design expertise of many collaborators. It requires in vitro testing, pharmacokinetic studies, safety, tolerability and adverse reaction evaluations, and a controlled clinical trial. This trial will be expensive, logistically complex, and ethically challenging if it involves placebo or withholding treatment from a control group of patients. There are virtually no financial incentives for the pharmaceutical industry to develop a program of research to evaluate Kaiser's treatment program. It is the kind of research that can only be done by the government.

Integration nearly always seems like a good idea because of the new synthesis that may emerge from the integration of Western and Eastern thought regarding the etiology, diagnosis, and treatment of human disease. As the philosopher Hegel promised us, out of the dialectic between seeming opposites (thesis and antithesis) comes a new and enlightening synthesis. It has been fascinating to watch medical students at Bastyr University who are being simultaneously trained in both naturopathic medicine and traditional Chinese medicine (TCM). For the first time in the United States, a new breed of physicians will be using both Eastern and Western medicine. Many of these students have received their most important clinical training in the HIV/AIDS integrated care clinics that have sprung up in major cities of the United States. We must continue to integrate the best parts of alternative medicine with the best parts of conventional molecular medicine. Out of it surely will come the best treatment for our patients and possibly greater understanding and therefore more humane and effective treatment for HIV/AIDS.

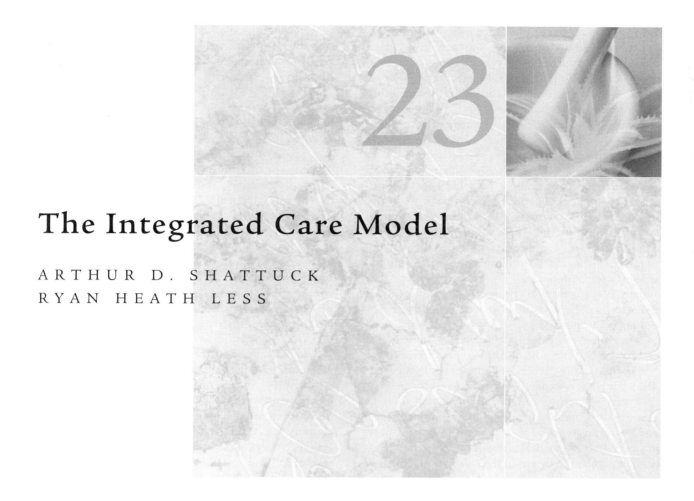

The Integrated Care Model

ARTHUR D. SHATTUCK
RYAN HEATH LESS

The integration of alternative and conventional medicine raises a number of complex and important issues. Although the overall climate has become increasingly favorable for integration, these issues remain a stumbling block. Integration has occurred, but progress still needs to be made. This chapter discusses the successes, failures, and obstacles involved in the integration of alternative and conventional medicine, specifically as they relate to the use of traditional Chinese medicine (TCM), the AIDS population, and method of delivery. The method of health care delivery can have a significant influence on promoting integration and improving the quality of life (QOL) of individuals with AIDS.

A BRIEF HISTORY

Unity between conventional and alternative health care practitioners was the exception rather than the rule during the early years of the AIDS epidemic. Although a number of clinics offering alternative treatments to AIDS patients requested the services of physicians and other conventional medical personnel, they invariably received negative answers. It is difficult to know exactly why this happened, but we can make some educated guesses.

A simple lack of communication could have been one factor. At a meeting of health care workers, a prominent physician, Renslow Shear, asked practitioners of alternative medicine what exactly they were doing for AIDS patients. They replied that the patients received acupuncture, massage, and herbal therapy at a number of alternative clinics and reported each week that they felt better. Dr. Shear responded by saying that such anecdotal information "did not count," which showed that conventional medical professionals were still waiting for scientific proof of the efficacy of alternative modalities. During the same meeting, the medical establishment, or at least some of its members, had the mistaken notion that practitioners of holistic medicine were attempting to cure AIDS. The holistic community clearly stated that this was not the case; they were trying to manage symptoms and provide relief. In short, the attitudes and inaccurate assumptions of the conventional medical establishment reflected the general lack of information about alternative medicine that existed a decade ago. Of course, this lack of information extended beyond medical personnel to the general population.

Over time, the gap between alternative medicine and conventional medicine has narrowed. There were two contributing factors. The first factor was that AIDS patients told their physicians about the benefits they received from holistic treatments, such as acupuncture, herbal therapy, and bodywork. The second factor was the referral of patients by holistic practitioners. Patients at alternative clinics told their practitioners which physicians in the conventional medical community seemed to work best with the AIDS population. The practitioners would then make repeated referrals to these physicians for health problems not amenable to alternative modalities, which created a connection between the two medical communities. Physicians became familiar with practitioners in the field of holistic therapy and vice versa. In fact, one physician, David Moore, actually began to visit the AIDS Alternative Health Care Project, which was located in Chicago. Looking back, this situation played a significant role in the promotion of alternative medicine in the United States. If the AIDS epidemic had never occurred, it is possible that the conventional medical establishment would have continued to ignore holistic medicine.

At any rate, an integrated health care model had not yet emerged. The clinic Dr. Moore visited regularly was a felonious institution because at the time, acupuncture, which was frequently used there, was illegal. Today, much has changed. Alternative medicine is widely used in a number of countries, and it has re-

ceived a slight nod of approval from various international and governmental institutions. Integration seems to be close; however, obstacles to true integration still remain.

THE CURRENT SITUATION: OBSTACLES AND PROMISE

The current situation here in the United States is the most auspicious yet. The National Institutes of Health (NIH), a branch of the United States Department of Health and Human Services, recently issued a consensus statement that favors the practice of acupuncture. It directly states, "The data in support of acupuncture are as strong as those for many accepted Western medical therapies" and that "incidence of adverse reactions is substantially lower than that of many drugs or other accepted medical procedures used for the same conditions" as acupuncture.[1] Furthermore, the World Health Organization (WHO) has long recognized the efficacy of acupuncture in treating a number of specific health conditions.

To some extent, integration has begun already. In California, the Daniel Freeman Marina Hospital has become the first hospital in the United States to offer acupuncture. California also makes acupuncturists eligible to work with individuals who are receiving worker's compensation benefits. However, the integration of alternative medicine into the health care system is spotty at best, with California being more the exception than the rule. The United States legislation generally does not favor practitioners of Chinese medicine.

Even in US states that favor acupuncture, attitudes of disrespect are hinted at within the legislation. California, which is perhaps the most acupuncture-friendly state in the country, not only allows board-certified acupuncturists to practice acupuncture, but it also allows physicians who have no acupuncture training to practice acupuncture. With a bit of extrapolation, one might come to the conclusion that the state legislature of California believes that physicians without any training in acupuncture possess the same skills as acupuncturists who have gone through 3 academic years of schooling and roughly 800 hours of clinical internship. This idea is almost as absurd as thinking that an acupuncturist could practice Western medicine without attending medical school. Either the legislators have little respect for the education provided by acupuncture schools, or they are unaware of the statement that such legislation makes, or the decision to create this legislation is based on less-than-desirable motives. This last topic is discussed later in the chapter.

In the state of Illinois, acupuncture has recently become legal, which is a definite step toward integration. Once again, however, legislation fails to fully respect the education necessary to properly and effectively practice acupuncture. Not only are physicians able to legally practice acupuncture without any training, but dentists are allowed to practice acupuncture as well. It would be difficult for most trained acupuncturists to accept such legislation as knowledgeable, safe for the public, or truly respectful of acupuncture.

Perhaps the reason for this legislation can be gleaned from the laws of the state of Alabama, where it is legal for physicians, osteopaths (DOs), and chiropractors to engage in the practice of acupuncture. Of these three, only chiropractors are required to receive any training (100 hours). This law tells us little except that Alabama recognizes only the conventional medical establishment as having the ability to administer health care. However, if other factual information is added, much can be surmised.

As recently as 1983, the American Medical Association (AMA) was found guilty of illegally boycotting the chiropractic profession. The court ordered the AMA to be prohibited from "restricting, regulating, or impeding . . . the freedom of any AMA member or any hospital or institution to make an individual decision as to whether or not that member, institution or hospital shall professionally associate with chiropractors, chiropractic students, or chiropractic institutions."[2] The AMA was also required to publish the court order in their medical journal. Other defendants, the American College of Surgeons and the American College of Radiology, settled with the chiropractic profession before the court issued its decision.

Unfortunately, this court order can only do so much. The laws of Alabama almost give one the impression that the conventional medical establishment is still on unfriendly terms with the chiropractic profession and the field of alternative medicine. After all, physicians and DOs may practice acupuncture without training, whereas chiropractors are required to receive 100 hours of training, and board-certified, trained acupuncturists may not even practice acupuncture. The question that arises is: How can one say that the AMA (which is, in our opinion, equivalent

to the conventional medical establishment) is implicated in the creation of such laws?

It would be nearly impossible to directly implicate the conventional medical establishment. Statistics, however, point out that legislation does not always have pure and clear motives. Consider that the AMA contributed $772,042 to political action committees (PACs) between 1993 and 1994.[3] It is difficult to believe that any organization contributing such a hefty financial sum to the political machinery of the United States does not exert a great amount of influence on which laws will be created.

The power of lobbying often interferes with the ability and desire of politicians to create laws that reflect the attitudes of their constituents and are based on the welfare of the public. Moreover, the equality of each individual's voice in the creation of legislation is something of a historical truth, which exists no longer. How many organizations have the financial ability to expend the $750,000 spent by the AMA? The pharmaceutical industry also made over $4 million in contributions to PACs since 1991. A significant number of members of Congress (or their immediate family members) held assets in the pharmaceutical industry during 1993.[3] The list of statistics on health care issues is long, but even these few examples paint a somewhat questionable picture about who decides how laws on alternative medicine will be written.

Under the present legislation, a true integration of alternative and conventional medicine cannot take place for obvious reasons. First, it is difficult to integrate the two medical systems when one is illegal in many states or when the laws reflect a much less-than-desirable attitude on the part of the conventional medical establishment. Second, the issue of health insurance coverage must be addressed. The integration of acupuncture and other holistic therapies necessitates coverage by health insurance companies. One cannot say that true integration has taken place or posit that it will if alternative medicine is not readily available to the public. Also, a large segment of the population cannot afford acupuncture, let alone conventional treatment, without health insurance. To some extent, positive legislation on alternative medicine will spur the health insurance industry to increase coverage, and on some level, health insurance and legislation are tied together.

The present policy of health insurance organizations, which we have just briefly discussed, is a stumbling block on the path leading to an integrated care model. Although health insurance occasionally covers acupuncture, many other modalities are not covered at all or are covered to an insignificant degree. Nutritional supplements, herbal therapy, and many types of bodywork are generally not covered by health insurance. In Chinese medicine, herbal therapy is often an integral part of treatment, and failure to cover its costs (which are usually quite low) limits the practitioner's effectiveness. Although $21 for a bottle of herbs is relatively inexpensive, particularly if it benefits the patient, it adds up over time. In a study at the Wisconsin Institute of Chinese Herbology, certain Chinese herbal formulas appeared to greatly benefit children with attention deficit disorder (ADD). Unfortunately, many of the parents who wished to continue treatment for their children after the study ended found it financially difficult. The group hit hardest was single mothers and low-income individuals.

Paradigms and Jargon

The second obstacle to an integrated care model arises as a direct result of converging paradigms. Imagine that a female patient walks into her physician's office and states, "My acupuncturist says that he can help my menstrual pain. He is giving me an herb formula called *Xue Fu Zhu Yu Tang (Drive Out Stasis in the Mansion of Blood Decoction),* because he says I have blood stasis." The physician's first response may be one of outright bewilderment, mixed perhaps with suspicion, since the physician knows of no static blood in this woman's arteries. Blood is defined quite differently in Chinese medicine than it is in allopathic medicine. In fact, the terminologies of TCM and Western medicine are in no way compatible; they vary greatly in every way.

If conventional physicians and practitioners of Chinese medicine each are ignorant of what the other does and their terminology is different, they cannot refer patients to each other, which precludes any integration. For example, AIDS patients often suffer from severe night sweats, but their physicians may not be able to alleviate this problem. If the physicians know something about Chinese medicine, they may feel comfortable referring their patients to alternative medical providers. However, if physicians do not know anything about Chinese medicine, their patients may never seek a practitioner of Chinese medicine, which is unfortunate, since TCM is often able to reduce the frequency and severity of night sweats.

This problem does not occur within a given system of medicine but only when integrating systems are founded on different premises. General practitioners of Western medicine gladly refer patients with recurring chest pains to a cardiologist because they know what a cardiologist does. They both work from a similar base of knowledge, and they understand the language that the other physician speaks.

Presently schools of Oriental medicine in the United States have already begun to include courses in Western sciences. These often include Western pathology courses, physical examinations (i.e., how to take blood pressure, simple methods of neurological testing, and so forth), survey of pharmacology, and invariably anatomy and physiology. This inclusion of Western medicine has closed the gap. The practitioner of Chinese medicine has at least a basic understanding of the human body from a Western medical framework and has some knowledge of the patient's medications and side effects and knowledge about the conditions for which they are prescribed. To expect Western-style physicians to take courses in TCM theory and pathology would not be reasonable. However, some education is necessary.

This obstacle may seem minor, but it is one that will probably not be resolved within 10 years. The attitudes of conventional health care providers vary greatly. Some will gladly educate themselves about alternative medicine, whereas others will fight against it. If we consider the judicial decision regarding the AMA and the chiropractic profession, we can surmise that this conclusion is probably not inaccurate.

However, the speediness with which this obstacle is resolved may increase in proportion to the proliferation of scientific studies on acupuncture and perhaps wind down even sooner than the 10 years we have estimated. If the NIH continues to fund studies, and the findings are positive, this is a possibility. However, herbal therapy studies will take longer to resolve.

Unlike Western medicines, which generally consist of a single chemical constituent with a specific biochemical action, herbs contain many chemical constituents, which may have a number of actions in the human body. In addition, single herbs are rarely used in Chinese medicine but are combined into herbal formulas, which may contain anywhere from 2 to over 15 herbs. Furthermore, over 400 herbs are commonly used in Chinese herbal therapy. It would be impossible to thoroughly study the effects of each chemical constituent in the Chinese pharmacopeia, let alone the effects of all the common combinations, within the next 100 years, even if that amount of time is sufficient.

This difficulty of scientific study of Chinese medicine is the final major foreseeable obstacle to integration. As mentioned, Chinese herbal therapy does not readily lend itself to such testing. Acupuncture, which may be more amenable, has its own brand of difficulty. For example, groups of fake points, known as *sham points,* are often used in control groups when studying the efficacy of acupuncture. However, these sham points create a physiological reaction in the subject similar to that produced by real acupuncture points. Furthermore, subjects often feel much greater pain with the insertion of a needle into a sham point, whereas proper acupuncture point location usually allows for insertion with minimal pain. It would be reasonable to assume that this pain has a negative effect on the subject over time and might create a poor response to treatment (i.e., a negative reinforcement is created).

A Difference of Attitudes

Although we may not consider it to be exactly an obstacle, it is important to note the different attitudes of the conventional medical establishment and holistic medicine. Before contrasting the two, we would like to qualify our following statements by stating that individuals within either camp vary greatly in their attitudes and behavior. We cannot make a blanket statement regarding allopathic physicians or holistic practitioners. However, there does seem to be an overall difference between the two, which has been noticed by lay persons and medical professionals alike.

This difference in attitude was blatantly obvious during the early years of the AIDS epidemic. "Hospitals and Western medical personnel were still very frightened by AIDS, and the patients felt the results of that fear,"[4] often being treated more as personified diseases than as human beings. The hospital wards where AIDS patients stayed were often cold, uncaring places. Activists attempted to rectify this situation by providing items such as afghans, hoping to make the wards more cheerful and comfortable, as did the holistic community. Bob King, the owner of a massage school, brought in massage therapists to work with AIDS patients. On one occasion, a nurse spotted King and his group. She informed them that, "we don't touch the patients." Mr. King replied, "Yes, I know. That is why we have come."

Perhaps holistic practitioners can spend more time directly relating to their patients because they are not burdened by the routine of conventional medical personnel. Holistic practitioners do not make rounds in hospitals nor do they spend their time running laboratory tests or worrying about following the status quo. (Many practitioners of holistic medicine do read laboratory tests, but this usually does not take most of their time. Furthermore, holistic practitioners should not be seen as a group unconcerned with the scientific side of health. However, they work in paradigms that take other aspects of health into account). Instead, they can be more creative in their approach to working with patients. They generally do not work in hospitals, and they use procedures and techniques that are noninvasive and have a low potential for side effects. These paradigms allow holistic practitioners more time to look at the big picture. This is a luxury not easily afforded by allopathic physicians, who must keep a close eye on the adverse reactions of medications and the newest lab test results and who have the prolongation of life as their primary goal.

Even if practitioners of alternative medicine worked in conventional settings such as hospitals, the situation they face is different, which relates to the basic views and philosophies that exist at the core of their medical model. To truly understand the difference in attitudes between alternative and conventional medicine, we must further explore these philosophies.

Consider that terminally ill patients are legally barred from suicide, even if that life is nothing more than intense and excruciating pain. Society, through the legal system, has stated what is acceptable behavior and what is not. Why have we done this? Two possible reasons seem very plausible. First, Western culture with its technology and scientific prowess has lost touch with the natural order of life. No matter who we are, we are born, we will at some point become ill, and eventually we will die. However, we fear death and reject it. We seek above all else to prolong life and to defy Mother Nature, which is an absolutely dysfunctional attitude. We prefer to ignore our own mortality, and by doing this we become far removed from the process of life.

This attitude leaves us in a bind. The average person knows little about what to say to dying persons or how to behave around them. Furthermore, when it is time for an individual to face his or her own mortality, he or she is often lost and bewildered. This is not the case in other parts of the world. In Tibet, death is viewed from a quite different perspective. It is accepted wholly as a natural part of life, rather than being separate from life. The Tibetan culture has crafted rituals to be carried out at the end of an individual's life. Family and friends gather around the dying person, connecting that individual with all aspects of his or her life.

The second reason why suicide is legally forbidden is that our view of human life, or life in general, is quite narrow, defined mostly in terms of biochemical reactions. We become sick because of a failure in the body to continually run these reactions properly. In essence, we have reduced life to a chemical equation. Viewing life and illness from this perspective, we attempt to find therapies based on the same perspective, which that we test and improve with mathematical precision. Again, the underlying drive for such activity is our fear, and thereby our desire, to control outcomes. There is certainly something noble about working to save lives, but the situation is a bit too heroic. Medical professionals have come to be viewed as superheroes in laboratory coats. Just as people often use religion as a crutch, seeing God as a gigantic babysitter who protects us, we have deified physicians and health professionals, hoping that they can stop the procession of life that inevitably leads to illness and death. In fact, the conventional medical establishment has accepted the public's high opinion of them. As one gentleman wrote, "Orthodox medicine means to give people the illusion it is handling everything."[5]

Thus the medical profession is limited to dealing with patients as walking bags of chemicals, with no recourse for addressing the mental and spiritual crises that occur during illness. (Even psychiatrists, who deal with the mind, have accepted a biomedical model and commonly administer drugs as the primary method of treatment). Physicians can help patients with *Pneumocystis carinii* pneumonia, but they cannot reconcile patients with their approaching death, or the anger they might experience about having AIDS.

Holistic medicine works from a different group of assumptions. For example, in Chinese medicine, a person is viewed as a complex flow of Qi (vital energy) which, when balanced, allows one to remain healthy and contented. Illness is the expression of the loss of harmony and balance. Therefore the physician should seek to understand the patient's disharmony and at-

tempt to promote the return of harmony. Two things can be extrapolated from this concept. First, illness is viewed as a reminder that the patient is not taking proper care of his or her life (or that something in the environment is amiss, such as being in an abusive relationship or living in a toxic location). This idea is radically different from the notion that illness is a bad thing, which is already an advantage. How we view illness in ourselves or others will shape our attitude when dealing with that illness. We could view it as an opportunity to heal some unattended aspect of ourselves, or we could view it as a harbinger of ill fortune. The choice is ultimately ours. Second, the physician points out the nature of the imbalance to the patient and offers ways to address it. The patient must play an active role in restoring harmony and must not rely solely on the physician's skill. (The degree of AIDS patients' proactivity is an important indicator of how they will fare and therefore should be fostered during treatment).

Chinese medicine also differs from conventional medicine in that it considers mental and physical health to be directly related. According to TCM, a patient with chronic menstrual pain who is depressed may suffer from Qi stagnation. In this paradigm, Qi stagnation is a pattern of disharmony that is at the root of both the physical and mental complaints. From another angle, we can say that in Chinese medicine there is no mind-body connection, because the two were never separated in the first place. This idea allows practitioners of this healing system to address both the physical symptoms of AIDS and emotional issues simultaneously. Another example is the AIDS patient who suffers from night sweats, weight loss, and severe anxiety. Chinese medicine describes all these symptoms as deficient Yin. Therapy that addresses this particular imbalance will (if the system works) improve all the symptoms, since they are related. In our experience, Chinese herbal therapy is effective for this symptom picture.

Therefore each medical system is limited by its own assumptions about reality. Because alternative medicine does not deal only with cells and chemical reactions, it is not limited to working solely on this level. It may also attempt to treat mental and spiritual aspects of illness, which is what makes it a *holistic* medicine. Thus the practitioner is often more observant of such phenomena and is in a better position to address such concerns. In addition, the attitudes of practitioners of various alternative medical systems differ. (We will revisit this concept in relation to methods of health care delivery.) Conversely, physicians are in a much better position to quickly check an opportunistic infection (OI), and they can monitor biological functions that cannot be measured by the diagnostic processes of acupuncturists.

In summary, alternative medicine has the potential to create humane practitioners who can affect many areas of a patient's life that may not be addressed by conventional physicians. Alternative medicine places a greater emphasis on the person as a whole. Physicians must, by the very nature of the establishment in which they work (and according to society's expectations), limit themselves to amelioration of symptoms and prolongation of life. Because of the difference in their predicaments, squabbles may arise. One practitioner may feel that what the other does is lacking and thus feel falsely superior. If the two medical systems can be integrated, each can use its strength while its weaknesses are offset by the presence of the other.

Why Should We Integrate?

One may wonder whether attempting to overcome these significant obstacles to an integrated care model is a worthwhile venture. The answer is an unquestionable yes; integrated care can derive a great deal of benefit.

AIDS brings with it a plethora of difficult issues, not the least of which are emotional hardship and turmoil. This is one area in which alternative medicine can be quite helpful. Chinese medicine is well equipped to deal with the mental health of AIDS patients. At its core, it is a paradigm that considers the effects of emotions on health and vice versa. Early in their academic careers, students of Oriental medicine are taught that one of the causes of disease is an excess of emotions. TCM theory even posits specific ways in which emotion can affect a patient's Qi. Scientific evidence supports the idea that the tools of Oriental medicine are efficacious for treating problems of the psyche.

Various studies show that acupuncture can improve a person's sense of well-being. In fact, some studies have shown that it directly affects levels of neurotransmitters in a positive manner. Although this effect is widely touted for its usefulness in drug rehabilitation, it appears to have a positive impact on mood

disorders as well,[6] which NIH studies seem to confirm. Perhaps the weightiest testimony on the subject, however, is from Dr. Leon Hammer, who is both a psychiatrist and acupuncturist. He states:

> When practiced at its best, acupuncture promotes and enhances awareness. The growing awareness is often painful as well as gratifying, since awareness is the antithesis of denial, as well as a detoxifier of all that deadens the feelings and senses. From the first encounter with needles, that side of a person that wants most to feel fully alive is engaged in unraveling the enigma of an avoidance of one's own life.[6]

Acupuncture is not the only alternative therapy that can help AIDS patients grappling with psychological issues; herbal therapy is equally helpful. Although some of the herbs in the Chinese pharmacopeia, such as Suan Zao Ren (Semen Zizyphi Spinosae), have been shown to exert a particular influence on neurochemistry, knowledge is limited. According to one authority on the subject:

> Biochemical action of herbs on the nervous system is extraordinarily complex. It is not even good enough to identify a neurologically active constituent in an herb. The responses are dose-dependent, and the herb in question might not offer enough of the constituent to produce the effect. When herbs are provided in complex formulas, the question of active ingredients and their effects becomes fuzzy at best.[7]

Nonetheless, we have seen a number of patients who, with the help of herbal therapy, have overcome feelings of despair and anger. Herbal therapy often greatly affects sleep cycles as well. If we consider that Chinese herbs are generally quite safe when used by a qualified practitioner, then their use in treating emotional difficulties seems to be a wise choice.

Even with such success, we fully recognize that any system of medicine has its limits. Therefore we suggest that AIDS patients seek the help of a psychotherapist or an appropriate mental health professional. From our experience, TCM practitioners working with mental health professionals can do a great deal to improve the QOL of AIDS patients, which is undoubtedly a reason for the integration of alternative practitioners into the health care model that seeks to treat the AIDS population. If a working rapport between the psychiatric community and the alternative medical community can be created, AIDS patients will benefit immensely.

A second principal reason for integrating holistic therapy into the conventional health care model is symptom management. Western medicine often offers little in the way of symptom management treatment. For example, night sweats, fatigue, aching muscles, and various other symptoms can often be abated through holistic therapy, with little-to-no incidence of side effects, whereas physicians may have virtually nothing that can alleviate these uncomfortable circumstances (and those methods that are employed generally have a much higher occurrence of adverse reactions). This problem is particularly true if the symptoms do not have an easily identifiable disease pattern.

Western medicine has greatly improved its management of OIs. *P. carinii* pneumonia, for example, is now treatable and is even preventable. With the advent of protease cocktails, a number of AIDS symptoms have been reduced, and the death toll has dropped significantly. However, many individuals do not have either insurance or the financial means to receive a regimen of the new drugs. Of those who can afford them, some do not respond well to the treatment. Some studies show an increase in viral loads despite administration of protease inhibitors (PIs). This situation further emphasizes the need for medicinal substances, herbal or otherwise, to improve the plight of AIDS patients.

Substances found in Chinese herbs (such as Baicalin, which occurs in *Scutelaria*) have inhibitory actions on HIV. Common sense indicates that these remedies would be a welcome addition in the fight against AIDS. Formulas made up of anti-HIV herbs have been created by various herb companies and organizations. The Institute of Traditional Medicine produces a formula, Composition-A, which includes a number of herbs.

Chinese medicine can also be a boon to an AIDS patient's immune system. Enhancement of immune functioning has been shown to result from the administration of a number of herbs. *Atractylodes macrocephala,* a common Chinese herb, has been shown to enhance cellular immunity, raise the white blood cell (WBC) count, and promote phagocytosis. *Isatis,* another widely used Chinese herb, is known to have marked antimicrobial effects, as does *Andrographitis paniculata*. The benefit of using these herbs is obvious. It is worth noting that 50% of the prescription medications used in the United States have their chemical basis in a natural substance.[8] The idea of using herbs for AIDS is not foreign to the pharmaceutical industry.

Another strength of Chinese medicine is its ability to ameliorate the side effects produced by Western medications. In the early years of the AIDS epidemic, when zidovudine (AZT) was the only choice, herbs were used to treat the bone marrow suppression that resulted from its use. Although new medications are now in use, their side effects can also be ameliorated; thus drugs can often be used in larger doses or for a longer period of time. A marriage of the two medical systems would greatly benefit AIDS patients.

Aside from the efficacy of alternative medicine, another reason for an integrated health care model is safety. Although holistic therapies are safe, the practitioners of these therapies lack the knowledge of a physician with respect to diagnosis. For instance, an acupuncturist is in no position to detect a carcinoma buried deep within a patient's body. Thus alternative medicine has definite limitations, which would be much less of a problem if integration occurred. A clinic offering both allopathy and Chinese medicine would be less likely to miss a diagnosis of severe dysfunction than a clinic offering only alternative treatment. Furthermore, since the condition of a weakened AIDS patient can change quickly, it would be logical to have conventional physicians on staff who can deal with emergency situations (e.g., the onset of meningitis).

Method of Delivery

We have already mentioned the difference in attitudes and situations of conventional and alternative medicine. However, the methods for delivery of health care have not yet been discussed, although they are, to some extent, an outgrowth of the very different ways in which these two systems operate. We have reserved this discussion until now, since it has implications related to not only attitudinal differences but also to the promotion of an integrated care model and improvement in the QOL of AIDS patients.

First, let us look at some of the nuances of the conventional method of health care delivery. In a physician's office (or hospital), the patient is separated from the receptionist, often by a wall with a window. The patient is then led into a room where he or she waits for an indefinite period of time. This separation and waiting can easily lead to feelings of anxiety, sending a hidden message that the patient is only one of the physician's many wards and can hope to receive only a bit of the physician's time. Of course, the office visit is usually short, since the office is filled with other patients, and things must run on schedule. Finally, the patient goes home, takes his or her medication, and receives little to no support from the medical field. Anyone who has ever gone to a hospital for tests, facing the unknown, knows that the situation is anxiety-provoking and lonely. The following specific example illustrates what we are describing.

A young lady we know recently suffered from a kidney infection. She was given Bactrim, which caused an allergic reaction, and ended up in the hospital. Throughout her stay, nurses would periodically come in and take blood samples. This was done in a very impersonal manner, with the young lady often being rudely roused from sleep so the blood could be drawn. She was never told either the purpose of the blood tests or their result. She stayed in the hospital for 4 days. She received intravenous (IV) drips, which contained a substance unknown to her and was never fully explained. Furthermore, the placement of the IV needle was painful, but the nursing staff refused to attempt to adjust it. When she was asked what her impressions of this experience were, she stated, "The whole thing was so impersonal. Everyone was rude except for the nurse's aides. It was that experience in the hospital which drove me to alternative medicine." Imagine how much worse it must be for a patient with a terminal illness, such as an AIDS patient who is in and out of hospitals frequently.

When establishing the Northside HIV clinic in Chicago, one of our primary goals was to avoid such a negative method of health care delivery. AIDS was scary enough, and patients did not need to be in any situation that increased anxiety or isolation. To create a better system, we looked at the medical system used in China. Patients there are often treated together in one big room, which had many advantages. Since the population of patients we treated were all gay males suffering from AIDS, treatment in a large room allowed an instant support group to evolve. Each week when the patients came, they received not only holistic treatment but support, friendship, and good conversation. It was a great stress reliever for patients to be in the company of others who shared so much in common; they could share stories and jokes that might not be understood by someone who was not part of the gay community.

Patients also shared information on conventional medical treatments that they were receiving. This flow of information helped gay men with AIDS become an extremely knowledgeable patient population, and it put them in a position to know which treatments they preferred, based on success and adverse reactions.

This method of delivery also greatly affected the alternative medical profession. Practitioners were able to educate themselves about which treatments were used in other forms of alternative medicine and their effect on AIDS patients. The naturopath could better understand the acupuncturist, and the Western herbalist could learn about Chinese herbs. Everyone gained knowledge, and treatment selection for AIDS improved. Practitioners realized the limits of their chosen modality and learned when to send a patient to a different practitioner for treatment.

The situation also created an atmosphere that was almost indescribable. Patients might come to the clinic not because it was their day for treatment but just to "hang out." It was a place where gay male AIDS patients felt they belonged. Interestingly, each patient used a pseudonym, since persons with AIDS often lost their jobs and homes. Thus practitioners did not treat "John Smith," they treated "Diana Ross" and "Liberace." The patients transformed a miserable situation into something more fun and enjoyable. People were not dying of AIDS; they were living with AIDS.

One of the most important aspects of our method of delivery was that the clinic was free. Because revenue was not generated by treatment, other sources had to be found. Patients donated time, money, and office supplies, and they were invested in seeing the clinic work. Instead of playing a passive role in their own health care, they became proactive. We feel that proactivity was crucial because it stopped the patients from ruminating about their situation and feeling sorry for themselves and empowered them instead. They no longer were concerned with only their plight but with that of their peers as well. Being proactive had definite positive therapeutic value. When we compared statistics from Northside with those from a hospital in San Francisco, we found that patients at the alternative clinic had fewer hospital stays, their recovery time was shorter, and their life expectancy was longer. It makes sense that patients will live longer and recover more quickly when they have friends and a community to visit (which Northside at least partially provided).

The question that arose was whether this type of delivery system would work for other populations. Later, when it was tried with elderly persons, women with endometriosis, and others, it worked equally well.

Homogeneity of patient population was the main factor of the delivery system's success. The AIDS population does not consist of only gay males; it consists of heterosexuals, sex workers, IV drug users—practically everyone. If we put gay males and female sex workers in the same room, the commonality among them would be almost nonexistent. Thus an alternative clinic set up in this fashion would need to have a day for gay males, a day for sex workers, and so on. In this way, patients with similar backgrounds have the opportunity to develop the instant support group mentioned earlier.

This method of health care delivery can also help promote the integration of alternative and conventional medicine. If we place practitioners from both systems in a similar model, allopaths would be exposed to holistic therapy firsthand. Physicians would see what acupuncturists do for their patients and that their treatment worked. They might even go under the needle themselves and find it relaxing. Just working side by side would lead to a rapport. Whether such a situation will ever arise is difficult to say, but it does happen occasionally. The Immune Enhancement Project in Portland, Oregon has both alternative and conventional practitioners on staff, as does the Quan Yin Healing Arts Center in San Francisco. Still, these places are the exception rather than the rule. Because the recent NIH consensus statement on acupuncture was so positive and more funds were designated for its study, perhaps things will change.

AN EYE TOWARD THE FUTURE

We have discussed the obstacles to an integrated care model, reasons for promoting such a model, and how method of delivery plays a role. But is integration really possible? Integrated care models already exist in other parts of the world. China uses Western medicine, Chinese medicine, and a number of other traditional healing systems (although the latter are not often discussed). Patients may receive whatever form of treatment they wish and often choose both.

Surprising as it may be, Chinese medicine is used for quite severe situations. For instance, the herb ginseng is administered in cases of shock resulting from hemorrhage. Herbal therapy is also used in cases of hepatitis, stroke, and various other medical conditions. The Chinese are an eminently practical people. With well over a billion people to treat, they use whatever resources they have. The bottom line is if something works, use it. Thus they have no qualms about using TCM with antibiotics, surgery, and x-rays.

China is not the only place where integration has occurred. Other countries, which lack financial resources to buy Western drugs and hospital equipment, have turned to traditional systems of medicine. Thailand, which has over 800,000 HIV-positive citizens, cannot afford Western treatment for everyone. Therefore they have made do with what they have, which is a form of alternative medicine known as traditional Thai medicine. To treat thrush, for example, they use a paste made from the herb Galangal, which has proven quite effective. In Nambia, an African country, traditional healers are considered to be every bit as legitimate as Western physicians.

Although these countries do not have the time or money to test every traditional therapy they use, they are as practical as the Chinese. If therapy works, they use it. In developed countries, the situation is quite different. Health care needs are not nearly as pressing, which allows us to drag our feet regarding finding out whether alternative therapies are worthwhile. Acupuncture had been in the United States for over a decade before the NIH decided to take a closer look.

However, things are changing. Demographically speaking, health care demands will increase greatly in the coming years. The aging population will be much larger than that of individuals who work, since life expectancy has increased. A great deal of money will need to be spent caring for the elderly. Add to this the large AIDS population, and one can see where the economy and the health care industry will be strained. If ever there was a time to look for cost-effective means of treatment, it is now; alternative medicine provides such means. The cost of acupuncture is far lower than that of surgery for back pain or the electroconvulsive therapy sometimes used for depression.

The greatest asset of alternative medicine may be its emphasis on prevention. It is far cheaper to maintain health than to address it once it has gone. As one Chinese medical text says, it is foolish to forge weapons after a battle has already begun. Although studies on Chinese medicine have focused on its ability to treat symptoms (e.g., nausea from chemotherapy, postsurgical pain) few if any have studied its efficacy in health maintenance. If such studies are undertaken, and the results are positive, it will be hard to explain to the public why it is not used in hospitals or covered by health insurance.

A health care model encompassing different paradigms is possible. It has been done, it is currently being done, and it is not impossible to imagine it occurring here in the West. As people continually turn to alternative medicine for a wide range of health problems, the reality of an integrated care model will continually come into clearer focus. In fact, the education of conventional medical personnel regarding holistic therapies happens mainly via patients who have used them and who pass the positive results along to their physicians. As we have mentioned, the AIDS epidemic may have done more to thrust alternative medicine onto center stage than anything else. It was the early AIDS patients who communicated to their physicians that alternative medicine had definite benefits.

Our best guess is that true integration will not occur for at least 10 years. However, before that happens, a pseudointegration will occur. A portion of the medical establishment will begin to refer patients to holistic practitioners on a regular basis. We have already begun to see this happen. As positive results from further NIH studies trickle down into hospitals and physician's offices and are reported by the media, this trend will grow from a small stream to a swelling river.

Dilemmas on the Horizon

As integration occurs, it will bring new dilemmas to be faced. For example, the method of delivery for alternative medicine may be forced to change. If holistic practitioners find themselves in hospital settings or conventional health clinics, time spent with patients may shorten. Increasing patient load could possibly contribute to this problem as well, which would be a disadvantage, since the client-patient relationship is considered an important part of the healing process. Reducing this relationship in any way would erase some of what makes alternative medicine unique. Practitioners might have to behave more like physicians and add an extra layer of formality. Alternative medicine could conceivably be forced to go down the same road as allopathy and become homogenized until it resembled conventional medicine.

There is also the possibility that holistic practitioners will end up being at the whim of physicians. Imagine a hospital in which the physician decides which alternative modality the patient will receive, which takes power away from patients and holistic practitioners alike. This idea is not so far-fetched.

Health insurance company policies might state that alternative treatment is covered only when recommended by a physician. Thus a patient desiring herbal therapy may be given a massage instead. It could happen, although it would be counterproductive. Alternative medicine works partly because patients come to holistic practitioners because they want to. They are at the acupuncturist's office because *they* felt it would help, not because someone told them it would be best. Besides, a physician cannot possibly have the ability to know all the alternative modalities and their strong points and weaknesses.

Another problem, which we have already faced, is cross-fertilization. For example, some chiropractors use muscle testing as a way to select Chinese herbs for patients, which defeats the whole purpose. Each paradigm has its own inherent logic, and mixing them is not particularly good. A practitioner of Chinese medicine should no more adjust someone than a chiropractor with no training should prescribe Chinese herbs. We would not expect a neurosurgeon to perform open-heart surgery, so it should not be any different for alternative health care providers.

Some individuals feel that integration will allow Western medicine to engulf alternative modalities. Already physicians can practice acupuncture without any formal training. Thus it is possible to fathom the medical establishment promoting the use of alternative medical treatments only by conventional medical professionals, and some physicians have already expressed this attitude. Such a monopoly can only serve to reduce the quality of treatment and the patient's freedom of choice.

Conversely, providers of alternative care may need to increase their knowledge of Western pathology. Chiropractors have already had this experience. As physicians, they are saddled with the responsibility of making proper and timely referrals, which is predicated on recognition of symptomatology of Western disease categories. This may become true for bodyworkers, acupuncturists, and others, as they become less of a last resort and more like primary care providers.

Finally, education of the public will need to be addressed. The average person generally lacks the information to make a decision about which treatment to pursue. Should an individual with arthritis see an acupuncturist, a bodyworker (of which there are numerous types, such as acupressurists and massage therapists), or a naturopathic physician? There is no absolutely correct decision, but patients need to decide which treatments they prefer, and they need to know what these different practitioners do. The process of educating the public will undoubtedly take a fair amount of time, since we are starting from the beginning. Things may be different for AIDS patients, since this particular population is quite proactive about educating themselves and seeking alternative care. Since AIDS is a disease for which the conventional medical field has no cure, and it is generally terminal, patients are trying anything that might help.

SUMMARY

Someone once said that trying to understand the principles on which the universe operates is like trying to pour the Atlantic Ocean into a small reed basket. Nonetheless, human beings are creatures of curiosity. For all our curiosity, we have grasped only a few of the body's mysteries. AIDS is a constant reminder of that concept. We cannot predict who will live asymptomatically with AIDS for years and who will succumb quickly to the disease, just as we cannot explain why PIs work for one person and not another.

Research efforts yield slow and often minimal improvements in therapy. As Subhuti Dharmananda has articulated, although growing evidence supports the efficacy of various herbal therapies in the treatment of AIDS, no plans to implement their use have been unveiled. There seems to be an overall attitude that we should focus our attentions on more research. Certainly this is necessary. However, we should also be concerned with the financial inability of many individuals to obtain proper treatment. Alternative medicine provides cost-effective means for improving QOL of the AIDS population through both physical and mental symptom management.

We are at a crossroads. Will the conventional medical establishment finally incorporate alternative medicine in the face of an ever-increasing epidemic? The choice should be a simple one. Other countries have adopted the use of traditional medicines for treating AIDS and have enjoyed a fair amount of success. As the health care system becomes more strained and financial reserves are depleted, it seems that an integrated care model will emerge as an obvious next step in the evolution of health care here in the West. We can only hope that this next step comes about sooner rather than later.

References

1. NIH Consensus Statement on Acupuncture, Volume 15, Number 5, November 3-5, 1997.
2. Order of Permanent Injunction, *Wilk v AMA* No. 76: 3777, ND Ill, August 27, 1987.
3. Bohm et al: Well-healed: inside lobbying for health care reform, Center for Public Integrity, Washington, DC, 1995 (online).
4. Ryan MK, Shattuck AD: *Treating AIDS with Chinese medicine,* San Francisco, 1994, Pacific View Press.
5. Grossinger R: *Plant medicine,* Berkeley, Calif, 1995, North Atlantic Books.
6. Hammer L: *Dragon rises, red bird flies,* Barrytown, NY, 1990, Station Hill Press.
7. Dharmananda S: Personal communication, 1997.
8. Spencer R et al: *Clinical pharmacology and nursing management,* Philadelphia, 1986, JB Lippincott.

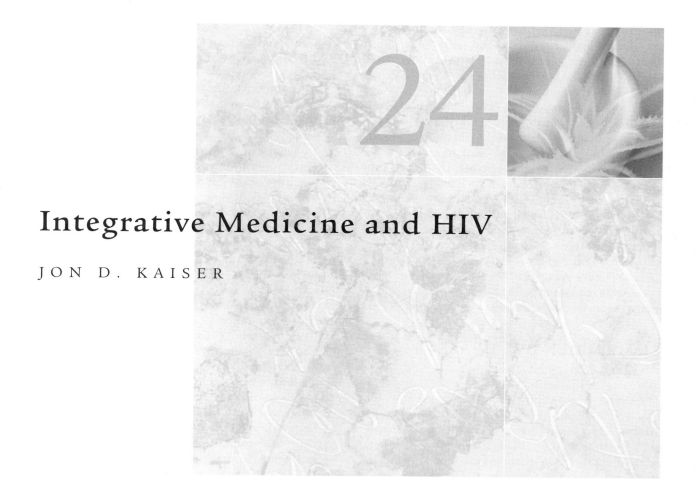

Integrative Medicine and HIV

JON D. KAISER

While attending medical school during the early 1980s, I quickly became frustrated with the highly mechanistic model of disease care that I was being taught. I use the term *disease care* instead of *health care* because learning how to care for one's health was not a significant part of the curriculum.

If a patient was diagnosed with a specific disease, I was taught how to treat his or her disease using an illness-oriented model that included drugs, surgery, and/or chemotherapy. The medical school curriculum had no interest in naturally supporting the patient's own immune system using diet, nutrient supplementation, stress reduction, herbs, or other complementary therapies.

In fact, the two most frequent modes of disease care that I was taught in medical school were (1) how

to kill bacteria, viral particles, fungi, or cancer cells with potentially toxic chemicals, and (2) how to suppress a patient's symptoms (i.e., pain, nausea, inflammation, shortness of breath) with drugs.

In response to my frustration with this narrow-minded philosophy, I strived to learn more healthful ways to care for my future patients. My search quickly led me to a local health food store. While working as a part-time manager, I learned that drugs and surgery were not the only ways to treat illness. Drawing from a wide range of books, clients, and the wonderful aroma of 10 lb bags of fresh peppermint, *uva-ursi,* comfrey root, and Egyptian chamomile, a door opened to the realm of natural therapies that almost lured me away from standard medicine completely. However, despite the allure of treating patients solely with natural forms of healing, I knew that my purpose in life was not to be relegated to either extreme but to continue my standard medical training and, with the credibility of my medical degree, to teach patients how to integrate the best of both modalities into personalized treatment programs.

Most infections in both HIV-positive and HIV-negative individuals are opportunistic. That is, they require a weakness of the body's immune defenses to gain a foothold. In HIV-positive patients, when the CD4 lymphocyte count decreases to below 200 cells/mm^3, specific infections, such as *Pneumocystis carinii* pneumonia (PCP), are much more common. Many infections in HIV-negative individuals are also promoted by a transient weakening of the immune system. These transient defects may be caused by poor nutrition, emotional distress, lack of exercise, or other lifestyle factors. As Louis Pasteur is reported to have finally realized late in his life, it is not primarily the germ responsible for disease, "It's the terrain!"

COMPREHENSIVE HEALING PROGRAM FOR HIV

The essence of a comprehensive healing program for HIV is to enable an HIV-positive individual's immune system to play a significant role in the battle against HIV, which is accomplished through diet, nutrient supplementation, the elimination of intestinal parasites, mind-body techniques, and other immune-strengthening therapies. Then, with strong and vital host defenses in place, an HIV-positive individual can use the least amount of antiviral (AV) medication possible while still remaining healthy and stable throughout a normal lifespan.

There are several reasons why I recommend that HIV-positive patients moderate their use of standard medications in the treatment of HIV disease. These include:

1. To avoid short-term side effects: Most AV medications have a wide range of side effects that can occur soon after treatment has begun. These include diarrhea, rash, peripheral neuropathy (PN), liver abnormalities, diabetes, and anemia. Taking AV medication only when absolutely necessary helps avoid these effects.

2. To avoid long-term side effects: Two of the three currently available classes of AV medications have been approved for the treatment of HIV only during the past 5 years. We have no idea what long-term toxicity these medications may possess. Already thousands of patients have developed long-term toxicities from these medications, including diabetes, osteoporosis, heart disease, and liver failure. Although these effects should not discount the enormous benefits these drugs have brought to thousands of HIV-positive individuals, their indiscriminate use should be strongly discouraged.

3. To avoid using medication options too quickly: This is probably the most important reason to practice the philosophy of moderating AV usage in treating HIV. It is necessary that patients keep important medications in reserve so they can continue to maintain a surplus of powerful and effective AV options well into the future. One's goal should be to remain healthy and stable over the long term, not to blast HIV to undetectable levels in the short term, only to realize that there are no additional treatment options when the virus develops multidrug resistance. Going through the list of currently available AV medications as slowly as possible also allows many newer and potentially more effective therapies to be released during the interim.

4. To minimize costs: It is obvious that, if current trends continue, sooner or later we will need to ration access to the number and types of HIV medications available to our patients. Already some patients with multidrug-resistant HIV are taking six or seven AV drugs in a last-ditch attempt to treat their infection. When the standard treatment of this condition is coupled with a comprehensive program of natural therapies, the need for expensive medications is lessened.

THE MIDDLE PATH

The basic premise that underlies an integrative medicine treatment program is that HIV must be addressed with the long-term health of the individual in mind. Taking AV medication can help achieve this goal, but these medications must be used with great care. Adding them to a patient's program as they truly become necessary allows that person to walk a middle path, which I define as taking just the right combination of natural therapies and standard medications that is best suited for each patient's needs. This approach allows an individual living with HIV to live the longest lifespan while maintaining the highest level of vitality possible.

When deciding whether to recommend AV medication for the first time or whether to change an AV program in any significant way, I always ask a patient the following three questions:

1. Are you asymptomatic?
2. Is your CD4 count greater than 300 cells/mm³ *and* stable or improving?
3. Is your viral load low (*at least* under 20,000 and preferably less)?

If patients can answer yes to all three of these questions, they are currently in what I call the *middle zone* of good health and stability. This means that the program they are presently following is working well, and they do not need to make any changes to their AV medications at this time. If it is determined that they are currently in the middle zone, they should relax and enjoy their life for a while. It is important for patients to not always worry that they are missing out on a new drug or therapy, especially if the above three questions can be answered in the affirmative.

If the patient can answer yes to only two of the above questions, they are still within the middle zone, but they need to monitor their condition closely. Of course, this is a very general version of my guidelines, and every case needs to be carefully individualized.

There is one exception to these recommendations. If a patient has recently started an AV treatment program that contains either a protease inhibitor (PI) or a nonnucleoside reverse transcriptase inhibitor (NNRTI) drug *for the first time,* and an undetectable viral load has not been achieved, intervening early and switching medications is warranted. High-level resistance to these two classes of drugs can occur quickly and may eventually limit the future efficacy of other drugs in the same class.

Clearly stated, the goal of staying in the middle zone is to ensure that an individual is using the minimum amount of medication necessary at any point in time to continue feeling well and remain clinically stable over the long term.

By following an aggressive natural therapies program, patients can lessen the amount of AV medication needed to help them remain stable. These medications will also work better and have a greater duration of effect when combined with a strong natural therapies program. I see these results in my practice every day.

The following patient story provides an example of how to use an integrated HIV treatment program.

About 5 years ago, a charming and attractive young woman came into my office for her initial consultation. Her name was Karen, and she had been exposed to HIV in 1988 through a heterosexual relationship. Karen was European, worked as a flight attendant, and was currently asymptomatic. She had started taking a combination of zidovudine (AZT) and didanosine (ddI) a few months before coming to see me and was tolerating her medications well. However, her CD4 count was continuing to fall and was now only 110 cells/mm³.

My initial recommendations to Karen were to significantly increase her protein intake, to begin acupuncture, to increase her intake of immune-enhancing herbs, and to begin prophylaxis for PCP with Septra DS 3 times/week. Not surprisingly, intestinal parasites were found on her initial stool analysis, and these were treated with the parasite elimination program in Table 24-3. I also advised her to change her AV medications with the hope of better suppressing her viral infection.

During the next couple of years, Karen was able to maintain her CD4 count in the 100 to 200 range with a variety of AV combinations. During this time, Karen felt extremely well, continued to work full-time, and began studying to be an acupressurist. She continued to experience no symptoms of ill health whatsoever.

In addition to her AV and prophylaxis program, Karen continued to eat a healthy diet, get regular exercise, maintain a positive attitude, and get frequent acupuncture treatments.

At the beginning of 1996, Karen's CD4 count again fell to 97 cells/mm³, accompanied by a viral load of 80,000 copies/ml. I recommended that she begin triple combination therapy with stavudine (d4T), lamivudine (3TC), and ritonavir (ABT-538; the most effective PI available at the time).

During the next 12 months, Karen's CD4 count increased to 350 cells/mm³, and her viral load became undetectable. She also became involved in a very nurturing relationship and got married.

Karen and I are extremely pleased with her progress. While one may attribute the majority of her improvement to the inclusion of a PI to her treatment regimen, I would like to highlight her positive attitude and fighting spirit. She never gave up hope or gave in to her illness. She maintained her smile, balanced outlook, and charm without letting HIV prevent her from achieving her goals. She fell in love, got married, improved her living situation, and changed her career. She is presently happy, healthy, and planning on being alive for a very long time. Karen is a shining example of a successful comprehensive treatment program for HIV.

The suppression of chronic viral infections is a role that the immune system is well suited to perform. Over 90% of adults possess chronic viral infections that their immune systems are able to completely suppress but not eradicate. These chronic viral infections include varicella-zoster virus (VZV; chicken pox), Epstein-Barr virus (EBV; mononucleosis), and multiple strains of herpes viruses. Although HIV is admittedly more virulent and serious than these other viral infections, the human immune system possesses the ability to significantly suppress it as well. In fact, the progression of HIV has been prevented in several of my patients for over 15 years without any need for AV medication.

PRIVATE PRACTICE DATA

It is not an exaggeration to say that I care for one of the healthiest groups of HIV-positive individuals around. They experience a very low rate of progression from this condition. I attribute this success to my "Middle Path" philosophy, which strikes a delicate balance between the *excessive* use of drugs and an *excessive reliance* on natural therapies.

My program also ensures that the body is provided with the natural support it needs to live healthfully with HIV for an entire lifespan. AV medication is used only when the body's immune system is not sufficiently able to stabilize HIV on its own. This approach enables my patients to make as few changes as possible to their AV program while continuing to remain healthy and stable. It also allows many newer, and potentially more effective, medication options time to be released during this period.

As a means of highlighting the level of AV medication use among my HIV-positive patients, I recently conducted a survey of my private practice. The following sampling of my long-term HIV-positive patients shows an interesting breakdown of medication usage (these are patients whom I have followed for a minimum of 2 years, $n = 74$):

On 0 AV medications: 12%
On 1 AV medication: 0%
On 2 AV medications: 31%
Less than triple therapy: 43%
On 3 AV medications: 37%

On 4 AV medications: 15%
On 5 AV medications: 5%
Triple therapy or more: 57%

Although 57% of my patients are taking at least a standard triple combination of AV medications, 43% are taking two AVs or less. More importantly, the patients taking two AVs or less are by far the healthier, more stable group. In general, they are more active and have fewer medication side effects. Also, fewer patients in this group have needed to go on medical disability.

Important point: It is currently not recommended that anyone take one AV medication for any amount of time because of the almost-certain emergence of resistance. I also do not recommend that patients decrease the number of AV medications they are currently taking.

The question that I am usually asked at this point is, "Although they are stable now, how long will patients on two or fewer AV medications remain stable?" The answer to this question, based on the past 5 years of my clinical experience using the Healing HIV program, is clear:

As long as these patients utilize their antiviral medication in combination with an aggressive natural therapies program as described in this book, they will remain healthy and stable for a very long time.

At our clinic, double combination AV therapy with two reverse transcriptase inhibitors (dual RTI therapy), instituted in patients with mild-to-moderate HIV disease (CD4 counts greater then 300 cells/mm³ *and* viral loads less than 50,000 cells/ml) lasts at least 2 years, *and often longer,* in at least 90% of the patients who use it. This allows our patients to go through the present list of AV medications more slowly than patients who are following a more aggressive treatment philosophy. This conservative approach allows safer and potentially more potent treatment options to be developed and released during this period of time. Remember, it is the aggressive natural therapies program that I prescribe to my patients that allows this strategy to work. It accomplishes this goal by encouraging the immune system to become a strong partner in the treatment of HIV.

The aggressive natural therapies program I recommend to my HIV-positive patients includes a seamless blend of the following treatment modalities:
1. Nutritional counseling
2. Antioxidant nutrient supplementation

3. Acupuncture and herbs
4. Regular exercise
5. Hormone balancing
6. Stress reduction/psychospiritual interventions
7. Standard medical therapies

Although each therapeutic intervention contained in the above list achieves a positive effect on its own, the Healing HIV program's overall ability to rebuild immune systems is maximized when all of them are combined. Immune reconstitution can then occur even in patients who have been declining or experiencing symptoms for years.

While using the Healing HIV program during the past 4 years, not one patient starting with a CD4 count greater than 300 cells/mm³ has progressed below that number. Additionally, not one patient starting with a CD4 count of greater than 50 cells/mm³ has become seriously ill or died from an HIV-related illness during this same time period. This experience encompasses the treatment of more than 300 HIV-positive individuals.

HEALING HIV RESEARCH STUDY

I know these statistics sound incredible; many colleagues have told me so, which is why I recently conducted a controlled, retrospective analysis of my HIV patient population (The Healing HIV Research Study). The data for this study was collected by an independent observer who reviewed the charts of all of the HIV-positive patients receiving continuous primary care at my practice during the past 2 years. A total of 74 patients met all of the inclusion criteria and were accrued. The majority of these patients live in San Francisco and have been exposed to the HIV virus for more than 10 years.

Each patient was given the same aggressive natural therapy and AV medication recommendations per the approach described in this book. Patients accepted or rejected my recommendations based on their personal philosophies and socioeconomic abilities. The extent to which they followed my program was not a criteria for admission to the study.

The control group for this study consisted of 74 HIV-positive individuals cared for by a similar HIV-specialty medical practice located within the same medical institution. The patients lived in the same geographical area, belonged to the same socioeconomic group, and were similarly aggressive about their care *except* that this group was provided with a more standard HIV treatment program with an emphasis on AV therapy and little if any counseling on the use of diet, vitamins, intestinal health, stress reduction, and so on. The control group individuals met the same inclusion criteria, and their charts were randomly selected from this practice's charts by a neutral party without prior knowledge of the study's purposes or goals.

Analysis of the study data revealed that the mean number of *AV* medications in use at the end of the 2-year study period was 2.58/patient in the study group (range: 0 to 5) and 3.08/patient in the control group (range: 0 to 5). Additionally, 43% of the patients in the study group were taking *less than triple combination therapy* compared with only 18% of patients in the control group who were taking less than triple combination therapy. This confirms the assumption that significantly *less AV medication* was prescribed to the study group participants.

Additionally, the mean number of *total* medications in use at the end of the 2-year study period was 5.96/patient in the study group (range: 2 to 12) and 8.46/patient in the control group (range: 2 to 22). This confirms that significantly *less total medication* was prescribed to the study group participants.

HEALING HIV STUDY RESULTS

1. The study group participants used less AV medication and less total medication than the control group participants.
2. When compared with the control group participants, the study group participants experienced:
   - A greater average rise in CD4 cells (45% versus 25%)
   - A greater average drop in viral load (−86% versus −72%)
   - Fewer opportunistic infections (OIs) (1 versus 3)
   - Fewer hospitalizations (0 versus 1)
   - Fewer hospital days (0 versus 5)

The results of this study are summarized in Table 24-1. The study group achieved as good or better outcomes using less AV and total medications. The results of this important study are currently being readied for submission to a peer-reviewed journal.

Additionally, since a level of 300 CD4 cells/mm³ usually signifies a normally functioning immune system, I thought it would be interesting to identify how many patients from both groups improved from below a level of 300 CD4 cells to above this level during

TABLE 24-1

Healing HIV Research Study: Data Summary

	Study group	Control group
Patients (no.)	74	74
Male/female ratio	69/5	73/1
Mean age	44	41
Baseline mean CD4 cell count	291	361
Ending mean CD4 cell count	423	451
Baseline mean viral load	101,627	31,828
Ending mean viral load	13,840	8894
Average CD4 cell change	+45%	+25%
Average viral load change	−86%	−72%
Mean antiviral medications (no.)	2.58	3.08
Mean total medications (no.)	5.96	8.46
Total opportunistic infections (no.)	1	3
Total HIV-related hospitalizations (no.)	0	1
Total HIV-related hospital days (no.)	0	5

the 2-year study period. I also looked at how many patients declined below this level. The results of this analysis are illustrated in Table 24-2.

DISCUSSION

This study concludes that:

The Healing HIV treatment program can potentially help HIV-positive individuals achieve as good or better outcomes using less AV medication than is commonly recommended. Although not specifically measured in this study, it was observed that the study group participants

TABLE 24-2

Healing HIV Research Study: Rebuilding the Immune System

	Study group	Control group
Patients (no.)	74	74
Improving from <300 CD4 cells to >300 CD4 cells	21	11
Declining from >300 CD4 cells to <300 CD4 cells	0	3

experienced fewer medication side effects and had an overall lower cost of care.

Despite the differences in the outcomes of these two groups, a second important conclusion can be drawn from this study: HIV-positive patients treated by an HIV specialist can remain extremely healthy over a 2-year period. When data from the two groups are examined together, 148 HIV-positive patients experienced only four OIs and one HIV-related hospitalization during a 2-year period. Many of these patients had severe HIV disease at the onset of this study, with 31% having CD4 counts below 200 CD4 cells/mm^3. This fact highlights the high level of care that can be delivered to HIV-positive individuals by physicians who commonly treat this condition. It also provides hope that patients at any stage of HIV disease today can be kept stable and healthy to benefit from newly emerging treatments.

Finally, I would like to thank the HIV treatment physicians who allowed us to use their practice as the control group for this study. I very much respect the care that they provide, and if I were HIV-positive, I would not hesitate to be treated at their practice. As one might expect, however, I would add a more aggressive program of natural therapies to my treatment program.

The following is another case history illustrating the significant benefits conferred by our integrative healing program for HIV.

When Keith and his wife came to my office for their initial consultation, they were extremely anxious. Keith is heterosexual and was probably exposed to HIV from a blood transfusion that he had in 1984 after a car accident. Thankfully his wife Karen had tested HIV-negative.

TABLE 24-3

Dr. Kaiser's Parasite Elimination Program*

Treatment	Frequency	Duration

Paromomycin (Humatin)†
   2 capsules (250 mg)
   And/or
	tid	10-14 days

Iodoquinol (Yodoxin)† 1 capsule (650 mg)	tid	10-20 days
Psyllium seed husks 2 tsp; add to water or juice‡	tid	10-14 days
Black walnut tincture 2 drops; add to water or juice‡	tid	10-14 days

tid, Three times/day; *tsp*, teaspoon.

*Extremely effective against *Blastocystis hominis, Endolimax nana, Iodamoeba butschlii, Entamoeba histolytica*, and *Entamoeba coli.*

†Paromomycin and iodoquinol are prescription medications that are very effective and better tolerated than the more commonly prescribed metroidazole (Flagyl). If two or more parasites are present, which is frequently the case, taking both paromomycin and iodoquinol concurrently for at least 10 days and then continuing iodoquinol alone for an additional 10 days is recommended.

‡Add to water or juice and take together with paromomycin and/or iodoquinol on an empty stomach (either ½ hour before or 2 hours after meals). All of the above must be taken together for maximum efficacy. Do not follow this program without medical supervision.

Keith learned about his HIV infection through a routine life insurance physical examination less than 1 month before his office visit. His initial CD4 count was 465 cells/mm³, but his viral load had not yet been done. At the time, Keith felt well and had no symptoms. His examination was normal, and his demeanor belied nothing out of the ordinary.

One week later, Karen and Keith returned to the office to review his lab tests. Although his CD4 count remained stable in the 400s, his baseline viral load came back at 221,000 copies/ml. A repeat of this test yielded similar results.

Despite a healthy CD4 count and the lack of any significant symptoms, it has been my experience that extremely high viral loads usually lead to an uncontrolled spread of HIV throughout the body and an eventual decline in one's immune function and CD4 count. Several research studies support this hypothesis. Therefore I initially recommended to Keith that he begin combination AV therapy with d4T 40 mg bid and ddI 200 mg bid.

This combination is one of the most effective two-drug combinations presently available, and it is also fairly well tolerated. The drug ddI now comes in pleasant-tasting, orange-flavored, chewable tablets that can be dissolved in cold water and cause fewer gastrointestinal (GI) symptoms than previous formulations. In addition, Keith began taking dehydroepiandrosterone (DHEA) 200 mg once a day because of a less-than-optimal DHEA sulfate (DHEAS) level of 207 ng/dl (the optimal DHEAS level for HIV-positive males is 300 to 600 ng/dl). With this program, I believed that Keith's viral load could be brought down to a healthier level and that more potent medications, such as PIs, could be saved for future use.

Finally, two intestinal parasites were identified with a comprehensive stool analysis, and they were appropriately treated using the parasite elimination protocol described in Table 24-3.

It is evident from Keith's treatment program that integrative HIV treatment does not stop with the prescription of AV medications. Hormone levels, optimum intestinal health, and the installation of hope and confidence (working with a patient's mental attitude) are all integral parts of a comprehensive approach to HIV care. As the results show, the comprehensive treatment of HIV works extremely well.

After 6 months on the comprehensive treatment program using dual RTI therapy, Keith's laboratory tests showed a rise in his CD4 count from 482 to 811, with a subsequent lowering of the viral load from 221,000 copies/ml to less than 500 copies/ml. Three months later, his CD4 count rose to 872 cells/mm³ with a continued undetectable viral load. Now, 2 years after first beginning this program, his CD4 cell count has risen to over 1000 cells/mm³ with a continued undetectable viral load. He feels extremely well and has had no side effects or symptoms from his treatment program.

It is important to point out that the notable success of a two-drug AV combination in this patient is due to the comprehensive nature of Keith's program. It includes a healthy diet, vitamin supplementation, parasite elimination, and stress reduction. When these complementary therapies are combined with an effective AV strategy, they can keep a patient healthy and stable for much longer than if they are not used. I anticipate that Keith's good health and stability will last a long time and that he will continue to preserve useful treatment options, such as PIs, for a long time to come.

In summary, an integrative approach to HIV treatment helps:

1. Minimize the need for standard medications
2. Allow standard medications to work more effectively
3. Minimize the occurrence and severity of medication side effects
4. Maximize an HIV-positive individual's quality of life (QOL)

In a landmark study, one out of three respondents reported receiving at least one unconventional therapy, but 75% of the respondents chose not to inform their conventional physician about the treatments they received.[1] In my experience, the percentage of HIV-positive individuals who use unconventional therapies is even higher. Physicians should become informed about the potential benefits and risks these therapies possess. It is only with experience and scientific study, not defensiveness or bias, that these interventions will have the opportunity to prove their effectiveness.

SUMMARY

I would like to make the following important closing points:

1. Natural therapies are most effective when used as part of a comprehensive program: Since individual natural therapies do not possess the strength or effect that are commonly seen with drugs, programs using nutrition, vitamins, stress reduction, hormone balancing, herbal therapies, parasite elimination, and other treatments should be evaluated as whole programs, not as individual interventions.

2. Integrative medicine does not mean choosing between natural and standard therapies: By definition, integrative health care means combining both natural and standard medical therapies into the best treatment program currently available. Because HIV is such a challenging condition, all treatment options should be considered.

3. A strong natural therapies program will help an allopathic, medication-oriented treatment program work better: By supporting the body's immune system, it can become a more potent force in the battle against HIV. A stronger immune system allows medications to work better and last longer. Many natural therapy interventions also support the body in ways that minimize medication-related side effects, such as hepatitis (alcohol avoidance), diabetes (dietary modification), and PN (micronutrient supplementation, massage, and acupuncture).

Finally, I truly believe that HIV has become a manageable illness and that through diligence, hard work, faith, and a little luck, HIV-positive individuals with currently intact immune systems can look forward to enjoying healthy, normal lifespans.

References

1. Eisenberg D, Wesson M: The most highly amphiphilic alpha-helices include two amino acid segments in human immunodeficiency virus glycoprotein 4l, *Biopolymers* 29(1):171-177, 1990.

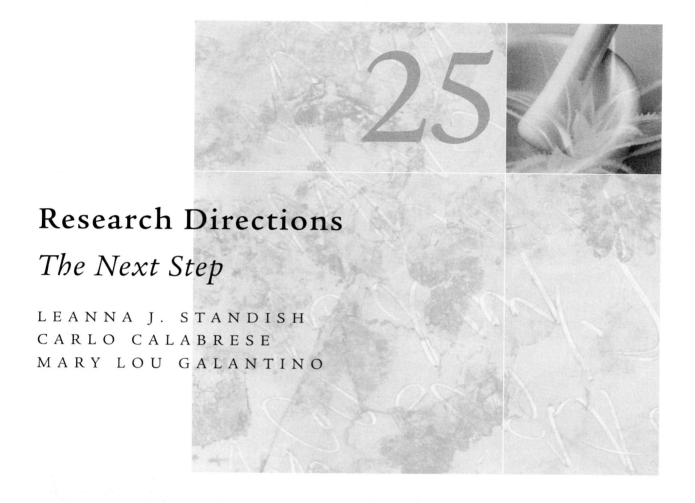

Research Directions

The Next Step

LEANNA J. STANDISH
CARLO CALABRESE
MARY LOU GALANTINO

There are already sufficient data to urge the inclusion of some of the less controversial and more competently researched alternative modalities in the comprehensive care of HIV-positive and AIDS patients. The specific benefits of nutrition, exercise, and physical therapy have been documented and are integrated into progressive HIV/AIDS conventional health care centers. Throughout the United States, a number of clinics that offer integrated health care have opened, often combining conventional care, Chinese medicine, and other CAM systems and approaches. CAM and conventional medicine integrated care models were pioneered in AIDS clinics in Portland, Seattle, San Francisco, New York, Miami, and Chicago. The trend toward integrated care in HIV/AIDS also has paved the way for integra-

ted health care programs for people with other serious chronic diseases.

In light of the evidence and substantial utilization of CAM, other serious chronic disease research in CAM in the treatment of HIV/AIDS should not only continue but accelerate. We need innovative treatments for this hitherto nearly intractable disease. The diversity of CAM approaches may provide insight into conventional therapeutic developments. As rates of HIV infection in Africa and Asia grow, therapies must be accessible and affordable. Recent admirable commitments by pharmaceutical companies to reduce the cost of highly active antiretroviral therapy (HAART) to $300/year in developing countries helps, but delivery remains unrealistic in countries where that price is comparable to the average annual income. The potential of traditional medicine practices—as well as their recent evolution in industrialized conditions in the twentieth century—have not been adequately mined by medical researchers. However, development of plant medicines in Western medicine nearly came to a halt with the advent of the "better living through chemistry" phase of pharmaceutical industrialization. The development of synthetic organic molecules has been the focus of most of pharmaceutical medicine since World War II.

There is still reason to believe that botanical medicine has both principles of practice and specific molecules to offer in the treatment of HIV/AIDS. Substantial data on the antiretroviral activity of a wide variety of plants justifies a research program whose aim is to develop and evaluate combination botanical anti-HIV therapy. These therapies may be in complex combinations of plant molecules within one plant or in combinations of plant products that produce viral suppression with a more tolerable set of side effects than those experienced with conventional pharmaceutical antiretroviral therapy (ART). Botanical medicine is also a fertile area in which to explore clinically effective immunomodulation. A major problem of AIDS treatment is immune system restoration. The potent effects of ART on both HIV RNA viral load and clinical health strengthens the HIV hypothesis of the pathogenesis of the 30 diseases that comprise AIDS. Suppression of HIV has led to enormous clinical benefits. Despite measurable and dramatic suppression of viral burden in patients receiving HAART, immune function is not restored to normal. The immunomodulatory potential of numerous families of plant chemical constituents has just begun to be evaluated. As conventional medicine and CAM are combined in practice, interactions are inevitable. Recently the negative results of interactions of botanicals and drugs—with the prime example of *Hypericum* and indinavir—have been highlighted. However, positive interactions are also likely, if not yet quite as well quantified, perhaps joining the mild antiviral (AV) effects via a broader selection of mechanisms in effective treatments with fewer side effects or by combining AV approaches with immune support via medical foods or botanicals.

For many CAM researchers, the future frontiers of CAM are the most interesting and include homeopathy, bioelectromagnetic therapies, and remote biological effects. They are frontier areas because widespread skepticism exists that nonmaterial doses of molecules, nonionizing electromagnetic (EM) fields, or conscious intention can exert effects on biological systems. National Institutes of Health (NIH) funding for the study of CAM frontier areas is now available in 2001. Brewitt attempted to conduct a double-blind, placebo-controlled study of a homeopathically prepared growth factor (GF) in the treatment of AIDS wasting through a grant from the NIH-funded Bastyr University AIDS Research Center. This study was stalled for 2 years despite the priority set by the reviewers and the agreement to fund it. The study was delayed for multiple reasons, including (1) NIH requirements for an investigational new drug (IND) number from the Federal Drug Administration (FDA) to conduct a clinical trial of an experimental therapy and (2) the misunderstanding of the homeopathic medical and scientific community toward ultrahigh dilutional (UHD; containing essentially no molecules of the original substance) biology and pharmacology. The FDA's inability to swiftly develop policies and procedures for UHD experimental medicines has also been detrimental.

Nevertheless, UHD biology and pharmacology should be explored. Sufficient evidence exists that extremely low concentrations of certain substances can exert biological effects. The periodicity of low-dose antigen levels in the induction of oral tolerance is one example. Biological effects have been observed when substances are diluted beyond Avogadro's constant (i.e., the probability of even a single molecule being present in dilutions of 10^{-24}, or 12 C in homeopathic terminology, is minuscule). UHD biology and pharmacology may become a promising area of research.

Remote biological effects also need to be further examined, both as a primary effect and as a confounder in studies of other therapies. Evidence is slowly accruing that thought patterns may alter biological systems, including those of human beings, at a distance. Some preliminary data suggest that these effects do not follow the inverse square law, which describes the relationship between energy and distance for other types of energy, such as light. Elizabeth Targ's data are intriguing (see Chapter 17). In a well-designed controlled study, she shows clinical effects in AIDS patients who were exposed to healing intention by a group of experienced "healers." AIDS is a good system for the scientific study of such controversial phenomenon. Early in the epidemic, researchers developed and agreed on reasonable surrogate markers. Progression to more serious disease and clinical outcomes is correlated with CD4$^+$ T-cell count and HIV RNA viral load. Consensus remains strong that CD4$^+$

T-cell count, HIV RNA viral load, and progression to one or more of 30 AIDS-defining illnesses are reasonably good measures by which to evaluate the efficacy of any therapy, whether remote healing effects or protease inhibitors (PIs).

Another reason to pursue research in CAM is that we can learn much about the efficacy and possible mechanisms of action of some innovative medical strategies of the CAM community—which may have repercussions well beyond CAM—by studying and developing these therapies in vitro and in vivo. Alternative approaches are a healthy challenge to an orthodoxy that has not yet achieved perfection. Many conventionally trained physicians are using at least one aspect of CAM as an effective complement to the pharmaceutical mindset, which they have concluded is incomplete. Alternative medicine research in AIDS should therefore continue for the benefit of both the HIV-positive and the medical and scientific communities.

For these reasons, the editors of this book believe that rigorous science can and should be done in the most promising areas of alternative medicine. Furthermore, we do not believe that alternative medicine requires alternative science. At the same time, the particular difficulties of studying CAM need to be respected as treatment methods validly and reliably evolve. Some of the research issues inherent in studying alternative medicine have been described in Chapter 1. Creative and workable solutions to the variety of problems confronting CAM research are needed, such as nonstandard interventions, nonmaterial interventions, combination treatments, individualized treatment, treatments not based on Western disease nosology, and the holism of interventions and outcomes. These treatments also should not be distorted to the point that they lose their potential effectiveness. For some of these issues, the research advances necessary for large-scale studies have yet to be made or generally accepted (either by the conventional or relevant CAM community). In the meantime, the accumulation of relevant data to form the right hypotheses is proceeding via all of the domains of medical science—laboratory, epidemiological, and clinical.

As more research programs and centers for alternative medicine are developed in the area of HIV/AIDS, it becomes increasingly important to define a better-56 focused research agenda. We must be efficient, and we must choose our research questions carefully. After all, more than 1000 CAM therapies are currently used by HIV-positive persons in the United States alone. We know virtually nothing about the efficacy of most of these therapies, and in many cases, we know little about their safety. Priority research directions and agendas should be articulated in more detail at the national level. For the investigators at the NIH Office of Alternative Medicine (OAM)-established Bastyr University AIDS Research Center, the research agenda includes (1) in vitro development and clinical evaluation of AV botanical/nutritional medicine combinations, (2) in vitro development and clinical evaluation of an immune therapy using combination immunomodulatory botanicals and nutrition, (3) further evaluation and exploration of acupuncture (both efficacy and mechanism of action), (4) evaluation and exploration of UHD effects of cytokines and GFs known to control immune function, and (5) controlled clinical trials of integrated treatment programs that use both CAM and conventional therapy. Only well-designed and adequately funded studies can answer relevant questions about the use of CAM in the treatment of HIV/AIDS.

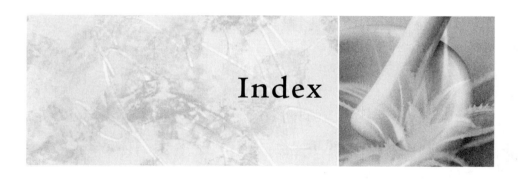

Index

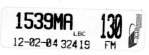